Cyanide in Biology

Cyanide in Biology

Edited by

B. VENNESLAND

Forschungsstelle Vennesland
der Max-Planck-Gesellschaft
Berlin, West Germany

E. E. CONN

University of California
Davis, California, USA

C. J. KNOWLES

University of Kent
Canterbury
Kent, UK

J. WESTLEY

University of Chicago
Chicago, Illinois, USA

F. WISSING

Royal Dental College
Aarhus, Denmark

1981

ACADEMIC PRESS

A Subsidiary of Harcourt Brace Jovanovich, Publishers

London New York Toronto Sydney San Francisco

ACADEMIC PRESS INC. (LONDON) LTD.
24/28 Oval Road,
London NW1

United States Edition published by
ACADEMIC PRESS INC.
111 Fifth Avenue
New York, New York 10003

British Library Cataloguing in Publication Data
Cyanide in biology.
1. Metabolism 2. Cyanides 3. Biological chemistry
I. Vennesland, B.
574.19'2 QD415.A1A

ISBN 0-12-716980-6

LCCCN 81-67912

Printed in Great Britain by
Whitstable Litho Ltd., Whitstable, Kent

CONTRIBUTORS

K. ALEXANDER *Department of Biochemistry and Biophysics, University of Hawaii, Honolulu, Hawaii 96822, USA*

K.S. ANDERSEN *Department of Biochemistry, The Royal Dental College, DK-8000 Aarhus C, Denmark*

A.W. BUNCH *Biological Laboratory, University of Kent, Canterbury CT2 7NJ, UK*

K.F. CASTRIC *Department of Biological Sciences, Duquesne University, Pittsburgh, Pennsylvania 15219, USA*

P.A. CASTRIC *Department of Biological Sciences, Duquesne University, Pittsburgh, Pennsylvania 15219, USA*

P. CHAMBERLAIN *Department of Molecular and Life Sciences, Dundee College of Technology, Bell Street, Dundee DD1 1HG, UK*

P.A. COLLINS *Biological Laboratory, University of Kent, Canterbury CT2 7NJ, UK*

E.E.CONN *Department of Biochemistry and Biophysics, University of California, Davis, California 95616, USA*

R.D. COOKE *Tropical Products Institute, 56/62 Gray's Inn Road, London WC1X 8LU, UK*

D.G. COURSEY *Tropical Products Institute, 56/62 Gray's Inn Road, London WC1X 8LU, UK*

R.H. DAVIS *Wye College, University of London, Wye, Ashford, Kent TN25 5AH, UK*

S.S. DUFFEY *Department of Entomology, College of Agricultural and Environmental Sciences, University of California, Davis, California 95616, USA*

N. ERB *Fachbereich Botanik der Universität des Saarlandes, D-6600 Saarbrücken, West Germany*

W.E. FRY *Department of Plant Pathology, Cornell University, Ithaca, New York 14853, USA*

H.-S. GEWITZ *Forschungsstelle Vennesland der Max-Planck-Gesellschaft, Harnackstrasse 23 D-1000 Berlin 33, West Germany*

M.-F. HENRY *Laboratoire de Biochimie (CNRS-ER 235 et INSERM U.191), Départment de Recherche Fondamentale, Centre d'Etudes Nucleaires, 85X, 38041 Grenoble cedex, France*

W. HÖSEL *Lehrstuhl für Biochemie der Pflanzen der Westfälischen Wilhelms-Universität, Hindenburgplatz 55, D-4400 Münster, West Germany*

M.A. HUGHES *Department of Genetics, Ridley Building, The University, Newcastle upon Tyne NE1 7RU, UK*

S. HUQ *Department of Botany, University of Dacca, Dacca, Bangladesh*

D.A. JONES *Unit of Genetics, University of Hull, Hull HU6 7RX, UK*
C.J. KNOWLES *Biological Laboratory, University of Kent, Canterbury CT2 7NJ, UK*
H. KRUTZ *Institute for Water Research Laboratorien, 5840 Schwertze 1, Geisecke, Dortmund Stadtwerke AG, West Germany*
A. LAZCANO-ARAUJO *Instituto de Astronomia, Universidad Nacional Autonoma de Mexico, Mexico 20, D.F., Mexico*
G. LEDUC *Department of Biological Sciences, Concordia University, Montreal, Quebec, Canada*
R.M. MACKENZIE *Department of Molecular and Life Sciences, Dundee College of Technology, Bell Street, Dundee DD1 1HG, UK*
R. MEGANATHAN *Department of Biological Sciences, Duquesne University, Pittsburgh, Pennsylvania 15219, USA*
B.L. MÖLLER *Department of Physiology, Carlsberg Laboratory, 10 Gamle Carlsberg Vej, DK-2500 Copenhagen Valby, Denmark*
D.F. MYERS *Department of Plant Pathology, University of California, Davis, California 95616, USA*
A. NAHRSTEDT *Institut für Pharmazeutische Biologie der Technischen Universtät, D-3300 Braunschweig, West Germany*
F. NARTEY *Division of Biochemistry, Institute of Plant Physiology, University of Copenhagen, Ø. Farimagsgade 2A. DK-1353 Copenhagen, Denmark*
N. NAZLY *Biological Laboratory, University of Kent, Canterbury CT2 7NJ, UK*
J. ORÓ *Departments of Biophysical Sciences and Chemistry, University of Houston, Houston, Texas 77004, USA*
J.M. PALMER *Department of Botany, Imperial College, London SW7 2AZ, UK*
E.K. PISTORIUS *Forschungsstelle Vennesland der Max-Planck-Gesellschaft, Harnackstrasse 23, D-1000 Berlin 33, West Germany*
P.B. RODGERS *Department of Biochemistry, University of Liverpool, P.O. Box 147, Liverpool L69 3BX, UK*
D.S. SEIGLER *Department of Botany, University of Illinois, Urbana, Illinois 61801, USA*
L.P. SOLOMONSON *Department of Biochemistry, University of South Florida, College of Medicine, Tampa, Florida 33612, USA*
A.M. SPEHAR *Department of Biochemistry, University of South Florida, College of Medicine, Tampa, Florida 33612, USA*
T. STELMASZYNSKA *Instytut Biochemii Lekarskiej, Akademia Medyczna, Kraków, Poland*
A.H. SYKES *Wye College, University of London, Ashford, Kent TN25 5AH, UK*
B. VENNESLAND *Forschungsstelle Vennesland der Max-Planck-Gesellschaft, Harnackstrasse 23, D-1000 Berlin 33, West Germany*

M. VOLINI *Department of Biochemistry and Biophysics, University of Hawaii, Honolulu, Hawaii 96822, USA*
J.L. WAY *Department of Pharmacy, Washington State University, Pullman, Washington 99164, USA*
J. WESTLEY *Department of Biochemistry, The University of Chicago, Chicago, Illinois 60637, USA*
F. WISSING *Department of Biochemistry, The Royal Dental College, DK-8000 Aarhus C, Denmark*
J.M. ZGLICZYNSKI *Instytut Biochemii Lekarskiej, Akademia Medyczna, Kraków, Poland*
H.-D. ZINSMEISTER *Fachbereich Botanik der Universität des Saarlandes, D-6600 Saarbrücken, West Germany*

PREFACE

In August 1978, a small group of investigators gathered for a European Molecular Biology Organisation workshop hosted by C.J. Knowles at the University of Kent in Canterbury. The title of that workshop was "HCN Metabolism", which was interpreted very broadly to mean everything that had a bearing on cyanide in biology. The present volume grew out of that meeting, but in line with the feelings of the delegates at the conference, it is much more than a record of the proceedings. The range of topics covered has been expanded to include authors not present at the meeting; and all authors have been encouraged to bring their material up to date (as of June 1980).

Like the meeting, this book comprises a mixture of reviews and experimental papers. Though an effort has been made to be comprehensive, we are painfully aware of gaps, such as the failure to cover *lathyrism* even superficially. In fact, except for the subject of cyanogenic glucosides and nitrile degradation by microorganisms, the topic of the nitriles in biology has not here been covered systematically. Demarcation lines must be drawn to keep length within bounds, and the drawing of boundaries is rather arbitrary. We apologize to those who are disappointed in our choice of topics.

Part of our subject matter, the cyanogenic glycosides, have a history that reaches back to the beginning of organic chemistry, and our knowledge of them has acquired a richness of chemical detail that attests to the long hard labour of a small group of devotees. Other areas, such as the generation of HCN by bacteria, fungi and algae, have only been opened up more recently, and our chemical knowledge in these areas is relatively sketchy and primitive. Intermediate in both its history and its stage of scientific development is our understanding of the biological mechanisms of protection against cyanide. We hope that this book does justice to the present stage of knowledge in all these areas of HCN metabolism, and that it can serve as an introduction for the uninitiated as well as a handbook for those whose interests are already engaged.

The subject of HCN-resistant respiration has been included, to controvert the facile argument, frequently heard, that HCN is such a strong respiratory inhibitor that its metabolic production would be suicidal. Not always, as the reader can readily learn.

Perhaps because of its reputation as a poison, little attention has previously been given to possible roles of HCN in normal metabolism. It is our hope that this book will contribute to placing cyanide in its proper biochemical perspective: a poison, yes; a polluter of our endangered environment, sometimes; but also a microconstituent of our "unpolluted" streams, a byproduct of phagocytosis by our own lymphocytes, and a metabolic product of a wide variety of species, including some of the world's important food plants. Cyanide has a history that includes a role in many a villainous act, but, stretching into the distant pre-biotic past, perhaps even a leading role in biogenesis.

August 1981

The Editors

CONTENTS

EARLY STUDIES ON THE TOXICOLOGY OF CYANIDE

A.H. SYKES

Wye College (University of London),
Ashford, Kent TN25 5AH, UK.

I. INTRODUCTION

The recognition of cyanide as a poison in bitter almonds, cherry laurel leaves, or cassava goes back to antiquity. An inscription on an Egyptian papyrus in the Louvre Museum, Paris refers to "the penalty of the peach" and Dioscorides in the first century AD was aware of the poisonous properties of bitter almonds. But it was not until the establishment of experimental science in the eighteenth century that any real understanding of its chemical nature or physiological action became possible. The mode of action of cyanide, and of other poisons for that matter, was investigated before the chemical constitution was known; crude extracts from plants ultimately gave place to increasingly pure chemical preparations but the advent of synthesis itself did not in fact mark any major step forward in the physiological investigation of cyanide and therefore purely chemical aspects of its history can be dealt with separately.

II. THE CHEMISTRY OF CYANIDE

It is generally agreed that HCN was first prepared by Scheele (1786), the Swedish chemist, in 1782 although he did not name it nor make any reference to its poisonous properties since he was more interested in the chemistry of the dye Prussian blue which had been well known since the beginning of the century. After describing his method of preparation of HCN from Prussian blue Scheele remarks that "this matter has a peculiar but not disagreeable smell, a taste somewhat approaching to sweet, and warm in the mouth, at the same time exciting cough"; had he been aware of its toxic nature he might have been less willing to take his biological examination as far as he did! In a later letter (1783) he refers to his new preparation as *acidum berolissense* and it was another chemist, Guyton de

Morveau who, in 1789, first used the name prussic acid (Partington, 1962). The next major step was the establishment of its proximate composition by Berthellot (Partington, 1962) who showed in 1787 that it consisted of hydrogen, carbon and nitrogen but did not contain oxygen, formerly believed to be an essential component of all acids. Schrader (1802) first showed that cyanide could be obtained from bitter almonds and Vauquelin (1803) also demonstrated the natural occurrence of cyanides and showed that Prussian blue could be prepared from apricots or almonds. The new acid was examined pharmacologically by Emmert in 1805 who referred to it as *acid borussici* (Earles, 1961).

A better understanding of the cyanides was achieved by Gay-Lussac who, in 1815, prepared HCN in a semi-pure form and named it hydro-cyanic acid; he also proposed the term cyanogen for the radical CN (Partington, 1962).

The inorganic chemistry of the cyanides was thus launched and before long the naturally occurring forms were also being investigated. Robiquet and Charland (1830) prepared from bitter almonds the substance which they named amygdalin from which they obtained HCN, a sugar and benzoic acid. In the same year (1830) Riccord-Mandiana (Miller, 1973) isolated manihotoxin, the cyanogenic glucoside in cassava and Henry and Charland (1836) identified the toxin itself as HCN. Thus it was established that HCN was present in plants in a bound form and it was suggested by Robiquet and Charland (1830) that some further process was required if free HCN were to be obtained. This suggestion was examined by Wöhler and Liebig (1837) who showed that there existed in plant tissues an active "principle" (the concept of an enzyme was not then established), called emulsin, which split amygdalin into HCN, benzaldehyde and sugar. From these beginnings there followed a period of very active investigation into the nature and distribution of cyanogenic plants of which there are now more than 800 species known. Of particular interest is the identification of linamarin with manihotoxin (Jorissen and Hairs, 1891) and the demonstration of emulsin-like activity in a number of plant tissues by Armstrong and Horton (1910). The subsequent history of cyanide in relation to cassava, a major world food crop, has been well described by Coursey (1973). By the end of the nineteenth century cyanide was no longer looked upon as an unusual poison but as a somewhat commonplace plant metabolite; Greshoff (1909) had found so many cyanogenic plants at Kew that he remarked "Indeed, in the ordinary plane tree of the London streets there is so much hydrocyanic acid present that the amount from every plane leaf would kill a London sparrow". By this time there was a much better understanding of the mode of action of cyanide as a result of experimental investigations which had been proceeding both before and after its chemical characterization.

III. THE RISE OF EXPERIMENTAL TOXICOLOGY

A. PHYSIOLOGICAL INVESTIGATIONS

The first account of experiments with dogs on the administration of extract of bitter almonds, and other poisons, dates from 1679 by Wepfer (Earles, 1963) a physician from Basle who had previously made important contributions to surgical pathology. He made careful observations on the symptoms of poisoning and on the post-mortem appearance of the organs after the administration of oil of almonds.

Two fatal cases of poisoning in Ireland caused by drinking cherry laurel water, used as a flavouring agent in cooking and to dilute brandy, led to the experiments of Maddern (1731). He showed that cherry laurel water contains "a poison never before known to be so though it has been in frequent use among us"; given orally, into the rectum or by injection it rapidly killed dogs. He compared the convulsions with those of epilepsy and noted that the more violent they were the more chance there was of subsequent recovery. The experiments were confirmed by Mortimer (1731), then acting Secretary of the Royal Society to whom Madden had sent his communication. Browne Langrish, a physician in London, in his book *Physical Experiments upon Brutes* (1746) gives an account of dosing horses and dogs with cherry laurel water. He noted that the blood became "beautiful" (fully oxygenated and therefore bright red?) when the extract was added. In addition to its acute toxic action he showed that small doses could be given over long periods without harm and even with apparent benefit. He also used a crude method of measuring the effect of laurel water on the tone of the resistance vessels "in imitation of my very ingenious friend the Rev. Dr Hales". The rate at which water entered the circulation through a cannula in the aorta of a freshly killed dog was found to increase when the laurel extract was added. (Since vasomotor tone is an active, metabolic process and thus subject to inhibition by cyanide.) Although his book was not published until 1746, Langrish read an account of his work to the Royal Society in 1734 and so followed shortly after Maddern and Mortimer.

The Abbé Felix Fontana studied poisons over many years from about 1767 onwards and wrote a two volume *Treatise on the venom of the viper; on the American poisons and on the cherry-laurel and some other vegetable poisons*. This was first published in Florence in Italian (1781) and was translated into English in 1795 but an account of some of his experiments on the cherry-laurel appeared, in Italian followed by a translation, in the Philosophical

Transaction of the Royal Society for 1780 - a point of forensic interest to be considered later.

He showed that mammals, birds, reptiles, amphibians, fish and insects could all be killed with small doses of laurel water and that after death the heart stopped beating much sooner than after decapitation or other poisons. His work showed the interest that was developing into the mode of action of poisons, in particular whether or not nerves were directly affected. He showed that there was no action when the sciatic nerve was covered with the extract and he inferred from this that the poison had to be transported by the circulation to be effective but he then, surprisingly, found no response following injection into the jugular vein. There is no ready explanation of this other than having an unusually weak extract but there were, then, no procedures for standardizing the preparations.

It was at this time that a celebrated murder case occurred in which cyanide was the lethal agent. John Donellan was tried and convicted for the murder of his brother-in-law, Sir Theodosius Boughton, at Warwick Assizes in March 1781. It was alleged that Donellan substituted a quantity of cherry laurel water for another medicine regularly taken by Sir Theodosius. John Hunter, the anatomist then at the Royal College of Surgeons, was called as a witness for the defence and his refusal to give unequivocal answers angered the judge and made a poor impression but by today's standards he was probably right in affirming no more than could be deduced from very tenuous evidence. After the trial it was stated that in Donellan's house had been found a copy of the *Philosophical Transactions* which fell open at an article giving instructions for distilling laurel water. The accounts do not specify this article but it could well have been that by Fontana who had submitted a paper to the Royal Society in advance of the first publication of his book in Italian. The paper appeared in volume 70 for 1780 and the murder took place on the 29th August, 1780. The instructions for preparing the extract were not very specific; it states only that a water extraction of the leaves is rather ineffective "but if the infusion be distilled *in balneo mariae* the distilled liquor becomes then a most powerful poison and proves fatal in a very short time". Possibly it was the arrival of this journal at Lawford Hall which suggested the idea of murder to Donellan. The case is memorable for the picture it presents of forensic medicine at that time and for the light it throws on Hunter's character as a scientist (Kobler, 1960).

Brodie (1811) was among the last to use plant extracts, in this instance the oil of bitter almonds which he gave orally or rectally to cats or applied to wounds in rabbits and mice. He concluded that the action was directly upon the central nervous system, a conclusion to be challenged later by Addison and Morgan. He also showed that recovery from a lethal dose was possible if artificial respiration was introduced, a procedure suggested by its successful use after curare poisoning. Although we know now that the modes of action of cyanide and curare are different, the experiment shows that both poisons are reversible; given time their effects wear off and normal respiration recommences.

From about this time preparations of hydro-cyanic acid replace extracts of cherry laurel or bitter almonds; Schrader (1802), guided by the characteristic smell of the extracts, suggested that HCN was the toxic ingredient and showed that it rapidly killed small birds when given orally. Emmert made similar observations on dogs in 1805 (Earles, 1961) and then Magendie (1817) carried out his systematic analysis of the action of several poisons, including HCN, with all his customary authority. He demonstrated the lethal action of the new acid recently (1815) synthesised from inorganic compounds by his fellow countryman Gay-Lussac. It was shown to be highly toxic in very small quantities and acted with great rapidity when given orally, intravenously or via the eye.

With these developments in the chemistry and toxicology of cyanide came a renewed interest in its use therapeutically. The detailed history of cyanide in medicine up to its final removal from the British Pharmacopoeia in 1948 has been well described by Earles (1967) and only the principal events will be related here.

At the start of Magendie's work (1817) cyanide was already employed in the treatment of pulmonary diseases but the preparations were not standardized and hence were hazardous in use. Magendie thought that the adoption of Gay-Lussac's new method of preparation would make for more accurate dispensing. He prepared the acid himself and treated one of his patients with it for a dry cough, with apparent success. Further cases were studied and the results published in his 1817 article. The remedy was later included in his Formulaire of 1821 which had several editions and was translated into English (1828). Meanwhile Granville, an eminent London physician and Italian patriot, had been travelling in Italy and in Paris and he may have heard of the therapeutic use of cyanide from Magendie. He mentions in his book that he advocated the use of cyanide for chest complaints in 1815, before Magendie had published. Granville vigorously promoted its use in his own practice, including treatment of his children, and publicized it by translating Magendie's 1817 article into English (1817) and by writing a small book (1819) on his clinical experiences. A second, greatly enlarged edition appeared the following year (1820). Magendie's article was also translated and published in America in 1820. There was, therefore, considerable publicity for this new remedy for asthma, catarrh, coughs, as a palliative in tuberculosis and as a sedative. In the early days considerable quantities were prepared for this purpose but its use declined as new, more specific and safer drugs were discovered.

This extension of interest into cyanide from physiological to practical medicine was empirical, unscientific and out of line with the main historical trend which has, on the whole, followed a logical, systematic path of investigation. Magendie was of course anxious to promote the status of physiology and that his experimental studies should result in a new clinical remedy was a triumph for his scientific approach to medicine. As a fashionable London physician and a Fellow of the Royal Society it is understandable that Granville should associate himself with what he considered to be a successful new advance.

The study of poisons had by now become an established discipline and had acquired, in the works of Orfila (1814) and Christison (1829), authoritative treatises. The treatment of cyanide by these authors is modern in their appreciation of the need for references, the use of quantitative information and the clear description of cases. Addison and Morgan (1829) published the first book in English on the action of poisons on the living body. It is mainly a short account of their own experiments which include the observations that cyanide was fatal when injected below the level of a spinal section but not when injected into a leg with the circulation, but not the sciatic nerve, ligated. They criticised Brodie's view that the poison acts directly on the brain but then came to the rather strange conclusion that an intact circulation is required, as shown above, in order to allow the poison access to "the sentient extremities of the nerves". They discuss in a modern way the nature of poisons and are aware of the need for sound experimental techniques (crossed circulation is used at one stage) but their final judgements have not stood the test of time and the book, sadly, falls just short of being a masterpiece.

A further step forward in understanding the mode of action of cyanide was made by James Blake, a former pupil of Magendie but by then working at University College, London, under what he acknowledges to be the stimulating leadership of William Sharpey, the first professor of physiology and anatomy in England. Blake (1839, 1840) used Poiseuille's haemodynamometer (mercury manometer) to measure blood pressure and the speed with which it was affected by cyanide given by different routes. He found that although cyanide acted quickly it still required an appreciable time, 30-45 seconds, to show its effects, which was compatible with his estimate of the circulation time. This argued strongly against any direct and immediate action on nerves. He further showed that cyanide placed in a dog's stomach had no effect if the portal vessels were ligated. On removal of the ligature for one minute respiration ceased but could be restored by artificial ventilation. Blake went on to have a picturesque medical career in the United States, a great loss to English physiology.

B. BIOCHEMICAL INVESTIGATIONS

Blake's work in a sense closes a phase in this history of cyanide which illustrates the development of experimental toxicology. The active chemical component of a natural poison had been identified, synthesized and shown to act on the body by its rapid absorption into the circulation. The next phase is dominated by the growing knowledge of biochemistry and sees the conclusion of the search for the mode of action of the poison.

Linking these two phases is one of the giants of physiology, Claude Bernard. He follows in the footsteps of his former teacher Magendie at the Collège de France in his technique but his experiments on cyanide connect him quite clearly with the developing interest in blood gas transport and the nature of cellular oxidation. He showed in 1857 that the cyanogenic glycoside amygdalin was harmless when injected intravenously and so too was the enzymic extract emulsin but the two when injected together were fatal. He also showed that when an animal died suddenly after breathing HCN gas the blood on both sides of the heart retained its bright red colour. This was similar to carbon monoxide poisoning except that with cyanide exposure to the air was necessary. He did not draw the correct conclusions from his work since it was still a few years before the discovery of the role of haemoglobin in oxygen transport. It was Hoppe-Seyler (1876) who showed that cyanide inhibited tissue oxidation and therefore oxyhaemoglobin was not reduced to its darker coloured form on passing to the veins and the right side of the heart. This conclusion was confirmed by others including Battelli and Stern (1907) who showed that cyanide poisoning of tissue respiration was a reversible process, thus recalling the earlier observations on the use of artificial ventilation. Cyanide was subsequently used by a number of biochemists to inhibit oxidative enzymes from plant and animal tissues and this led to the work of Warburg (1925) who demonstrated that cyanide inhibits oxidations catalysed specifically by iron salts. Finally Keilin (1929) showed that it combines with the trivalent iron atom in the tissue enzyme cytochrome oxidase, which forms a vital link between the tricarboxylic acid cycle and the formation of metabolic water.

During this chemical phase another aspect of cyanide poisoning emerged. Lang (1894) showed that the presence of cyanide resulted in the formation in the body of greater amounts of thiocyanate, a process which was helped if additional thiosulphate was supplied. Thiocyanate is relatively harmless and its formation, by a reaction between thiosulphate and cyanide, was seen as an example of the process of detoxification first discovered by Jaffe in 1877. This was an important step forward since it showed that the body is equipped to dispose of a poison which might be ingested accidentally or in the diet. Furthermore Pascheles (1894) showed that this transformation took place *in vitro* and was possibly enzymic. This last point was subsequently proved by (another) Lang (1933) who isolated an enzyme which he called rhodanese, meaning an enzyme which formed rhodanide, the German for thiocyanate (rhodanase would mean an enzyme which split thiocyanate).

The existence of an endogenous defence mechanism suggested possible ways of improving upon nature in cases of acute poisoning. Thiosulphate was an obvious choice of antidote and this was investigated by Meurice (1900) who extended the range of compounds undergoing detoxification to include a nymber of organic nitriles.

About this time Kobert (1891) showed that the oxidized form of haemoglobin, methaemoglobin, rapidly formed a stable compound with cyanide; the affinity was so great that as little as 2 μg HCN could be detected spectroscopically. Thus any increase in the amount of methaemoglobin would lower the concentration of free cyanide in the blood. Nitrites e.g. sodium or amyl nitrite, were known to induce methaemoglobin formation and hence could be used as a possible antidote. Thus a knowledge of haemoglobin chemistry enabled the iron-binding capacity of cyanide to be exploited in a hitherto unforseen but entirely scientific manner. Finally a suggestion (Autal, 1894) that cobalt, which has marked cyanide binding properties, might be useful as an antidote subsequently proved to have a sound theoretical basis and in the form of hydroxycobalamin (vitamin B12) or as cobalt edetate, is still in use as an antidote today.

REFERENCES

Addison, T. and Morgan, J. (1829). "An Essay on the Operation of Poisonous Agents on the Living Body". Longmans, London.

Antal, J. (1894). *Lancet* 1, 1521.

Armstrong, H.E. and Horton, E. (1910). *Proc. Roy. Soc. B* 82, 349-367.

Batelli, F. and Stern, L. (1907). *J. Physiol. Pathogen.* 9, 228-240.

Bernard, C. (1857). "Lecons sur les Effets des Substances Toxiques et Médicamenteuses". Bailliere et Fils, Paris.

Blake, J. (1839). *Edin. Med. Surg. J.* 51, 330-345.

Blake, J. (1840). *Edin. Med. Surg. J.* 53, 35-49.

Brodie, B.C. (1811). *Phil. Trans.* 101, 178-208.

Christison, R. (1829). "Treatise on Poisons". Black, Edinburgh.

Coursey, D.G. (1973). *In* "Chronic Cassava Toxicity". (B. Nestel, ed.) I.D.R.C., Ottawa.

Earles, M.P. (1961). *Ann. Sci.* 17, 97-110.

Earles, M.P. (1963). *Ann. Sci.* 19, 241-254.
Earles, M.P. (1967). *Med. Hist.* 11, 305-313.
Fontana, F. (1780). *Phil. Trans.* 70, appendix, ix-xlv.
Fontana, F. (1795). "Treatise on the Venom of the Viper; on the American Poisons; and on the Cherry Laurel and Some Other Vegetable Poisons". (J. Skinner, Trans.). London.
Granville, A.B. (1818). *J. Sci.* IV, 347-358.
Granville, A.B. (1820). "Further Observations on the Internal Use of the Hydro-Cyanic (Prussic) Acid". 2nd edn. Burgess and Hill, London.
Greshoff, M. (1909). *Kew Bull. Misc. Inform.* 10, 396-411.
Henry, O. and Charlard, A.F.B. (1836). *Mem. Acad. Med. Paris* 5, 212-220.
Hoppe-Seyler, F. (1876). *Pflug. Arch. ges. Physiol.* 12, 1-17.
Jorissen, A. and Hairs, E. (1891). *Acad. Roy. Belg.* 3 21, 529-540.
Keilin, D. (1929). *Proc. roy. Soc. B.* 104, 206-252.
Keilin, D. (1966). "The History of Cell Respiration and Cytochrome". Cambridge University Press,Cambridge.
Kobert, R. (1891). Cited by Keilin, 1966.
Kobler, J. (1960). "The Reluctant Surgeon". Heinemann, London.
Lang, S. (1894). *Arch. exp. Path. Pharm.* 34, 247-258.
Lang, K. (1933). *Biochem. Z.* 259, 242-256.
Langrish, B. (1746). "Physical Experiments upon Brutes". Henry, London.
Maddern, T. (1731). *Phil. Trans.* 37, 84-99.
Magendie, F. (1817). *Ann. Chim. Phys.* 6, 347-360.
Magendie, F. (1828). "Formulary for the Preparation and Employment of Several New Remedies". 6th edn. Trans. Houlton, J., London.
Meurice, J. (1900). *Arch. intern. Pharmacodyn.* 7, 11-53.
Miller, L.P. (1973). "Phytochemistry I". Academic Press, London.
Mortimer, C. (1731). *Phil. Trans.* 37, 163-173.
Orfila, M.J.B. (1814). "Traité des Poisons". Crochard, Paris.
Partington, J.R. (1962). "History of Chemistry". Vol. 3, p. 511, 527. McMillan, London.
Pascheles, W. (1894). *Arch. exp. Path. Pharm.* 34, 281-288.
Robiquet, F. and Charlard, A.F.B. (1830). *Ann. Chim. Phys.* 44, 352-382.
Scheele, C.W. (1786). "Chemical Essays" pp. 238-255. Trans. Beddoes, T., Reprint 1966. Dawson, London.
Schrader, J.C.C. (1802). *J. phys. chem. hist. nat.* 56, 224-226.
Vauquelin, P. (1803). *Ann. Chim.* 45, 206-212.
Warburg, O. (1925). Cited by Keilin, 1966.
Wöhler,F. and Leibig, J. (1837). *Ann. Phys., Lpz.,* 41, 345-366.

CYANIDE AS A METABOLIC INHIBITOR

LARRY P. SOLOMONSON

Department of Biochemistry, University of South Florida, College of Medicine, Tampa, Florida 33612, USA

I. INTRODUCTION

Cyanide has long held a prominent position amongst metabolic poisons. Perhaps the best known effect of cyanide is as an inhibitor of respiration. Indeed, the lethality of cyanide results directly from the inhibition of the terminal oxidase (cytochrome oxidase) of the mitochondrial respiratory chain. A number of other enzymes, some of which are listed in Table I, are also inhibited by low levels of cyanide and are in many cases as sensitive or more sensitive to cyanide than is cytochrome oxidase. There have been literally thousands of reports in the literature concerning the inhibition of various enzymes by cyanide. In some cases, such as the cytochrome P_{450} system, the sensitivity of the enzyme is so low as to be of little or no biological significance. In other cases, however, sensitivity to cyanide is high enough to result in substantial inhibition under conditions of sub-acute or chronic poisoning. In the case of assimilatory nitrate reductase, the sensitivity to cyanide is extremely high and cyanide has been proposed to have a regulatory role in this system.

In this review, I will review evidence that cyanide is a common and dynamic metabolite and will then briefly consider certain toxicological aspects of cyanide before considering the major metabolic effects of cyanide and where possible, the molecular bases for these effects. Special emphasis will be given to the action of cyanide on assimilatory nitrate reductase. References cited in this review are illustrative rather than exhaustive. For further references on toxicological aspects, see Way, this volume.

II. SOURCES

Cyanide and cyanide precursors are ubiquitous in nature.

Table I Sensitivities of various enzymes to cyanide

Enzyme	$K_d^{(a)}$, $I_{50}^{(b)}$, or $K_i^{(c)}$ (Moles/liter)	References
Cytochrome Oxidase (ox)	$1 \times 10^{-6(a)}$	(Van Buuren *et al.*, 1972 a,b; Wilson *et al.*, 1972)
Cytochrome Oxidase (red)	$1 \times 10^{-4(a)}$	(Van Buuren *et al.*, 1972 a,b; Wilson *et al.*, 1972)
Horseradish Peroxidase	$3 \times 10^{-6(a)}$	(Ellis and Dunford, 1968)
Yeast Cytochrome *c* Peroxidase	$4 \times 10^{-6(a)}$	(Erman, 1974)
Lactoperoxidase	$3 \times 10^{-5(a)}$	(Dolman *et al.*, 1968)
Catalase	$5 \times 10^{-6(b)}$	(Galston, 1955)
Myoglobin (ox)	$8 \times 10^{-7(a)}$	(VerPloeg, 1971)
Cytochrome P-450	$5 \times 10^{-3(b)}$	(Matsubara and Touchi, 1977)
Superoxide Dismutase	$2 \times 10^{-5(b)}$	(Rotilio *et al.*, 1972)
Acyl CoA Desaturase	$1 \times 10^{-4(b)}$	(Kader, 1977)
Ribulose Diphosphate Carboxylase	$6 \times 10^{-6(b)}$	(Marsho and Kung, 1976)
Nitrite Reductase	$5 \times 10^{-6(c)}$	(Lafferty and Garrett, 1974)
Nitrogenase	$2 \times 10^{-5(c)}$	(Biggins and Kelly, 1970)
Nitrate Reductase (ox)	$2 \times 10^{-5(c)}$	(Garrett and Greenbaum, 1973)
Nitrate Reductase (red)	$4 \times 10^{-10(a)}$	(Lorimer *et al.*, 1974)

$^{(a)}K_d$ = dissociation constant for enzyme-cyanide complex.

$^{(b)}I_{50}$ = concentration of cyanide which gives 50% inhibition.

$^{(c)}K_i$ = inhibition constant.

Cyanide ingestion in man and animals is principally from vegetables containing cyanogenic glycosides (Ermans *et al.*, 1972). Dietary foodstuffs which contain moderate to high levels of cyanogenic glycosides include cassava, a dietary staple in several regions of Africa (Cooke and Coursey, this volume) as well as other common foods such as lima beans, sorghum, linseed, kernels of fruits, sweet potatoes, maize, millet, and bamboo shoots. The maximum yield of cyanide from some of these sources can be as high as 100-300 mg per 100 gm of tissue (Montgomery, 1969) so the amount of cyanide ingested from these sources can be substantial, especially in comparison with the lethal dose range for humans, which is in the range of 0.5-3.5 mg/kg body weight (Ermans *et al.*, 1972). Normal food preparation processes, however, reduce the content of cyanide and cyanide precursors in these foods to tolerable levels provided such foods are not the major dietary component.

There are also several non-dietary sources of cyanide. Tobacco smoke is one common source and can lead to higher levels of blood cyanide and thiocyanate in smokers as compared to non-smokers (Pettigrew and Fell, 1973; Thomson and Anderson, 1980). Laetrile, a controversial preparation which has been used in the treatment of cancer, can give rise to high levels of cyanide, especially if ingested together with foods which containe enzymes that degrade laetrile to cyanide (Schmidt *et al.*, 1978). Amygdalin, a cyanogenic glycoside which is the principal component of laetrile, can be degraded in the gut to cyanide and benzaldehyde. Several cases of cyanide poisoning resulting from ingestion of laetrile given either orally or as an enema have recently been reported (Humbert *et al.*, 1977; Smith *et al.*, 1977; Ortega and Creek, 1978; Braico *et al.*, 1979). Carter *et al.* (1980) have shown in experiments with germ-free rats that the gastro-intestinal flora are obligatory for the release of toxic amounts of cyanide from amygdalin.

Other potential sources of cyanide in man and animals include sodium nitroprusside ($Na_2Fe(CN)_5NO$), succinonitrile ($NC-CH_2-CH_2-CN$) and organic thiocyanates (RSCN). Sodium nitroprusside is a potent hypotensive agent which has been widely used to treat severe hypertension and to minimize bleeding during surgery. Patients receiving sodium nitroprusside had considerable increases in both red blood cell and plasma cyanide levels (Vesey *et al.*, 1976; Cottrell *et al.*, 1978). Cyanide generated in animals following nitroprusside treatment appears to react mainly with hemoglobin to form cyanomethemoglobin (Smith and Druszyna, 1974). Free cyanide would then be slowly liberated from the latter complex. Cyanide production from nitroprusside also appears to require a reductant. Reduced glutathione and ascorbate were more effective than NADH or NADPH in stimulating the production of cyanide from nitroprusside in a mitochondrial suspension from rat liver (Nakemura *et al.*, 1977).

Cyanide can also be liberated from succinonitrile, a widely used antidepressant. Liver slices catalyze this formation but cyanide was not formed in homogenates or crude fractions of mitochondria, microsomes or cytosol or by liver slices treated with Triton X-100 (Contessa and Santi, 1973). More recently it has been shown that acute or chronic ethanol treatment significantly increased cyanide formation from succinonitrile in rat liver slices, thereby increasing the toxicity of the drug (Contessa *et al.*, 1978). This increase in toxicity appeared to be due to a stimulation of cyanide formation rather than to an inhibition of detoxifying enzymes.

Cyanide can also be formed from organic thiocyanates which are commonly employed as insecticides. The liberation of cyanide from organic thiocyanates appears to be catalyzed by the enzyme, glutathione S-transferase (Ohkawa and Casida, 1971).

Cyanide formation from several endogenous compounds other than cyanogenic glycosides has been found to occur in higher plants and microorganisms. Glycine, for example, is the principal source of cyanide in cyanogenic bacteria (Castric, this volume; Nazly *et al.*, this volume; Wissing, this volume). Glyoxylate plus hydroxylamine (Solomonson and Spehar, this volume) and histidine or the aromatic amino acids (Vennesland *et al.*, this volume) have been proposed as potential sources of the cyanide utilized for the reversible inactivation of assimilatory nitrate reductase in photosynthetic organisms. Cyanide formation from histidine and the aromatic amino acids is catalyzed by amino acid oxidase supplemented with peroxidase or cytochrome *c*. Either D-amino acid oxidase or L-amino acid oxidase will catalyze this reaction with the appropriate substrate. The "yield" of cyanide can be as high as 70% under optimal conditions (Gewitz *et al*, 1980). The physiological significance of this reaction is not yet established, but considering the wide distribution of the amino acid oxidases, it is quite likely that some cyanide would be formed via these reactions.

From the foregoing evidence, it can be concluded that, rather than being a metabolic anomaly, cyanide is a rather common metabolite which can be formed from a variety of precursors which are widely distributed in nature.

III. TOXICITY AND DETOXIFICATION

Although cyanide is generally considered to be a potent poison, it is perhaps less toxic, on a molar basis, than some "essential" vitamins and minerals. The intraperitoneal LD_{50} in mice is about 0.1 mmole per kg body weight (Smith and Gosselin, 1966) while a lethal dose for man is in the range of 0.02-0.13 mmole per kg body weight when ingested orally (Montgomery, 1969). Cyanide is rapidly absorbed from the upper gastrointestinal tract. Low levels of ingested cyanide are normally rapidly converted to thiocyanate in a reaction between cyanide and thiosulfate catalyzed by the enzyme, rhodanese (Westley, this volume). Rhodanese is widely distributed in nature and is particularly active in mammalian liver tissue (mitochondrial fraction). Thiocyanate is less toxic than cyanide and is the major excretion product of cyanide metabolism (Pettigrew and Fell, 1972). Some thiocyanate can apparently be oxidized to sulfate and cyanide in the blood in a reaction catalyzed by hemoglobin acting as a peroxidase (Chang and Wood, 1971), suggesting that cyanide and thiocyanate may be in dynamic equilibrium. A report by Vesey and Wilson (1978) suggests that this apparent "thiocyanate oxidase" activity may be due in part to an artifact of the assay. Cyanide, however, is a normal constituent of blood and is usually present at concentrations below 12 μM (Thomson and Anderson, 1980). The ratio of cyanide to thiocyanate is normally about 1:1000 in body fluids (Pettigrew and Fell, 1973).

Acute doses of cyanide will lead to death from respiratory failure if not treated promptly. Antidotes for cyanide poisoning include thiosulfate, nitrite and hydroxycobalamin (Way, this volume). Thiosulfate is a substrate for the enzyme rhodanese, which converts cyanide to thiocyanate. Nitrite converts hemoglobin to methemoglobin which has a high affinity for cyanide. The HCN-methemoglobin complex then slowly releases cyanide, which is converted to thiocyanate via rhodanese. Cyanide reacts with hydroxycobalamin in a non-enzymic reaction to form cyanocobalamin (Reenstra and Jencks, 1979).

The principal effects associated with chronic cyanide poisoning include demyelination, lesions of the optic nerve, decrease in sulfur-containing amino acids, increase in thiocyanate, goiter, ataxia, hypertonia and depressed thyroid function (Ermans *et al.*, 1972). These symptoms may develop in individuals who ingest significant quantities of cyanide or cyanogenic precursors in their diet or as a result of cyanogenic drugs. These toxic effects of chronic, sublethal doses of cyanide are especially common in parts of the world which depend on cassava as a major dietary component (Cooke and Coursey, this volume, Way, this volume).

Cyanide is toxic to most higher plants and microorganisms. Besides being converted to thiocyanate via rhodanese in these organisms, cyanide can also condense with a three-carbon unit such as cysteine or serine to form β-cyanoalanine. β-Cyanoalanine can then be converted to either asparagine or other derivatives such as γ-glutamyl-β-cyanoalanine (Blumenthal-Goldschmidt, 1963; Fowden and Bell, 1965; Oaks and Johnson, 1972). The ultimate fate of cyanide is different for different species but it appears that the β-cyanoalanine pathway may be a major pathway for cyanide detoxification in many non-mammalian organisms. Cyanide can also be detoxified to CO_2 by some fungi (Fry and Myers, this volume; Bunch and Knowles, this volume).

IV. METABOLIC EFFECTS

A. RESPIRATION

The inhibition of respiration by cyanide is attributable

to the binding and inactivation by cyanide of cytochrome oxidase, the terminal component of the mitochondrial electron transport chain. Other components of the mitochondrial chain have a relatively low affinity for cyanide.

Cytochrome oxidase is a multimeric enzyme complex containing two heme *a* components and two copper ion oxidation-reduction centers (Hartzell *et al.*, 1978). The nature of the interaction of cyanide with cytochrome oxidase has been extensively studied (VanBuuren *et al.*, 1972a, b; Nicholls *et al.*, 1972; Wilson *et al.*, 1972; Wilson and Erecinska, 1978). One mole of cyanide binds tightly to one mole of cytochrome oxidase (cytochrome aa_3). Both the rate of binding and the tightness of binding are dependent on the oxidation state of the enzyme. Although cyanide binds to both the fully oxidized and the fully reduced forms of cytochrome oxidase, its affinity for the oxidized form is about two orders of magnitude higher than that for the fully reduced form (Table I). The reaction rate for the binding of cyanide to the oxidized form of cytochrome oxidase, however, is about two orders of magnitude less than the reaction rate for the binding of cyanide to the reduced form. Thus, cyanide binds more tightly but reacts more slowly with the oxidized form of cytochrome oxidase. When cyanide is added during active turnover, the apparent K_d is only slightly higher than that for the fully oxidized enzyme. The rate of binding is also higher. It therefore appears that, when added during active turnover, cyanide reacts with the reduced enzyme which is then oxidized to the more stable oxidized cytochrome aa_3-cyanide complex. The oxidized cytochrome oxidase-cyanide complex is extremely stable but in the presence of reducing equivalents, cyanide readily dissociates from the enzyme to form active cytochrome aa_3.

It was earlier suggested that the inhibition of cytochrome oxidase by low concentrations of cyanide may involve binding of cyanide to one of the copper ions in the oxidase (Antonini *et al.*, 1971). X-ray absorption edge studies on cyanide-bound cytochrome oxidase, however, indicated that cyanide has no effect on the Cu edge spectrum of the oxidized protein while the intensity of the 1s-3d transition in the Fe edge spectrum was enhanced. This was attributed to π-bonding of cyanide to iron (Hu *et al.*, 1977). Also, the addition of cyanide to partially reduced cytochrome oxidase results in the appearance of a low spin electron spin resonance signal at g=3.58 which was ascribed to the ferricytochrome aa_3-cyanide complex (DerVartanian *et al.*, 1974). Cyanide did not significantly affect the EPR spectrum of fully oxidized cytochrome oxidase.

Although the predominant toxicological effect of cyanide is considered to be due to the inhibition of cytochrome oxidase, Isom and Way (1976) reported that cyanide lethality could occur with no apparent inhibition of liver cytochrome oxidase activity. To explain these results they suggested that brain cytochrome oxidase may be the site of lethal action of cyanide, as judged from the tissue distribution of cyanide, thiosulfate and rhodanese. Earlier studies indicated that brain cytochrome oxidase is inhibited *in vivo* by cyanide (Olsen and Klein, 1947). Thus *in vivo* sensitivity to cyanide is dependent not only on the affinity of cytochrome oxidase for cyanide but on the activity and distribution of competing detoxification reactions.

B. GLUCOSE METABOLISM

Isom *et al.*, (1975) studied the effect of sublethal doses of cyanide on glucose catabolism in mice by use of radiorespirometric techniques. Cyanide caused an approximately 100% increase in catabolism of glucose via the pentose phosphate pathway and an approximately 50% decrease in the catabolism of glucose via the glycolytic pathway. Sublethal doses of cyanide cause an increase in blood glucose and lactic acid levels and a decrease in the ATP/ADP ratio resulting from a shift from aerobic to anaerobic metabolism (Handler, 1945; Albaum *et al.*, 1946; Olsen and Klein, 1947). Isom *et al.* (1975) suggested that the increased catabolism of glucose via the pentose phosphate pathway and accompanying increase in NADPH and pentose phosphate production may reflect a compensating mechanism of the cell to maintain a balanced redox state since an increased conversion of pyruvate to lactate would result in a decrease in the NADH/NAD ratio. A special type of diabetes associated with pancreatic calcification and loss of β-cell function has been linked to cyanide ingestion (McMillan and Geevarghese, 1979). Jakob and Diem (1974) found that glucose production and phosphorylase activity in isolated perfused rat livers were increased by cyanide. Cyanide activated glycogenolysis to about the same extent as did glucagon but the effects of the two agents were additive. Sublethal doses of cyanide, therefore, may alter the intermediary metabolism of carbohydrates by causing an increase in glycogen breakdown and a shunting of glucose to the pentose phosphate pathway while decreasing the rate of glycolysis and inhibiting the TCA cycle.

Of possible relevance to the effects of cyanide on carbohydrate metabolism is the promotion of seed germination by cyanide (Taylorson and Hendricks, 1973; Hendricks and Taylorson, 1975). The promotion of seed germination was accompanied by an inhibition of catalase and a stimulation of the pentose phosphate pathway. Hendricks and Taylorson (1975) suggested that this stimulation of the pentose phosphate pathway and promotion of seed germination occurred via the metabolic network shown in Fig. 1.

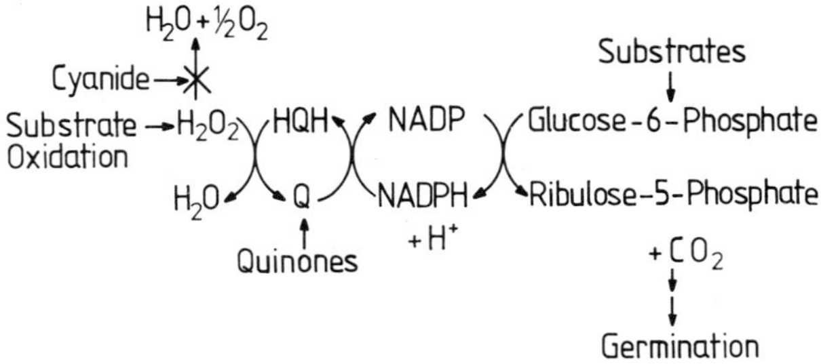

Fig. 1

C. THYROID FUNCTION

Cyanide affects thyroid function indirectly through its major detoxification product, thiocyanate. Thiocyanate is relatively non-toxic at levels normally found in blood. The increased levels of thiocyanate resulting from subacute cyanide poisoning however, may be sufficient to depress thyroid function markedly, especially if accompanied by an iodine deficiency. Iodine plays an essential role in the occurrence of endemic goiter and cretinism. Kreutler *et al.* (1978) showed that thiocyanate can affect thyroid growth and function in the neonatal rat. Both cyanide and thiocyanate caused goiter formation and elevation of thyroid stimulating hormone (TSH) in iodine-deficient animals but not in iodine-sufficient animals, suggesting that thiocyanate may be a factor in the etiology of endemic cretinism and goiter in areas where iodine intake is marginal and precursors of thiocyanate appear in the diet. Thiocyanate inhibits both the active uptake of iodine by the thyroid and the organic binding (as monoiodotyrosine and diiodotyrosine residues of thyroglobulin) of iodide which does enter the cell. The concentration of thiocyanate which inhibited iodide uptake by 50% was approximately 10^{-4} M while the concentration which inhibited organic binding was about 10^{-3} M (Greer *et al.*, 1966). Uptake of iodide therefore appears to be more sensitive to thiocyanate than organic binding. Michajlovikij and Langer (1974) have reported that thiocyanate also causes a competitive displacement of thyroxin from serum thyroxin-binding proteins, resulting in a transient increase in serum thyroxin levels. This would also render thyroxin more susceptible to degradation. Thus thiocyanate appears to affect thyroid function at several different levels, most or all of which can be prevented by sufficient iodine intake.

D. MOLYBDOENZYMES

The molybdoenzymes are a class of enzymes which include

nitrogenase, nitrate reductase, xanthine oxidase and sulfite oxidase. All of these enzymes contain other prosthetic groups in addition to molybdenum. Nitrogenase and xanthine oxidase contain non-heme iron/labile sulfide centers. Nitrate reductase and sulfite oxidase contain no non-heme iron but do contain heme in the form of a b-type cytochrome. Nitrate reductase and xanthine oxidase contain FAD as a third prosthetic group. In all cases the molybdenum is associated with a low molecular weight cofactor which has been only partially characterized but appears to be similar or identical for all molybdoenzymes (Ketchum *et al.*, 1970; Nason *et al.*, 1971). The cofactor from nitrogenase contains 8 Fe and 6 acid-labile sulfides per molybdenum (Shaw and Brill, 1977). Another type of molybdenum cofactor which contains no iron appears to be common to nitrate reductase, xanthine oxidase and sulfite oxidase. The cofactor associated with these enzymes has recently been shown to contain a pteridine moiety as a structural component (Johnson *et al.*, 1980).

Cyanide acts as a substrate for nitrogenase (Biggins and Kelly, 1970) and inhibits all other molybdoenzymes. In the case of assimilatory nitrate reductase from photosynthetic organisms, this inhibition by cyanide is of possible importance in the metabolic control of nitrate assimilation (Solomonson, 1974; Gewitz *et al.*, 1974; Pistorius *et al.*, 1976; Solomonson and Spehar, 1977, 1979). Cyanide reacts with nitrate reductase in the presence of NADH (reduced form of enzyme) to give an inactive product which resembles an inactive enzyme precursor found in crude extracts (Vennesland and Jetschmann, 1971; Vennesland and Solomonson, 1972; Solomonson and Vennesland, 1972; Solomonson, 1974). Garrett and Greenbaum (1973) also observed that the sensitivity of assimilatory nitrate reductase from *Neurospora crassa* to inhibition by metal binding agents such as cyanide is dependent on the oxidation state of the enzyme. The oxidized form of the enzyme was less sensitive to inhibition by cyanide. Inhibition of the oxidized form was freely reversible and competitive with respect to nitrate. If the enzyme was reduced by preincubation with its natural reductant, NADPH, however, its sensitivity to cyanide was increased and the inhibition was not competitive with respect to nitrate (Garrett and Greenbaum, 1973).

The amount of cyanide needed to effect a reversible inactivation of *Chlorella* nitrate reductase in the presence of excess NADH was in the same concentration range as that of the enzyme (Solomonson, 1974). This inactivation by cyanide could, in fact, be used as a sensitive bioassay for cyanide (Gewitz *et al.*, 1974). Both forms of nitrate reductase are stable. The enzyme remains in the inactive form after removal of excess cyanide and NADH by gel filtration, although the cytochrome *b* associated with nitrate reductase reverts back to the oxidized form when the gel filtration is done under aerobic conditions. Thus there was no apparent correlation between the state of activation and the state of oxidation of the cytochrome *b* associated with nitrate reductase (Solomonson, 1974). Furthermore, there were no detectable changes in the reduced or oxidized cytochrome absorption spectrum or in molecular size associated with the inactivation-activation reactions. Although no significant conversion from the inactive form to the active form of the enzyme took place upon removal of excess NADH and cyanide, the enzyme was rapidly and fully activated by treatment with an oxidant such as ferricyanide (Jetschmann *et al.*, 1972; Solomonson *et al.*, 1973; Solomonson, 1974). It was postulated that cyanide may complex with the molybdo-moiety of the enzyme and alter its properties in such a way as to allow reduction to a lower oxidation state such as Mo III, which would not participate in O-atom transfer reactions and thus would not be able to reduce nitrate (Solomonson, 1974).

Subsequent work showed that the binding of cyanide to the enzyme was linearly proportional to the amount of inactivation and the bound cyanide was released (as cyanide) upon reactivation of the enzyme (Lorimer *et al.*, 1974). Upon complete inactivation, there was one cyanide bound per molybdenum center (Solomonson *et al.*, 1975). The Mo V EPR signal observed upon reduction with NADH disappears upon inactivation of the enzyme with cyanide (Solomonson, 1979). The dissociation constant measured for the inactive nitrate reductase-cyanide complex was 3.6×10^{-10} M (Lorimer *et al.*, 1974), which is about three orders of magnitude lower than the dissociation constant for cyanide complexes of other enzymes, such as cytochrome oxidase, which are sensitive to inhibition by cyanide.

The extreme sensitivity of nitrate reductase to cyanide and the reversibility of the inhibition made cyanide an ideal candidate for a physiological regulator of nitrate reductase. Evidence that cyanide may indeed be a natural regulator of nitrate reductase activity came from the demonstration that the inactive form of nitrate reductase isolated from cells which had been treated with ammonia to convert the enzyme to the inactive form *in vivo*, contained a stoichiometric amount of bound cyanide which was released upon conversion to the active form (Lorimer *et al.*, 1974; Gewitz *et al.*, 1978). This demonstration has so far been done only with *Chlorella*. It is not known whether such conversions take place in other nitrate assimilating organisms as well. The relative importance of this *in vivo* inactivation by cyanide in the cellular regulation of nitrate reductase has also not been established. It is not known, for example, whether cyanide is involved in the formation of a stable, storage form of the enzyme. It is known, however, that the process is rapidly and fully reversible, *in vivo* as well as *in vitro* (Solomonson and Spehar, 1977) and that O_2, CO_2, Mn, light and adenylate energy charge are all involved in the process (Pistorius *et al.*, 1976; Solomonson and Spehar, 1977, 1979). Recent work in this area has been concerned primarily with defining conditions for and elucidating possible pathways for the formation of cyanide utilized in the formation of the inactive enzyme-cyanide complex (Pistorius *et al.*, 1976, 1977, 1978, 1979; Solomonson and Spehar, 1977, 1979; Gewitz *et al.*, 1976, 1980). The latter subject is discussed in more detail elsewhere (see Vennesland *et al.*, this volume).

The general features of the reversible inactivation by cyanide are similar for other molybdoenzymes. There is, however, a several-fold difference in sensitivity to cyanide inhibition and only in the case of assimilatory nitrate reductase could cyanide have a regulatory function. Cohen *et al.* (1971) reported that incubation of hepatic sulfite oxidase with cyanide in the presence of its natural reductant, sulfite, resulted in a slow, progressive and apparently irreversible inactivation of the enzyme. This inactivation was accompanied by a concomitant and proportional loss of the MoV EPR-signal. The oxidized form of sulfite oxidase was not inhibited by 1 mM cyanide whether it was pre-incubated with cyanide prior to assay or not (Cohen and Fridovich, 1971). In more recent work, Coughlan *et al.* (1980) have shown that the reduced form of the molybdoenzymes, sulfite oxidase, xanthine oxidase, xanthine dehydrogenase, and aldehyde oxidase, are all reversibly inhibited by cyanide. The concentrations of cyanide required to achieve approximately 50% inactivation in 30 minutes ranged from 0.5 mM for hepatic xanthine oxidase to 50 mM for hepatic sulfite oxidase. These concentrations are several orders of magnitude higher than those required for the reversible inactivation of nitrate reductase (Solomonson, 1974). As was found with nitrate reductase, however, the inactive forms of these molybdoenzymes remained in the inactive state following removal of excess reductant and cyanide by gel filtration, and reactivation was achieved by incubation with suitable oxidants. Coughlan *et al.* (1980) showed that stoichiometric binding of cyanide is required for the onset of inactivation but its continued binding is not required for the maintenance of inactivation. EPR studies and difference absorption spectra were consistent with the molybdenum centers being the binding site for cyanide. Reactivation of the inactive forms of these molybdoenzymes by ferricyanide under anaerobic conditions required 3 to 4 moles of ferricyanide per active site, indicating that the molybdenum center in the inactive enzyme had been reduced below the oxidation states attained during catalysis. As pointed out by Coughlan *et al.* (1980), the overreduced state of molybdenum appears to render the molybdenum center incapable of participating in electron transfer to the natural carriers or acceptors.

Only the molybdenum-containing hydroxylases, xanthine oxidase, xanthine dehydrogenase and aldehyde oxidase appear to be inactivated by cyanide in the oxidized state. In contrast to the inactivation of the reduced molybdoenzymes, this inactivation is irreversible and is accompanied by the formation of a stoichiometric amount of thiocyanate (Massey and Edmonson, 1970; Branzoli and Massey, 1974; Cleere and Coughlan, 1974; Coughlan, 1977; Coughlan *et al.*, 1980). Massey and Edmonson (1970) showed that oxidized xanthine oxidase, inactivated with cyanide, could be partially reactivated by incubation with sodium sulfide. They also demonstrated the incorporation into the reactivated enzyme of ^{35}S from $Na_2{}^{35}S$ which was removed as $^{35}SCN^-$ upon re-inactivation of the oxidized form of the enzyme by cyanide. They postulated that the sulfur released following cyanide treatment originated with a persulfide (RSS^-) group associated with the molybdenum center. Coughlan (1977) proposed an alternative interpretation in which an active center cysteine residue was the source of the cyanolysable sulfur. In support of this alternative explanation is the finding of a dehydroalanine residue associated with the inactive form of xanthine dehydrogenase (Cleere and Coughlan, 1974). Coughlan proposed that sulfide would react with the dehydroalanine residue to regenerate the active center cysteine residue instead of reacting with a sulfhydryl group to regenerate active center persulfide as proposed by Massey and Edmundson (1970).

Thus, cyanide can inactivate molybdoenzymes in one of two ways: either by reaction with the reduced molybdoenzyme to form an inactive enzyme-cyanide complex which can be readily reactivated by treatment with an oxidant, or by reaction with oxidized forms of the molybdo-hydroxylases to form an inactive enzyme plus thiocyanate which can be partially reactivated by treatment with sodium sulfide.

E. OTHER METALLO-ENZYMES

Cyanide inhibits a number of metallo-enzymes besides those containing heme or molybdenum and thereby may perturb metabolic processes involving these enzymes. These enzymes include those containing zinc or copper. The inhibition of the cytosolic Cu/Zn superoxide dismutase by cyanide (Rotilio *et al.*, 1972), for example, can be used to distinguish this enzyme from the cyanide insensitive manganese superoxide dismutase associated with the mitochondrial matrix.

The zinc metallo-enzymes, alkaline phosphatase and carbonic anhydrase are also sensitive to inhibition by cyanide. Leucocyte alkaline phosphatase was shown to be rapidly inhibited upon infusion of rabbits with sub-acute doses of cyanide (Thorling and Niazy, 1973). The activity gradually returned to normal values 25-30 days after cessation of the cyanide infusion. Thus, the inhibition is apparently long acting and not freely reversible. Cyanide forms a 1:1 inhibition complex with carbonic anhydrase and binding is directly to the zinc moiety of the enzyme (Feeney and Burgen, 1973).

Cyanide blocks photosynthetic electron transport through interaction with the copper protein, plastocyanin, which functions as an electron carrier between photosystems I and II (Ouitrakal and Izawa, 1973; Berg and Krogmann, 1975). Cyanide, at a concentration of 10^{-5} M, removes the copper from plastocyanin leaving the inactive apoplastocyanin which is unable to transfer electrons to photosystem I (Berg and Krogmann, 1975). The blue copper protein, ascorbate oxidase, is also inactivated by cyanide, probably by removal of copper from the enzyme (Strothkamp and Dawson, 1977).

Iron-sulfur proteins such as clostridial ferredoxin can be inactivated and bleached by cyanide (Wallace and Rabinowitz, 1971). This treatment with cyanide is accompanied by the formation of thiocyanate. Sulfide was released prior to SCN^- formation, suggesting that the thiocyanate formed from ferredoxin and cyanide results from production of a persulfide bond between the apoprotein and the released sulfide (Wallace and Rabinowitz, 1971).

Cyanide can also remove selenium from seleno-enzymes. Treatment of highly purified sheep glutathione peroxidase with cyanide at concentrations as low as 0.1 mM resulted in loss of enzyme activity and release of selenium from the enzyme (Prohaska *et al.*, 1977). The inactivation was time-dependent and the rate of inactivation was influenced by temperature, pH andthe oxidation state of the enzyme. Prior reduction of the enzyme with reduced glutathione or other reductants prevented the inactivation by cyanide. Other related inhibitors such as thiocyanate or azide did not cause inactivation or removal of selenium. The Se-CN interaction can explain the partial prevention by cyanide of selenium poisoning (Palmer and Olson, 1979) and the ability of the cyanogenic glycosides of linseed meal to protect animals against selenium toxicity (Smith *et al.*, 1980).

F. NON-METALLO-INTERACTIONS

Low concentrations of cyanide can inhibit a number of enzymes through interactions not involving a metal. These interactions have in some cases been shown to involve reaction between cyanide and a Schiff base intermediate or between cyanide and a substrate to form an inhibitory compound. An example of the latter case is the indirect inhibition of ribulose diphosphate carboxylase/oxygenase by cyanide. This enzyme is the key enzyme in the Calvin cycle of photosynthetic CO_2 fixation. Kinetic studies suggested that the active inhibitory substance is the cyanohydrin derivative formed from the reaction between cyanide and ribulose diphosphate (Marsho and Kung, 1976). The reaction is time-dependent and is greatly enhanced by the mixing of equimolar quantities of cyanide and ribulose diphosphate before the assay. Under these conditions approximately 50% inhibition was observed with 6 μM cyanide.

All enzymic reactions which involve Schiff base intermediates are potentially susceptible to inhibition by cyanide. An example of the reaction between cyanide and a Schiff-base intermediate is that between hepatic 2-keto-4-hydroxyglutarate aldolase and cyanide (Hansen and Dekker, 1976). This enzyme catalyzes the terminal step in the catabolism of hydroxyproline by mammals. Inactivation is apparently due to cyanide addition to the Schiff base aldimine and consequent stable formation of an amino-nitrile as shown in Fig. 2.

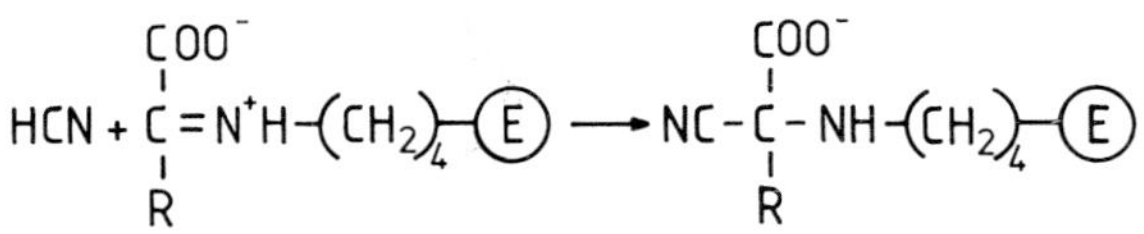

Fig. 2

Cyanide, at concentrations as low as 1 μM, also inhibits clostridial acetoacetate decarboxylase by forming an adduct with a Schiff base intermediate at the active site (Autor and Fridovich, 1970). Enzymes which contain pyridoxal phosphate go through a Schiff base intermediate. As might be expected, therefore, these enzymes are also sensitive to inhibition by cyanide. An example is the inhibition of rat brain glutamate decarboxylase and γ-aminobutyric acid (GABA) transaminase (Tursky and Sajter, 1962). Fifty percent inhibition of glutamate decarboxylase was achieved with 6.5×10^{-4} M cyanide. GABA transaminase was inhibited 50% by 6.5×10^{-3} M cyanide. These results suggested that the decreased concentration of GABA in brains of rats following cyanide treatment was due to the inhibition of glutamate decarboxylase (Tursky and Sajter, 1962).

Although cyanide generally acts as an enzyme inhibitor, in some cases it acts as an apparent stimulator. For example, cyanide stimulated guanylate cyclase activity in a wide range of tissues including liver, lung, stomach, colon and kidney (Vesely *et al.*, 1979). The effective concentration range was 0.1 to 3 mM and the degree of stimulation was about two-fold. Cyanide can also mimic the effects of ethylene, which is a plant hormone involved in fruit ripening (Solomos and Laties, 1974, 1975, 1976).

Both agents appear to act by stimulating cyanide-insensitive respiration and are attended by an enhancement in the rate of glycolysis. Cyanide-resistant respiration is discussed by Palmer, this volume.

V. CONCLUDING REMARKS

From the foregoing evidence it is apparent that cyanide may have a multiplicity of effects on metabolism arising from the fact that it is a potential inhibitor of several metallo-enzymes as well as enzymes involving Schiff base intermediates. The metabolic response to cyanide will depend not only on the concentration of cyanide but also on a number of other factors, including levels of B_{12}, iodine, sulfur amino acids and levels and distribution of detoxifying enzymes such as rhodanese. It also appears that cyanide toxicity may be a rather common occurrence and may be exacerbated by other dietary deficiencies mentioned above. It is not yet possible to explain with certainty all of the toxic effects of cyanide in metabolic terms but knowledge of the relative sensitivities of various enzyme systems to cyanide should facilitate a better understanding of both the toxic effects of cyanide and possible physiological functions of cyanide and its metabolites.

ACKNOWLEDGEMENTS

Research from the author's laboratory was supported in part by a grant from the National Institutes of Health (GM23407). I am grateful to those authors who supplied me with manuscripts before publication.

REFERENCES

Albaum, H.G., Tepperman, J. and Bodanzky, O. (1946). *J. Biol. Chem.* 164, 45-51.

Antonini, E.A., Brunori, M., Greenwood, C., Malstrom, B.G. and Rotilio, G.C. (1971). *Eur. J. Biochem.* 23, 396-400.

Autor, A.P. and Fridovich, I. (1970). *J. Biol. Chem.* 245, 5214-5222.

Berg., S.P. and Krogmann, D.W. (1975). *J. Biol. Chem.* 250, 8957-8962.

Biggins, D.R. and Kelly, M. (1970). *Biochim. Biophys. Acta* 205, 288-289.

Blumenthal-Goldschmidt, S., Butler, G.W. and Conn, E.E. (1963). *Nature* 197, 718-719.

Braico, K.T., Humbert, J.R., Terplan, K.L. and Lehotay, J.M. (1979). *New Engl. J. Med.* 300, 238-239.

Branzoli, U. and Massey, V. (1974). *J. Biol. Chem.* 249, 4346-4349.

Carter, J.H., McLafferty, M.A. and Goldman, P. (1980). *Biochem. Pharmacol.* 29, 301-304.

Chang, J. and Wood, J.L. (1971). *J. Biol. Chem.* 246, 555-560.
Cleere, W.F. and Coughlan, M.P. (1974). *Biochem. J.* 143, 331-340.
Cohen, H.J. and Fridovich, I. (1971). *J. Biol. Chem.* 246, 367-373.
Cohen, H.J., Fridovich, I. and Rajagopalan, K.V. (1971). *J. Biol. Chem.* 246, 374-382.
Contessa, A.R. and Santi, R. (1973). *Biochem. Pharmacol.* 22, 827-832.
Contessa, A.R., Floreani, M., Bonnetti, A.C. and Santi, R. (1978). *Biochem. Pharmacol.* 27, 1135-1138.
Coughlan, M.P. (1977). *FEBS Lett.* 81, 1-6.
Coughlan, M.P., Johnson, J.L. and Rajagopalan, K.V. (1980). *J. Biol. Chem.* 255, 2694-2699.
DerVartanian, D.V., Lee, I.Y., Slater, E.C. and VanGelder, B.F. (1974). *Biochim. Biophys. Acta* 347, 321-327.
Dolman, D., Dunford, H.B., Chowdhury, D.M. and Morrison, M. (1968). *Biochemistry* 7, 3991-3996.
Ellis, W.D. and Dunford, H.B. (1968). *Biochemistry* 7, 2054-2062.
Erman, J.E. (1974). *Biochemistry* 13, 39-44.
Ermans, A.M., DeLange, F., VanDerVeldern, M. and Kinthaert, J. (1972). *Adv. Exp. Med. Biol.* 30, 455-486.
Feeney, J. and Burgen, A.S.V. (1973). *Eur. J. Biochem.* 34, 107-111.
Fowden, L. and Bell, E.A. (1965). *Nature* 206, 110-112.
Galston, A.W. (1955). *Methods in Enzymol.* 2, 789-791.
Garrett, R.H. and Greenbaum, P. (1973). *Biochim. Biophys. Acta* 302, 24-32.
Gewitz, H.S., Lorimer, G.H., Solomonson, L.P. and Vennesland, B. (1974). *Nature* 249, 79-81.
Gewitz, H.S., Pistorius, E.K., Voss, H. and Vennesland, B. (1976). *Planta* 131, 149-153.
Gewitz, H.S., Piefke, J. and Vennesland, B. (1978). *Planta* 141, 323-328.
Gewitz, H.S., Piefke, J., Langowska, K. and Vennesland, B. (1980). *Biochim. Biophys. Acta* 611, 11-26.
Greer, M.A., Stott, A.K. and Milne, K.A. (1966). *Endocrinol.* 79, 237-247.
Handler, P. (1945). *J. Biol. Chem.* 161, 53-63.
Hansen, B.A. and Dekker, E.E. (1976). *Biochemistry* 15, 2912-2917.
Hartzell, C.R., Beinert, H., vanGelder, B.F. and King. T.E. (1978). *Methods Enzymol.* 53, 54-66.
Hendricks, S.B. and Taylorson, R.B. (1975). *Proc. Natl. Acad. Sci. USA* 72, 306-309.
Hu, V.W., Chan, S.I. and Brown, G.S. (1977). *FEBS Lett.* 84, 287-290.
Humbert, J.R., Tress, J.H. and Braico, K.T. (1977). *J. Am. Med. Assoc.* 238, 482.
Isom, G.E. and Way, J.L. (1976). *Biochem. Pharmacol.* 25, 605-608.
Isom, G.E., Liu, D.H.W. and Way, J.L. (1975). *Biochem. Pharmacol.* 24, 871-875.
Jakob, A. and Diem, S. (1974). *Biochim. Biophys. Acta* 362, 469-479.
Jetschmann, K., Solomonson, L.P. and Vennesland, B. (1972). *Biochim. Biophys. Acta* 275, 276-278.
Johnson, J.L., Hainlain, B.E. and Rajagopalan, K.V. (1980). *J. Biol. Chem.* 255, 1783-1786.
Kadar, J.C. (1977). *Biochim. Biophys. Acta* 486, 429-436.
Ketchum, P.A., Cambier, H.Y., Frazier, W.A., III, Madansky, C.H. and

Nason, A. (1970). *Proc. Natl. Acad. Sci. USA* 66, 1016-1023.
Kreutler, P.A., Varbanov, V., Goodman, W., Olaya, G. and Stanbury, J.B. (1978). *Am. J. Clin. Nutrition* 31, 282-289.
Lafferty, M.A. and Garrett, R.H. (1974). *J. Biol. Chem* 249, 7555-7567.
Lorimer, G.H., Gewitz, H.S., Volker, W., Solomonson, L.P. and Vennesland, B. (1974). *J. Biol. Chem.* 249, 6074-6079.
Marsho, T.V. and Kung, S.D. (1976). *Arch. Biochem. Biophys.* 173, 341-346.
Massey, V. and Edmonson, D. (1970). *J. Biol. Chem.* 245, 6595-6598.
Matsubara, T. and Touchi, A. (1977). *Japan. J. Pharmacol.* 27, 701-708.
McMillan, D.E. and Geevarghese, P.J. (1979). *Lancet* 2, 341-342.
Michajlovskij, N. and Langer, P. (1974). *Acta Endocrinol.* 75, 707-716.
Montgomery, R.D. (1969) *In* "Toxic Constituents of Plant Foodstuffs" (I.E. Liener, ed.), pp. 143-157. Academic Press, New York and London.
Nakamura, S., Shin, T., Hirokata, Y. and Shigematsu, A. (1977). *Br. J. Anaesth.* 49, 1239-1244.
Nason, A., Lee, K.Y., Pan, S.S., Ketchum, P.A., Lamberti, A. and DeVries, J. (1971). *Proc. Natl. Acad. Sci. USA* 68, 3242-3246.
Nicholls, P., VanBuuren, K.J.H. and Gelder, B.F.V. (1972). *Biochim. Biophys. Acta* 275, 279-287.
Oaks, A. and Johnson, F.J. (1972). *Phytochem.* 11, 3465-3471.
Ohkawa, H. and Casida, J.E. (1971). *Biochem. Pharmacol.* 20, 1708-1711.
Olson, N.S. and Klein, J.R. (1947). *J. Biol. Chem.* 167, 739-746.
Ortega, J.A. and Creek, J.E. (1978). *J. Pediatrics* 93, 1059.
Ouitrakal, R. and Izawa, S. (1973). *Biochim. Biophys. Acta* 305, 105-118.
Palmer, J.S. and Olson, O.E. (1979). *Biochem. Biophys. Res. Commun.* 90, 1379-1386.
Pettigrew, A.R. and Fell, G.S. (1972). *Clin. Chem.* 18, 996-1000.
Pettigrew, A.R. and Fell, G.S. (1973). *Clin. Chem.* 19, 466-471.
Pistorius, E.K., Gewitz, H.S., Voss, H. and Vennesland, B. (1976). *Planta* 128, 73-80.
Pistorius, E.K., Gewitz, H.S., Voss, H. and Vennesland, B. (1977). *Biochim. Biophys. Acta* 481, 384-394.
Pistorius, E.K., Funkhauser, E.A. and Voss, H. (1978). *Planta* 141, 279-282.
Pistorius, E.K., Jetschmann, K., Voss, H. and Vennesland, B. (1979). *Biochim. Biophys. Acta* 585, 630-642.
Prohaska, J.R., Oh, S.H., Hoekstra, W.G. and Ganther, H.E. (1977). *Biochim. Biophys. Res. Commun.* 74, 64-71.
Reenstra, W.W. and Jencks, W.P. (1979). *J. Am. Chem. Soc.* 101, 5780-1791.
Rotilo, G., Bray, R.C. and Fielden, E.M. (1972). *Biochim. Biophys. Acta* 268, 605-609.
Schmidt, E.S., Newton, G.W., Sanders, S.M., Lewis, J.B. and Conn, E.E. (1978). *J. Am. Med. Assoc.* 239, 943-947.
Shah, V.K. and Brill, W.J. (1977). *Proc. Natl. Acad. Sci. USA* 74, 3249-3253.
Smith, C.R., Jr., Weisleder, D., Miller, R.W., Palmer, J.S. and Olson, O.E. (1980). *J. Org. Chem.* 45, 507-510.
Smith, F.P., Butler, T.P., Cohan, S. and Schein, P.S. (1977). *J. Am.*

Med. Assoc. 238, 1361.
Smith, R.P. and Gosselin, R.E. (1966). *Toxic Appl. Pharmac.* 8, 159.
Smith, R.P. and Kruszyna, H. (1974). *J. Pharmacol. Exp. Ther.* 191, 557-563.
Solomonson, L.P. (1974). *Biochim. Biophys. Acta* 334, 297-308.
Solomonson, L.P. (1979). *In* "Nitrogen Assimilation of Plants" (E.J. Hewitt and C.V. Cutting, eds), pp. 199-205. Academic Press, New York and London.
Solomonson, L.P. and Spehar, A.M. (1977). *Nature* 265, 373-375.
Solomonson, L.P. and Spehar, A.M. (1979). *J. Biol. Chem.* 254, 2176-2179.
Solomonson, L.P. and Vennesland, B. (1972). *Biochim. Biophys. Acta* 267, 544-557.
Solomonson, L.P., Jetschmann, K. and Vennesland, B. (1973). *Biochim. Biophys. Acta* 309, 32-43.
Solomonson, L.P., Lorimer, G.H., Hall, R.L., Borchers, R. and Bailey, J.L. (1975). *J. Biol. Chem.* 250, 4120-4127.
Solomos, T. and Laties, G.G. (1974). *Plant Physiol.* 54, 506-511.
Solomos, T. and Laties, G.G. (1975). *Plant Physiol.* 55, 73-78.
Solomos, T. and Laties, G.G. (1976). *Biochem. Biophys. Res. Commun.* 70, 663-671.
Strothkamp, R.E. and Dawson, C.R. (1977). *Biochemistry* 16, 1926-1929.
Taylorson, R.B. and Hendricks, S.B. (1973). *Plant Physiol.* 52, 23-27.
Thomson, I. and Anderson, R.A. (1980). *J. Chromatography* 188, 357-362.
Thorling, E.B. and Niazy, M.S. (1973). *Acta Med. Scand.* 194, 271-276.
Tursky, T. and Sajter, V. (1962). *J. Neurochem.* 9, 519-523.
VanBuuren, K.J.H., Zuurendonk, P.F., VanGelder, B.F. and Muijsers, A.O. (1972a). *Biochim. Biophys Acta* 256, 243-257.
VanBuuren, K.J.H., Nicholls, P. and VanGelder, B.F. (1972b). *Biochim. Biophys. Acta* 256, 258-276.
Vennesland, B. and Jetschmann, K. (1971). *Biochim. Biophys. Acta* 227, 554-564.
Vennesland, B. and Solomonson, L.P. (1972). *Plant Physiol.* 49, 1029-1031.
VerPloeg, D.A., Cordes, E.H. and Gurd, F.R.N. (1971). *J. Biol. Chem.* 246, 2725-2733.
Vesely, D.L., Benson, W.R., Sheinin, E.B. and Levey, G.S. (1979). *Proc. Soc. Exp. Biol. Med.* 161, 319-321.
Vesey, C.J. and Wilson, J. (1978). *J. Pharm. Pharmacol.* 30, 20-26.
Vesey, C.J., Cole, P.V. and Simpson, P.J. (1976). *Br. J. Anaesth.* 48, 651-660.
Wallace, E.F. and Rabinowitz, J.C. (1971). *Arch. Biochem. Biophys.* 146, 400-409.
Wilson, D.F. and Erecinska, M. (1978). *Methods in Enzymology* 53, 191-201.
Wilson, D.F., Erecinska, M. and Brocklehurst, E.S. (1972). *Arch. Biochem. Biophys.* 151, 180-187.

PHARMACOLOGIC ASPECTS OF CYANIDE AND ITS ANTAGONISM

JAMES L. WAY

Department of Pharmacology, Washington State University, Pullman, Washington 99164, USA

I. HISTORY

The early history of hydrocyanic acid and of its use in toxicology and medicine has been reviewed (Earles, 1967; Sykes, this volume). Cyanide is believed to have been one of the more frequently employed preparations for homicides and suicides during the nineteenth century. Hydrogen cyanide probably has accounted for more human fatalities than any other chemical known, particularly because of its application in legal executions and as a genocidal agent during World War II.

One of the most widespread potential applications of cyanide is by the military, because hydrogen cyanide has many properties of a practical chemical weapon to be employed in gas warfare (SIPRI, 1971, 1972). In addition to its quick-kill properties, the potential mask-breaking effect of HCN is advantageous, as small molecules are not readily adsorbed on charcoal. Napoleon III is reported to have employed some form of hydrogen cyanide as a tactical military weapon; however, it was not until World War I that this application received widespread consideration. Approximately eight million pounds of hydrogen cyanide were manufactured by France as a chemical weapon and it was used in various mixtures called Manganite and Bincennite. These mixtures contained hydrogen cyanide and various stabilizers, dilutents and smoke markers as well as arsenic trichloride. The military application of hydrogen cyanide in World War I was not highly successful, partly due to the limitation of projectile size and partly because the relatively high vapor pressure of hydrogen cyanide limits its persistency. During World War II, various countries tested and manufactured hydrogen cyanide in larger payloads, as the vaporization of large quantities caused cooling and thus eventually decreased evaporation. The Japanese were armed with 50 kg bombs, and the United States employed 500 kg bombs. It was estimated that during World

War II, hydrogen cyanide was produced as a chemical weapon in Japan, the USSR and the United States in quantities from 500,000 to over 1,000,000 pounds (SIPRI, 1972).

Hydrogen cyanide frequently has been discussed as a poison for clandestine use, primarily because of its quick-kill potential. Cyanide projectiles and spring-loaded devices have reportedly been employed against individuals, and canisters of hydrogen cyanide that may be shattered by an explosive charge detonated by a radio-controlled fuse have been manufactured to be employed against groups of people in buildings or vehicles. In addition to the above uses of cyanide, other past applications directly related to its toxicity are use as a fumigant and as a control agent for predators (e.g. coyotes) by the use of solutions containing cyanide in livestock collars or spring-loaded devices to spray cyanide (Sterner, 1979). Surprisingly, human fatalities from accidental exposure to hydrogen cyanide are relatively infrequent, probably because it is generally recognized for its high toxicity and rapid onset of action; therefore, it is handled with caution.

As a pharmaceutical preparation (cherry laurel), hydrocyanic acid was used fairly extensively until the early parts of the twentieth century as a sedative and cough suppressant, and for gastric pains. This pharmaceutical preparation derived from peach stones and almond(s) was also employed as a flavoring agent, with occasional lethal effects. For details of the early history, see Sykes, this volume.

II. SOURCES

Ingestion of cyanide-containing staple foods, such as cassava (B. Osuntokun, 1970) and forage plants (Schoeder, 1976), probably has accounted for most instances of cyanide exposure in man and range animals. However, in the past few decades the industrial production of hydrogen cyanide has been accelerating. For example, in the United States production was over 700 million pounds per year by 1977 and is rapidly increasing. The predominant uses of cyanide are in the metal industries and for the production of monomers, such as acrylonitrile for use in plastics. Cyanide wastes are generated by these industries in increasing quantities and attempts have been made to control this waste cyanide, but an appreciable amount is still being discharged into the environment.

A particularly difficult problem occurs in the electroplating industries, where the aqueous waste streams may contain initially up to 20 per cent cyanide. It is estimated that approximately 20 million pounds of aqueous cyanide is discharged each year by the electroplating industry in the United States. Other industries which generate cyanide wastes in our waterways are the paint, steel and mining industries. These are relatively well-known sources of contamination; however, newer sources of cyanide contamination have evolved in the past decade. An aluminum company was found to have contaminated the underground water table from aluminum waste products near Mead, Washington. Whether this cyanide contamination in aluminum sludge is world-wide or only a local problem has not been investigated. Probably the greatest future potential sources of HCN-contamination of our water supply are coal gasification processes for making synthetic gas from coal. Many of these procedures produce high concentrations of cyanide. The cyanide concentration in waste waters from these processes are of such a magnitude that procedures have been sought to recover the cyanide for sale as a by-product. If coal gasification should become a major alternative utilized in meeting our energy needs, the production of cyanide from this source would dwarf the total present cyanide input into our environment.

In present practice cyanide effluent from industrial processes usually does not escape in any appreciable amounts into the environment, primarily due to proper waste management procedures which degrade the cyanide before it is discharged. The treatment techniques employed are the complete destruction of the cyanide ion or its conversion to less toxic forms. The procedure most frequently employed is alkaline chlorination, but other oxidizing methods, such as treatment with ozone or permanganate also are employed. There are also various other methods employed in cyanide disposal; electrolytic decomposition, exposure to ionizing radiation, acidification, reaction with an aldehyde, ion exchange, evaporation, lagooning, and biologic degradation are all used.

Nonindustrial sources of HCN in air include automobile pollution control devices with malfunctioning catalytic converters (Voorhoeve *et al.*, 1975) and home fires, especially as the plastic content in the home increases the potential for the liberation of hydrogen cyanide by the combustion of various plastic materials, particularly polyurethane (Jellinek and Takada, 1977). Lastly, one of the major contributors of hydrogen cyanide in air that affects man is tobacco smoke. It should be noted that the use of low tar filter cigarettes does not necessarily decrease the hydrogen cyanide concentration of tobacco smoke.

A different source of potential HCN exposure is from the ingestion of cyanogenic foods. Various food products contain naturally occurring substances that can release cyanide. This is of considerable concern, as some cyanogenic plant materials form the major dietary constituents in certain countries (see Cooke and Coursey, this volume). Toxicity from cyanogenic plants is also a problem for various range animals and wildlife. The incidence of poisoning is more prevalent during drought, as animals become less selective in their forage. Furthermore, a higher concentration of cyanogenic glycosides is formed in certain plants during these drought periods. Besides cyanogenic compounds, plant foods may contain cyanide residues resulting from fumigation with HCN; such residues can persist for an extensive time. There are tolerances listed for HCN residues in various food products in the United States, and these limits vary from 25 p.p.m. in beans to 250 p.p.m. in spices.

With increasing use of cyanide in various industrial processes, the amount of cyanide dispersed into our environment has greatly accelerated. Although it is generally recognized that cyanide has relatively low persistence in air and water under normal circumstances, it should be emphasized that when cyanide contaminates underground water, its persistence is prolonged. In future years the potential for cyanide contamination of our underground drinking water, leading to cyanide toxicity, will be increased. Improper management of industrial cyanide effluent occasionally has resulted in fish kills and contamination of ground water. The disposal of cyanide in waste water is still a significant problem for various industries. It is of interest to note that the U.S. Environmental Protection Agency recently filed a Refuse Act suit against the ARMCO Steel Company for discharging cyanide-containing effluents into the Houston shipping channels. The discharge was in the form of a continuous-process generated effluent stream and the case of the United States versus the ARMCO Steel Company (C.A. 70-H-1335) was prosecuted successfully by the government.

III. PHARMACODYNAMICS AND PHYSIOLOGY

The discussion of the physiologic effects of cyanide will be confined only to those effects which are obtained with reasonable doses, with an emphasis on effects on the intact animal. Studies that have employed overwhelming doses of cyanide to elicit a response, as in some *in vitro* systems, are not considered in this discussion, since they bear little relevance to the pharmacology and toxicology of cyanide.

In concert with experiments on the effect of cyanide on cell respiration (Keilin, 1929; Warburg, 1931), studies were conducted (Gesell and Hertzman, 1927) on the effects of cyanide on the regulation of respiration and blood flow in the intact animal. Much of the knowledge on the inhalation toxicity of hydrogen cyanide (Barcroft, 1931) and the effects of cyanide on tissue respiration in various species and organs were reported about 50 years ago (Dixon and Elliott, 1929). The responses to cyanide of the respiratory and cardiovascular system have been studied rather intensively over the past two decades. Bradycardia caused by cyanide in the dog has been attributed to the activation of the chemoreceptors in the carotid body (Jacobs *et al.*, 1971). Cyanide is also known to stimulate the peripheral chemoreceptors to promote a stimulation of ventilation. Apparently, this can occur by extracranial and carotid and aortic chemoreceptor mechanisms. However, the site(s) where these extracranial receptors are located have not been identified (Levine, 1975). The increased afferent discharges from the carotid body produced by cyanide were abolished by oxygen (von Euler *et al.*, 1939). This phenomenon has been adapted into a clinical pulmonary function test, as oxygen abolishes the inspiratory gasp produced by cyanide in normal individuals, whereas those who have impaired gaseous diffusion continue to exhibit this gasp (Cope and Abramowitz, 1960). Some of the most consistent changes produced by cyanide are electroencephalographic (Ivanov, 1959) and electrocardiographic (Cope, 1961). These changes can be antagonized with oxygen (Burrows *et al.*, 1973). It is emphasized that the mechanism involved in antagonizing the lethal effects of a compound may be quite different from those involved in the blocking of a physiologic or biochemical response induced by a sublethal dose. Such considerations may explain the differences reported (Burrows *et al.*, 1973; Cope, 1961), concerning the effect of oxygen in reversing the action of cyanide on the EKG. Other studies of cardiovascular responses to cyanide have focused primarily on the effects of cyanide on chemoreceptor reflexes and on their action on the central nervous system (Paulet, 1960; Calvelo *et al.*, 1970; Offterdinger, 1970; Krasney, 1971). The marked increase in arterial blood pressure could be attributed to such reflex activities, whereas the increase in central venous pressure may be due to a more direct action, producing a relative cardiac insufficiency as shown by parallel alterations in EKG rhythm.

In electroencephalographic (EEG) recordings, cyanide can produce neuroelectrical changes which correlate with alterations in cellular energy. Cyanide (1-10 mg/kg) can produce an abrupt loss of electrical activity followed by a prolonged period of depressed wave amplitude (Burrows *et al.*, 1973). These periods of electrical silence, as well as EEG abnormalities, can be antagonized with oxygen and can be correlated with the role of oxygen in antagonizing cyanide lethality.

The respiratory changes produced by cyanide appear to occur in the same manner as the cardiovascular responses, i.e. primarily as a result of reflex activity of chemoreceptors. Direct effects of small doses of cyanide on the activity of respiratory neurons *in vivo* have been reported (Brodie, 1959).

Solomonson (this volume) discusses the interaction of cyanide with cytochrome oxidase *in vitro*. There have been very few studies on the effect of cyanide on brain cytochrome oxidase *in vivo*. The toxicity of cyanide has always been attributed to its production of a decrease in the tissue utilization of oxygen or to the production of a "histotoxic" anoxia. Albaum *et al*. (1946a, b) reported that rats receiving sodium cyanide (5 mg/kg, ip) displayed a 50 per cent decrease in brain cytochrome oxidase activity These studies indicated that tissue anoxia induced by the inactivation of cytochrome oxidase resulted in a shift from aerobic to anaerobic metabolism and a depletion of energy-rich compounds, as indicated by a decrease in the concentration of glycogen, phosphocreatine, and adenosine triphosphate, with a concomitant increase in inorganic phosphate, lactic acid, phosphopyruvate, phosphoglycerate, and hexose diphosphates. *In vivo* studies by Schubert and Brill (1968) showed that rodents receiving potassium cyanide intraperitoneally produce a maximal inhibition of cytochrome oxidase within 5-10 minutes. Subsequently, Ballantyne *et al*. (1972) correlated the tissue concentrations of cyanide with cytochrome oxidase activity and showed that animals killed by injection of HCN had both higher tissue levels of cyanide and lower levels of cytochrome oxidase activity than did those killed by injection of KCN.

IV. PATHOLOGY

The pathology of cyanide intoxication varies according to the dose, route and duration of cyanide administration. Ballantyne (1970) conducted studies on pigs which indicated that no specific gross or histopathological changes were caused by captive bolt and intramuscular injection of hydrogen cyanide. The animals to which lethal doses of cyanide were administered had no autopsy characteristics to permit a specific diagnosis of "death from cyanide poisoning". It is of interest to note that no cyanide odor could be detected on opening the body cavity and that the color of the blood was variable. The cytochrome oxidase in the spinal cord was markedly inhibited; but the cytochrome oxidase in the liver and kidneys was not significantly affected. These findings do not imply that in other cases of cyanide poisoning the odor of "bitter almonds" may not be detected on opening the body cavities or that the blood may not be a slight pink color, but only that these findings can be variable. Hurst (1940) reported that in monkeys receiving potassium cyanide (i.m.) the most apparent lesion in the brain was in the white matter, and that necrosis was more frequent than demyelination. These results could be produced by a single dose of potassium cyanide, but were more apt to occur on chronic administration. Experimental cyanide encephalopathy has been studied in rats (Levine and Stypulkowski, 1959; Levine, 1967; Hirano *et al*., 1967) by single brief exposure, and lesions were found to develop in both the gray and white matter. Lesions in the white matter, which were more apt to occur in less severe cyanide poisoning involved particularly the corpus callosum, optic nerves, and optic chaisma, as well as the corpus striatum and ventral hippocampal commisure. These studies concluded that the lesions of cyanide encephalopathy were caused by the direct effect of histotoxic anoxia, and that these lesions were not secondary to neuronal difunction and edema.

Pathological changes also occur in the myocardium. Suzuki (1968) reported that large doses of cyanide exert a direct effect not only on metabolism, but also on the contractile components of the myocardium. The pathology in the myocardium was not surprising, as Wexler *et al.* (1947) had found that cyanide causes extensive alterations in cardiac physiology.

There has been a series of reports on the tropical neuropathies produced by cassava. One of these studies, by Osuntokun (1972), demonstrated the demyelination of peripheral nerves and decreased conduction velocity in these nerves. Cassava is strongly implicated in tropical neuropathic ataxia, with cyanide as a presumptive etiological agent. Recent clinical field studies indicate a clinical, biochemical, electrophysiological, and histopathologic picture that is consistent with chronic cyanide poisoning. It is always difficult to draw unequivocal conclusions about the relationships in this type of study, as other factors hitherto unknown may be a contributing cause; however, the implication of cyanide on the basis of present evidence is reasonable.

V. CYANIDE POISONING

A. SIGNS AND SYMPTOMS

The clinical signs and symptoms of cyanide poisoning were described over 150 years ago by Francois Magendie, and because of the widespread use of cyanide, its toxic effects are well known (Polson and Tattersal, 1969). Although cyanide has been known as a rapidly acting poison, this effect, like those of all chemicals, is dose dependent. There are reports that cyanide in sublethal doses may produce severe toxic effects which persist for days with the ultimate recovery of the individual. Because cyanide has received a deserved reputation for its rapid lethal action, partly from its use in mass and criminal executions, and in suicides and homicides, it is not usually recognized that low level chronic intoxication from cyanide does exist and can be quite incapacitating.

B. ACUTE AND SUBACUTE TOXICITY

Acute and subacute toxic effects of poisoning with cyanide

can vary from dramatic events such as convulsions, screaming, vomiting, and bloody frothing, to a slow, quiet onset of coma and subsequent death. Although many authors separate the effect of hydrogen cyanide by inhalation from those observed when administration is by another route, the clinical manifestations do not vary appreciably except that with inhalation the local irritating effect of cyanide on the membranes of the eyes, oropharynx, and pulmonary tissue are more apt to be manifested. There are no distinguishing signs and symptoms which are pathonomonic for cyanide other than possibly the smell of cyanide in the breath of the victim, frequently described as a burnt almond-like odor. The predominant effect which one would observe initially is a hyperpnea followed by dyspnea, and subsequently convulsions. Although cyanide is usually described as producing a "histotoxic anoxia". it is generally forgotten that in cyanide poisoning there probably is an anoxic anoxia component. The lethal effects in low lethal doses are probably directed towards cytochrome oxidase in the central nervous system, with associated cardiovascular signs at higher doses. It has been noted often that the electrical activity of the brain may be silent when the heart is still functioning.

Gettler and St. George (1934) have described the signs and symptoms of cyanide poisoning in as great detail as any other authors. Their report arbitrarily divides these signs and symptoms into three stages. In the dyspneic stage subsequent to the hyperpnea there is associated headache, vertigo, weak and rapid pulse, nausea and vomiting, and a staggering gait. In the second stage there are convulsions and the victim falls; his pupils dilate; the skin is cold, clammy and moist; and the pulse becomes weaker and more rapid. There are associated opisthotonus, trismus and urination. In the final stage (asphyxia) the heartbeat becomes irregular and slow. The body temperature falls and cyanosis is manifested in the lips, face and extremities. The victim then sinks into a coma, and frothy bloody saliva flows from the mouth.

With regard to exposure levels, experience with cyanide has been sufficient to provide some human toxicity data. Inhalation of HCN at a concentration of 110-135 p.p.m. (0.12-0.15 mg/liter) (Fassett, 1963) has been reported to produce fatalities within a few hours, whereas HCN at a concentration of 270 p.p.m. (0.3 mg/liter) will produce immediate fatalities (Prentiss, 1937). Ingestion of a spoonful (1-5 g) of sodium or potassium cyanide usually will produce death, as the minimal lethal dose has been estimated to be approximately 0.2 g/adult (approximately 3 mg/kg). The actual toxicity will of course be dependent on the rate of absorption and the ability of the body to dispose of cyanide.

C. CHRONIC EFFECTS

Most of the literature on cyanide is focused on the acute effects, and the chronic effects have been almost ignored. Perhaps this is because most of the reports of chronic effects are clinical or field reports. In practice it is difficult to ascribe the effects specifically to cyanide, because a mixture of chemicals is usually involved. The effects of long-term exposure to low concentrations of cyanide probably produces clinical signs of intoxication which are not yet clearly understood. It is becoming increasingly probable that there is a series of signs and symptoms which can be ascribed to a chronic cyanide syndrome. In the past two decades there have been various correlations which implicate the effects of chronic low cyanide in specific diseases. These include: Nigerian nutritional neuropathy, Leber's optical atrophy, retrobulbar neuritis, pernicious anemia, tobacco amblyopia, cretinism and ataxic tropical neuropathy. Recent epidemiological studies also implicate the adverse effects of chronic exposure to cyanide in occupational (El Ghawabi *et al.*, 1975), dietary (Osuntokun, 1970) and environmental conditions. Also, various diseases have been inferred to have a correlation with chronic low level exposure to cyanide. Projections suggest that there will be a greater exposure to cyanide in the future because of newer industrial advances. The present potential for chronic poisoning may be dwarfed by future developments in an effort to seek alternative energy supplies to replace petroleum.

The diet in some tropical areas consists mainly of cassava as the staple food, and this plant has a high content of cyanogenic glycosides (linamarin). Tropical neuropathies can develop into a characteristic syndrome which is characterized by nerve deafness, optic atrophy and an involvement of the sensory spinal nerve that produces ataxia (Money, 1958). Other signs and symptoms include stomatitis, glossitis and scrotal dermatitis. The correlation between the pathology and the clinical manifestation of this disease is relatively consistent.

In many field studies, it is difficult to assess the contribution of cyanide to these lesions due to the lack of experimental controls. However, the evidence accumulating is consistent with the hypothesis that cyanide intoxication is a major cause, although this may be an oversimplification of a complex problem. Osuntokun and co-workers (1969) have contributed significantly to studies in this area. In some villages cassava represents approximately two-thirds of the diet, so that in addition to cyanide, there are various complicating nutritional factors. For example, Osuntokun and co-workers (1968) indicated that a lack of substrate for cyanide detoxification may occur because of a deficiency of sulfur containing amino acids in the diet. Although most investigations have focused on the chronic cyanide intoxication (Monekosso and Wilson, 1966; Osuntokun *et al.*, 1970), some studies also indicate that deficiencies in protein and in water-soluble vitamins may be important contributing factors.

There are other neuropathies in which cyanide is a possible cause. These include West Indian amblyopia, tobacco amblyopia and Leber's optic atrophy, diseases which are characterized by a disturbance in the visual field. One finding which indicated that chronic cyanide intake is a contributing factor in these visual disturbances is that administration of cyanocobalamin or hydroxocobalamin in tobacco amblyopia improved vision rather dramatically (Chrisholm *et al.*, 1967). Hydroxocobalamin was more effective than cyanocobalamin, as one would expect (Foulds *et al.*, 1970).

The activity of cyanide as an etiologic agent in producin human neuropathies has been investigated experimentally (Lessell, 1971; Lessell and Kuwabara, 1974). These studies indicated that cyanide lesions produced in rats were similar to those of human disorders. However, it was pointed out that the cyanide dose necessary to produce experimental nerve damage in rats was in the lethal range, and the corpus callosum was more sensitive to cyanide than the optic nerve. This is quite different from human disorders, in which optic disturbances are frequently the only involvement of the central nervous system.

Finally, there is very little information on the carcinogenic, teratogenic, and mutagenic properties of cyanide, and the evidence that is available warrants additional examination. Cyanide has been employed in cancer chemotherapy in experimental animals and in man (Brown *et al.*, 1960). There has been a longstanding hypothesis for an anticancer effect of the cyanogenic glycosides (Morrone, 1962; Krebs, 1970). These claims have been refuted by other laboratories (Greenberg, 1975; Lewis, 1977). The basis for the putative antitumor effect of the cyanogenic glycoside, amygdalin (also called laetrile), is its postulated selective hydrolysis by a beta glucosidase, liberating cyanide and benzaldehyde at the neoplastic site. The cyanide then selectively attacks the cancer cell which is presumed to be low in rhodanese, whereas normal cells are assumed to possess both sufficient rhodanese and sufficient sulfur donor to detoxify the cyanide. Some of the opponents of this theory have indicated (Greenberg, 1975; Lewis, 1977) that many tumor tissues are not selectively enriched in beta-glucosidase nor are they low in rhodanese. Also, there are various studies indicating a lack of antitumor activity of amygdalin in model tumor cells (Hill *et al.*, 1976; Laster and Schnabel, 1975; Levi *et al.*, 1965; Wodinsky and Swiniaski, 1975).

VI. CYANIDE ANTIDOTES

Since the time when cyanide poisoning was documented in

the nineteenth century, various antidotes have been proposed. It is rather a paradox that some of the cyanide antagonists proposed in the nineteenth century were quite effective, whereas some of the cyanide antagonists still recommended at present are ineffective. There are various reports on the development of "new" cyanide antidotes, which would be considered quite efficacious compared to other chemical poisonings. However, such reports may be considered relatively trivial because of the highly effective antidotal combinations already available for protection against cyanide poisoning. Many of these studies also become questionable when subjected to statistical analysis. With cyanide, unlike most chemicals, it is always necessary to differentiate between the antidotal effects produced with a minimal lethal dose and those produced with massive poisoning, as the results obtained can be quite different.

A. BIOTRANSFORMATION OF CYANIDE

Subsequent to the demonstration of the existence of a thiosulfate sulfurtransferase (rhodanese) in liver to convert cyanide to thiocyanate it became fairly apparent that this would be an effective mechanism to detoxify cyanide (Lang, 1933a, b). Independent studies in Argentina (Hug, 1933) and the United States (Chen *et al.*, 1933) incorporated thiosulfate into an antidotal combination to antagonize cyanide intoxication. The use of sodium thiosulfate as the sulfur donor is ideal in many aspects, as the enzyme is present in large amounts (Himwich and Saunders, 1948), has a high turnover number and catalyzes a reaction that is essentially irreversible (Sorbo, 1953a, b). One of the limitations of this antagonist is that the selective distribution of hydrogen cyanide does not parallel that of the antagonist. Furthermore, the enzyme is localized in the mitochondria in various tissues, and the penetration of sodium thiosulfate to these sites is relatively limited. In a successful attempt to minimize these distribution problems, crystalline enzyme was injected intravenously in combination with the sulfur donor. This represents the first report of the use of an enzyme directly as an antidote to antagonize the toxic effects of a chemical. Various other sulfur donors have been studied (Sörbo, 1953a, b) and some have been employed in the treatment of cyanide poisoning (Clemedson *et al.*, 1955).

B. CYANIDE BINDING

1. *Methemoglobin Generating Chemicals*

a. Methylene blue Earlier studies on cyanide poisoning utilized methylene blue as a cyanide antagonist. The basis for methylene blue action was related to the formation of methemoglobin, which reacts with cyanide to form cyanmethemoglobin (Wendel, 1933). Although methylene blue is still being advocated as a cyanide antagonist, it really is not an effective antidote (Chen *et al.*, 1933) because it is a poor methemoglobin former (Bodansky, 1950). The main contribution of methylene blue to cyanide poisoning is that it stimulated research to discover more effective cyanide antagonists.

b. Nitrites The first study of the efficacy of nitrites against cyanide poisoning in dogs was conducted with amyl nitrite (Pedigo, 1888). The report of this research went relatively unnoticed, as it was published in a journal which was not widely circulated. Subsequent studies employing sodium nitrite in anesthetized and unanesthetized dogs showed that nitrite could protect against an amount of KCN equal to several lethal doses (Chen *et al.*, 1933). Cyanide has a low affinity for hemoglobin but a relatively high affinity for methemoglobin. Nitrite generates methemoglobin which combines with cyanide to form cyanmethemoglobin. Methemoglobin does not have a higher affinity for cyanide than does cytochrome oxidase, but there is a much larger potential source of methemoglobin than there is of cytochrome oxidase. Therefore the efficacy of methemoglobin is primarily a mass action effect.

c. Other chemicals which generate methemoglobin Under conditions in which amyl nitrite normally would be used, it is doubtful that it would contribute substantially to the formation of methemoglobin. Moreover, the efficacy of amyl nitrite in combating cyanide poisoning has been challenged (Jandorf and Bodansky, 1946). This has led to a search for agents which would form methemoglobin more rapidly than sodium nitrite. The first of these agents was p-aminopropiophenone, which was shown to form methemoglobin rather rapidly (Jandorf and Bodansky, 1946). Subsequently, a series of studies by Kiese and Weger (1969) led to the development of a 4-dimethylaminophenol as the agent of choice among the aminophenol derivatives. The development of a more rapid methemoglobin former is important, as Albaum *et al.* (1946a, b) have reported the reactivation of cyanide-inhibited cytochrome oxidase by methemoglobin in studies *in vitro*. Moreover, various other laboratories (Paulet *et al.*, 1960; Weber *et al.*, 1962) have reported that limitations on the use of nitrites in cyanide intoxication may be attributed to the slow rate of formation of methemoglobin.

2. Cobalt compounds

Cobalt nitrate was first used in the treatment of cyanide poisoning in the nineteenth century (Antal, 1894). Its efficacy was confirmed (Meurice, 1900) in pigeons and rabbits; however, the use of cobalt at a cyanide antagonist did not receive widespread support predominantly because it was felt that the cobalt salts were themselves too toxic. It was over fifty years later that interest revived in using cobalt compounds in the treatment of cyanide poisoning (Mushett *et al.*, 1952). These studies employed hydroxocobalamine to antagonize potassium cyanide intoxication in mice. Subsequent to these studies, many laboratories have used various cobalt-containing compounds as cyanide antagonists. Compounds tested include hydroxocobalamine and its derivatives (Mushett *et al.*, 1952; Rose *et al.*, 1965; Evans, 1964), cobalt histidine (Schwarzkopf and Friedberg, 1971; Mercker and Bastian, 1959), cobalt chloride (Burrows and Way, 1979; Isom and Way, 1973), and dicobalt ethylenediamine tetra-acetic acid (Co_2EDTA) (Paulet, 1958). Various laboratories have reported on the successful use of cobalt-EDTA in cyanide poisoning under both experimental and clinical conditions (Paulet, 1958; Mercker and Bastian, 1959; Bartelheimer *et al.*, 1962; Nagler *et al.*, 1978).

The use of cobalt EDTA has a good pharmacologic basis, as cobalt ions form stable complexes with cyanide. The principal reason for advocating the use of cobalt is that the reaction is rapid, whereas methemoglobin-generating compounds, by the very nature of their action, provide a protection that is delayed at a time when a rapid onset of action is essential.

3. *Carbonyl Compounds*

In addition to various agents which would accelerate the formation of methemoglobin to bind cyanide and cobalt-containing agents to form metal ion complexes of cyanide, other chemicals which would bind directly with cyanide have been tested as antidotes. Cyanide is known to interact with the carbonyl groups of various compounds to form cyanhydrins. One laboratory reported that sodium pyruvate can reverse the inhibitory effects of cyanide on tumor cells and that this compound is also effective in antagonizing the lethal effects of cyanide (Cittadini *et al.*, 1971, 1972). The minimal protective effect of sodium pyruvate alone was subsequently confirmed by Schwartz *et al.* (1979), and these studies were extended in mice. Although sodium pyruvate is not as effective as sodium nitrite and does not appear to enhance the effect of sodium nitrite, it does potentiate the antidotal effect of sodium thiosulfate. Moreover, although the sodium pyruvate-sodium thiosulfate combination is not as effective as the classic sodium nitrite-sodium thiosulfate combination, the addition of sodium pyruvate to the sodium nitrite-sodium thiosulfate combination further enhances the antidotal effect. The use of sodium pyruvate as a cyanide antagonist has theoretical advantages, as it would not be dependent on forming a second compound for activity. Also, pyruvate is transported by an active mechanism; therefore, pyruvate has the potential of being a cyanide antagonist which is superior to the methemoglobin formers, as it can distribute to sites of cyanide localization. Lastly, as a possible supplement to the nitrite-thiosulfate combination, it may provide a basis for decreasing the dose of sodium nitrate, an antagonist that has caused fatalities.

C. OXYGEN AS AN ANTAGONIST

Since cyanide is believed to exert its toxic effects by the inhibition of cytochrome oxidase (Keilin, 1930), oxygen transport and oxygen tension in cyanide poisoning are expected to be normal; only the cellular utilization of oxygen should be depressed. Therefore, the administration of oxygen might serve no useful purpose in antagonizing cyanide intoxication. Nevertheless, it was reported that oxygen is useful as an integral part of the treatment (Way *et al.*, 1966, 1972; Way and Sheehy, 1968), rather than simply as an adjunct (Cope, 1961; Gordh and Norberg, 1947). Oxygen potentiation was demonstrated not only prophylactically but therapeutically (Sheehy and Way, 1968). The most striking potentiation observed is when oxygen is administered in combination with sodium nitrite and sodium thiosulfate, but the mechanism for this potentiation is still not apparent.

VII. TREATMENT OF CYANIDE POISONING

The treatment of cyanide poisoning at the present state of the art can be summarized as follows: (1) removal from the site of contamination; (2) supportive treatment; (3) antidotal combinations which will not only bind but also detoxify cyanide.

The treatment of cyanide poisoning, in contrast to the treatments of most chemical poisonings, can be managed with any of a variety of efficacious agents. Under these circumstances, different particular regimens have been recommended and there is no unanimity of opinion with regard to which is best. This is not surprising, as different species of animals have been employed in testing the efficacies of the various antidotes. Moreover, cyanide poisoning occurs with sufficient frequency that there have been various reports of the "successful" treatment of cyanide intoxication by a variety of methods.

The inhibition of enzymes such as cytochrome oxidase by cyanide is discussed by Solomonson in this volume. Cytochrome oxidase is the terminal oxidative respiratory enzyme in the mitochondria, and it is an essential catalyst for the tissue utilization of oxygen. Therefore, when this enzyme is inhibited by cyanide, a histotoxic anoxia occurs as aerobic metabolism is inhibited. The organism attempts to compensate by shifting to anaerobic metabolism, with the accumulation of such products as lactate, pyruvate, glucose, etc. Essentially, in the underlying pathologic mechanism, the tissues have sufficient oxygen but are unable to utilize it in tissue metabolism. The brain is probably the organ most sensitive to cyanide and therefore most of the attention has focused on brain cytochrome oxidase. It should be emphasized that other organs, such as the heart, can be affected. The primary focus on cytochrome oxidase is attributable to both the sensitivity of this enzyme to cyanide and to its location in the biochemical metabolic chain.

The discussion on the treatment of cyanide poisoning can be separated into three arbitrary areas.

A. THE GENERAL SUPPORTIVE TREATMENT

Since there are various effective specific antidotes for the treatment of cyanide poisoning, the importance of general supportive treatment frequently is overlooked. Because of the rapidity of action of cyanide, there are very few complete clinical studies on acute cyanide poisoning. As indicated earlier, various reports and textbooks describe in detail the signs and symptoms of cyanide poisoning, but the fact remains that in the absence of a suitable history, the diagnosis of cyanide poisoning is difficult. These points are stressed by one case report of a single incident of a man ingesting potassium cyanide. The only treatments employed were supportive as diagnosis of cyanide poisoning was not established until later (Graham *et al.*, 1977). These studies represent a clinically well-documented study on cyanide poisoning in man. The dose of cyanide was established at 600 mg, and the blood level of cyanide was reportedly 2.0 μg/ml, 12 h after admission to the hospital. The predominant importance of these studies (Graham *et al.*, 1977) is to reemphasize the fact that even though effective antidotes are available, the general supportive treatment of any poisoning should not be ignored. It may be lifesaving, particularly when the diagnosis of cyanide poisoning has not been established.

B. NITRITE-THIOSULFATE-OXYGEN

Various combinations of proposed cyanide antagonists have been reported to have varying efficacies in animals receiving cyanide. The reports on the synergistic protective effect of the nitrites with sodium thiosulfate were reported independently by investigators in Argentina and the United States (Hug, 1933; Chen *et al.*, 1933). Each of these drugs had been known for quite some time to antagonize cyanide intoxication; however, these were the first trials of this antidotal combination. It is still one of the most efficacious antidotes against cyanide poisoning. The nitrites were employed to oxidize hemoglobin to methemoglobin so that cyanide could form cyanmethemoglobin.

This treatment was based on early studies (Bernard, 1932) which indicated that cyanmethemoglobin is much less toxic than free cyanide, and that cyanide has a much higher affinity for methemoglobin than for hemoglobin.

The proprietary mixtures of sodium thiosulfate and sodium nitrite which are employed in cyanide poisoning, in veterinary practices, contain too low a dose to obtain maximal antidotal efficiency. Nevertheless, these mixtures can protect against 6 LD-50 doses of cyanide. With adjustment of the dose of sodium nitrite and sodium thiosulfate, it has been possible to raise the protection over that of the proprietary mixture by almost threefold. These studies were conducted in sheep, as they are among the animals most apt to be poisoned by cyanide (Burrows and Way, 1979). The cyanide was administered orally, and a five minute waiting period was instituted prior to initiation of the antidote so that the toxic effects of cyanide poisoning could be fully elicited.

It must be pointed out that the sodium nitrite-sodium thiosulfate combination is not without its own toxic effects. As noted by Berlin (1970), care must be taken in the administration of the sodium nitrite and sodium thiosulfate combination, particularly in children. It is recommended that children under 25 kg should have the dose of sodium nitrite adjusted; if the adult dose is employed, it can be potentially lethal. Experience with use of sodium nitrite and sodium thiosulfate as an antidotal combination in the treatment of cyanide intoxication and in clinical cases of poisoning has been summarized for human medical practice (Chen and Rose, 1952) and for veterinary practice in sheep and cattle (Clawson *et al.*, 1934).

There appears to be no hazard in the use of oxygen in combination with sodium nitrite and sodium thiosulfate, and the procedure could be lifesaving; its adaptation as a routine measure appears justified.

C. COBALT

There are various proponents for the use of cobalt EDTA in the treatment of cyanide poisoning (Paulet, 1960). Although cobalt salts were among the earliest antidotes employed to antagonize the lethal effects of cyanide (Antal, 1894), they did not receive widespread acceptance, because of their toxicity, until hydroxocobalamine and cobalt EDTA were introduced. Whether these compounds have appreciably lower toxicity on a molar basis with regard to cobalt is still an open question. Recent studies (Nagler *et al.*, 1978; Hilman *et al.*, 1974; Naughton, 1974) appear to relate the ventricular arrhythmias primarily to cobalt EDTA itself. Many studies on cobalt compounds suggest that cobalt should be employed with sodium thiosulfate, as in most cases the thiosulfate enhances the antidotal effects of cobalt (Friedberg, 1968; Schwarzkopf and

Friedberg, 1971; Isom and Way, 1973). However, cobalt EDTA is usually employed alone and the proprietary mixture contains no sulfur donor. Various investigators have suggested that cobalt EDTA should be employed as one of the cyanide antagonists, with the implication that a cobalt chelate or an aminophenol derivative in combination with sodium thiosulfate might replace the classic antidotal nitrite-thiosulfate combination. Objections to the nitrite-thiosulfate combination relate to its slow onset of action and low detoxifying capacity (Friedberg, 1968). These conclusions were based on the rate of methemoglobin formation (Kiese and Weger, 1969) and measurement of the physiological effects of cyanide and/or rate of cyanide excretion. On the other hand, Burrows and Way (1973) indicated that some of these measurements may not necessarily be reliable parameters in assessing the therapeutic efficacy of the antidotal potential against the lethal effects of cyanide. It is of interest to note that there is a species specificity with regard to the susceptibility to cobalt. Whereas cobalt-thiosulfate combinations were much more effective than nitrite-thiosulfate in mice (Isom and Way, 1972), tolerance to cobalt salts was much lower in sheep. Since cobalt evidently exerts its effect primarily by combining directly with cyanide ion, its action is dependent on the molar ratio of cobalt to cyanide. When the dose of cobalt was adjusted to a level which could be tolerated in sheep, the cobalt-thiosulfate combination was not as efficacious as the nitrite-thiosulfate combination in mice or sheep (Burrows and Way, 1977, 1979). Such observations indicate that in investigations conducted by various laboratories there are differences in experimental conditions, animal species and doses of antagonists employed which make the comparison of relative efficacy difficult.

Unlike the addition of oxygen to the nitrite-thiosulfate antidotal combination, the addition of cobalt compounds may involve a substantial hazard. Even though cobalt could be lifesaving, a careful study of the toxicity of cobalt is essential. Its use under clinical conditions may lead to signs of cobalt toxicity such as ventricular arrhythmias.

VIII. ASSESSMENT OF THE TREATMENT OF CYANIDE INTOXICATION: SUMMARY

In most cases of chemical poisoning there is very little that can be done, other than supportive treatment or the use of antagonists with only a minimal degree of efficacy. However, the treatment of cyanide intoxication has been blessed with a variety of agents which are quite efficacious, and for this reason there have been differences of opinion with regard to how these intoxications should be treated. The classic nitrite-thiosulfate treatment of cyanide poisoning developed almost fifty years ago (Chen *et al.*, 1933; Hug, 1933) on a rational pharmacologic basis is one of the antidotal combinations still employed. The only unambiguous improvement to this antidotal combination is the addition of oxygen therapy (Way *et al.*, 1966; Sheehy and Way, 1968), as it potentiates the effectiveness of the nitrite-thiosulfate combination. Some concerns have been raised with regard to the use of the nitrite-thiosulfate combination, and this is partly because of the toxicity of nitrite (Berlin, 1970). Also some questions have been raised about the timeliness of its onset of action, particularly with regard to sodium nitrite (Friedberg, 1968; Kiese and Weger, 1969). Various agents have been employed which yield a faster rate of methemoglobin formation, and there are proponents for replacing sodium nitrite with 4-dimethylaminophenol (Kiese and Weger, 1969). Proponents of the use of cobalt-containing compounds to bind cyanide have focused predominantly on cobalt EDTA (Paulet, 1960) which is widely used. An argument in support of this treatment stresses the rapid, direct action to form a stable cyanide complex, in contrast to the action of other less directly acting antidotes which are dependent on the generation of methemoglobin. However, concern has been expressed with regard to the toxicity of this cobalt compound, and the issue has not been fully resolved.

ACKNOWLEDGEMENT

This research was supported by funds from the National Institute of Environmental Health Sciences, National Institute of General Medical Sciences, Department of the Army and U.S. Army Medical Research and Development Command.

REFERENCES

Albaum, H.G., Tepperman, J. and Bodansky, O. (1946a). *J. Biol. Chem.* 163, 641-647.

Albaum, H.G., Tepperman, J. and Bodansky, O. (1946b). *J. Biol. Chem.* 164, 45-51.

Antal, J. (1894). *Arch. Med.* 3, 117-128.

Ballantyne, B. (1970). "Medicine, Science and the Law", pp. 171-78. Sweet and Maxwell, London.

Ballantyne, B., Boardman, S.P., Bright, J., Coffee, D.J., Webber, T.D. and Williams, P. (1972). *Br. J. Pharmacol.* 44, 382-383.

Barcroft, J. (1931). *J. of Hygiene* 31, 1-34.

Bartelheimer, E.W., Friedberg, K.D. and Lendle, L. (1962). *Archs. int. Pharmacodyn. Ther.* 139, 99-108.

Berlin, C.M. (1970). *Pediatrics* 46, 193-6.

Bodansky, O. (1951). *Pharmacol. Rev.* 3, 144-196.

Brodie, D.A. (1959). *J. Pharmacol. Exp. Therap.* 126, 264-269.
Brown, W.E., Wood, C.D. and Smith, A.N. (1960). *Am. J. Obstet. Gynecol.* 80, 907-918.
Burrows, G.E., Liu, D.H.W. and Way, J.L. (1973). *J. Pharmacol. Exp. Ther.* 184, 739-748.
Burrows, G.E. and Way, J.L. (1977). *Amer. J. Vet. Res.* 38, 223-227.
Burrows, G.E. and Way, J.L. (1979). *Amer. J. Vet. Res.* 40, 613-617.
Calvelo, M.G., Abboud, F.M., Ballard, D.R. and Abdel-Sayed, W. (1970). *Circ. Res.* 27, 259-276.
Chen, K.K., Rose, C.L. and Clowes, G.H.A. (1933). *Proc. Soc. Exp. Biol. Med.* 31, 250-252.
Chen, K.K. and Rose, C.L. (1952). *J. Am. Med. Ass.* 149, 113-119.
Chisholm, I.A., Bronte-Stewart, J. and Foulds, W.S. (1967). *Lancet* ii, 450-451.
Cittadini, A., Galeotti, T. and Terranova, T. (1971). *Experientia* 27, 633-635.
Cittadini, A., Caprino, L. and Terranova, T. (1972). *Experientia* 28, 943-944.
Clawson, A.B., Bunyea, H. and Couch, J.F. (1934). *J. Wash. Acad. Sci.* 24, 369-385.
Clemedson, C., Hulfman, H.I. and Sörbo, B. (1955). *Acta Phys. Scand.* 35, 31-35.
Cope, C. and Abramowitz, S. (1960). *Am. Rev. Resp. Dis.* 81, 321-328.
Cope, C. (1961). *J. Am. Med. Ass.* 175, 1061-1064.
Dixon, M. and Elliott, K.A.C. (1929). *Biochem. J.* 23, 812-830.
Earles, M.P. (1967). *Med. Hist.* 11, 305-313.
El Ghawabi, S.H., Gaafar, M.A., El-Saharti, A.A., Ahmed, S.H., Malash, K.K. and Fanes, R. (1975). *Br. J. Ind. Med.* 32, 215-219.
Estler, C.J. (1966). *Arch. exp. Path. Pharmak.* 252, 305-313.
Evans, C.L. (1964). *Brit. J. Pharmac. Chemother.* 23, 455-475.
Fassett, D.W. (1963). *In* "Industrial Hygiene and Toxicology" (D.W. Fassett and D.D. Irish, eds) Vol. 2, 2nd edn, pp. 191-2036. John Wiley, New York.
Foulds, W.S., Cant, J.S., Chisholm, I.A., Bronte-Stewart, J. and Wilson, J. (1968). *Lancet* i, 896-897.
Friedberg, K.D. (1968). *Arch. Toxikol.* 24, 41-48.
Gesell, R. and Hertzman, A.B. (1927). *Am. J. Physiol.* 83, 420-444.
Gettler, A.O. and St. George, A.V. (1934). *J. Clin. Pathol.* 4, 429-437.
Gordh, T. and Norberg, B. (1947). *Acta Physiol. Scand.* 13, 26-34.
Graham, D.L., Lamar, D., Theodore, J. and Robin, E.D. (1977). *Arch. Int. Med.* 13, 1051-1055.
Greenberg, D.M. (1975). *West. J. Med.* 122, 345-348.
Hill, G.J., Shine, T.E., Hill, H.Z. and Miller, C. (1976). *AKR Leukemia Cancer Res.* 36, 2102-2107.
Hilmann, B., Bardham, K.D. and Bain, J.T.B. (1974). *Postgrad. Med. J.* 50, 171-174.
Himwich, W.A. and Saunders, J.P. (1948). *Am. J. Physiol.* 153, 348-354.
Hirano, A., Levine, S. and Zimmerman, H.M. (1967). *J. Neuropathol. Exp. Neurol.* 26, 200-213.
Hug, E. (1933). *Revta. Soc. Argent. de Biol.* 9, 91-97.
Isom, G. and Way, J.L. (1972). *Toxicol. and Appl. Pharmacol.* 24, 449-456.

Isom, G.E., Liu, D.H.W. and Way, J.L. (1975). *Biochem. Pharmacol.* 24, 871-875.
Ivanov, J.P. (1959). *Pharmacol. and Toxicol. (USSR)* 22, 476-479.
Jacobs, L., Sampson, S.R. and Comroe, J.H. (1971). *Am. J. Phys.* 220, 472-476.
Jandorf, B.J. and Bodansky, O. (1946). *J. Ind. Hyg. a Toxicology* 28, 125-132
Jellinek, H.H.G. and Takada, K. (1977). *J. Polymer Sci.* 15, 2269-2288.
Keilin, D. (1929). *Proc. Roy. Soc. B* 104, 206-252 (1929).
Kiese, M. and Weger, N. (1969). *Europ. J. Pharmacol.* 7, 97-105.
Krasney, J.A. (1971). *Amer. J. Physiol.* 220, 1361-1366.
Krebs, E.T., Jr. (1970). *J. Appl. Nutr.* 22, 75-86.
Lang, K. (1933a). *Biochem. Z.* 259, 243-256.
Lang, K. (1933b). *Biochem. Z.* 263, 262-267.
Laster, W.R. and Schnabel, F.M. (1975). *Cancer Chemothe. Rep. Part 1* 50, 951-965.
Lessell, S. (1971). *Arch. Ophthalmol.* 86, 194-204.
Lessell, S. and Kuwabara, T. (1974). *Invest. Ophthalmol.* 13, 748-756.
Levi, L., French, W.D., Bickis, I.J. and Henderson, I.W.D. (1965). *Can. Med. Assoc. J.* 92, 1057-1061.
Levine, S. and Stypulkowski, W. (1959). *Am. Med. Ass. Arch. Path.* 67, 306-323.
Levine, S. (1967). *J. Neuropath. Exp. Neurol.* 26, 214-222.
Levine, S. (1975). *J. Appl. Phys.* 39, 199-204.
Lewis, J.P. (1977). *West. J. Med.* 127, 55-62.
Mercker, H. and Bastian, G. (1959). *Arch. exp. Path. Pharmakol.* 236, 449-458.
Meurice, J. (1900). *Arch. int. Pharmacodyn.* 7, 12-53.
Monekosso, G.L. and Wilson, J. (1966). *Lancet* i, 1062-1064.
Money, G.L. (1958). *W. Afr. Med. J.* 7, 58-62.
Morrone, J.A. (1962). *Exp. Med. Surg.* 20, 299-308.
Mushett, C.W., Kelley, K.L., Boxer, G.E. and Rickards, J.C. (1952). *Proc. Soc. Exp. Med.* 81, 234-237.
Nagler, J., Provoust, R.A. and Parizel, G. (1978). *J. Occ. Med.* 20, 414-416.
Naughton, M. (1974). *Anaesth. Intens. Care* 4, 351-356.
Offterdinger, H. (1970). *Naunyn-Schmiedberg Archiv. Pharmakol.* 266, 416.
Osuntokun, B.O., Durowoju, J.E., McFarlane, H. and Wilson, J. (1968). *Br. Med. J.* 3, 647-649.
Osuntokun, B.O., Monekosso, G.L. and Wilson, J. (1969). *Br. Med. J.* 1, 547-550.
Osuntokun, B.O. (1970). *Br. J. Nutr.* 24, 797-800.
Osuntokun, B.O., Aladetoyinbo, A. and Adeuja, A.O.G. (1970). *Lancet* ii, 372-373.
Osuntokun, B.O. (1972). *Plant Foods Hum. Nutr.* 2, 215-266.
Paulet, G. (1957). *Presse Med.* 65, 573-576.
Paulet, G. (1958). *J. Physiol. (Paris)* 50, 438-442.
Paulet, G. (1960). "L'intoxication cyanhydrique et son treatment", pp. 48-51. Masson and Co., Paris.
Pedigo, L.G. (1888). *Tr. M. Soc. Virg.* 19, 124-131.
Polson, C.J. and Tattersall, R.N. (eds) (1969). "Hydrocyanic Acid and Cyanides, Clinical Toxicology", 2nd edn., pp. 128-159. J.B.

Lippincott Co., Philadelphia.
Prentiss, A.M. (1937). "Systemic Toxic Agents, Chemicals in War", pp. 170-176. McGraw-Hill, New York.
Rose, C.L., Worth, R.M., Kikuchi, K. and Chen, K.K. (1965). *Proc. Soc. Exp. Biol. Med.* 120, 780-783.
Schroder, U.N. (1976). *Proc. Soil and Crop Sci. Soc., Florida* 36, 195-197.
Schubert, J. and Brill, W.A. (1968). *J. Pharmacol.* 162, 352-359.
Schwartz, C., Morgan, R.L., Way, L.M. and Way, J.L. (1979). *Toxicol. Appl. Pharmacol.* 50, 437-441.
Schwarzkopf, H.A. and Friedberg, K.D. (1971). *Arch. Toxicol.* 27, 111-123.
Sheehy, M. and Way, J.L. (1968). *J. Pharmacol.* 161, 163-168.
SIPRI (Stockholm Int. Peace Res. Inst.) (1971). "Problems of Chemical and Biological Warfare, I. The Rise of CB Weapons". Humanities Press Inc., NJ.
SIPRI (1972). "Problems of Chemical and Biological Warfare, II. CB Weapons Today". Humanities Press Inc., NJ.
Sörbo, B.H. (1953a). *Acta Chem. Scand.* 7, 1129-1136.
Sörbo, B.H. (1953b). *Acta Chem. Scand.* 7, 1137-1145.
Sterner, R.T. (1979). *Bull. Env. Contam. Toxicol.* 23, 211-217.
Suzuki, T., (1968). *Tohoku J. Exp. Med.* 95, 271-287.
Von Euler, U.S., Liljestrand, G. and Zotterman, Y. (1939). *Scand. Arch. Physiol.* 83, 132-152.
Voorhoeve, R.J.H., Patel, C.K.W., Trimble, L.E. and Kerl, R.J. (1975). *Science* 190, 149-151.
Warburg, O. (1931). *Biochem. Z.* 231, 493-497.
Way, J.L., Gibbon, S.L. and Sheehy, M. (1966). *J. Pharmacol. Exp. Ther.* 153, 381-385.
Way, J.L., End, E., Sheehy, M.H., Miranda, M., Feitknecht, U.F., Burrows, G.E., Gibbon, S.L. and Bachand, R. (1972). *Toxicol. and Appl. Pharmacol.* 22, 415-421.
Weber, D., Friedberg, K.D. and Lendle, L. (1962). *Arch. exp. Path. u. Pharmak.* 244, 1-16.
Wendel, W.B. (1933). *J. Am. Med. Ass.* 100, 1054-1055.
Wexler, J., Whittenberger, J.L. and Dumke, P.R. (1947). *Am. Heart J.* 34, 163-173.
Wodnisky, I. and Swiniarski, J.K. (1975). *Cancer Chemother. Rep. Part 1* 59, 939-950.

CYANIDE DETOXICATION IN THE DOMESTIC FOWL

R.H. DAVIS

Wye College (University of London), Wye, Ashford, Kent, TN25 5AH, UK

I. INTRODUCTION

With the increasing use of cassava and rapeseed meal in animal feeding there is greater exposure to dietary toxins, from cyanogenic glucosides in the former and glucosinolates in the latter. It is generally accepted that the toxicity of cyanogenic glucosides is due entirely to the release of free cyanide, but the mechanism of glucosinolate toxicity is more complex. The goitrogenic effects of rapeseed meal are well documented (e.g. Van Etten and Tookey, 1979) but it has been observed that nitriles are major products in the digestive tract (Smith and Campbell, 1976) and release of cyanide from these could contribute to the detrimental effects which can occur when intake of this food is not held at a low level. Consequently aspects of the release of cyanide within the body and the ability to detoxify cyanide by conversion to thiocyanate are being investigated, using the domestic fowl as a suitable species.

Thiocyanate is the major detoxication product of cyanide. As early as 1894, Lang demonstrated increased thiocyanate excretion following administration of nitriles to dogs and rabbits (see also Sykes, this volume). This has subsequently been confirmed by other workers for a wider range of nitriles and for other species. It is now clear that there is considerable variation between animal species in both the extent to which thiocyanate is formed and the rate at which it is eliminated from the body. For example, Gut *et al.* (1975) concluded that free cyanide plays only a minor role in acrylo-nitrile toxicity in rats but may play quite an important one in mice.

With respect to birds, there do not appear to have been any studies with the domestic fowl and the only information is derived from some early studies with pigeons by Meurice (1900). He tested the toxicity of a range of nitriles and also detected thiocyanate in their excreta, but only when thiosulphate was also given as a sulphur donor. It appears that pigeons may be more resistant to nitriles than rabbits, mice or frogs, even the α-hydroxynitriles which readily release cyanide non-enzymically in an aqueous medium. It does not follow that chickens are equally resistant but Barcroft (1931) has shown that they are more resistant to atmospheres containing hydrogen cyanide than are pigeons.

In 1952, Stern *et al.* showed that rat liver homogenates could convert the aliphatic dinitrile, malononitrile, to free cyanide but no reaction was observed with other nitriles tested. More recently, Ohkawa *et al.* (1972) apparently demonstrated cyanide release from several nitriles by a microsomal preparation from mouse liver. The activity of the microsomes was attributed to the presence of the mixed function oxidase system.

$$R.CH_2CN \xrightarrow[\text{NADPH}]{\text{mfo}} R.CH\ (OH).CN \xrightarrow{\text{non-enzymic}} R.CHO + HCN$$

This report deals with two aspects of nitrile and cyanide toxicity in the domestic fowl; the release of cyanide from nitriles by liver homogenates and the excretion of thiocyanate after cyanide administration, with and without simultaneous administration of sulphur compounds.

II. RELEASE OF CYANIDE FROM NITRILES

Although activity of the mixed function oxidase system is located in microsomes, some activity is lost in the preparation of the microsomal fraction. Consequently a procedure has been developed for determination of cyanide release following incubation of nitriles with whole liver homogenates. It differs from the method used by Ohkawa *et al.* (1972) in several respects. The NADPH concentration was reduced to correspond to its optimum for this enzyme system, and activity was greatly increased by inclusion of manganous ion, previously shown to be required for α-hydroxylation of nitriles in plants (Liljegren, 1978). Estimations of cyanide released on incubation were made by the Epstein (1949) procedure. One problem that is encountered when using whole liver homogenates is that recovery of cyanide is variable due to binding, notably to haemoglobin. It is necessary, therefore, to include a range of standards as a routine measure. The difficulty is minimized if animals are sacrificed by exsanguination.

The substrate giving the greatest release of cyanide to date has been phenylacetonitrile (benzyl cyanide). The mean percentage breakdown from the standard amount of 500 nmoles when incubated with homogenate from 50 mg of liver tissue was 22.3 ± 4.8% for determinations from 4 different livers. Thus phenylacetonitrile has been used as a control and all other values related to it. Release of cyanide from aliphatic nitriles is shown in Table I. For the simple

Table I Release of cyanide from aliphatic nitriles (Relative to phenylacetonitrile as 100)

Simple mononitriles		Simple dinitriles		Others	
Aceto-, CH_3-	0.0	Malono-, -CH_2-	0.0	Acrylo-, CH_2 = CH-	0.0
Propio-, C_2H_5-	0.5	Succino-, -C_2H_4-	0.0	Allyl- CH_2 = CH.CH_2-	2.0
Butyro-, C_3H_7-	4.0	Glutaro-, -C_3H_6-	0.0	Dehydromucono- -CH_2.CH = CH.CH_2-	6.8
Valero-, C_4H_9-	5.8	Adipo-, -C_4H_8-	0.0	Chloraceto-, Cl CH_2.-	3.3
Capro-, C_5H_{11}-	7.7	Pimelo-, -C_5H_{10}-	1.9	β-aminopropio-, $H_2N.CH_2.CH_2$-	0.0
Caprylo-, C_7H_{15}-	15.0	Subero-, -C_6H_{12}-	34.7	β-cyanoalanine CN.CH_2.CH(NH_2).COOH	0.0
				Ethylcyanoacetate, CN.CH_2.$COOC_2H_5$	3.7

mononitriles there is a clear progression, with more cyanide being released as chain length increases. Despite the availability of the second nitrile group in the dinitriles, it is necessary to have a longer carbon chain before free cyanide is produced than in the mononitriles. Malononitrile is an exception because there was a non-enzymic release of cyanide, which gave a relative value of 14.5. A double bond between β and γ carbon atoms enhances cyanide release but when located between α and β carbons, as in acrylonitrile, it is without effect. Substitution of a chlorine atom into acetonitrile resulted in some cyanide production. No cyanide was obtained from either of the naturally occurring nitriles, β-aminopropionitrile and β-cyanoalanine, but some was released with ethyl cyanoacetate as substrate.

Of other nitriles tested, indolylacetonitrile gave the highest relative value, 36.4. Little or no cyanide is released when the nitrile group is attached directly to an aromatic ring. The cyanogenic glycoside, amygdalin, was also tested without any clear result.

These resulte agree well with the observations of Meurice (1900) on the toxicity of nitriles to pigeons. Chain length is important for alkyl nitriles, with the exception of malononitrile from which cyanide is released by some mechanism that does not involve the NADPH-dependent mixed function oxidase. In general it would appear that alkyl nitriles release cyanide much less readily than aryl alkyl nitriles such as phenylaceto- or indolylaceto-, accounting for their lower toxicity, and the toxicity of aryl nitriles does not appear to result from the formation of free cyanide.

With respect to naturally occurring nitriles that might

arise from glucosinolates, *Cruciferae* containing both benzyl and 3-indolylmethyl glucosinolates occur (Van Etten and Tookey, 1979) but in rapeseed meal, which is the major cruciferous material included in poultry diets, the predominant glucosinolates yield nitrile derivatives of butene in the digestive tract (Smith and Campbell, 1976). These have yet to be tested for cyanide release but one would not predict that they would be good substrates for the enzyme system. Other naturally occurring nitriles, such as β-aminopropionitrile, have been implicated in the condition known as lathyrism. This nitrile may be converted to cyanoacetic acid and excreted as such, without loss of the nitrile group (Ehrhart *et al.*, 1963). Cyanoacetic acid has not been tested for cyanide release but the ethyl ester, slightly the more toxic of the two according to Meurice (1900), did yield cyanide to a small extent.

In many instances the yield of cyanide was rather low and detoxication to thiocyanate might not present any real difficulty following ingestion of many of these nitriles at the levels which might be encountered in practice. If this is so, the major concern would be chronic rather than acute toxicity, with greater emphasis upon the effects of increased thiocyanate ion rather than the direct effect of free cyanide. The cyanide giving rise to thiocyanate need not necessarily arise from nitriles. Chicken tissues also contain glutathione-S-transferase activity which results in the release of cyanide from organic thiocyanates. There is much evidence for disturbance of thyroid function following the consumption of glucosinolate-containing materials which does implicate thiocyanate, but the nitriles which can arise from glucosinolates have been shown to be acutely toxic also (Van Etten *et al.*, 1969), and their fate and effects within the body merit further investigation.

III. URINARY EXCRETION OF THIOCYANATE

The excretion of thiocyanate by hens following dosage with cyanide has been studied in acute experiments in which urine flow was increased by means of a diuretic. In the first series of tests, both ureters were cannulated, by the technique of Sperber (1948), with the birds under deep anaesthesia induced by barbiturates. The diuretic was a 15% solution of mannitol, infused into the brachial vein. Test compounds were given by the same route unless stated otherwise. The urinary thiocyanate was determined spectrophotometrically as the ferrithiocyanate complex.

The rate of thiocyanate excretion following the infusion of mannitol alone was found to be almost constant over a 6.5 h period. In subsequent tests, therefore, each bird acted as its own control, urine samples being taken to establish the control rate of excretion for 30 min prior to administration of test compounds. A single dose of

50 μmoles of potassium cyanide was found to be lethal, so 30 μmoles was the standard dose used, equivalent to approximately 0.9 mg/kg body weight.

Following an intravenous injection of 30 μmoles of potassium thiocyanate the excretion of thiocyanate increased rapidly to 10 times the control level after 10 min. A rapid decline followed and the rate had returned to the control level after 3.5 h. The recovery of thiocyanate, i.e. the excess excreted above control level during the whole 6 h collection was equivalent to 85% of the dose. This demonstrated the extent to which rapid elimination from the body was possible under the experimental conditions.

There was a similar rapid rise in thiocyanate excretion following a single injected dose of cyanide with a peak excretion rate (after 30 min) which was 4.5 times the control level. The rate then declined until, after 3 h, it became almost constant but still more than double the control level. A 50% recovery was obtained over 6 h, the majority during the first 4 h as shown in Table II. Little cyanide was excreted directly, 2.4 x 10^{-2} μmoles in 6 h, less than 0.1% of the dose. There was a marked decrease in thiosulphate excretion to approximately one quarter of the control level after 30 min, suggesting that thiosulphate had contributed the sulphur for cyanide detoxication. In Fig. 1 the patterns of excretion of thiocyanate, cyanide and thiosulphate are illustrated. A similar pattern of thiocyanate excretion was observed following cyanide administration by intramuscular and intraduodenal routes. A recovery of 42% over 6 h was obtained after injecting cyanide into the leg muscles while 30% of a dose of 48 μmoles was recovered in 4 h after introducing it into the duodenum.

Table II Recovery of thiocyanate (%) over different periods

Collection period (min)	Recovery (%)
240	40.7 ± 2.42
300	42.7 ± 0.50
360	49.7 ± 1.28
420	52.4 ± 2.88

Single dose of cyanide (30 μmoles) given intravenously

In the following tests cyanide was given more slowly by infusion over an extended period, 30 μmoles at 0.35 μmoles /min. When cyanide was given alone the recovery was 53.1 ± 1.62% and, when given together with sulphur compounds in varying amounts, the results given in Table III were obtained. Thiosulphate did not enhance thiocyanate excretion, even though previous results had indicated that it might be a natural sulphur donor. On the contrary, recovery

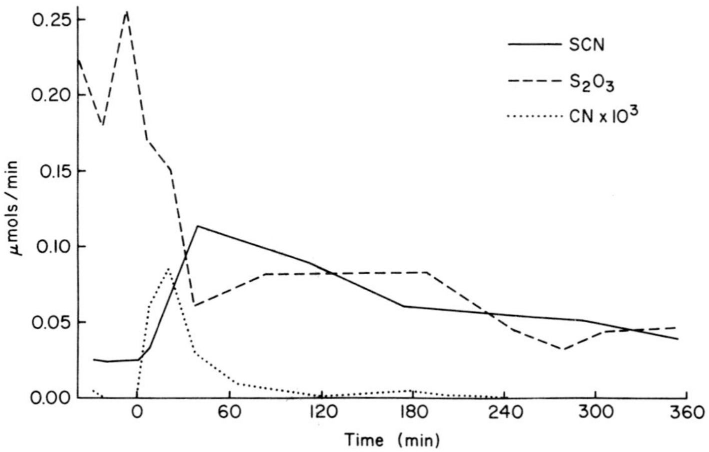

Fig. 1 Excretion rates of thiocyanate, thiosulphate and cyanide following intravenous injection of 30 μmoles cyanide.

decreased as the amount of thiosulphate given was increased. Nor did methionine or cysteine increase excretion, and elevation of the methionine dosage served only to depress thiocyanate recovery. A more marked depression occurred when sulphite was given, but the pattern of thiocyanate excretion remained the same as in the other tests, rising to a definite peak, at least 3 times the control rate in this instance, followed by a steady decline. This was unlike the response to simultaneous infusion of sodium nitrite with cyanide, when the excretion rate reached a plateau at little more than twice the control level. With cyanide and nitrite at a ratio of 1:22 recovery of thiocyanate was only 34% over the same 6 h period.

Table III Recovery of thiocyanate (%) in anaesthetized birds

CN/S ratio	Thiosulphate	Sulphite	Methionine	Cysteine
1:2	48.2 ± 0.32	42.2 ± 2.88	52.5 ± 1.62	54.1 ± 0.08
1:4	46.3 ± 0.98		47.9 ± 0.98	
1:22	32.0*			

*Single estimate

Simultaneous infusion of cyanide and sulphur compounds. 30 μmoles cyanide infused at 0.35 μmoles/min together with sulphur compounds in varying proportions.

A further series of tests was carried out under different conditions to see if the observations and trends observed would be repeated. By use of a cloacal cannula to separate urine and faeces (Bokhori, 1961), urine was collected over 3.5 h periods from unanaesthetized birds. The birds were fasted for 24 h prior to experiments to minimize contamination of urine by faeces and blockage of the cannula. In this case the diuretic was hypotonic saline, 0.5%, infused into the brachial vein. Sulphur compounds were given in the saline so that the total amount given over 3.5 h gave pre-determined cyanide : sulphur ratios but cyanide, 30 μmoles, was injected into the leg muscles, thus avoiding immediate mixing with the administered sulphur compounds. Again the urine collected over the first 30 min was used to establish the control rate of thiocyanate excretion and so the recovery values obtained apply to a 3 h period.

Table IV Recovery of thiocyanate (%) from unanaesthetized birds

CN/S ratio	Thiosulphate	Sulphite	Mercaptopyruvate
1:2	52.5 ± 1.4	55.0 ± 2.7	64.8 ± 0.9
1:4	55.2 ± 1.4	46.0 ± 5.1	61.4 ± 9.9
1:8	42.0 ± 2.2	-	49.0 ± 11.7
1:16	29.6 ± 6.9	-	36.4 ± 1.6

30 μmoles cyanide given intramuscularly, sulphur compounds given by intravenous infusion to give varying cyanide:sulphur ratios.

The results given in Table IV show some differences from those obtained in the first series of tests. They should be compared with the recovery of 47.2 ± 2.85%, a mean value for 4 birds, after dosage with cyanide alone. Recovery tended to increase at the lower levels of thiosulphate but, again, higher levels caused a depression. When an attempt was made to increase the level still further to give a 1:32 ratio the bird died and, in fact, one bird was lost at the 1:16 ratio. It would appear that mercaptopyruvate is a better sulphur donor than thiosulphate, higher recoveries being obtained at each level of dosage. Nevertheless, the trend was the same; increased recoveries at lower dosage levels but diminished recoveries at the higher levels.

In view of the results in the first series, it was surprising that thiocyanate recovery increased at the lowest level of sulphite dosage. However, it fell when sulphite dosage was raised and two attempts to increase sulphite to the next level resulted in the loss of both birds. In all instances in which fatalities occurred the symptoms were those of cyanide poisoning and subsequent tests confirmed that in the absence of cyanide, birds could tolerate the doses of thiosulphate or sulphite given without any obvious sign of distress. This suggests that the reduced recoveries are the result of reduced thiocyanate formation rather than of any hindrance in its excretion. It also appears to indicate that the metabolism of cyanide by other routes is restricted and that much remains as free cyanide if it cannot be converted to thiocyanate.

The results were broadly similar for the two series of experiments. The main difference was the increased thiocyanate recovery that occurred in the second series, but not the first, at low dosage levels of sulphur compounds. A possible explanation for this is that the sulphur compounds were administered for 30 min prior to the injection of cyanide in the second series whereas they were given together with cyanide in the first. Alternatively the difference in the rate at which the cyanide was given, i.e. injection versus infusion, may be the cause. However, the trend on increasing the dose of sulphur compounds was the same and so both series can be considered together.

The excretion of thiocyanate may differ between diuretic and normal chickens but all the indications are that, in these experiments, it is thiocyanate formation that is limited, not its excretion. It has long been recognized that detoxication of cyanide is not limited by the availability of the sulphur transferring enzymes necessary for its conversion to thiocyanate. It has also been customary to allocate the primary role to rhodanese (thiosulphate sulphurtransferase, EC 2.8.1.1) rather than to 3-mercaptopyruvate sulphurtransferase, EC 2.8.1.2. This may be correct (see Westley, this volume). Thiosulphate excretion certainly fell, following dosage with cyanide alone, when this was checked at an early stage in these investigations, suggesting that it was being utilized; but mercaptopyruvate is clearly an efficient sulphur donor also. Rhodanese can use other sulphur compounds as donors if sulphane sulphur is present. Unfortunately there appear to be no available procedures whereby the amount of sulphane sulphur present could be assessed, but it seems unlikely that the amount of transferable sulphur could be the limiting factor, in view of the extremely low doses of cyanide that are lethal. The limiting factor rather appears to be the extent to which the sulphur which is present can be drawn upon.

The key results may be those obtained with sulphite. Sulphite is a product in the rhodanese reaction when thiosulphate is the donor and is also formed during the catabolism of sulphur amino acids. Experiments with partially purified rhodanese from chicken liver have shown sulphite to be a more efficient acceptor of sulphane sulphur than cyanide and it also accepts sulphur from mercaptopyruvate. In both cases thiosulphate is the product. This might be expected to enhance thiocyanate formation. However, sulphite is an inhibitor of the rhodanese reaction when cyanide is the sulphur acceptor. Thus it is tentatively suggested that the administration of thiosulphate, mercaptopyruvate or sulphur amino acids elevates sulphite concentration *in situ* to a sufficient extent to depress thiocyanate formation. Some of the metabolic interactions are illustrated in Fig. 2. A greater flux through alanine sulphinate will increase sulphite formation and this could occur by a feedback mechanism, following dosage with sulphur amino acids or following mercaptopyruvate dosage. How thiosulphate administration influences thiocyanate

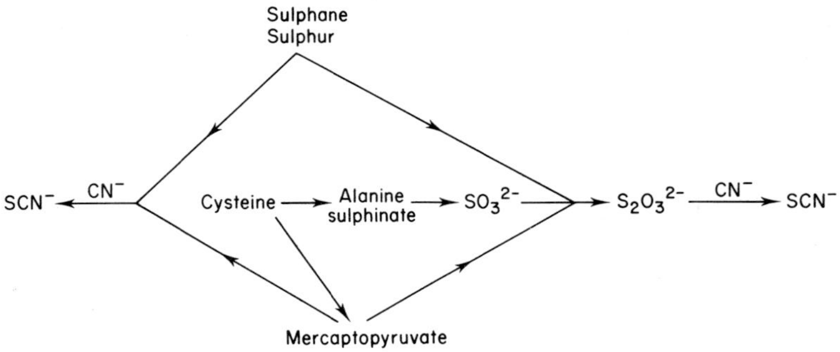

Fig. 2 The interactions of cyanide with metabolism of sulphur compounds

excretion is not clear. More information is required on the concentrations and intracellular location of metabolites, and also on the extent to which they can be transported across membranes.

IV. CONCLUSION

Although some of the breakdown products from glucosinolates may have specific toxic effects, the wide range of compounds that may be formed after ingestion of cruciferous foods includes some that would be good substrates for those enzyme systems which release free cyanide. Prolonged ingestion of such foods could present the same threat of chronic cyanide poisoning as has been found to result from continued consumption of foods such as cassava, that contain cyanogenic glucosides. For both glucosinolates and cyanogenic glucosides there is a need for further studies both at the enzyme level and in whole animals to assess the nature and extent of the problem.

It is also clear that studies of cyanide detoxication need to be related more closely to the metabolism of sulphur compounds. Consumption of cassava is known to reduce the plasma levels of sulphur amino acids in humans and several studies with farm animals have indicated that dietary supplements of sulphur amino acids, above the levels normally required, may be needed to achieve high levels of performance. The amount of sulphur directed towards thiocyanate production in detoxication of liberated cyanide is insufficient to account for the changes in plasma level or in the dietary requirement of sulphur amino acids. It would be helpful to have more quantitative information on the effect of cyanide on amino acid requirements and on its interaction with their metabolism.

Differences between animal species need to be considered also. The chicken has proved to be a suitable animal for the present studies, and is of economic importance, but it is not known if the results obtained are generally applicable. In particular, it is not known how far they can be related to chronic cassava toxicity in human populations, a problem which is so extensive. However, they do indicate areas where comparative studies could be helpful.

ACKNOWLEDGEMENTS

The studies on cyanide release from nitriles has been supported by a grant from the Agricultural Research Council. I also wish to thank Dr S. Y. Oh, now at University Pertanian Malaysia, P. R. Adams, M. M. Hassan and J. H. Scofield for their help in the investigations and Dr A. H. Sykes for helpful comments and discussion.

REFERENCES

Barcroft, J. (1931). *J. Hyg.* 31, 1-34.

Bokori, J. (1961). *Acta vet. Med. Hung.* 11, 415-422.

Ehrhart, L.A., Lipton, S.H. and Strong, F.M. (1963). *Biochemistry* 2, 300-304.

Epstein, J. (1949). *Anal. Chem.* 19, 272-274.

Gut, I., Nerudová, J., Kopecký, J. and Holoček, V. (1975). *Arch. Toxicol.* 33, 151-161.

Lang, S. (1894). *Arch. exp. Path. Pharmak* 34, 247-258.

Liljegren, D.R. (1978). *Phytochem.* 17, 1695-1699.

Meurice, J. (1900). *Arch. int. Pharmacodyn.* 7, 11-53.

Ohkawa, H., Ohkawa, R., Yamamoto, I. and Casida, J.E. (1972). *Pest. Biochem. Physiol.* 2, 95-112.

Smith, T.K. and Campbell, L.D. (1976). *Poult. Sci.* 55, 861-867.

Sperber, I. (1948). *Zool. Bidrag. Upps.* 27, 429-448.

Stern, J., Weil-Malherbe, H. and Green, R.H. (1952). *Biochem. J.* 52, 114-125.

Van Etten, C.H. and Tookey, H.L. (1979). *In* "Herbivores: Their Interaction with Secondary Plant Metabolites" (G.A. Rosenthal and D.H. Janzen, eds), pp. 471-500. Academic Press, New York.

Van Etten, C.H., Wolff, I.A. and Daxenbichler, M.E. (1969). *J. Agric. Food Chem.* 17, 483-491.

CYANIDE AND SULFANE SULFUR

JOHN WESTLEY

Department of Biochemistry,
The University of Chicago,
Chicago, Illinois 60637,
USA

I. SULFANE SULFUR

The thing most likely to happen to cyanide biologically is its irreversible reaction with sulfane sulfur to form thiocyanate. This assertion states the central point of the following presentation; to understand it fully we need a definition of "sulfane sulfur". This is provided in Fig. 1, which shows the partial ionization of a generalized member of the class of compounds known as sulfanes (Roy and Trudinger, 1970). The fully ionized sulfanes, familiar under the name "inorganic polysulfides", consist entirely of sulfane sulfur atoms - divalent sulfur covalently bonded only to other sulfur.

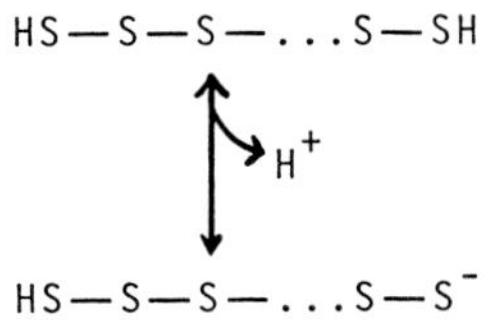

Fig. 1 Sulfanes

The foregoing definition of sulfane sulfur also fits certain atoms in compounds other than the sulfanes themselves. Figure 2 shows a number of these. The organic analogs of sulfanes, the persulfides ($R\text{-}S\text{-}S^-$) and polysulfides ($R\text{-}S\text{-}S_x\text{-}~S\text{-}R'$), contain sulfur chains in which one or more atoms are sulfane sulfurs. So also do inorganic thiosulfate ($S_2O_3^{2-}$) and its organic analogs, the thiosulfonates (RSO_2S^-), as well as the polythionates ($O_3S\text{-}S_x\text{-}SO_3^{2-}$). Even elemental sulfur in its most usual forms (for example, the staggered eight-membered ring) consists of sulfane atoms according to our definition.

It must be obvious, however, that fitting an arbitrary definition is not the point; sulfane atoms so defined are grouped into a common category because they share a common

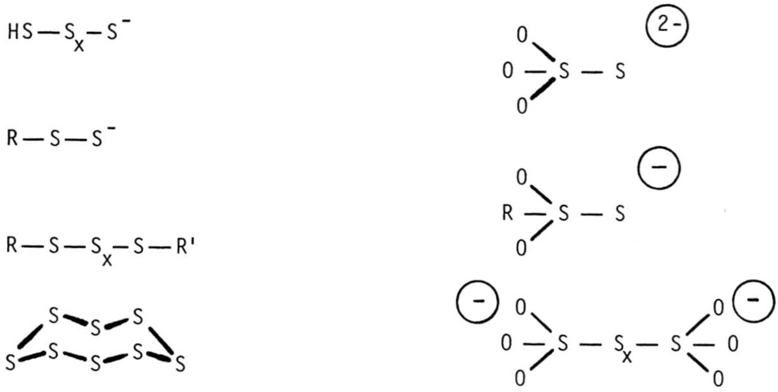

Fig. 2 Compounds with sulfane sulfur atoms

$$R{-}S{-}SH + Y^- \rightleftharpoons R{-}SH + YS^-$$

Thiophilic series of Y^- species:

Carbanions, HS^-, $R\text{-}S^-$ > ϕS^- > CN^- > SO_3^{2-} > OH^- > RSO_2^- > SSO_3^{2-} > SCN^-

Fig. 3 Reaction between a persulfide and a thiophilic anion, Y^-.

chemical reactivity. This is illustrated in Fig. 3 with the reaction between a persulfide and a generalized nucleophile, Y^-. The sulfane atom is removed from the persulfide essentially as an atom of zero valence sulfur, leaving a thiol behind and forming YS^-.

A reactivity series for sulfur nucleophiles, which resembles but is not identical to the nucleophilic series for carbon, is shown below the reaction in Fig. 3. Cyanide anion is a powerful thiophile, ranking behind only the carbanions and various thiolate anions and ahead of sulfite, hydroxide, and the other common nucleophiles.

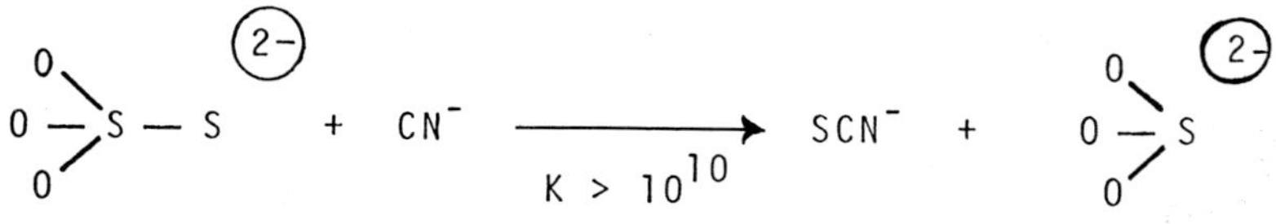

Fig. 4 Reaction between thiosulfate and cyanide

This much, then, tells us what sulfane atoms are and something about what we may expect of them in the presence of cyanide. Next we must consider the question of the irreversibility of the reaction, both chemically and biologically. Figure 4 shows that the reaction of cyanide with the sulfane atom of thiosulfate has an equilibrium constant in excess of 10^{10} - this despite the fact that the product sulfite is itself a rather good thiophile. The equilibrium constant is in fact too large to measure; the reverse reaction has not even been detected. Chemically, the assertion of practical irreversibility is on solid ground.

It happens, however, that the *biological* ground appears less solid. Biologically, cyanide has a history of arising from its own ashes, so to speak. No sooner has one safely detoxified cyanide, by the irreversible reaction with sulfane sulfur to form thiocyanate, than some of it reappears as cyanide again. This occurs not by reversal of the forming reaction, however, but by way of the oxidative reaction of thiocyanate shown in Fig. 5. This reaction is catalyzed by peroxidases very generally, and by both methemoglobin and oxyhemoglobin as well (Wood, 1975; Vesey and Wilson, 1978).

$$SCN^- + 3\ H_2O_2 \longrightarrow CN^- + SO_4^{2-} + 2\ H_3^+O$$

Fig. 5 Peroxidation of thiocyanate.

Plainly, this reaction is a nuisance for all organisms that must detoxify cyanide. Further, it is a nuisance exacerbated by the rather low rate of excretion of thiocyanate ion. The kidneys filter out SCN^- well enough in the glomeruli but, unfortunately, also reabsorb it well in the tubules.

We might summarize what has been said to this point by noting simply that there is a cyanide-reactive form of sulfur to which biologists may wish to pay some attention. What remains to be done here is to investigate the reported biological occurrence of such material and especially of the enzymes that catalyze its reactions.

II. RHODANESE

The best known of these enzymes is rhodanese (thiosulfate: cyanide sulfurtransferase, EC 2.8.1.1), which catalyzes reactions of the kind shown in Fig. 6 (Westley, 1973; Sörbo, 1975). The sulfur-donor substrate $[RSO_xS]^-$ can be practically any sulfane-containing anion. The acceptor substrate can be any of a number of thiophiles, including cyanide, dihydrolipoate, and sulfite. Monothiols such as cysteine and glutathione are relatively poor acceptors.

Efforts to place the rhodanese-catalyzed reactions into a physiological setting have given rise to the notion of a mixed metabolic pool of sulfane sulfur, indicated in Fig. 7 as "the sulfane pool" (Westley, 1973, 1977, 1980). When an experimental animal is injected with sulfane sulfur - say, thiosulfate with ^{35}S in the sulfane position - subsequent analysis of the animal's plasma shows the

$[RSO_xS]^-$ + Thiophilic Anion $\rightleftharpoons$ $[RSO_x]^-$ + Thiolated Anion
(e.g., CN^- or dihydrolipoate) (e.g., SCN^- or lipoate persulfide)

Fig. 6 Generalized reaction of the kind catalyzed by rhodanese. R may be an aryl or alkyl residue or O^-. X is an integral value in the range 0 - 2.

presence of a variety of sulfane-containing materials, including various polythionates and what behaves like protein-associated elemental sulfur as well as thiosulfate itself. On closer examination, the protein-associated sulfur turns out to be just that - elemental sulfur carried by the serum albumin (Schneider and Westley, 1969).

There is some evidence to suggest that these sulfane materials, which are in rapid equilibrium with each other physiologically, can also equilibrate with the protein persulfide generated in the endoplasmic reticulum of cells that detoxify parathion and other sulfur-containing pesticides (Kamataki and Neal, 1976; Seawright *et al.*, 1976). There is also clear evidence that the small molecular per- and poly-sulfides shown in Fig. 7 are formed in enzymic reactions, although the former are too unstable to permit isolation (Hylin and Wood, 1959; Flavin, 1962; Cavallini *et al.*, 1962; Villarejo and Westley, 1963; Crewe and Ross, 1975).

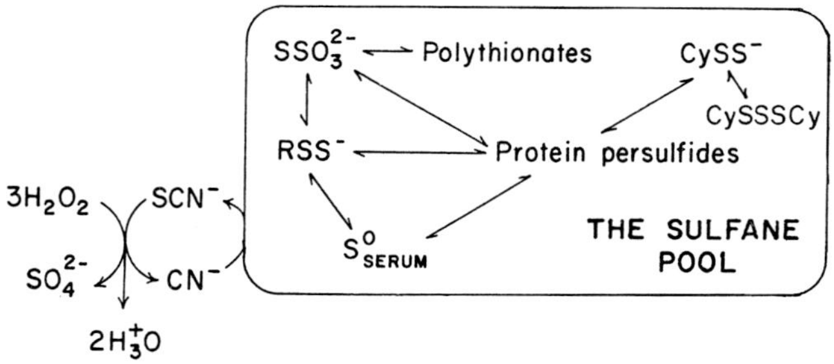

Fig. 7 The sulfane pool: biological materials containing sulfur atoms.

All of the foregoing sulfane-containing materials can be sulfur-donor substrates for rhodanese. To put it another way, rhodanese can catalyze the interconversions of all of these compounds as well as the transfer of sulfane sulfur to cyanide, the reaction for which the enzyme is best known.

Rhodanese is very nearly ubiquitous in biology. Figure 8 records the fact that it has been definitely established to occur in plants (Chew and Boey, 1972), fungi (Oi, 1973), actinomycetes (Yamamoto and Oi, 1977), and various bacteria*

* See the reviews of Sörbo (1975) and Westley (1973).

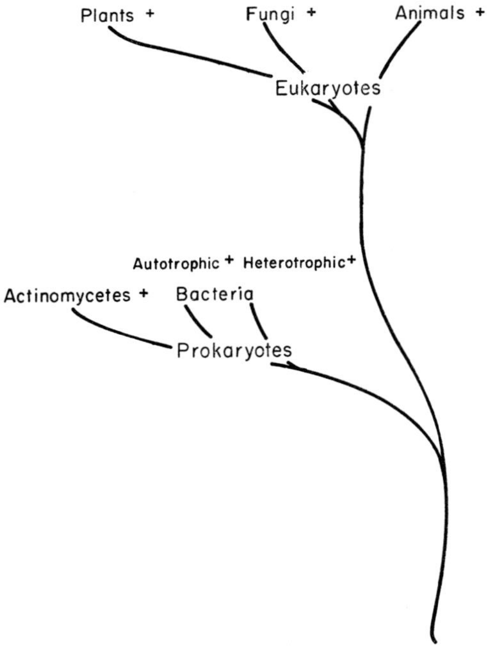

Fig. 8 Phylogenetic distribution of rhodanese. + indicates occurrence.

as well as in all phyla of the animal kingdom (Schiewelbein *et al.*, 1969). In mammals it occurs most richly in liver tissue, with a smaller amount in kidney and generally much less in other organs (Koj *et al.*, 1977). In liver, at least, it is exclusively an enzyme of the mitochondrial matrix (Koj *et al.*, 1975).

A great deal is known about rhodanese. Its fundamental formal mechanism (Fig. 9) shows that the free enzyme reacts with a sulfane-containing compound to cleave the S-S bond of the donor substrate and form a sulfur-substituted enzyme (ES), which then can react with a thiophilic acceptor. Considerable chemical detail, at the level of what chemical group in the enzyme does what in the catalysis, is known (Westley, 1977). Some six years ago, a completely detailed chemical mechanism for the action of rhodanese was proposed on the basis of the chemical and kinetic data available to that time (Schlesinger and Westley, 1974). Very recently

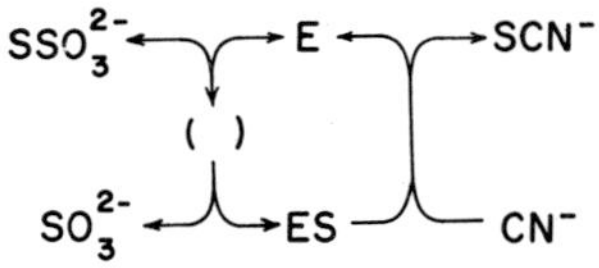

Fig. 9 Formal mechanism of rhodanese action. E is the free enzyme; ES is the sulfur-substituted enzyme.

both the total primary structure (Russell *et al.*, 1978) and the high resolution X-ray crystallographic structure (Ploegman *et al.*, 1978) of one form of the enzyme have been completed; they are in accord with the mechanism of action inferred previously. The substantial puzzles remaining for investigators of rhodanese are structural (and perhaps physiological - see Volini and Alexander, this volume); mechanistically, rhodanese has become one of our best known enzymes.

III. 3-MERCAPTOPYRUVATE SULFURTRANSFERASE

From the foregoing account it may be concluded that biology has a widespread, efficient and well understood mechanism for transfers of sulfane sulfur atoms. This leaves us wondering how sulfane sulfur originates. That is, how is sulfur at the level of sulfhydryl groups converted to sulfane sulfur? Largely by the reaction given in Fig. 10, as far as we know. The enzyme that catalyzes this reaction is mercaptopyruvate sulfurtransferase (EC 2.8.1.2); it cleaves a carbon-sulfur bond (Meister *et al.*, 1954; Vachek and Wood, 1972). When a thiol is the acceptor substrate, a persulfide is the immediate product (Jarabak and Westley, 1978). Alternatively, when cyanide is the acceptor, thiocyanate is formed directly (Jarabak and Westley, 1980).

$$HS{-}CH_2C(=O)COO^- + RS^- \text{ or } CN^- \rightleftharpoons H_3CC(=O)COO^- + RSS^- \text{ or } SCN^-$$

Fig. 10 Reaction catalyzed by 3-mercaptopyruvate sulfurtransferase

These reactions, like those catalyzed by rhodanese, can be placed into their physiological setting. Figure 11 shows the reactions catalyzed by mercaptopyruvate sulfurtransferase in relation to the components of the sulfane pool discussed previously and to the common reactions of cysteine metabolism.

Mercaptopyruvate is formed by transamination of cysteine. However, cysteine may also be oxidized to cysteine sulfinate [$^-O_2S{-}CH_2CH(NH_3^+)COO^-$], which is at a central crossroads of sulfur metabolism. It may be further oxidized to cysteic acid and then decarboxylated, or first decarboxylated and then oxidized, in either case yielding taurine [$^-O_3S{-}CH_2CHNH_3^+$]. Alternatively, cysteine sulfinate may be transaminated to yield sulfinyl pyruvate [$^-O_2S{-}CH_2CO(COO^-)$], which is cleaved to sulfite and pyruvate. The sulfite so produced may be oxidized to sulfate or it may react with mercaptopyruvate in a further reaction catalyzed by mercaptopyruvate in a further reaction catalyzed by mercaptopyruvate sulfurtransferase to form thiosulfate, another member of the sulfane pool. This reaction is thought to be the principal source of the thiosulfate found in mammalian tissues and urine (Sörbo, 1957).

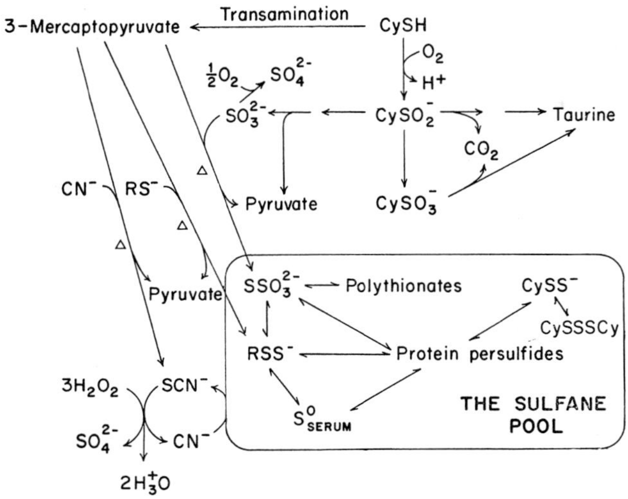

Fig. 11 Reactions catalyzed by mercaptopyruvate sulfurtransferase (indicated as △) in context of reactions of cysteine metabolism and the sulfane pool.

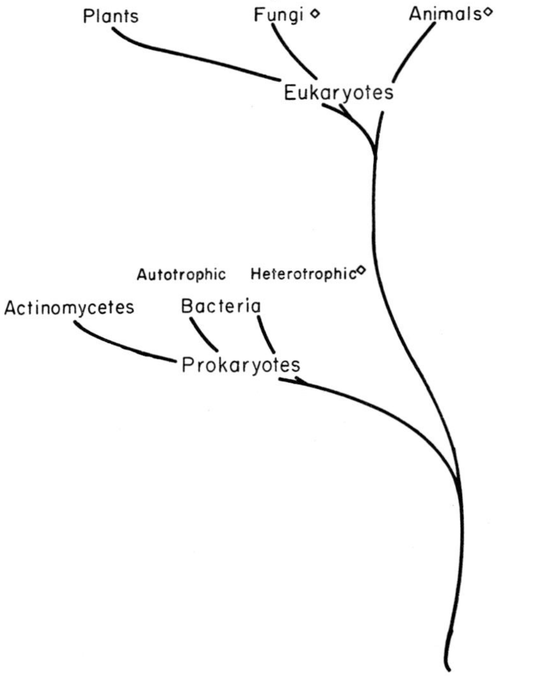

Fig. 12 Phylogenetic distribution of mercaptopyruvate sulfurtransferase. ◇ indicates occurrence.

The established biological distribution of mercaptopyruvate sulfurtransferase is indicated in Fig. 12. Mammalian erythrocytes (Van Den Hamer *et al.*, 1967), liver (Fanshier and Kun, 1962) and kidney (Jarabak and Westley, 1978) tissue are good sources for preparation of the enzyme, as is also *E.coli* (Vachek and Wood, 1972). This sulfurtransferase also occurs in yeast but no procedure for its purification from this source has been reported.

Much less is known about the chemical mechanism and structure of this enzyme than is known about rhodanese. However, the formal mechanism of the mercaptopyruvate sulfurtransferase from bovine kidney has recently been studied. As shown in Fig. 13, this mechanism differs substantially from that of rhodanese. There is no sulfur-substituted enzyme as an intermediate in the reaction cycle; the formation of a ternary complex of the enzyme with both intact substrates is required; the order of substrate combination is random. Furthermore, the fact that mercaptopyruvate is itself a thiol enables this compound to act both as an acceptor and as a donor. This gives rise to the autotransfer "bridge" across the middle of the reaction diagram and lends some interesting features to the kinetic results on which the diagram is based (Jarabak and Westley, 1978).

One might possibly guess that this experimental situation could be simplified by substituting cyanide anion for the thiol acceptor substrate. Such a guess, however, would be mostly wrong. Cyanide does serve as a sulfur-acceptor substrate but of course mercaptopyruvate must still be present as donor and it therefore can continue to serve as an alternate acceptor. Furthermore, cyanide and mercaptopyruvate are involved in a rapid equilibrium formation of mercaptopyruvate cyanohydrin. The one simplification that is achieved resides in the fact that with cyanide as acceptor substrate, the kinetic mechanism is of the rapid equilibrium-ordered form with the donor as the leading substrate, rather than the random form shown in Fig. 13 (Jarabak and Westley, 1980).

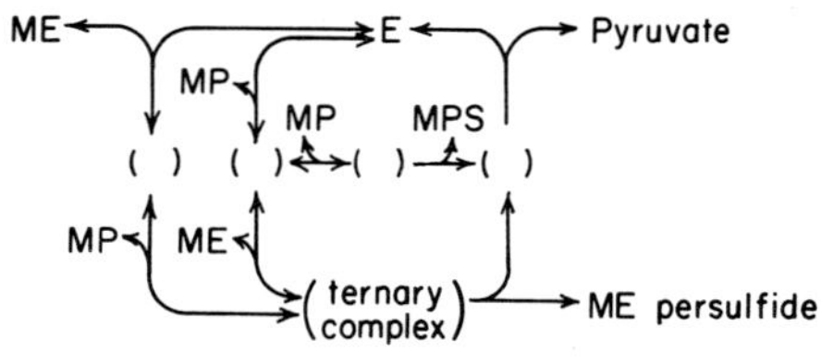

Fig. 13 Formal catalytic mechanism of mercaptopyruvate sulfurtransferase with a thiol acceptor substrate. ME, 2-mercaptoethanol; MP, 3-mercaptopyruvate; MPS, 3-mercaptopyruvate persulfide.

There is currently a controversy regarding a possible role of mercaptopyruvate sulfurtransferase in the thiolation of some pyrimidine nucleotide residues in transfer

Table I Sulfur-donor specificities of tRNA sulfurtransferase

Preferred or exclusive donor	Source	Reference
3-Mercaptopyruvate	*B.subtilis*	T.-W. Wong *et al.*, *Biochemistry* 9, 2376 (1970)
	Rat brain	T.-W. Wong *et al.*, *Biochemistry* 13, 2805 (1974)
	Morris hepatoma	T.-W. Wong *et al.*, *B.B.R.C.* 65, 1137 (1975)
Cysteine	*E. coli*	J.W. Abrell *et al.*, *J. Biol. Chem.* 246, 294 (1971)
	Rat liver	C.L. Harris *et al.*, *Cancer Res.* 35, 3608 (1975)
	Rat brain	C.L. Harris, *Nucleic Acids Res.* 5, 599 (1978)

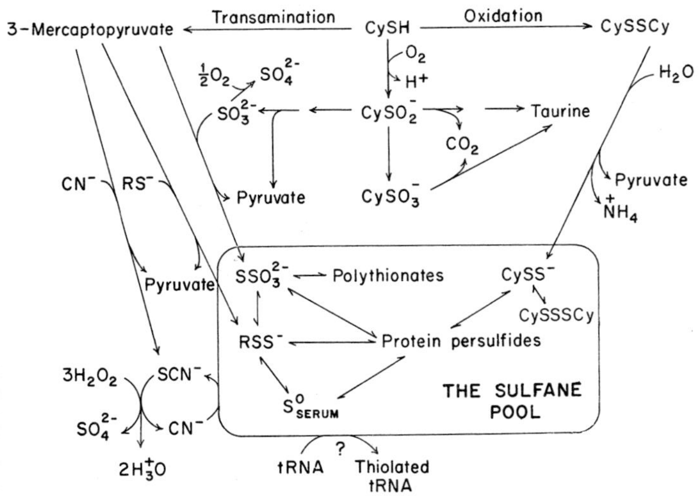

Fig. 14 Reactions of sulfur biochemistry related to the sulfane pool, including the possible participation of tRNA sulfurtransferase and of cystathionase.

RNA. As shown in Table I, Wong and her collaborators have found mercaptopyruvate to be a far better donor for the thiolation of tRNA than is cysteine. Other investigators, however, have found exactly the reverse. The present considerations suggest that this thiolation may be achieved at the expense of the general sulfane pool, as shown at the bottom of Fig. 14. The specificity differences seen in the various reported experiments probably relate mainly to the detailed balance of the various enzymes and metabolites present in the crude supernatants used as "tRNA sulfurtransferase" preparations.

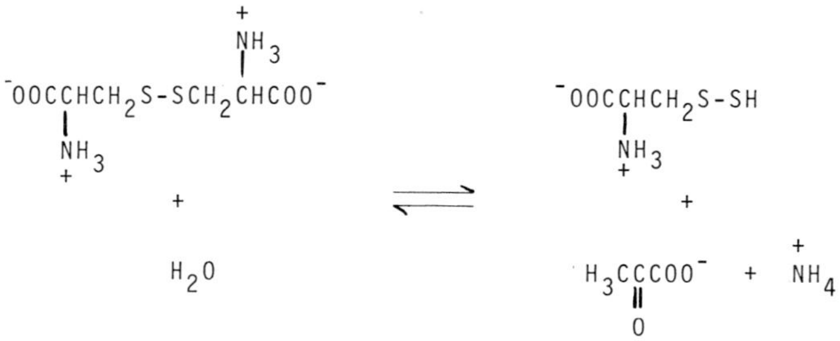

Fig. 15 Cleavage of cystine by cystathionase

IV. γ-CYSTATHIONASE

Figure 14 also shows one further possible source of sulfane sulfur. Oxidation of cysteine to cystine can be followed by asymmetric hydrolytic cleavage by γ-cystathionase (cystathionine γ-lyase, EC 4.4.1.1) to yield cysteine persulfide (Flavin, 1962; Cavallini *et al.*, 1962). The trisulfide thiocystine has been shown to accumulate when this reaction is conducted *in vitro* (Szczepkowski and

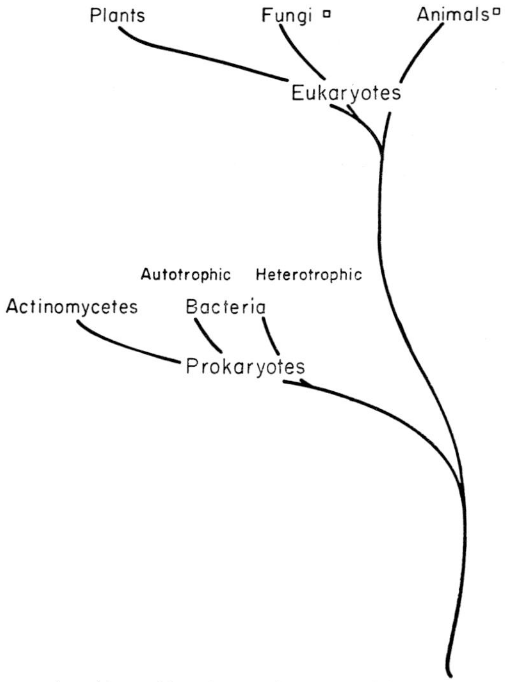

Fig. 16 Phylogenetic distribution of cystathionase. □ indicates occurrence.

Wood, 1967; see also Abdolrasulina and Wood, 1980). The reaction of cystine catalyzed by cystathionase is shown in Fig. 15. A carbon-sulfur bond is cleaved and the persulfide product is formed. Some doubts have been expressed concerning this reaction as a significant source of sulfane sulfur, however, since the concentration of free cystine in cells is normally very low.

As indicated in Fig. 16, γ-cystathionase is known to occur in both fungi (Segal, 1964) and animals (Matsuo and Greenberg, 1958) but not in any prokaryotic organisms (Greenberg, 1975).

The mechanism of the cystathionase-catalyzed reaction of cystine might have been expected to resemble either that of rhodanese-catalyzed reactions or, more likely, that of the mercaptopyruvate sulfurtransferase-catalyzed cleavage of the carbon-sulfur bond of mercaptopyruvate. This is clearly not the case, however, at least at the level of mechanistic resolutions so far reached. Cystathionase is a pyridoxal phosphate enzyme, unlike the others discussed

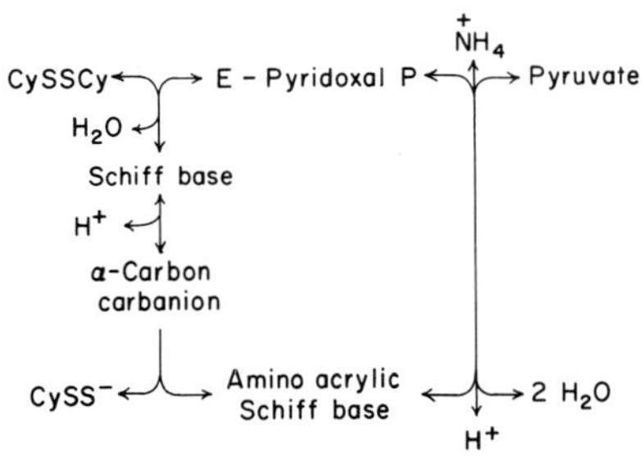

Fig. 17 Catalytic mechanism of cystathionase

above, and its mechanism is a typical pyridoxal phosphate-dependent mechanism (Fig. 17). Cystine reacts with enzyme-bound pyridoxal phosphate to form a Schiff base, which can deprotonate to yield a stabilized α-carbon carbanion, a form in which several bonds are labile. The enzyme directs the cleavage to the carbon-sulfur bond and the complex can then discharge the cysteine persulfide product, leaving an animoacrylic Schiff base. This in turn hydrolyzes to regenerate the free enzyme-bound pyridoxal phosphate, ready for another substrate molecule (Flavin, 1962; Dunathan, 1971).

V. SULFANE REDUCTASE

Finally, let us ask whether there are any other known enzyme-catalyzed reactions that either contribute to or utilize the sulfane pool components. There appear to be just two additional users. One of these is indicated by the results of the sulfane-labeling experiments *in vivo* mentioned earlier (Schneider and Westley, 1969). There, the ^{35}S present initially as sulfane pool components in the plasma could be detected at later times incorporated into the cystine of hair. Studies *in vitro* (Schneider and Westley, 1963) have also shown that lysed rat liver mitochondria will incorporate radioactive sulfane sulfur into cysteine if supplied with serine and pyridoxal phosphate. However, no results of this sort with purified systems have yet been reported, and the identity of the enzyme(s) involved is not known.

The last of the enzymes known to utilize sulfane sulfur has been called thiosulfate reductase or sulfane reductase.* Its over-all reaction is the reduction of sulfane sulfur to the sulfide level, and it may be responsible for furnishing the inorganic sulfur used in the synthesis of iron-sulfur proteins. If iron-sulfur proteins must be synthesized in the peripheral tissues using inorganic sulfur at the sulfide level, it would make great biological sense to have such a catalyst present to produce the sulfide as required locally from sulfane sulfur carried in the circulation bound to serum albumin. Certainly, inorganic sulfide cannot be transported around the body as such; it is as toxic as cyanide, and for very much the same reasons.

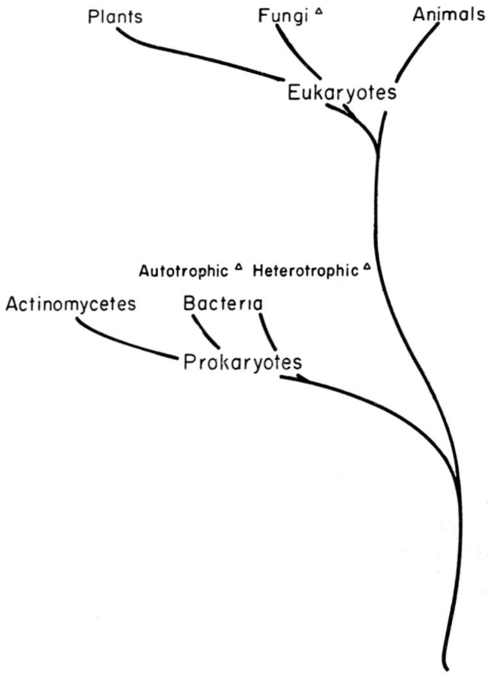

Fig. 18 Phylogenetic distribution of sulfane reductase (thiosulfate reductase). △ indicates occurrence.

* The more general term acknowledges the fact that organic thiosulfonates can also serve as sulfur-donor substrates for this enzyme (T. Chauncey and J. Westley, unpub. obsv.).

As shown in Fig. 18, the reductase activity has been established to occur in fungi (Kaji and McElroy, 1959) as well as in animals (Sörbo, 1964; Koj, 1968; Sido and Koj, 1972) and also in various bacteria (Peck and Fischer, 1962; Nakatasukasa and Akagi, 1969; Haschke and Campbell, 1971; Oltmann and Stouthamer, 1975; Hatchikian, 1975). Animal sulfane reductase has proved to be very difficult to purify, as it is extraordinarily evanescent and unstable, but the enzyme in some other eukaryotes has been a bit easier to work with. It has recently been found possible to purify the enzyme from yeast to apparent homogeneity (Uhteg and Westley, 1979).

Whether or not the chief physiological function of sulfane reductase is in the synthesis of iron sulfur proteins, the recent work on its mechanism of action indicates that the enzyme may catalyze only the first of the two reactions shown in Fig. 19 - two reactions that sum up to the overall reaction observed (Uhteg and Westley, 1979). Viewed in this way, sulfane reductase is seen to be a sulfurtransferase differing from rhodanese only in acceptor-substrate specificity. Like rhodanese, the reductase cleaves the S-S bond of thiosulfate; unlike rhodanese, the reductase will not accept cyanide but prefers as acceptor substrates such monothiols as cysteine and glutathione. In the presence of excess thiol, the persulfide product can react spontaneously to yield inorganic hydrosulfide and an organic disulfide, as shown in Fig. 19.

$$SSO_3^{2-} + GS^- \overset{E}{\rightleftharpoons} SO_3^{2-} + GSS^-$$

$$GSS^- + GS^- \rightleftharpoons GSSG + S^{2-}$$

$$SSO_3^{2-} + 2\,GS^- \overset{E}{\rightleftharpoons} SO_3^{2-} + GSSG + S^{2-}$$

Fig. 19 Reaction catalyzed by sulfane reductase.

A formal kinetic mechanism analogous to those given above for the other enzymes discussed here is shown in Fig. 20. Surprisingly (to us, anyhow), here again the reaction sequence is unlike that of the rhodanese mechanism. There is no sulfur-substituted enzyme but random addition of substrates to form a ternary complex from which the products are discharged (Uhteg and Westley, 1979). Whether there is an underlying commonality of mechanism at the chemical level, as there could easily be despite the formal mechanistic differences, is not yet known.

VI. CONCLUSION

Figure 21 summarizes what is known about the sulfane pool in terms of the enzyme-catalyzed reactions related to it;

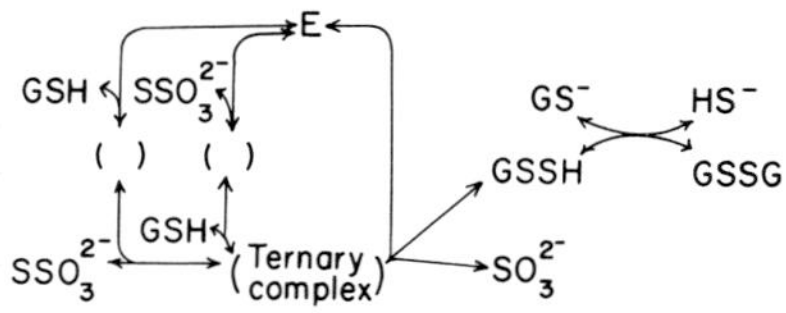

Fig. 20 Formal catalytic mechanism of sulfane reductase.

let us try to extract some central messages. Certainly for people interested in the biological *fate* of cyanide, there is significance in the near ubiquity of biological sulfane-containing materials and of the enzymes that catalyze their reactions. Similarly, for those with a primary focus on the biological *effects* of cyanide, the message must be that cyanide is very likely indeed to deplete the sulfane pool. The consequent impairment of all the normal functions of this pool (whatever these are ultimately shown to be) must surely be counted among the potential effects of cyanide *in vivo*.

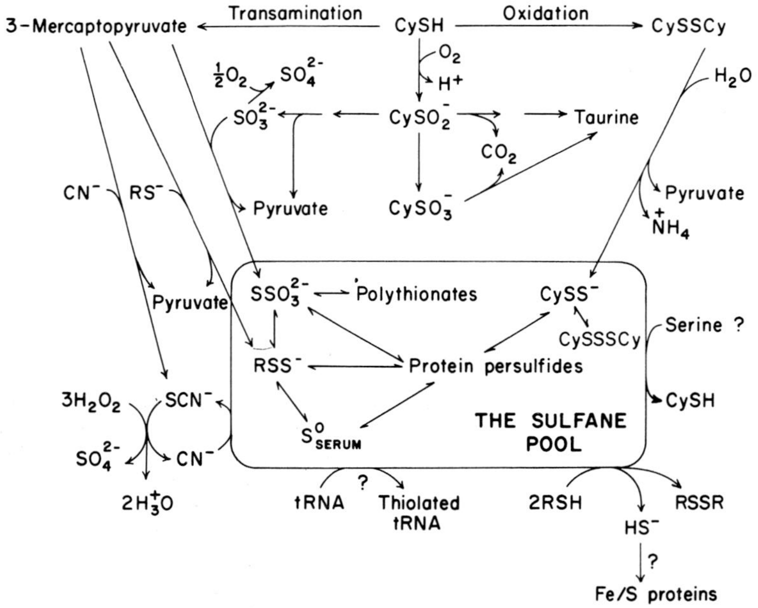

Fig. 21 Summary of all reactions known or thought to involve sulfane pool components.

ACKNOWLEDGEMENT

Current support of research in this laboratory on topics related to the subject matter of this review is from National Science Foundation Grant PCM 77-26861 and the United States Public Health Service Grant GM-18939.

REFERENCES

Abdolrasulina, R. and Wood, J.L. (1980). *Bioorganic Chemistry* 9, 253-260.

Cavallini, D., Mondovi, B., De Marco, C. and Scioscia-Santoro, A. (1962). *Enzymologia* 24, 253-266.

Chew, M.Y. and Boey, C.G. (1972). *Phytochemistry* 11, 167-169.

Crewe, R.M. and Ross, F.P. (1975). *Nature* 254, 448-449.

Dunathan, H.C. (1971). *Adv. Enzymol.* 35, 79-133.

Fanshier, D.W. and Kun, E. (1962). *Biochim. Biophys. Acta* 58, 266-278.

Flavin, M. (1962). *J. Biol. Chem.* 237, 768-777.

Flavin, M. and Segal, A. (1964). *J. Biol. Chem.* 239, 2220-2227.

Greenberg, D.M. (1975). *In* "Metabolic Pathways" (D.M. Greenberg, ed.) 3rd edn, Vol. 7, pp. 505-528. Academic Press, New York.

Haschke, R.H. and Campbell, L.L. (1971). *J. Bacteriol.* 106, 603-607.

Hatchikian, E.C. (1975). *Arch. Microbiol.* 105, 249-256.

Hylin, J.W. and Wood, J.L. (1959). *J. Biol. Chem.* 234, 2141-2144.

Jarabak, R. and Westley, J. (1978). *Arch. Biochem. Biophys.* 185, 458-465.

Jarabak, R. and Westley, J. (1980). *Biochemistry* 19, 900-904.

Kaji, A. and McElroy, W.D. (1959). *J. Bacteriol.* 77, 630-637.

Kamataki, T. and Neal, R.A. (1976). *Mol. Pharmacol.* 12, 933-944.

Koj, A. (1968). *Acta Biochim. Polon.* 15, 161-169.

Koj, A., Frendo, J. and Wojtczak, L. (1975). *FEBS Lett.* 57, 42-46.

Koj, A., Michalik, M. and Kasperczyk, H. (1977). *Bull. Acad. Polon. Sci., Ser. Sci. Biol.* 25, 1-6.

Matsuo, Y. and Greenberg, D.M. (1958). *J. Biol. Chem.* 230, 545-560.

Meister, A., Fraser, P.E. and Tice, S.V. (1954). *J. Biol. Chem.* 206, 561-575.

Nakatsukasa, W. and Akagi, J.M. (1969). *J. Bacteriol.* 98, 429-433.

Oi, S. (1973). *Agric. Biol. Chem.* 37, 629-635.

Oltmann, L.F. and Stouthamer, A.H. (1975). *Arch. Microbiol.* 105, 135-142.

Peck, H.D. and Fischer, E. (1962). *J. Biol. Chem.* 237, 190-197.

Ploegman, J.H., Drent, G., Kalk, K.H. and Hol, W.G.J. (1978). *J. Mol. Biol.* 123, 557-594.

Roy, A.B. and Trudinger, P.A. (1973). "The Biochemistry of Inorganic Compounds of Sulphur", pp. x-xiii. Cambridge University Press, London.

Russell, J., Weng, L., Keim, P.S. and Heinrikson, R.L. (1978). *J. Biol. Chem.* 253, 8102-8108.

Schiewelbein, H., Baumeister, R. and Vogel, R. (1969). *Naturwissenschaften* 56, 416-417.

Schlesinger, P. and Westley, J. (1974). *J. Biol. Chem.* 249, 780-788.

Schneider, J.F. and Westley, J. (1963). *J. Biol. Chem.* 238, PC 3516-3517.

Schneider, J.F. and Westley, J. (1969). *J. Biol. Chem.* 244, 5735-5744.

Seawright, A.A., Hrdlicka, J. and Matteis, F. (1976). *Br. J. Exp. Pathol.* 57, 16-22.

Sido, B. and Koj, A. (1972). *Acta Biol. Crac.* 15, 97-103.

Sörbo, B. (1957). *Biochim. Biophys. Acta* 24, 324-329.

Sörbo, B. (1964). *Acta Chem. Scand.* 18, 821-823.

Sörbo, B. (1975). *In* "Metabolic Pathways" (D.M. Greenberg, ed.) 3rd

edn., Vol. 7, pp. 433-456. Academic Press, New York.
Szczepkowski, T.W. and Wood, J.L. (1967). *Biochim. Biophys. Acta* 139, 469-478.
Uhteg, L.C. and Westley, J. (1979). *Arch. Biochem. Biophys.* 195, 211-222.
Vachek, H. and Wood, J.L. (1972). *Biochim. Biophys. Acta* 258, 133-146.
Van Den Hamer, C.J.A., Morell, A.G. and Scheinberg, I.H. (1967). *J. Biol. Chem.* 242, 2514-2516.
Vesey, C.J. and Wilson, J. (1978). *J. Pharm. Pharmacol.* 30, 20-26.
Villarejo, M. and Westley, J. (1963). *J. Biol. Chem.* 238, 4016-4020.
Westley, J. (1973). *Adv. Enzymol.* 39, 327-368.
Westley, J. (1977). *In* "Bioorganic Chemistry" (E.E. Van Tamelen, ed.) Vol. 1, pp. 371-390. Academic Press, New York.
Westley, J. (1980). *In* "Enzymatic Basis of Detoxication" (W.B. Jakoby, ed.) Vol. 2, pp. 245-262. Academic Press, New York.
Wood, J.L. (1975). *In* "Chemistry and Biochemistry of Thiocyanic Acid and Its Derivatives" (A.A. Newman, ed.) pp. 156-221. Academic Press, New York.
Yamamoto, T. and Oi, S. (1977). *J. Ferment. Tech.* 55, 560-569.

MULTIPLE FORMS AND MULTIPLE FUNCTIONS OF THE RHODANESES

MARGUERITE VOLINI and KEITH ALEXANDER

Department of Biochemistry and Biophysics, University of Hawaii, Honolulu, Hawaii 96822, USA

I. INTRODUCTION

When Lang first described rhodanese activity (Lang, 1933), he assumed that the enzyme functioned solely to detoxify cyanide. Since that time a number of other roles have been proposed (for example see Westley, 1973, 1977; Sörbo, 1975 and particularly Westley, this volume).

The classical definition of rhodanese activity is the protein-mediated catalysis of thiocyanate formation by sulfur transfer from thiosulfate to cyanide ions. In this paper we present experimental evidence for the occurrence in biological systems of several protein forms which by this definition are properly called rhodanese. We continue to use the trivial name rhodanese rather than that assigned by the Enzyme Commission (thiosulfate-cyanide sulfurtransferase, EC 2.8.1.1), since the enzyme catalyzes other reactions than the transfer of S to cyanide. For a discussion of the mechanism of rhodanese, see Westley, this volume.

II. CHARACTERIZATION OF RHODANESES

Rhodanese activity is widespread in the biosphere (Westley, 1973). Notably the enzyme activity from bovine liver has been studied by several groups of investigators resulting in an extensive literature (Westley, 1973, 1977; Sörbo, 1975). The studies described below, which originate in this laboratory, utilize two eukaryotic systems, bovine liver and heart tissue, and two prokaryotic systems, *Escherichia coli* and *Pseudomonas aeruginosa*.

A. THE TWO FORMS IN CRYSTALLINE PREPARATIONS

Kinetic, physical and chemical studies have been done on crystalline preparations of the bovine liver enzyme, including the amino acid sequence and X-ray crystallographic analyses of a single polypeptide chain of molecular weight 32,900 with one reaction center per molecule (Ploegman *et al.*, 1978). On the other hand, a large body of evidence has accumulated from solution studies that indicates the bovine liver enzyme is a dimer of $M_r \sim 37,000$ that is dissociable under certain conditions to similar, possibly identical subunits, with two catalytic sites per dimer. This evidence includes demonstrations of two active sites (Green and Westley, 1961; Westley and Nakamoto, 1962), two essential sulfhydryl groups (Wang and Volini, 1968), two independent binding sites for divalent metal ions (Volini *et al.*, 1967, 1978b; Bryant and Rajender, 1971), peptide maps (Volini *et al.*, 1967; Blumenthal and Heinrikson, 1971), fluorescence polarization studies (Horowitz and Westley, 1970), and gel filtration studies (Volini *et al.*, 1967).

Helping to reconcile these observations, sedimentation equilibrium studies carried out in this laboratory have demonstrated the presence of both rhodanese forms in crystalline preparations of full specific activity (equivalent to 720 units per mg where 1 unit is defined as the amount of enzyme that catalyzes the formation of 1 μmol of SCN^-/min at 25°C). Dissociation of rhodanese preparations to lower molecular-weight forms is readily detectable by the short column sedimentation method of Yphantis (1960), in which molecular weight is proportional to the midpoint height of the equilibrium schlieren pattern (Volini *et al.*, 1978a).

Properties of the rhodanese protein which complicate structural analyses are its tendency to autoxidize and its specialized interaction with thiols (Wang and Volini, 1968; Volini and Westley, 1966). Oxidation of protein sulfhydryls to form a disulfide bridge has been documented repeatedly (Wang and Volini, 1968; Baillie and Horowitz, 1976; Weng *et al.*, 1978; Ploegman *et al.*, 1978). These properties probably explain the fact that the low molecular-weight monomer, $M_r \sim 19,000$, is not usually resolved by SDS-mercaptoethanol incubation followed by SDS-gel electrophoresis. Further, the oxidized dimer and the nondissociable species are not readily distinguished on SDS gels since they have similar molecular weights ($\sim 37,000$ and $\sim 33,000$, respectively). However, they appear to be clearly observed on polyacrylamide gels in the absence of SDS, and depending on their relative proportions, in molecular exclusion chromatography (Volini *et al.*, 1967, 1978a).

B. THE MULTIPROTEIN COMPLEX

In recent investigations of rhodanese-associated synthesis of iron-sulfur centers, Volini *et al.* (1980a) have detected in liver mitochondrial extracts a high molecular-weight, multiprotein complex that exhibits rhodanese activity and forms iron-sulfur centres (Fig. 1, Fraction I). The complex

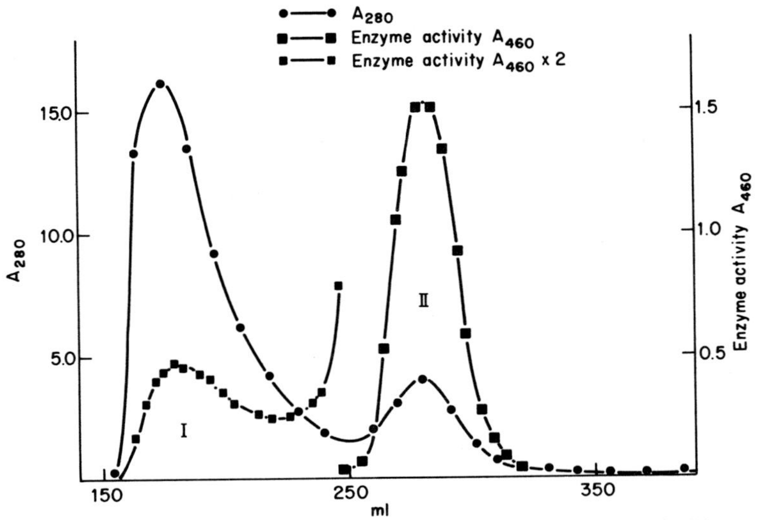

Fig. 1 Resolution of two rhodanese fractions from a partially purified liver mitochondrial extract on Sephadex G-100. For details see Volini *et al.* (1980a).

is characterized by a V_e/V_o value (i.e. ratio of elution volume to void volume) of 1.1 which by comparison with values for marker proteins implies a molecular weight near 90,000. Rechromatography confirms that rhodanese activity is an intrinsic property of the high molecular-weight form.

Apparently the complex can be reconstituted from subunit proteins of molecular weight 20,000-40,000. Concentration by ultrafiltration of the rhodanese and other proteins eluted in the low molecular-weight range (Fig. 1, Fraction II) gives rise to essentially pure complex of molecular weight ∿90,000. The rhodanese activity associated with the reconstituted preparation appears upon activation with mercaptoethanol.

Analysis of SDS-gel patterns suggests that the complex is composed of multiples of three polypeptide chains with approximate molecular weights of 19,000, 14,000 and 11,000. In addition, the complex is characterized by a visible absorption band with a maximum near 410 nm, which appears to arise from a pyridoxal-like moiety.*

A complex with properties identical to those described has also been partially purified from crude homogenates of heart tissue and whole bovine liver. The three low molecular-weight SDS-gel bands are also observed in these preparations. Bands common to all three preparations are also observed at higher molecular weights but these species appear to be different combinations of the three

---

* Data of Ogata, Blackburn, Hartman and Volini (Volini *et al.*, 1980b). A complete report of this work will appear elsewhere.

basic polypeptide chains.*

C. THE RHODANESES FROM *P. AERUGINOSA* AND *E. COLI*

Rhodanese activity is released from *P. aeruginosa* by a variety of methods including freeze-thaw, acetone extraction, sonication or, as recently reported by Ryan *et al.* (1979), cold shock treatment. We have used the former two methods primarily for release of both the *E. coli* and *P. aeruginosa* enzymes. The *E. coli* enzyme is readily accessible to the rhodanese substrates, thiosulfate and cyanide ions, in whole cell suspensions washed with dilute Tris buffers, pH 8.6, suggesting that the activity is localized in the periplasmic space as proposed for the enzyme from *P. aeruginosa* (Ryan *et al.*, 1979).

Two strains of *P. aeruginosa* have been used for most of this work. *P. aeruginosa* 9-D2 was obtained from P. Castric of Duquesne University. This strain produces cyanide during late log to stationary phase (Castric, 1977; Castric *et al.*, 1979; Kralik and Castric, 1979). *P. aeruginosa* 10145 was obtained from the American Type Culture Collection. This is the neotype strain of *P. aeruginosa* (Judicial Commission of the International Committee of Nomenclature of Bacteria, 1970). Reports of rhodanese in *E. coli* have varied but both Lang (1933) and Schievelbein (1969) have described strains with measurable activity. We have worked with two isolates from a culture of *E. coli* CSH61 (D7011). One of these isolates, CSH61-1, exhibits abundant rhodanese activity but the other, CSH61-3, displays only low levels of rhodanese activity under normal aerobic growth conditions (Table I).

Extracts from both strains of *P. aeruginosa* and from *E. coli* CSH61-1 have been chromatographed on Sephadex G-100 in order to obtain estimates of the molecular weights of their rhodanese proteins (Fig. 2). The strains of *P. aeruginosa* produce rhodanese proteins with V_e/V_0 values of 1.55 (9-D2) and 1.60 (ATCC). These values are close to the average values obtained for the crystalline bovine liver enzyme, 1.58, and also the major activity peak from crude liver and heart homogenates, 1.60. By comparison to values for marker proteins (Fig. 3), molecular weights for the *P. aeruginosa* enzymes of 33,000 (ATCC) and 30,000 (9-D2) are inferred. The *E. coli* rhodanese protein, on the other hand, exhibits the larger V_e/V_0 value of 2.05, implying a molecular weight of only 14,000. In fact the elution diagram of ribonuclease (M_r13,700) from the same column, when normalized, is virtually identical to that for the *E. coli* rhodanese protein. Chromatography of the *E. coli* enzyme was repeated several times on different

---

* Data of Ogata, Blackburn, Hartman and Volini (Volini *et al.*, 1980b). A complete report of this work will appear elsewhere.

Table I Rhodanese activity in *P. aeruginosa* and *E. coli*

Organism	Activity, (units/mg protein)[a] x 10 Nutrient broth[b]	Synthetic medium[b]
P. aeruginosa		
9-D2	3.3	4.8
	4.6	4.6
ATCC 10145	15.3	14.4
	14.3	
	13.8	
E. coli		
CSH61-1		
aerobic	28.5	
anaerobic	3.0	
CSH61-3		
aerobic	∿0.5[c]	

[a] One unit is defined as the amount of enzyme that catalyzes the formation of 1 μmol of SCN^-/min at 25°C. SCN^- formation was measured as described previously (Wang and Volini, 1968). Activity was released by freezing and thawing of washed cell suspensions. Supernatants obtained following centrifugation were chromatographed on Sephadex G-25 and void volume fractions were analyzed for protein by the method of Zamenhof (1955). Each value represents a different harvest (see Fig. 6).

[b] Incubations were at 37°C in a New Brunswick gyrotory shaker bath. The synthetic medium for *P. aeruginosa* was that described by Castric (1977). For anaerobic growth of *E. coli*, 0.2% glucose was added to nutrient broth.

[c] Protein was estimated by comparison of absorbance values and harvest weights with those for *E. coli* CSH61-1.

extracts from three cell growths. Full activity was recovered for the chromatogram in Fig. 2.

In contrast to the monomer of M_r∿19,000 from bovine liver preparations, the low molecular-weight form of rhodanese from *E. coli* appears to be stable in nonassociated form. Two low molecular-weight forms of rhodanese, M_r ∿ 17,500 and ∿12,600, have also been reported in rat liver (Oi, 1975) and there has been a report of low molecular-weight rhodanese forms from *Thiobacillus* (Bowen *et al.*, 1965). *P. aeruginosa* and *E. coli* were selected for study here rather than organisms that oxidize sulfur for energy since it is expected that their sulfur metabolism more closely resembles that in mammalian systems.

III. RHODANESE, METAL IONS AND SEWAGE TREATMENT

Early studies clearly showed that crystalline bovine liver

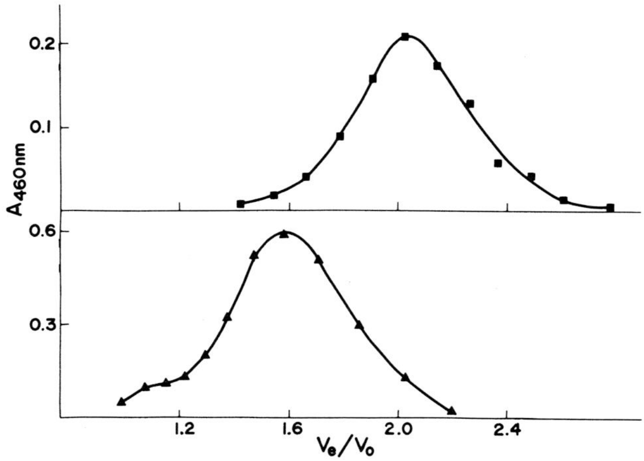

Fig. 2 Molecular exclusion chromatography of extracts from *P. aeruginosa* ATCC 10145 and *E. coli* CSH61-1 on Sephadex G-100. Upper diagram: an acetone powder of *E. coli* CSH61-1 was extracted with 10 mM potassium phosphate buffer, pH 7.0 containing 1mM thiosulfate and 0.5 ml was added to a column, 48.5 cm x 0.7 cm, preequilibrated with Tris acetate buffer, 0.05 I, pH 8.6 containing 50 mM thiosulfate. In other similar experiments the column was preequilibrated with the extraction buffer. Fractions, ∿0.8 ml, were collected in tared plastic vials and volumes were calculated using a specific gravity of 1.0. For activity measurements 0.2 ml aliquots were incubated in the standard assay system for 2 min. Recovery of activity was 100%.
Lower diagram: a 65% ammonium sulfate precipitate of *P. aeruginosa* combined extracts obtained by sonication and by freezing and thawing of washed cells was dissolved in potassium phosphate buffer, 0.01 M, pH 7.0. A 0.26 ml volume was added to a column, 47.9 cm x 0.7 cm, preequilibrated with the same buffer. For activity measurements, 0.1 ml aliquots were incubated for 10 min in the standard assay system. Recovery of activity was 87%. Other conditions were the same as for the *E. coli* enzyme.

rhodanese was not a metalloprotein, but that it contained two binding sites for divalent metal ions per 37,000 molecular weight (Sörbo, 1962; Volini *et al.*, 1967; Bryant and Rajender, 1971). Because solutions of the common substrates always contain some divalent metal ions, the question of whether the enzyme is metal-activated was at first left open.

Later studies combined equilibrium binding measurements with comprehensive analyses of the rate effects of both transition and alkaline earth metal ions, and showed that the dissociable form of bovine liver rhodanese is activated by various metals. Under the usual assay conditions

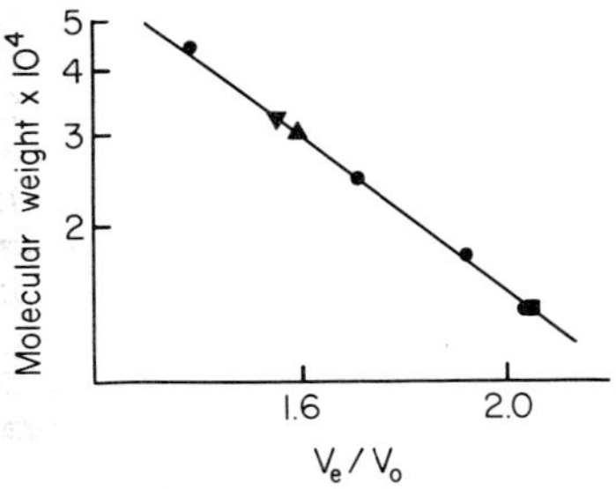

Fig. 3 The relationship between molecular weight and V_e/V_o for the bacterial rhodaneses. V_e is the elution volume of maximum activity for rhodanese or maximum absorbance at 280 nm for the marker proteins. V_o is the void volume of the column as determined by blue dextran. V_o values were 6.55 ml and 6.65 ml for the columns described in Fig. 3. ▼ *P. aeruginosa* 9-D2; ▲ *P. aeruginosa* ATCC 10145; and ■ *E. coli* CSH61-1. The marker proteins, ● , were ovalbumin (43,500), chymotrypsinogen (24,700), myoglobin (17,500) and ribonuclease (13,700).

the activator is a calcium ion (Volini *et al.*, 1978b).

The results with zinc, copper, nickel and iron were complicated by the fact that all of these metals form complexes with cyanide, one of the enzyme substrates of the assay system. Addition of any of these metals usually caused inhibition of the activity as measured by thiocyanate formation, but the degree of inhibition was dependent on the cyanide concentration. The net charge on the complex varies with the number of CN^- ions bound. Species with negative net charge, e.g. $[Zn^{2+}(CN^-)_4]^{-2}$, $[Cu^+(CN^-)_3]^{-2}$ and $[Ni^{2+}(CN^-)_4]^{-2}$, are inhibitors competitive with the substrate, thiosulfate ion. The copper cyanide complex with no net charge combines with the enzyme to form a functionally active complex. The zinc cyanide complex with net positive charge and the anomalous ferrocyanide anion exhibit inhibition competitive with the substrate cyanide ion (Volini *et al.*, 1977, 1978b).

Table II Rhodanese inhibition by metallocyanide anions[a]

Anion	K_I, M^{-1}	Enzyme complex	Rate effect
$Cu(CN)_3^{2-}$	∿500	$E{\cdot}Cu(CN)_3^{2-}$	Competitive with SSO_3^{2-}
$Zn(CN)_4^{2-}$	700	$E{\cdot}Zn(CN)_4^{2-}$	Competitive with SSO_3^{2-}
$Ni(CN)_4^{2-}$	19,000	$E{\cdot}Ni(CN)_4^{2-}$	Competitive with SSO_3^{2-}
$Fe(CN)_6^{4-}$	27,000	$ES{\cdot}Fe(CN)_6^{4-}$	Competitive with CN^-

[a] Data from Volini *et al.* (1977, 1978b).

Values of the inhibitor constants, K_I, for the bovine

enzyme interaction with metallocyanide anions are listed in Table II. Such studies have recently been extended to the *E. coli* rhodanese.*

Even when washed whole cell suspensions of *E. coli* were used as the enzyme, the results were very similar to those obtained with the purified enzyme from bovine liver. This is illustrated in Fig. 4 which compares some of the results obtained by adding zinc ion to the two different enzyme systems. At high levels of cyanide where the anionic zinc cyanide species is virtually the only metal species present, inhibition competitive with thiosulfate is observed, indicating that the enzyme-metal complex, $E{\cdot}Zn(CN)_4^{-2}$, is formed. At the lower cyanide concentrations, however, inhibition uncompetitive with thiosulfate is observed. This inhibition arises in part from uptake of cyanide ion to form a zero-valence metal-cyanide species and in part from formation of a nonproductive enzyme complex with net positive charge involving the enzyme-sulfur intermediate, $ES{\cdot}Zn^{2+}$. At the high level of cyanide, the value of the inhibitor constant, K_I, for the $E{\cdot}Zn(CN)_4^{2-}$ complex is 600 M^{-1} for *E. coli* rhodanese and 700 M^{-1} for the bovine enzyme. Data for copper ion with *E. coli* rhodanese (not shown) also exhibit the more complicated behaviour observed for this metal ion with the bovine enzyme. This inhibition effect on rhodanese of metal ion-cyanide complexes may be related to some results obtained by Pettet and Mills (1954) in a study of the inhibition of biological disposal systems which detoxify cyanide in synthetic electroplating wastes containing the same metallocyanide anions. In these experiments percolating filters were fed sewage to which cyanide and metal ion were added. The metal ions inhibited cyanide removal in proportion to the increasing order of the stability constants for the metallocyanide complexes. At 150 p.p.m. HCN, the order of inhibition was Cu < Zn < Ni << Fe, which is qualitatively the same as the increasing order of the inhibition constants (K_I) listed in Table II.

IV. RHODANESE-ASSOCIATED SYNTHESIS OF IRON-SULFUR CENTERS

A number of investigators have shown that apoproteins prepared from ferredoxin or adrenodoxin can be reconstituted by incubation with either rhodanese or 3-mercaptopyruvate sulfurtransferase in the presence of their respective substrates, iron ions and a reducing agent (for example, Finazzi-Agro *et al.*, 1971; Taniguchi and Kimura, 1974). If sulfide ions replace either sulfurtransferase and its substrate in the incubation mixtures, reconstitution is also observed, as judged from increasing

---

* Unpublished observations of K. Alexander and M. Volini. A complete report of the work will appear elsewhere.

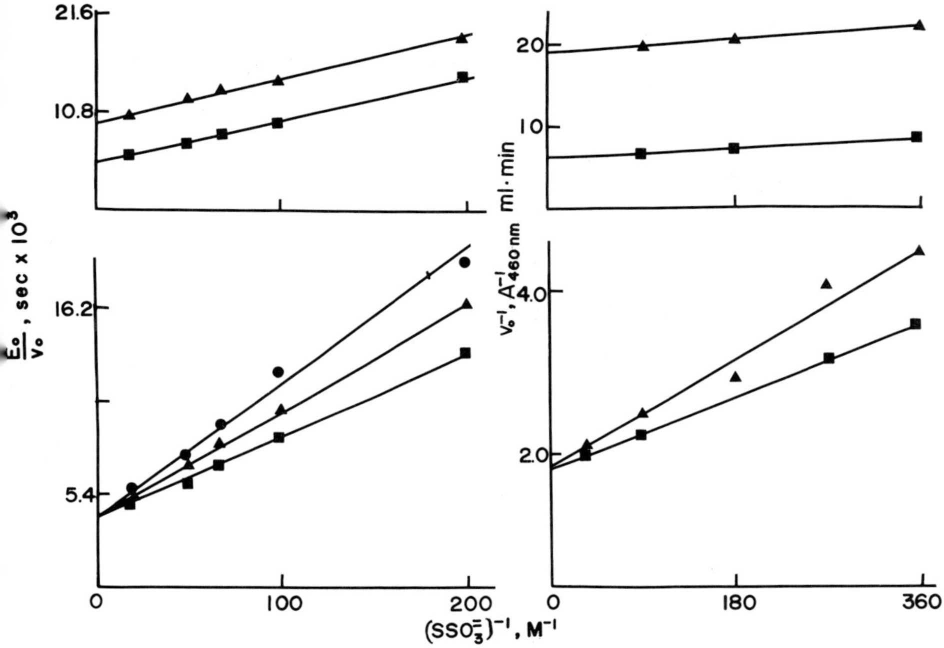

Fig. 4 Inhibition of eukaryotic and prokaryotic rhodaneses by zinc ion at different concentrations of the cyanide substrate. The double reciprocal plots at *left* represent rate data obtained in the presence of the bovine liver enzyme. The lower and upper plots were obtained at 20 mM CN_t and 1.25 mM CN_t, respectively: ■——■, control; ▲——▲, 0.5 mM Zn_t; ●——●, 1.0 mM Zn_t. CN_t and Zn_t are the total concentrations of cyanide and zinc ion respectively. Initial rates denoted as v_o, were measured in the absence of product; E_o is the total enzyme concentration. From Volini *et al.* (1978b). The double reciprocal plots at *right* represent rate data obtained with the enzyme from *E. coli* CSH61-1. Cells were washed once with Tris acetate buffer, 0.025 I, pH 8.6, and resuspended at a concentration of 0.26 g/ml in the same buffer. Aliquots of either 0.1 ml or 0.2 ml were used directly for rate measurements. The lower and upper plots were obtained at 28 mM CN_t and 1.4 mM CN_t, respectively: ■——■, control; ▲——▲, 0.56 mM Zn_t. Other conditions were the same as for the bovine enzyme.

absorbance near 420 nm. The apparent lack of specificity for the reaction raises the question of whether the sulfurtransferases serve in a direct donor capacity in these model systems or only to supply the necessary sulfide ions.

In liver cells rhodanese activity is localized in the mitochondria. Our investigations involve measurements of the iron- and sulfur-binding efficiencies of the two fractions exhibiting endogenous rhodanese activity that can be resolved from liver mitochondrial extracts (see Fig. 1 above). Time course data are presented in Fig. 5 for the uptake of iron and "labile" sulfur by the fraction containing the multiprotein complex (Fig. 1, Fraction I).

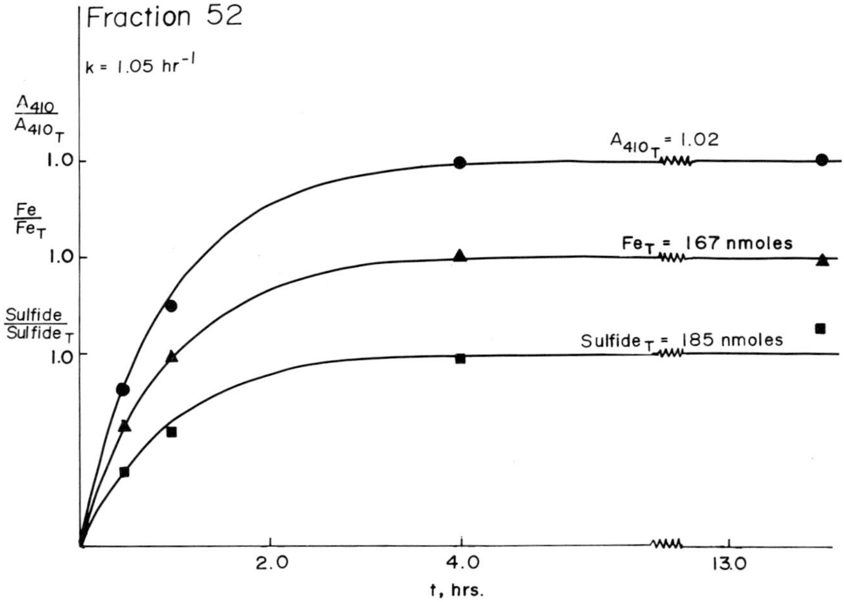

Fig. 5 The time course of iron binding, labile sulfur binding and increasing absorbance at 410 nm for a subfraction of the multiprotein complex resolved on Sephadex G-100 (Fig. 2, Fraction I). The midpoint elution volume of subfraction 52 from the G-100 column was 193 ml. Aliquots were incubated with 28 mM thiosulfate ion, 0.46 mM iron ions, and 0.18 M mercaptoethanol and chromatographed on Sephadex G-25 at the incubation times specified by the experimental points. The experimental values are superposed on theoretical first order curves (see text). From Volini *et al.* (1980a).

Aliquots of the fraction were incubated with iron ions, mercaptoethanol, and the rhodanese substrate, thiosulfate at 7°C. At the incubation times specified by the experimental points in Fig. 5, individual aliquots were chromatographed on Sephadex G-25 to stop the reaction and to remove excess iron ions, mercaptoethanol and thiosulfate. Both visible and ultraviolet absorption spectra of the resulting protein fractions were recorded. Their iron content was measured by atomic absorption spectrophotometry and their "labile" sulfur content was determined by a modification of the procedure of Chen and Mortenson (1977). Since known sample volumes were added to the G-25 column and recoveries were quantitated, the time course data shown in Fig. 5 could be calculated.

In the figure the experimental values are superimposed on a theoretical curve generated for a rate constant of 1.05 h^{-1}. The limiting values estimated at infinite time for the increase in absorbance at 410 nm, the iron content and the labile sulfur content are shown above their respective curves. It is of interest that the same rate constant is obtained for all three parameters, the concentration ratio of bound iron to bound sulfur is close to 1.0 and the extinction coefficient at 410 nm is close to 6000 $M^{-1}cm^{-1}$ per mole of bound iron. Together these results indicate that nonheme iron-sulfur centers are formed.

By the same criteria, the lower molecular-weight fraction containing the major part of the rhodanese activity (Fig. 1, Fraction II) also forms iron-sulfur centers, as does the multiprotein complex reconstituted from proteins in the lower molecular-weight fraction.

The conditions used for partial purification of rhodanese in the mitochondrial extract prior to molecular exclusion chromatography are those expected to release iron-sulfur centers from proteins (precipitation by high salt concentrations at acidic pH). Examination of supernatants from this purification step by atomic absorption spectrophotometry shows that they contain large amounts of iron. This finding could explain the fact that mainly apoprotein is present in the rhodanese-containing precipitate. Similar purification steps are used in the isolation of the crystalline enzyme from whole liver extracts. Successful crystallization of the enzyme in the latter preparations appears to be related to their content of nonheme iron protein (Volini *et al.*, 1977).

Succinic dehydrogenase is normally membrane-bound, but it can be released from the membrane by a variety of procedures, including treatment with cyanide. Bonomi *et al.* (1977) have reported that the reconstitutive capacity - by this is meant the capacity of the solubilized enzyme to recombine with the membrane - could be restored by direct sulfur transfer from rhodanese. They also found that the interaction of rhodanese with succinate dehydrogenase greatly reduces the catalytic activity of the sulfurtransferase with respect to thiocyanate formation. In our system, a similar interaction with an iron-binding protein in the high molecular-weight complex could account for the small amount of thiocyanate-forming activity observed. This activity corresponds to ∿2% of the total activity in semipurified mitochondrial extracts but it accounts for as much as 10% of the total in crude liver homogenates that have not been subjected to the partial purification procedure mentioned above*.

V. GROWTH AND RHODANESE ACTIVITY IN *P. AERUGINOSA* AND *E. COLI*

The cyanogenic capacity of *P. aeruginosa* 9-D2 increases to a maximum during the transition from exponential growth to stationary phase (Castric *et al.*, 1979). During the transition period, the rhodanese activity of this strain is some three-fold lower than that of *P. aeruginosa* ATCC 1014[illegible] (Table I). The latter organism gives a negative picrate paper test for cyanide production. Thus rhodanese activity seems unrelated to cyanide production.

Representative growth curves for both organisms are shown in Fig. 6 with harvest times indicated at which cells were analyzed for enzyme activity. The rhodanese content of the 9-D2 strain relative to that for the ATCC culture is significantly lower at all harvest times regardless of whether the cells are grown in nutrient broth or in synthetic medium (Table I). It may be that cyanogenesis also occurs in the ATCC culture, but is not measurable because of further metabolism in which rhodanese plays a role. The enzyme may function similarly in the 9-D2 strain but to a lesser degree in accordance with the reduced activity. In stationary phase where the cyanogenic capacity of the 9-D2 culture decreases (Castric *et al.*, 1979), the ratio of the enzyme activity to total protein is stable in both strains, suggesting that cyanide detoxication is not the only function of rhodanese in these organisms.

Both *Pseudomonas* cultures exhibit only limited accessibility of rhodanese to the substrates in washed whole cell suspensions. Under these conditions, virtually all of the enzyme activity can be measured in *E. coli* CSH61-1. The relative values observed prior to and after cell disruption for the aerobic harvest of CSH61-1 listed in Table I were 2.95 units/mg and 2.85 units/mg respectively. For this reason, this organism was selected as the model system for study with the metal-cyanide complexes.

Growth curves for *E. coli* CSH61-1 under aerobic and anaerobic conditions are presented in Fig. 6. Analyses of cells harvested at the times indicated in the figure showed that the rhodanese activity is decreased by an order of magnitude under anaerobic conditions (Table I)†. This observation indicates that rhodanese is in part involved in aerobic energy metabolism in this organism. It is in accordance with the behavior expected if, as proposed for

---

* Data of Ogata, Blackburn, Hartman and Volini (Volini *et al.*, 1980b) A complete report of this work will appear elsewhere.

† Unpublished observations of K. Alexander and M. Volini. A complete report of the work will appear elsewhere.

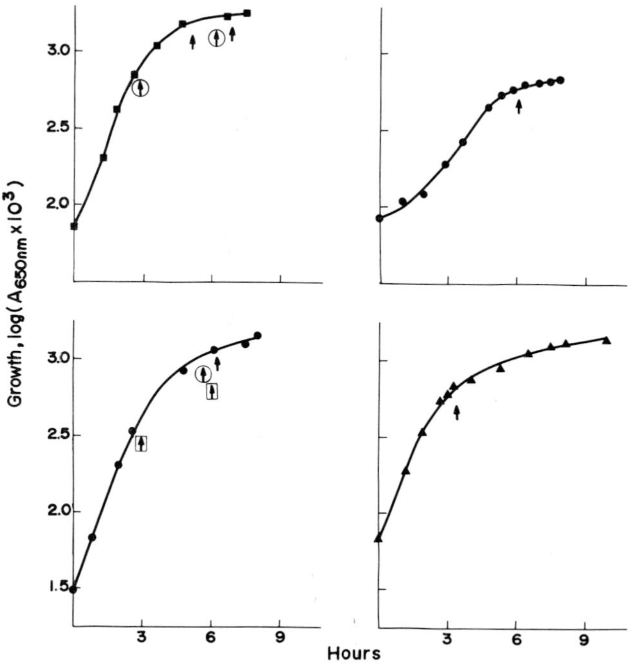

Fig. 6 Growth curves for *P. aeruginosa* and *E. coli* in nutrient broth showing harvest points for rhodanese analysis. The two curves at *left* were obtained with *P. aeruginosa* ATCC 10145 (lower, ●—●) and 9-D2 (upper, ■——■); those at *right* were obtained with *E. coli* CSH61-1 under aerobic (lower, ▲——▲) and anaerobic (upper, ●——●) conditions. The arrows, ↑, indicate when harvests were taken for growth in nutrient broth represented by the curves shown. The circled and boxed arrows, (↑) and [↑] , represent harvest times for other experiments in the synthetic medium or nutrient broth, respectively. In the latter experiments the growth curves were displaced somewhat from those shown by lag phases but limiting absorbances were nearly the same.

mammalian systems, the enzyme participates in the biosynthesis of iron-sulfur proteins, some of which are important for aerobic respiration. In this view, the sixty-fold lower value of enzyme activity observed with the SHC61-3 isolate may reflect decreased dissociation of a multiprotein complex similar to that observed in liver and heart tissue rather than a low rhodanese content *per se*.

The CSH61-1 strain, despite its high rhodanese activity in late exponential phase, shows the cyanide sensitivity typical of most *E. coli* strains. Preliminary experiments indicate, however, that the rhodanese activity as measured by thiocyanate formation is also low in early exponential phase (0.34 units/mg) and thus only marginally available for cyanide metabolism. Furthermore, though growth of *E. coli* CSH61-1 is inhibited by cyanide, the sensitivity to cyanide is a matter of degree rather than absolute. This organism, like other *E. coli* strains, can accommodate low levels of cyanide up to about 150 μM. This accommodation may be a direct consequence of the limited amount of rhodanese available for thiocyanate formation in the early growth phase.

In considering these results together with those described in the previous two sections, it seems probable that the traditional role proposed for rhodanese as sulfur donor to cyanide is complementary to its role as sulfur donor to other proteins. According to this view, cyanide detoxication is an accessory function occurring only to a minor extent when the enzyme is associated into complexes for iron-sulfur center synthesis.

ACKNOWLEDGEMENT

This research was in part supported by Grants BMS75-23299 and PCM79-07563 from the National Science Foundation.

REFERENCES

Baillie, R.D. and Horowitz, P.M. (1976). *Biochim. Biophys. Acta* 429, 383-388.

Blumenthal, K. and Heinrikson, R.L. (1971). *J. Biol. Chem.* 246, 2430-2437.

Bonomi, F., Pagani, S., Cerletti, P. and Cannella, C. (1977). *Eur. J. Biochem.* 72, 17-24.

Bowen, T.J., Butler, P.J. and Happold, F.C. (1965). *Biochem. J.* 97, 651-657.

Bryant, R.G. and Rajender, S. (1971). *Biochem. Biophys. Res. Commun.* 45, 532-536.

Castric, P.A. (1977). *J. Bacteriol.* 130, 826-831.

Castric, P.A., Ebert, R.F. and Castric, K.F. (1979). *Current Microbiology* 2. 287-292.

Chen, J.-S. and Mortensen, L.E. (1977). *Anal. Biochem.* 79, 157-165.

Finazzi-Agro, A., Cannella, C., Graziani, M.T. and Cavallini, D. (1971). *FEBS Letters* 16, 172-174.

Green, J.R. and Westley, J. (1961). *J. Biol. Chem.* 236, 3047-3050.

Horowitz, P. and Westley, J. (1970). *J. Biol. Chem.* 245, 986-990.

Judicial Commission of the International Committee on Nomenclature of Bacteria (1970). *International Journal of Systematic Bacteriology* 20, 15-16.

Kralik, C.A. and Castric, P.A. (1979). *Current Microbiology* 3, 71-74.

Lang, K. (1933). *Biochem. Z.* 259, 243-256.

Oi, S. (1975). *Biochem.* (Tokyo) 78, 825-834.

Pettet, A.E.J. and Mills, E.V. (1954). *J. Appl. Chem.* 4, 434-444.

Ploegman, J.H., Drent, G., Kalk, K.H., Hol, W.G.J., Heinrikson, R.L.,

Keim, P., Weng, L. and Russell, J. (1978). *Nature* 273, 124-129.
Ryan, R.W., Gourlie, M.P. and Tilton, R.C. (1979). *Can. J. Microbiol.* 25, 340-351.
Schievelbein, H., Baumeister, R. and Vogel, R. (1969). *Naturwissenschaften* 56, 416-417.
Sörbo, B. (1962). Proc. 1st Int. Pharmacol. Meet. 1961, Vol. 6, pp. 121-128.
Sörbo, B. (1975). *In* "Metabolic Pathways" (D.M. Greenberg, ed.) Vol. 7, pp. 433-456. Academic Press, New York.
Taniguchi, T. and Kimura, T. (1974). *Biochim. Biophys. Acta* 364, 284-295.
Volini, M. and Westley, J. (1966). *J. Biol. Chem.* 241, 5168-5176.
Volini, M., DeToma, F. and Westley, J. (1967). *J. Biol. Chem.* 242, 5220-5225.
Volini, M., Craven, D. and Ogata, K. (1977). *Biochem. Biophys. Res. Commun.* 79, 890-896.
Volini, M., Craven, D. and Ogata, K. (1978a). *J. Biol. Chem.* 253, 7591-7594.
Volini, M., van Sweringen, B. and Chen, F.-S. (1978b). *Arch. Biochem. Biophys.* 191, 205-215.
Volini, M., Ogata, K. and Craven, D. (1981a). *In* "Frontiers in Protein Chemistry" (D. Liu and K.T. Yasunobu, eds). Elsevier Publishing, New York (in press).
Volini, M., Blackburn, D., Ogata, K. and Hartman, R. (1980b). *Fed. Proc.* 39, 1628, abs.
Wang, S.-F. and Volini, M. (1968). *J. Biol. Chem.* 243, 5465-5470.
Weng, L., Heinrikson, R.L. and Westley, J. (1978). *J. Biol. Chem.* 253, 8109-8119.
Westley, J. and Nakamoto, T. (1962). *J. Biol. Chem.* 237, 547-549.
Westley, J. (1973). *Adv. Enzymol.* 39, 327-368.
Westley, J. (1977). *In* "Bioorganic Chemistry" (E.E. van Tamelen, ed.) Vol. 1, pp. 371-390. Academic Press, New York.
Yphantis, D.A. (1960). *Ann. N.Y. Acad. Sci.* 88, 586-601.
Zamenhof, S. (1955). *In* "Methods in Enzymology" (S.P. Colowick and N.O. Kaplan, eds) Vol. 3, p. 702. Academic Press, New York.

CASSAVA: A MAJOR CYANIDE-CONTAINING FOOD CROP

R.D. COOKE and D.G. COURSEY

Tropical Products Institute, 56/62 Gray's Inn Road, London WC1X 8LU, UK

I. INTRODUCTION

Cassava is one of the very few, and by far the most important, of the human food crops in which the content of cyanide creates nutritional problems. Since the crop is little known outside the tropics, and the only comprehensive treatment (Montaldo, 1979) is in Spanish, this chapter begins with a general description of the botany of the plant and its economic uses, as a background to the problem of its content of cyanogenic compounds.

A. NOMENCLATURE AND TAXONOMY

The cassava plant is correctly *Manihot esculenta* Crantz, but there has been much confusion over its nomenclature, partly on account of the great variability of the cultivated plant. It is often incorrectly referred to, especially in the older agricultural literature, as *Manihot utilissima* Pohl. The position is further confused by the incorrect use of taxa such as *M.aipi* Pohl, *M. palmata* (Pohl) Muell-Arg. and *M.dulcis* (J.F. Gmelin) Pax. to separate the so-called "sweet" and "bitter" forms which are considered later. The complex synonymy of the species has been discussed in some detail by Rogers and Appan (1973).

The genus *Manihot* lies within the family Euphorbiaceae and contains some 100 species, widely distributed throughout the New World tropics, but confined to the American continent. *M.esculenta* is, however, a cultigen, unknown in the wild except as an escape from cultivation, and its taxonomic position is somewhat obscure. The closest wild relatives, which have a generally similar erect habit of growth, and swollen roots, appear to be *M. aesculifolia* Pohl, *M.pringlei* Watson and *M.rubricaulis* Johnston, which are native to Mexico.

It is now generally accepted that these and probably

several other species have contributed to the genetic ancestry of *M.esculenta* (Rogers and Appan, 1973; Rogers and Fleming, 1973; Jennings, 1976). The variability of cultivars has probably also been enhanced by chance hybridization with several other wild species. Under early domestication, there was a selection for large roots; for enhanced ability to grow from stem cuttings; and possibly for a more erect and less branched habit of growth. The second of these factors would have favoured forms with swollen, prominent leaf scars providing additional food reserves, which feature is now a taxonomic criterion of *M.esculenta*, while the last would have favoured forms which produce fewer flowers, as branching occurs when inflorescences are formed, and thus partial sterility. Since the initiation of controlled breeding programmes, genetic material from *M.glaziovii* Muell-Arg. and *M.dichotoma* Ute has been introduced.

Many common names are in use in various parts of the world; the most commonly used English name is cassava, the similar cassave is used in Dutch. Manioc is also commonly used in English and in French, Maniok in German. It appears to be derived from the Brazilian Portugese mandioca, which is the name commonly used in Brazil and southern South America, although macaxeira and aipim (the latter for "sweet" cultivars only) are also used there. The plant and its products are usually called tapioca in Anglophone Asia, although in conventional English it is restricted to the grocery starch product. The usual name in Spanish-speaking Latin America is yuca, although guacamote (Mexico), caxcamote (Central America) and manoco (Puerto Rico) are also used (Montaldo, 1972).

B. ORIGINS AND DISPERSAL

M.esculenta is native to tropical America, and it was there that it emerged as an artefact of human cultivation. It was widespread in cultivation through most of South and Central America and the Caribbean at the time of the earliest European contacts in 1492 and relatively sophisticated methods for processing cassava roots into stable dried food products had been developed by many tropical American ethnic groups, for which there is ample historical evidence (Sturtevant, 1969; Dole, 1956; Renvoise, 1972) before that time.

There are archaelogical traces of cassava utilization in both Mexico and MesoAmerica (Rogers, 1963) dating back approximately 4,000 years, while linguistic evidence suggests that Mayan names for cassava are of similar antiquity (Renvoise, 1972). There is also evidence that cassava flour was a major item in long-distance trade in what are now Venezuela and Colombia, as early as 4,000 or 5,000 years ago (Lathrap, 1973).

It is impossible to say where within the crop's current

range from southern Mexico to northern Argentina it was first domesticated (Rogers, 1973; Renvoise, 1972). Separate origins for "sweet" and "bitter" strains have been suggested, as there appear to be differences in distribution between these groups, the former more widely distributed, but the latter more intensively grown in particular areas. In view of the probability that several *Manihot* species contributed to the ancestry of *M.esculenta*, the domestication of cassava should perhaps be regarded as a continuing evolutionary process, that took place in many small stages at many different locations - a pattern now regarded as fairly general for vegetatively propagated crop plants (Coursey, 1976).

The value of cassava as food was recognised by the earliest European visitors to America (Sturtevant, 1969) who transported it first to the area around the mouth of the Congo, and shortly after to other parts of West and South-West Africa, during the sixteenth century. It spread rapidly in cultivation across Angola and Southern Zaire, but in West Africa only more slowly, mainly after the introduction of Brazilian processing techniques in the mid-nineteenth century (Jones, 1959). Cassava was introduced to East Africa, the Indian Ocean islands, Southern India and the Far East during the later 1700s (Purseglove, 1968), but in most of the Old World it remained a rather secondary food crop until the beginning of the present century.

C. BOTANY AND PHYSIOLOGY

1. *The Cassava Plant*

The cassava plant is extremely variable in form and many thousands of cultivars are known, only a relatively small proportion of which have ever been properly classified (Rogers and Fleming, 1973). It is a short lived shrub, attaining anything from 1-5 metres in height. The leaves are petiolate with a palmate lamina usually of five to seven lobes, and are borne mainly towards the end of the stems; when they fall they leave very prominent scars. The small, usually not very conspicuous, white or cream flowers are normally borne in the same inflorescences, which are axilliary racemes near the ends of the branches. The female flowers are followed by dehiscent three-seeded capsules, though the rate of fertility is rather low. In cultivation, however, cassava is nearly always propagated by hardwood stem cuttings. Although seedlings initially form a tap root, the root system of plants grown from cuttings is basically fibrous but a proportion of the roots develop by a process of secondary thickening into root tubers, which are the main economic portion of the plant. The number, shape, size and angle of distribution of the root tubers, their colour and internal structure vary greatly between cultivars, though typically there are between five and ten tubers per plant of a cylindrical or tapering form, between 150-1000 mm long, 30-150 mm in diameter and occasionally bifurcated. The root tubers consist of an outer skin or periderm which may be rough or smooth and of colours ranging from light cream through pink or red to dark brown; a thin rind or cortex, usually white but occasionally tinged with pink or brown; and the main bulk consisting of a core or pith of parenchyma rich in starch but with bundles of xylem vessels and latex tubes running through the centre (Purseglove, 1968). The growth physiology of the cassava plant has recently been discussed in some detail by Hunt *et al.* (1977).

2. *The Function of the Roots*

The physiological function of the root tuber in cassava is somewhat obscure. Swollen roots occur in several *Manihot* species, especially those native to regions of seasonal drought (Rogers and Appan, 1973), and presumably function as reserves for the plant against periods of water stress. Other root and tuber crop plants, whether tropical or temperate, exhibit well-marked periods of dormancy in the dry or the cold season respectively, during which the epigeous parts of the plant die away completely, leaving the tuber as the entire surviving part of the plant, to resume active growth only after breakage of dormancy when climatic conditions are favourable. Cassava does not exhibit such dormancy: although under extreme water stress cassava plants can become defoliated, there is never total senescence leading to survival of the plant as isolated, dormant tubers. The tubers of cassava further do not constitute effective propagules, and do not bear bud primordia: they have been contrasted with those of other economic tuber crops as being organs of perennation rather than of propagation (Passam and Noon, 1977).

The domestication of cassava having progressively selected for large tubers, it could be argued that cassava root tubers have now become too large to have any significant biological function in the plant, and indeed should be regarded as abnormal or teratological forms. This, together with the lack of true dormancy, may account for the extreme perishability of cassava roots, which is much greater than that of other root and tuber crops (Coursey and Booth, 1977).

The roots cannot normally be kept in the fresh state for more than a few days. The nature of the post harvest deterioration processes is still poorly understood; the initial phase of discolouration, commencing from the vascular bundles appears to be physiological, but is rapidly followed by invasion by a wide range of micro-organisms (Booth, 1976; Noon and Booth, 1977). This has been a major constraint on the development of the crop and also has led to the custom of leaving the standing crop in the ground until required, a practice which is believed to tie up around three-quarters of a million hectares of agricultural land across the tropics, much of which could be used for alternative crop production. The quality and starch content of the root tubers also decline when left in the ground beyond the optimum harvest time (Ingram and Humphries, 1972).

D. ECOLOGICAL REQUIREMENTS AND CULTIVATION

Cassava is a most adaptable crop which is grown to some extent almost everywhere between 30°N and 30°S, at altitudes up to about 2000 m. Rainfall is adequate at above 500 or 600 mm per year, and temperatures above about 20°C, are required for active growth periods. It is tolerant of periods of drought and of extremely poor or exhausted soils (Cock and Howeler, 1978), but benefits from good soil, deep cultivation and manuring. Under favourable conditions, it is one of the biologically most efficient producers of edible carbohydrate. The combination of high productivity and tolerance of poor soils has led to cassava being criticized as being a soil-depleting crop.

Cassava can be grown as a monoculture in pure stands, but when grown by subsistence farmers it is often interplanted with annual food crops. The removal of weed competition in the early stages is especially beneficial, although many cultivars later form a sufficiently closed canopy to suppress weed growth. Cassava is tolerant of a wide range of soil pH, between the extremes of about 3.5 to 9.0, although mildly acid soils of pH 5.0 to 6.0 are optimal, but is highly sensitive to salinity or to waterlogging. Propagation under farming conditions is invariably by hard-wood cuttings normally 200 to 300 mm long and preferably taken from the middle part of the stems. There is much variation between cultivars in time to maturity. Most tend to fall into one of two main categories:

(1) short-season cultivars (often of low cyanide content) which may be mature enough to harvest in 6 to 9 months from planting, and whose root tubers frequently deteriorate if left in the ground for prolonged periods;

(2) long-season cultivars (more frequently of relatively high cyanide content) which take 12 months or more to harvest maturity, and whose tubers may be left in the ground for even several years with no deterioration other than increasing lignification (Purseglove, 1968).

II. ECONOMICS AND UTILIZATION

Cassava is one of the most important food crops of the

tropical world. Global production of roots is now estimated at some 100 million tons, representing a doubling of production in the last three decades. Table I indicates the distribution of production between the continents. Brazil produces almost a third of the world's total, and together with Indonesia, Zaire, Nigeria and India, about two thirds, but the crop is grown to some extent in almost all countries where ecological conditions permit.

Table I World cassava production (million metric tons) (after FAO, 1977)

Tropical America (incl. Caribbean)	32.761
Asia	32.932
Africa	44.263
Oceania	0.212
Total	110.167

Production is still largely within the subsistence sector of the economy, as the crop has many advantages for small farmers, who indeed have been mainly responsible for the expansion of its cultivation in recent decades. It is high yielding; tolerant of poor or exhausted soils; relatively free from pests and diseases; reliable as a food producer; drought resistant; and needs the use only of the stems for planting material. Above all, an extremely high return of food is produced per unit of energy input in its cultivation, which is a consideration of prime importance to the tropical subsistence farmer, who has no access to mechanized implements, and frequently none to draught animal power. Even in those districts where cassava is not popular as food, it is a valuable reserve against famine, on account of its great reliability (Cock and Howeler, 1978).

The roots are the main economically useful part of the plant, although the leaves are eaten as a green vegetable in many parts of the world, and are a valuable source of dietary protein (Rogers and Milner, 1963). The roots, however, are essentially carbohydrate or starch, typical analyses being given in Table II: it must be emphasized that the total dry matter content may differ greatly between roots according to cultivar, state of maturity and condition of growth, within the range approximately 20%-40%. Protein content varies but is never high enough to be nutritionally significant, and much of the little protein present is removed by processing. Assuming that the carbohydrate staple provides around half the total calorific intake in a normal diet, Coursey and Haynes (1970) and Nestel (1973) have calculated that cassava provides the staple food for some 200-300 million people across the tropical world. Phillips (1974) suggests that cassava may be even more extensively consumed than this, indicating that it provides 37% of the total calorific

Table II Composition of fresh cassava roots (after Jones, 1959)

Item	Unit	Composition of cassava roots per 1,000 g edible portion 1	2	3	4
Food energy	MJ	5.481	6.109	5.481	6.025
Water	g	600	625	647	620
Carbohydrate	g	320	347	327	350
Protein	g	7	12	11	7
Fat	g	trace	3	3	0
Calcium	mg	250	330	330	250
Phosphorus	mg	-	-	530	500
Iron	mg	10	7	8	5
Vitamin A	IU	0	trace	trace	-
Thiamine B_1	mg	0.2	0.6	0.7	0.2
Riboflavin B_2	mg	1	0.3	0.3	0.7
Niacin	mg	-	6	6	6
Vitamin C	mg	300	360	400	300

intake in Africa, 12% in Latin America and 7% in the Far East.

By far the greater part of the world's cassava crop, probably around 90%, is used as human food, in the countries of production. Substantial quantities are used as animal feeding stuff both in producer countries, and dried for export to temperate countries, mainly in Northern Europe, where it is used primarily in pig and poultry rations. Demand for cassava for this purpose has increased in Europe from 1½ to over 4 million tons of dried product in less than a decade (Anon., 1977). Similar quantities are consumed in the manufacture of industrial starch and starch products (Phillips, 1974). Recently, there has been much discussion of the use of cassava as a substrate for fermentation for production of power alcohol (de Menezes, 1978) or of microbial protein for animal feed (Gregory, 1977).

III. THE TOXICITY OF CASSAVA

A. THE NATURE AND EXTENT OF CYANIDE TOXICITY

The toxicity of cassava must have been recognized by the earliest Amerindian cultivators of the plant, who devised various processing methods, including sun-drying, leaching followed by drying, and soaking in running water with subsequent starch extraction or fermentation followed by drying or roasting (Coursey, 1973), to reduce the toxicity and at the same time convert the highly perishable fresh roots into stable products. The first report of the toxicity in Western literature is that of Clusius in 1601; the toxic principle was later identified as a cyanogenic glycoside, shown to be identical with flax linamarin:

2-(β-D-glucopyranosyloxy)-isobutyronitrile (Conn, 1969). Recently, it has been shown that the linamarin occurs together with small (10%) amounts of lotaustralin (methyl-linamarin, i.e. 2-(β-D-glucopyranosyloxy)methylbutyronitrile). All parts of the plant, except possibly the seeds, contain the glucosides together with the enzyme linamarase. This enzyme effects hydrolysis of the nitrile to free HCN when the tissue cellular structure is damaged (de Bruijn, 1971, 1973; Nartey, 1978).

As far as is known, all *Manihot* species contain cyanogenic glycoside, though only a few have been examined in detail (Rogers and Appan, 1973; Nassar and Fitchner, 1978) and it is presumed, although without published data, that it is linamarin and lotaustralin that are present. Within *M.esculenta*, there is a very wide range of cyanide levels between cultivars, from only a few ppm, to over 1000 ppm: no totally acyanogenic strain is known. Cultivars are often classified into "sweet" (low HCN) and "bitter" (high HCN). Some earlier authors regarded these as separate species, and classified them under names such as *M.dulcis* Pax, *M.palmata* Muell-Arg. and *M.aipi* Pohl. There is in fact no consistent correlation between cyanide level and morphological features, and only a very imperfect one with perceived sweetness or bitterness (Coursey, 1973; Sinha and Nair, 1968).

Cyanide toxicity in humans and animals on cassava diets is a well-recognized problem (Oke, 1968; Coursey, 1973), but understanding its extent is difficult at present because little of the published data permits one to relate the effect of cyanide intake on health parameters. A principal limitation is that existing assay methods for the total (potential) cyanide content of cassava and its products are inaccurate, irreproducible and very tedious (discussed in the next section). Monitoring the cyanide intakes in differing diets has therefore been very difficult and the majority of studies only detail the cassava contents in the diets.

Another difficulty is that the relative toxicities of free cyanide (non-glucosidic) and bound cyanide are unknown (Montgomery, 1969). This is an important factor since these two forms of cyanide have very different responses to cassava processing (see later). The toxicity of cassava and cassava products was until recently assumed to be associated with free cyanide, 50-60 mg of which constitutes a lethal dose for an adult man. The cyanogenic glucosides were at first thought to be of little consequence to mammals if cassava hydrolytic enzymes had been inactivated. The possibility of hydrolysis during digestion has latterly been considered and oral doses of pure linamarin have recently been shown to produce physiological and biochemical changes in rats without the simultaneous presence in the food of linamarase activity (Philbrick *et al.*, 1977).

A difficulty with human, as opposed to animal data, is that the populations studied were in a poor nutritional state which complicates attempts to differentiate the effects of cassava ingestion. Furthermore, chronic toxicity aspects are characterized by a number of strong interactions with other nutritional problems. Cyanide detoxification mechanisms (Westley, this volume) increase the requirement for sulphur containing essential amino acids. Moreover, thiocyanate, one of the detoxification products, inhibits iodine absorption and promotes goitre which is a common ailment in the developing world (Dorozynski, 1978). Fatalities, due to acute poisoning by cassava, though not unknown, are rare. Potentially more serious are long-term toxic effects such as ataxic neuropathy, goitre and cretinism that have been attributed to high cassava content in diets (Osuntokun, 1972; Delange *et al.*, 1976; Dorozynski, 1978; Ermans *et al.*, 1980).

In summary, gauging the extent of cyanide toxicity in animals has been difficult because of the problem of measuring cyanide intake. In human studies this problem is further complicated by the difficulty in measuring effects on health. The following sections describe a solution to the first of these problems i.e. the development of an accurate enzymatic assay for the cyanide contents of cassava and cassava products which readily permits measurement of the free and bound cyanide ratio.

B. THE LIMITATIONS OF CURRENT ASSAY METHODS

Existing assay methods for cassava cyanogenic glucosides depend on three stages:

(1) hydrolysis of the cyanogenic glucosides;
(2) isolation of cyanide released from the mixture (steam distillation or aspiration);
(3) determination of the cyanide.

The difficulties arise in the first two steps since there are many reliable techniques for cyanide determination. The first step is accomplished by either acid hydrolysis or by autolysis (by linamarase present in the cassava tissue). Chemical hydrolysis is subject to problems of incomplete hydrolysis caused by the relative stability of these β-glucosides, and to problems of amide and ammonia formation (Wood, 1966). Autolysis is sensitive to the variations in linamarase activity present in the plant tissue and the long incubations required (usually 12-24 hours) probably incur errors due to secondary reactions that may sequester the released cyanide. For example, both rhodanese (Boey *et al.*, 1976) and β-cyanoalanine synthase (Nartey, 1973) activities have been detected in cassava and could cause such interferences. Autolysis also can not be used with cassava products which have been heat processed in some manner. An autolytic procedure has recently been reported (Williams, 1979) using organic solvents to promote the breakdown of cell membranes and enhance enzyme-substrate interaction. No mention was made of likely solvent inhibition of linamarase or of competing enzyme activities and no linamarin recovery data were presented. Isolation of the cyanide from the substrate (step 2) is a tedious operation susceptible to many artefacts (Zitnak, 1973). The selection of a representative sample of cassava roots is hindered by variation between individual roots and by the cyanide gradients which exist within them, but this difficulty has often been completely ignored. Sampling problems are discussed in more detail later.

These problems explain the many conflicting reports (Coursey, 1973) describing the effects of different agronomic practices and different storage and processing conditions on the cyanide contents of cassava. An enzymatic assay, described in the following sections, was developed with the objectives of achieving a rapid and quantitative hydrolysis of the cyanogenic glucosides and obviating the need for steam distillation or aspiration (Cooke, 1978).

C. THE ENZYMATIC ASSAY FOR CASSAVA CYANIDE

1. Purification and Characterization of Cassava Linamarase from Parenchymal Tissue

Linamarase hydrolyses (Fig. 1) the cyanogenic glucosides to the corresponding cyanohydrin and Conn (1969) postulated by analogy with sorghum, that a second enzyme hydroxynitrile lyase, catalyses the dissociation of the cyanohydrin. The design of an enzymatic assay would be complicated (requiring both enzymes) if this cyanohydrin dissociation is rate limiting in the absence of such an

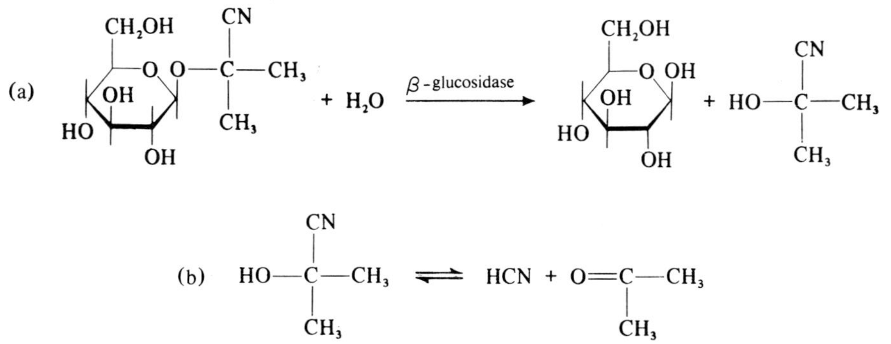

Fig. 1 The enzymatic degradation of linamarin (after Conn, 1969)

enzyme. The stability of acetone cyanohydrin at pH 6 and 30°C has been shown (Cooke, 1978) to correspond to a half-life of about 30 min and stopping the reaction shown in Fig. 1 with NaOH promptly dissociates the cyanohyrdin without the need for a secondary enzyme activity. Therefore the cyanide in cassava can be considered to be of two types, (a) bound cyanide (linamarin and lotaustralin) and (b) free cyanide (non-glucosidic).

Linamarase was initially extracted (Cooke *et al.*, 1978a) from cassava parenchymal tissue, i.e. peeled root, by homogenization in acetate buffer. Inclusion of dithiothreitol, EDTA, polyvinylpyrrolidone or diethyldithiocarbamate did not alter the activity of these crude extracts. Fractionation with ammonium sulphate was found to be an effective initial purification giving a 14-20 fold increase in specific activity. Subsequent chromatography on DEAE-cellulose (Fig. 2) resolved two peaks of linamarase activity. Analyses of 3 batches of parenchymal tissue indicated that peak 1 corresponded to between 10 and 40% of peak 2. The eluted activities were monitored by assaying with both linamarin and *p*-nitrophenyl β-D glucoside (PNP-glucoside) since it had been suggested (Butler *et al.*, 1965) that linseed linamarase is specific for linamarin/lotaustralin and that hydrolysis of other glucosides is due to different β-glucosidases. Figure 2 shows that in cassava these two activities follow one another.

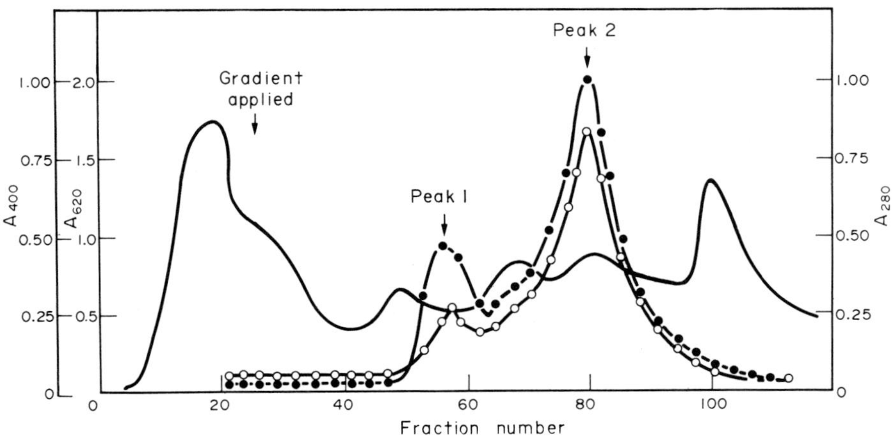

Fig. 2 Elution of linamarase from DEAE-cellulose by a linear NaCl gradient (Cooke *et al.*, 1978a). Key to symbols: ——— A_{280}; ●———● A_{620} (linamarase activity); O———O A_{400} (PNP-glucosidase activity).

The second peak eluted from the DEAE-cellulose column is found in the excluded volume from both Sephadex G-150 and

G-200. Gel filtration on Sepharose 6B(Fig. 3) gives a single peak with an apparent molecular weight of 600,000 which was not altered by the inclusion of 0.1 M NaCl in the buffer. This large apparent molecular weight may be caused by an enzyme - carbohydrate complex as has been suggested (Robinson, 1966) to explain the occurrence of different β-glucosidases in the same tissue. The final recovery after ammonium sulphate fractionation and chromatography on DEAE-cellulose and Sepharose 6B was 35% with a 350-fold increase in specific activity (Cooke *et al.*, 1978a).

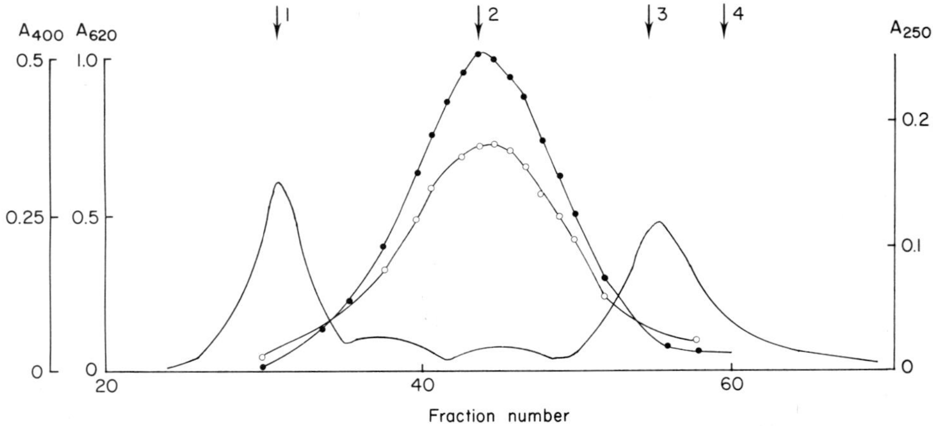

Fig. 3 Gel-filtration of a sample (0.9 ml) of Peak 2 (Fig. 2) on a column (50 x 1.3 cm) of Sepharose 6B (R.D. Cooke and G.G. Blake, unpub. obsv.). Symbols are as in Fig. 2. The elution position of the following molecular weight markers are also shown: 1, Dextran Blue; 2, Bovine thyroglobulin (699,000); 3, Lactate dehydrogenase (144,000); 4, Bovine serum albumin (67,000).

Wood (1966) reported the preparation of linamarase from cassava peel using acetone precipitation; the specific activity was only slightly greater than that of the crude extract. Linamarase has been prepared (Hughes, 1968) from white clover (*Trifolium repens* L.) by stepwise DEAE-cellulose chromatography, but no purification data was presented. The enzyme has also been prepared from linseed (*Linum usitatissimum* L.) meal by alcohol precipitation (Coop, 1940) and by stepwise DEAE-cellulose chromatography and Sephadex G-200 followed by analytical scale column electrophoresis on Sephadex G-25 (Butler *et al.*, 1965). Little purification resulted from the DEAE-cellulose and G-200 stages, but the analytical electrophoresis gave a 105-fold purification.

The K_m values of the purified cassava enzyme for

linamarin and PNP-glucoside are 1.45 mM and 0.46 mM, respectively, at pH 6 and the specific activity is the same for both substrates (Cooke *et al.*, 1978a). No data are available for the linseed, white clover or cassava peel preparations referred to above; but the β-glucosidases from sorghum (Mao and Anderson, 1967) and barley (Dey, 1977) have K_m values for PNP-glucoside in a similar range. The pH dependence peak of the purified cassava enzyme activity is rather broad, the optimum corresponding to pH 6 for linamarin and pH 6.4 for PNP-glucoside (Cooke *et al.*, 1978a) and the activity in phosphate buffer at pH 6 is almost independent of buffer molarity in the range 5-500 mM with both substrates.

The activity of the purified enzyme is unaffected by 10 mM glucose, KCN, EDTA, iodoacetate, dithiothreitol or cellobiose in the assay medium of either substrate. The lack of inhibition by cellobiose agrees with earlier studies (Butler *et al.*, 1965; Hutson, 1964) indicating separate roles for β-disaccaridase and β-glucosidase activities. The enzyme is inhibited competitively by glucono-(1-5) lactone with a K_i similar to that of other plant glucosidases (Mao and Anderson, 1967; Dey, 1977). The PNP-galactosidase (EC 3.2.1.23) activity of the crude enzyme is about 50% of the PNP-glucosidase activity, but this was not detectable in the purified enzyme (Cooke *et al.*, 1978a). In contrast, both galactosidase and glucosidase activities appear to be exhibited by multi-functional enzymes in almond (Grover *et al.*, 1977) and white clover (Maher and Hughes, 1971) whereas β-glucosidase fractions with and without PNP-galactosidase activities have been isolated from alfalfa (Robinson, 1966) and barley (Dey, 1977).

2. *Cassava Peel Linamarase*

The peel enzyme (i.e. derived from cassava cortex or rind) is precipitated by ammonium sulphate at the same concentration (60%) as the parenchymal enzyme, elutes from DEAE-cellulose in about the same position as peak 2 in Fig. 2 and elutes from Sepharose 6B in the same manner (Cooke *et al.*, 1978a). The peel enzyme also resembles the parenchymal enzyme closely in its pH and ionic strength dependence and K_m for limarin. The specific activity of the crude peel extract is about 5 times higher and a greater purification is achieved by the ammonium sulphate fractionation. Both the purified parenchymal enzyme and the ammonium sulphate concentrated peel enzyme are sufficiently active to hydrolyse quantitatively the dilute linamarin solutions present in cassava extracts.

3. *Development of the Enzymatic Assay*

The first problem was to choose an extraction medium in

which the cassava or cassava product could be homogenized to extract the free and bound cyanide present. Three requirements were defined for this extraction medium (Cooke, 1978):

(1) Endogenous cassava linamarase must be inactivated to prevent the conversion of bound to free cyanide during the extraction, thus allowing estimation of the ratio of bound to free cyanide in the sample.
(2) Cyanogenic glucosides and free cyanide must be stable in the solution, premitting processing of large numbers of samples prior to cyanide estimation.
(3) The solution must not require further fractionation (steam, distillation, etc.) before cyanide estimation.

Very basic or very acidic solutions are commonly employed to inactivate endogenous enzyme activities. Both free and bound cyanide are lost rapidly in sodium hydroxide extracts of cassava, presumably due to reaction with other components of the extracts, whereas extracts in orthophosphoric acid give solutions in which the free and bound cyanide concentrations are constant for at least 4 days at 4°C in stoppered bottles (Cooke, 1978). This has been confirmed with extracts of cassava parenchymal tissue, peel or fresh leaves from several different cassava cultivars. Different tissue homogenization treatments were tested to maximise cyanide extraction. Glass fibre filtration (GF/A paper) of these acid extracts yields fairly clear solutions that can be used directly, without further fractionation, for cyanide estimation using the specific pyridine/pyrazolone method of Jorgensen (1955).

Zitnak (1973) emphasized that existing autolytic or chemical assay methods have not been evaluated with regard to the essential criterion of measuring added linamarin recovery. Figure 4 shows the results of a linamarin recovery experiment in which linamarin was added to cassava tissue prior to homogenization; the extracts were then assayed using differing linamarase activities. A short enzyme incubation period (15 min) was chosen to minimize interference from any chemical or enzymatic side reactions that might occur. For routine analytical purposes 0.3 units of enzyme are used giving 95 ± 2% recoveries from cassava parenchyma, peel or fresh leaves i.e. the linamarase from 360 g of peel is sufficient for about 5,000 assays (Cooke, 1978). Analyses of different cassava products and mixtures should be preceded by a linamarin recovery experiment to check for chemical or enzymatic interference. The limit of assay sensitivity is about 0.01 mg of cyanide per 100 g fresh weight of parenchyma, and 40-50 samples per day can be readily processed by one person. A detailed description of this assay has recently been published (Cooke, 1979). The enzyme assay is more sensitive, reproducible and faster than existing quantitative methods.

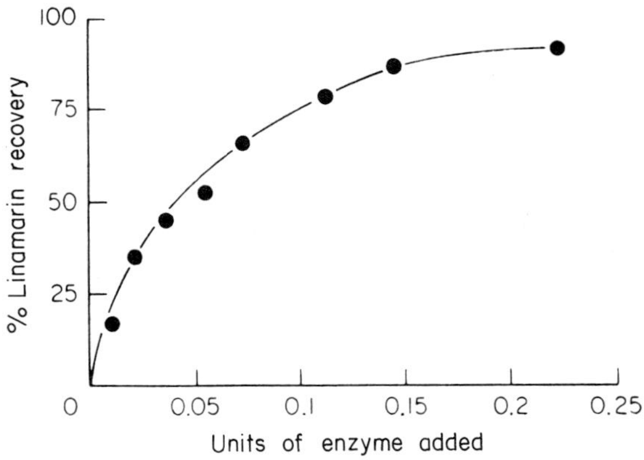

Fig. 4 The dependence of linamarin recovery on the activity of added enzyme (Cooke, 1978)

D. SAMPLING PROBLEMS

1. The Distribution of Cyanide Within Cassava Roots

There are many publications concerning the effects of differing agronomic practices on the cyanide contents of cassava, but few describe the sampling method used (Zitnak, 1973). Sinha and Nair (1968) suggested that there is a minimal variation in the cyanide contents of peeled tubers; Joachin and Pandittesekere (1944) reported a decrease from the proximal to the distal end of the roots in one cultivar. A study of 3 cultivars (de Bruijn, 1971) indicated both longitudinal and radial gradients in the peeled roots. This has been confirmed by an analysis of 8 cultivars (Cooke, 1978) showing that the radial gradient is especially marked. The outer parenchyma (near the peel) in some cases has over ten times the concentration of central portions. The longitudinal gradient is shallower, but sampling that ignores these two gradients can produce very misleading results.

2. The Inter-Root Variation in Cyanide Content

Analysis of 43 roots from 9 plants of 2 clones grown under the same conditions (Cooke *et al.*, 1978b) indicated that there is a considerable inter-root variation, conflicting with the earlier indication (Sinha and Nair, 1968) that there is little difference in the cyanide content of roots of about the same size from the same plant. Representative sampling of roots and plants is therefore essential in any agronomic study.

IV. CASSAVA BREEDING SCHEMES TO REDUCE TOXICITY

Extensive cassava screening programmes have failed to locate acyanogenic cultivars of cassava, but breeding programmes are continuing with the objective of producing low cyanide cultivars (Moh and Alan, 1972; CIAT, 1973; Sadik *et al.*, 1974). Breeding programmes require simple and rapid screening methods and the semi-quantitative sodium picrate method (AOAC, 1970) is commonly used for screening leaves. This is convenient because leaves are more accessible than roots. However, a recent study of 108 cassava clones emphasized the shortcomings of this very approximate method (Cooke *et al.*, 1978b) and suggested possible modifications. The effectiveness of the picrate leaf-test score as an indicator of root cyanide contents is limited by two possible factors. Firstly, the leaf score may not be directly proportional to the leaf cyanide content; it may also be a function of leaf linamarase and side-reactions sequestering the released hydrogen cyanide. Secondly, the relation between leaf and root cyanide contents may not be direct, but complicated by different transport and metabolic activities in the different clones. This aspect is receiving further study.

No evidence was found to support the earlier hypothesis that there is a correlation between cyanide content and root yield (Holleman and Aten, 1956). An analysis of the dry weight root yields of 50 clones revealed a correlation coefficient of only 0.18 (Cooke *et al.*, 1978b).

V. EFFECTS OF PROCESSING ON THE CYANIDE CONTENT OF CASSAVA

Cassava roots are traditionally processed by a diverse variety of different methods to reduce their toxicity, improve palatability and convert the perishable fresh roots into stable products. These methods comprise different combinations of drying, soaking, boiling and fermentation of the roots. All of these processes decrease the total cyanide content of the cassava, but the many earlier studies (reviewed by Coursey, 1973 and Nartey, 1978) are of doubtful value because of the shortcomings of the analytical procedures used.

The cyanide losses incurred by three of the processes involved in traditional methods, i.e. dehydration, leaching in water and boiling, have recently been investigated using the enzymatic assay (Cooke and Maduagwu, 1978) which permits differentiation between free and bound cyanide contents.

A. DEHYDRATION

Drying chips of peeled cassava roots in a forced air drier

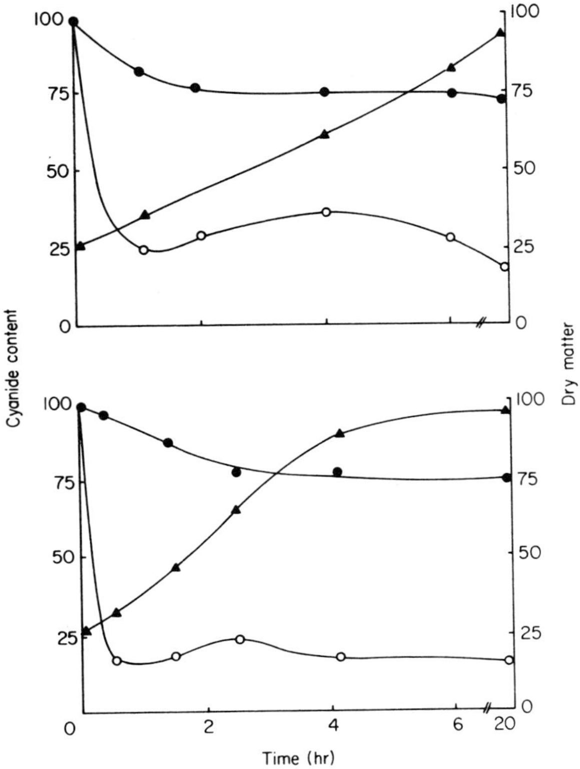

Fig. 5 The effect of drying cassava chips (a) at 47°C, (b) at 60°C on the cyanide concentrations in the chips (Cooke and Maduagwu, 1978). Free cyanide (O: percentage of initial concentration in the chips); bound cyanide (●); dry matter content (▲). The mean dimensions of the chips were 40 mm x 8.2 mm x 6.8 mm.

showed that about a third of the bound cyanide was removed at 47°C and 60°C (Fig. 5). The marginally greater loss at 47°C reflects the longer time spend in the intermediate moisture content range, under which conditions the enzyme is active. Faster drying at 80°C or 100°C incurred only a 10%-15% decrease in bound cyanide (Cooke and Maduagwu, 1978). The corresponding losses of free cyanide were 80%-85% at 47°C and 60°C (Fig. 5) and over 95% at the higher temperatures. The rate of loss of free cyanide is complex (Fig. 5) because it is a function of three types of process: (1) loss of the volatile hydrogen cyanide; (2) loss and degradation of the less volatile cyanohydrins; (3) production by endogenous linamarase of cyanohydrins during the initial stages of drying.

The non-glucosidic fraction of the total cyanide present in both fresh roots or chipped roots that have been stored several hours is usually 10% or less (Cooke, 1978). Consequently, the decrease in total cyanide content on air-drying is quite small. Preliminary experiments (Fernandez and Cooke, 1978; R.H. Booth and R.D. Cooke, unpub. obsv.) have shown that the slower drying rates of sun-drying produce greater losses in bound cyanide, consistent with the inverse dependence between drying rate and cyanide loss observed in air-drying experiments (Cooke and Maduagwu, 1978).

Losses of cyanide during dehydration as evaluated using the enzymic assay are generally smaller than those reported by earlier studies. For example, Paula and Rangel (1939) reported an 85% loss of cyanide in oven drying; 90% losses were quoted by Charavanapavan (1944). Tewe *et al.* (1978) reported losses of 43% and 94% on oven-drying sweet and bitter grated cassava samples.

The confirmation that only a small percentage of the total cyanide in cassava roots is present as free cyanide (Cooke, 1978) explains the common paradox arising out of Bolhuis' (1954) often-quoted classification of the toxicity of cultivars:

Innocuous: less than 50 mg/kg fresh peeled tuber.
Moderately poisonous: 50-100 mg/kg fresh peeled tuber.
Dangerously poisonous: more than 100 mg/kg fresh peeled tuber.

This classification was based on the lethal dose of hydrogen cyanide and common consumption levels, but with the assumption that all the cyanide is available as hydrogen cyanide. The latter assumption explains the observation that consumption even of the roots from cultivars classified as dangerously poisonous is rarely lethal.

B. SOAKING (LEACHING) AND BOILING

Rapid stirring in cold water produced a negligible decrease in bound cyanide after 4 h (Fig. 6), but 90% of the free cyanide was removed and most of this could be accounted for in the water. Stirring the chips overnight (18 h) at tropical ambient (Fig. 6) caused a marked decrease in bound cyanide accompanied by a drop in pH and a sour smell indicating the onset of fermentation (Akinrele, 1964). The free cyanide content had increased perhaps due to endogenous linamarase activity following cell disintegration or to microbial glucosidase activity. Preliminary experiments at the Centro Internacional de Agricultura Tropical, Colombia (Guillermo Gomez and R.D. Cooke, unpub. obsv.) also indicated that fermentation can markedly reduce bound cyanide contents. Cassava is traditionally fermented in West Africa, but in some cases this has been reported to decrease crude protein and increase crude fibre (Oke, 1966).

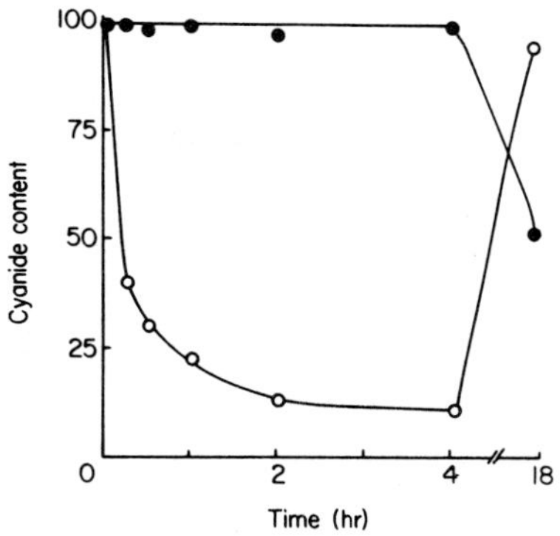

Fig. 6 The effect of soaking cassava chips in cold (24°C) water on the cyanide concentrations in the chips (Cooke and Maduagwu, 1978). Symbols are as described in Fig. 5.

The free cyanide content of fresh chips is rapidly removed in boiling water (over 90% removed within 15 min). The bound cyanide decreases at a much slower rate; 55% of the bound cyanide had been removed when the chips were thoroughly cooked, i.e. after 25 min (Cooke and Maduagwu, 1978). The literature data for cyanide losses on boiling are very variable, consistent with the shortcomings in the analytical procedures employed. Losses of 90-100% (Raymond *et al.*, 1941; Paula and Rangel, 1939), 50-80% (Joachim and Pandittesekere, 1944; Gondwe, 1974; Pieris *et al.*, 1974) and 10% (de Bruijn, 1971) have been reported.

These applications of the enzymatic assay to determine the free (non-glucosidic) and bound cyanide in cassava products indicate that the residual bound cyanide concentrations are greater than earlier studies suggest. The need to investigate the chronic toxicity implications of bound cyanide (cyanogenic glucosides) in cassava based foods is emphasized.

REFERENCES

Akinrele, I.A. (1964). *J. Sci. Fd. Agric.* 15, 589-594.

Anon. (1977). "Cassava: Export Potential and Market Requirements". International Trade Centre UNCTAD/GATT, Geneva.

AOAC (1970). "Methods of Analyses" (W. Horwitz, ed.) 11th edn. Association of Official Analytical Chemists, Washington D.C.

Boey, C.G., Yeoh, H.H. and Chew, M.Y. (1976). *Phytochemistry* 15, 1343-1344.

Bolhuis, G.G. (1954). *Neth. J. Agric. Sci.* 2, 176-185.

Booth, R.H. (1976). *Expl. Agric.* 12, 103-111.

de Bruijn, G.H. (1971). *Mededelingen Landbouwhogeschool (Wageningen)* 71, 1-140.

de Bruijn, G.H. (1973). *In* "Chronic Cassava Toxicity" (B.L. Nestel

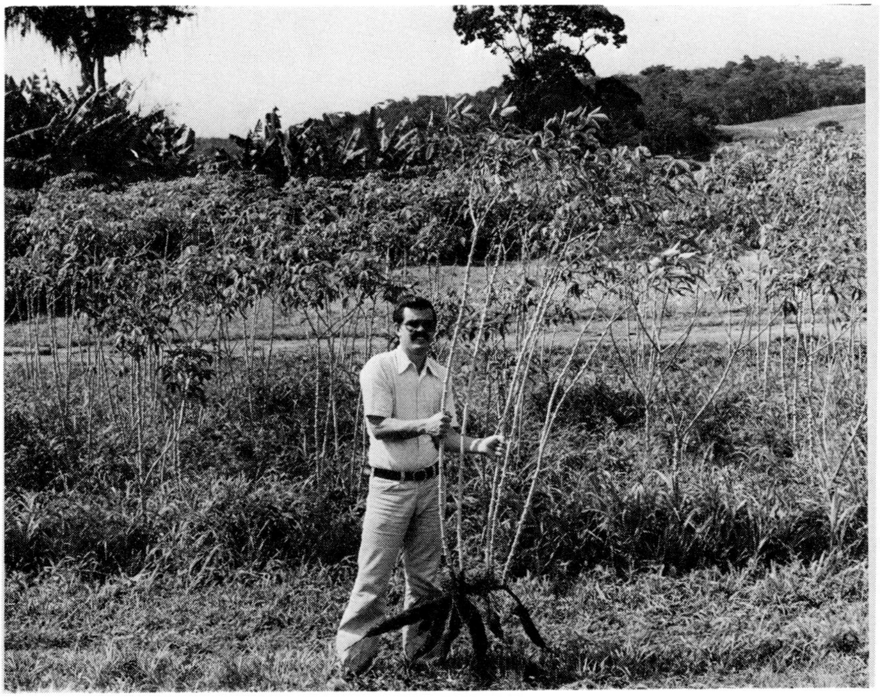

Fig. 7 Cassava growing in Costa Rica

and R. MacIntyre, eds) pp. 43-48. International Development Research Centre, Ottawa, Canada.
Butler, G.W., Bailey, R.W. and Kennedy, L.D. (1965). *Phytochemistry* 4, 369-381.
Charavanapan, C. (1944). *Trop. Agriculturist* 100, 164-168.
C.I.A.T. (1973). Annual Report. Centro Internacional de Agricultura Tropical, Cali, Colombia.
Cock, J.H. and Howeler, R.H. (1978). *In* "Crop Tolerance to Suboptimal Land Conditions" (J.A. Jung, ed.) pp. 145-154. American Society of Agronomy.
Conn, E.E. (1969). *J. Agric. Fd. Chem.* 17, 519-526.
Cooke, R.D. (1978). *J. Sci. Fd. Agric.* 29, 345-352.
Cooke, R.D. (1979). "Enzymatic Assay for Determining the Cyanide Content of Cassava and Cassava Products". Cassava Information Centre, C.I.A.T., Cali, Colombia.
Cooke, R.D. and Maduagwu, E.N. (1978). *J. Fd. Technol.* 13, 299-306.
Cooke, R.D., Blake, G.G. and Battershill, J.M. (1978a). *Phytochemistry* 17, 381-383.
Cooke, R.D., Howland, A.K. and Hahn, S.K. (1978b). *Expl. Agric.* 14, 367-372.
Coop, I.E. (1940). *New Zealand J. Sci. Technol.* 22B, 71-83.

Coursey, D.G. (1973). *In* "Chronic Cassava Toxicity" (B.L. Nestel and R. MacIntyre, eds) pp. 27-36. International Development Research Centre, Ottawa, Canada.
Coursey, D.G. (1976). *J. Root Crops* 2, 1-9.
Coursey, D.G. and Booth, R.H. (1977). *Acta Hort.* 53, 23-33.
Coursey, D.G. and Haynes, P.H. (1970). *World Crops* 22, 261-265.
Delange, F., Bordoux, P., Gamus, M., Gerard, M., Mafuta, M., Hanson, A. and Ermans, A.M. (1976). *Proc. 4th Int. Symp. Trop. Root Crops.* pp. 237-242. International Development Research Centre, Ottawa, Canada.
Dey, P.M. (1977). *Phytochemistry* 16, 323-325.
Dole, G.E. (1956). *In* "Man and Cultures" (A.F.C. Wallace, ed.) pp. 241-248. University of Pennsylvania Press, Philadelphia.
Dorozynski, A. (1978). *Nature* 272, 121.
Ermans, A.M., Mbulamoke, N.M., Delange, F. and Ahluwalia, R. (eds) (1980). "Role of Cassava in the Etiology of Endemic Goitre and Cretinism". IDRC 136e, International Development Research Centre, Ottawa.
F.A.O. (1977). "Production Statistics 1977". Food and Agriculture Organisation of the U.N., Rome, Italy.
Fernandez, R. and Cooke, R.D. (1978). *Cassava Newsl.* 4, 10-11.
Gondwe, A.T.D. (1974). *E. Afr. Agric. For. J.* 40, 161-167.
Gregory, K.F. (1977). *In* "Cassava as Animal Feed" (B.L. Nestel and M. Graham, eds) pp. 72-78. International Development Research Centre, Ottawa, Canada.
Grover, A.K., Macmurchie, D.D. and Cushley, R.J. (1977). *Biochim. Biophys. Acta* 482, 98-108.
Holleman, L.W.J. and Aten, A. (1956). "Processing of Cassava and Cassava Products in Rural Industries". F.A.O. Agric. Rev. Paper 54, Rome, Italy.
Hughes, M.A. (1968). *J. Exp. Bot.* 19, 427-434.
Hunt, L.A., Wholey, D.W. and Cock, J.H. (1977). *Field Crop Abs.* 30, 77-91.
Hutson, D.H. (1964). *Biochem. J.* 92, 142-146.
Ingram, J.S. and Humphries, J.R.O. (1972). *Trop. Sci.* 14, 131-148.
Jennings, D.L. (1976). *In* "Evolution of Crop Plants" (N.W. Simmonds, ed.) pp. 81-84. Longmans, London.
Joachim, A.W.R. and Pandittesekere, D.G. (1944). *Trop. Agriculturist* 100, 150-163.
Jones, W.O. (1959). "Manioc in Africa". Stanford University Press, Stanford, California.
Jorgensen, K. (1955). *Acta Chem. Scand.* 9, 548.
Lathrap, D.W. (1973). *World Archeol.* 5, 170-186.
Mao, C.H. and Andersen, L. (1967). *Phytochemistry* 6, 473-483.
Maher, E.P. and Hughes, M.A. (1971). *Phytochemistry* 10, 3005-3007.
de Menezes, T.J.B. (1978). *In* "Cassava Harvesting and Processing" (E.J. Weber, J.H. Cock and A. Chouinard, eds) pp. 41-45. International Development Research Centre, Ottawa, Canada.
Moh, C.C. and Alan, J.J. (1972). *Trop. Root Crops Newsl.* 6, 29-31.
Montaldo, A. (1972). "Cultivo de Raices y Tuberculos Tropicales". Instituto Interamericano de Ciencias Agricolas, Lima, Peru.
Montaldo, A. (1979). "La Yucao Mandioca". Instituto Interamericano de Ciencias, San Jose, Costa Rica.

Montgomery, R.D. (1969). *In* "Toxic Constituents of Plant Foodstuffs" (I.E. Liener ed.) pp. 143-157. Academic Press, New York.
Nartey, F. (1973). *In* "Chronic Cassava Toxicity" (B.L. Nestel and R. MacIntyre, eds) pp. 73-87. International Development Research Centre, Ottawa, Canada.
Nartey, F. (1978). "Cassava - Cyanogenesis, Ultrastructure and Seed Germination". Munksgaard, Copenhagen.
Nassar, N.M.A. and Fitchner, S.S. (1978). *Can. J. Plant Sci.* 58, 577-578.
Nestel, B.L. (1973). *In* "Chronic Cassava Toxicity" (B.L. Nestel and R. MacIntyre, eds) pp. 11-26. International Development Research Centre, Ottawa, Canada.
Noon, R.A. and Booth, R.H. (1977). *Trans. Br. Mycol. Soc.* 69, 289-290.
Oke, O.L. (1966). *Trop. Sci.* 8, 23-27.
Oke, O.L. (1968). *Wld. Rev. Nutr. Diet* 9, 227-250.
Osuntokun, B.O. (1972). *Plant Foods Human Nutr.* 2, 215-266.
Paula, R.D. de G. and Rangel, J. (1939). *Rev. Alimentar (Rio de Janeiro)* 3, 215-217.
Passam, H.C. and Noon, R.A. (1977). *Ann. Appl. Biol.* 85, 436-440.
Philbrick, D.J., Hill, D.C. and Alexander, J.C. (1977). *Toxicol. Appl. Pharmacol.* 42, 539-551.
Phillips, T.P.(1974). "Cassava Utilization and Potential Markets". International Development Research Centre, Ottawa, Canada.
Pieris, N., Jansz, E.R. and Kandage, R. (1974). *J. Natn. Sci. Coun. Sri Lanka* 2, 67-76.
Purseglove, J.W. (1968). "Tropical Crops - Dicotyledons". Longmans, London.
Raymond, W.D., Jojo, W. and Nicodemus, Z. (1941). *E. Afr. Agric. J.* 6, 154-159.
Renvoise, B.S. (1972). *Econ. Bot.* 26, 352-360.
Robinson, D. (1966). *Phytochemistry* 5, 699-705.
Rogers, D.J. (1963). *Bull. Torrey Bot. Club* 90, 43-54.
Rogers, D.J. (1973). *Trop. Root Crops Newsl.* 6, 4-10.
Rogers, D.J. and Appan, S.G. (1973). Flora Neotropica, Monograph No. 13 "Manihot Manihotoides (Euphorbiaceae)". Hafner Press, New York.
Rogers, D.J. and Fleming, H.G. (1973). *Econ. Bot.* 27, 1-113.
Rogers, D.J. and Milner, M. (1963). *Econ. Bot.* 17, 211-216
Sadik, S., Okereke, O.U. and Hahn, S.K. (1974). "Screening for Acyanogenesis in Cassava", Tech. Bull. 4. International Institute of Tropical Agriculture, Ibadan, Nigeria.
Sinha, S.K. and Nair, T.V.R. (1968). *Ind. J. Agric. Sci.* 38, 958-963.
Sturtevant, W.C. (1969). *In* "The Domestication and Exploitation of Plants and Animals" (P.J. Ucko and G.W. Dimbleby eds). Duckworth, London.
Tewe, O.O., Maner, J.H. and Gomez, G.G. (1977). *J. Sci. Fd. Agric.* 28, 750-756.
Williams, H.J. (1979). *Expl. Agric.* 15, 393-399.
Wood, T. (1966). *J. Sci. Fd. Agric.* 17, 85-90.
Zitnak, A. (1973). *In* "Chronic Cassava Toxicity" (B.L. Nestel and R. MacIntyre, eds) pp. 89-96. International Development Research Centre, Ottawa, Canada.

CYANOGENESIS IN TROPICAL FEEDS AND FOODSTUFFS

FREDERICK NARTEY

Division of Biochemistry, Institute of Plant Physiology, University of Copenhagen, Ø. Farimagsgade 2A, 1353-DK Copenhagen, Denmark

I. INTRODUCTION

Several plant species of immense agricultural significance to man and animals exhibit the phenomenon of cyanogenesis whereby HCN is liberated when the plants' tissues are damaged. The ability of these plants to release HCN depends on the synthesis and accumulation of cyanogenic materials in their leaves, stems, fruits, seeds, roots and tubers, coupled with the presence of hydrolytic enzymes which are capable of cleaving these materials. Since the cyanogenic materials are largely localized within the vacuoles of cyanophoric plant cells, while their hydrolytic enzymes are cytoplasmic, damaging the cells leads to disruption of cellular integrity and results in a situation where the enzymes come into contact with the cyanogenic materials with the concomitant evolution of HCN. Cyanogenesis is known to have a broad phylogenetic distribution, occurring in well over 1000 plant species representing some 80 families and 300 genera (Nartey, 1978a). Cyanogenesis also occurs in fungi, some bacteria and animals (see this volume).

Several cyanophoric plants play important economic, dietary and nutritional roles in the tropics and subtropics. Species such as *Manihot*, *Phaseolus*, *Sorghum*, *Dioscorea*, *Linum*, *Arachis*, *Pennisetum*, *Zea*, *Glycine*, *Colocacia*, *Acacia*, *Bambusa*, *Macrozamia*, (belonging to the families of *Euphorbiaceae*, *Leguminosae (Mimosoideae)*, *Aracaeae*, *Gramineae*, *(Cydaceae)*), are extensively incorporated into human diets and animal feeds. With particular reference to *Manihot esculenta* (Cassava), its leaves, tubers and fermented-tuber products are incorporated into the diets of well over 300 million people in the tropics and subtropics. Furthermore, leaves and tuber peel form common feed for domestic animals in these areas. Sorghums and millets, apart from contributing a substantial proportion of the dietary cereals of man in the tropics and subtropics, also form common animal feed. The *Acacia* species of Africa and

Australia are known to be fed to livestock, including cattle, sheep and goats. *Phaseolus* species are also common ceed (Göhl, 1975; Nartey, 1980a).

Various species of the above mentioned genera have been reported to be cyanophoric (Gibbs, 1974), and when incorporated into human diet or animal feed generate varying concentrations of HCN. It has been estimated that an adult in tropical regions where cassava forms the staple diet consumes as much as 750 g of cassava daily, a quantity capable of generating at least 35 mg HCN (see Table II). This value represents half the lethal dose of HCN (Williams *et al.*, 1967), so that humans and livestock maintained on high rations of foods and feedstuffs derived from such cyanophoric plants become exposed to calculated risks of cyanide poisoning.

II. TROPICAL FEEDSTUFFS

Tropical and subtropical fodder and feedstuffs consist of grasses, legumes, shrubs of miscellaneous plants, fruits and vegetables, root crops, cereal grains, oilseeds and oilseed cakes. The tropics rely mostly on natural grasslands in the arid and semi-arid regions and the savannas for grazing by cattle, game, ruminants, sheep, goats, pigs and other animals. However, certain plant species are grown intentionally to provide animal feed and fodder. This applies to *Saccharum*, *Sorghum*, *Triticum*, *Linum*, *Pennisetum*, *Alocasia*, *Xanthosoma*, *Diocorea* and *Manihot* species. *Vicia* species are also grown for animal feed, and in the cooler regions of the tropics, *Trifolium* species are grown and used for fodder. *Acacia* species, which are grown for reforestation of semi-arid and savannah zones, are used for fodder in several regions of Africa and Australia (Butterworth, 1967; Göhl, 1975; Nonguneirma A., 1977).

The naturally growing grasses are heavily grazed, and considered valuable and palatable fodder crops. A few of the grasses which are intentionally grown for animal feed yield cereal grains for human consumption. This applies to wild species of *Oryza*, *Sorghum*, *Paspalum*, *Panicum* and *Medicago*. The straw and stalks of these grasses are often used for hay used as forage and fodder.

In Nigeria, Southern and Eastern Africa, *Acacia* and *Colocacia* species are eaten by game and livestock, horses and camels. Frequently the pods of *Acacia* species are fed to domestic animals on account of their high protein content and palatability (Oyenuga, 1959; Irvine, 1961; Watt *et al.*, 1962).

Cassava tubers, apart from being incorporated into human diet, form a substantial part of animal feed. The tuberpeel and leaves are fed to, and browsed by livestock and game. In cassava growing areas where excess of the tuber is available, the flesh is also fed to livestock.

Table I Cyanide concentration of tissues of some African and Australian *Acacia* species

Plant species	Origin	Tissue analysed	mg HCN/100 g tissue
Acacia erioloba	South Africa	Leaves	180.7
A. erioloba	South Africa	Leaves, grown from seed in Copenhagen	115.9
A. erioloba	South Africa	Leaves	105.9
A. erioloba	South Africa	Unripe pod	88.2
Acacia hebeclada *susp. hebeclada*	South Africa	Leaves	192.4
Acacia sieberiana *var. villosa*	West Africa	Leaves	0.0
Acacia sieberiana			
var. woodii	South Africa	Leaves	139.4
var. woodii	South Africa	Ripe pod	113.4
var. woodii	South Africa	Unripe pod	110.0
var. woodii	South Africa	Leaves, grown from seed in Copenhagen	231.7
Acacia cheelii	Australia	Leaves	123.7
Acacia conninghamnii	Australia	Leaves	23.6
A. conninghamnii	Australia	Leaves, grown from seed in Copenhagen	11.8
Acacia doratoxylon	Australia	Leaves	23.4
Acacia glaucescence	Australia	Leaves	251.3

Industrial wastes from cassava and other starchy root crops also give products that are used for livestock feeds. Species of these genera have been shown to be cyanogenic and sometimes lead to loss of stock. Some of these grasses, legumes, shrubs, cereal grains and oleagenous plants therefore represent dangers to animals (Table I) unless the feeds derived from them are properly detoxified before use, or other species which are non-cyanogenic are used.

III. TROPICAL FOODSTUFFS

Most tropical foodstuffs are derived from plant origin, particularly in those areas where the production of livestock for food is limited. Most of the tropical plants used for food provide the starchy food products, which are processed before being incorporated into the diet. These include edible *Aroids* belonging to the genera *Alocasia, Colocasia, Cytosperma, Xanthomosa* and *Dioscorea*. In New Guinea, the Solomon Islands and Tonga the trunk of *Metroxylon sagu* provides basic starchy food and fermented food products (Standal, 1980).

All parts of *Cycads* are used for food, either unfermented or fermented (Whiting, 1963). Besides being used for animal

Table II Concentration of cyanide in some tropical foodstuffs (modified after Nartey, 1968a; Montgomery, 1969)

Plant/Tissue	mg HCN/kg
Cassava (bitter)/Dried root cortex	2450
Cassava (bitter)/Leaves	310
Cassava (bitter)/ Whole tubers	395
Cassava (sweet)/ Leaves	468
Cassava (sweet)/ Whole tubers	462
Sorghum/Whole immature plant	2500
Bamboo/Immature shoot tip	8000
Lima beans from Java (coloured)	3120
Lima beans from Puerto Rico (black)	3000
Lima beans from Burma (white)	2100

feed, the *Acacia* pods provide food at times of hunger, and are used medicinally (Irvine, 1961; Watt *et al.*, 1962). Sorghum, millets and maize are incorporated in the diet as porridge or fermented cakes.

In the tropics *Manihot esculenta* and *Dioscorea* species provide the major staple food, their starchy tubers being incorporated into the diet after cooking or fermentation to give various food derivatives (Cooke and Coursey, this volume). Fermentation yields food-products with high protein content, acceptable flavours and long storage life. Consumption of cassava and lima beans have been shown to cause poisoning in humans incorporating excessive quantities in the diet, on account of cyanide intoxication (Table II). Fermentation products such as "Akpo" and gari have also been suspected of causing cyanide toxicity. Cassava processed into flour is also incorporated in the diet as bread (Kim *et al.*, 1969). Tables III and IV give the cyanide content of some of the foodstuffs derived from processed cassava.

Total cyanide released in the presence of added β-glucosidase was determined quantitatively by the method of Epstein (1947), as modified by Jørgensen (1955). Qualitativ tests without the added β-glucosidase showed the presence of low levels of cyanide in all samples. This raises the question as to the origin of the free cyanide found in processed cassava food products. It has been shown that cyanide is bound in the form of *Linamarin* and *Lotaustralin* in the cassava plant throughout its life cycle (Nartey, 1968). Processing of root tuber for the production of gari, cassava flour and other various food derivatives for human consumption involves cutting the tuber into chips and drying in the sun, grating the tuber and allowing the pulp to ferment in bags, and soaking the tuber in water for several days. During these processes several microorganisms infect the cassava tuber, chips and pulp, utilizing the tuber starch and other constituents as substrates for their metabolic activities and synthesis of new product

Table III Concentration of cyanide in plants used as food in Nigeria

Cassava products	mg HCN/kg
Fermented (Purupuru/Lafun)	2.70
Fermented (Gari, Eba)	0.60 g
Diascorea sp.	0.16
Colocasia	15.2
Oryza sp.	0.16
Musa sp.	0.16
Zea sp.	0.14
Sorghum (dried pulp)	108.00
Sorghum (immature whole plant)	249.00
Vicia sp. (seeds)	51.30

(Modified after Osuntokun, 1980)

It is important to stress that although cassava root tubers form the most important staple food in the tropics, a considerable proportion of the 100 million tons produced annually is processed and fermented specifically to produce various food derivatives, which are used as the principal diets of tropical populations. Further, sundried or oven-dried chips are exported to the developed countries where they are used as compound animal-feed and in various industries.

It appears that during cassava processing, either for human consumption or for industry, a natural infection with the microflora of the atmosphere and the soil takes place, leading to the hydrolysis of linamarin and lotaustralin. This detoxification of cassava cyanogens by microbial β-glucosidases may lead to the generation of cyanide, which may be lost to the atmosphere, converted into other metabolic products by microbial enzymic processes, or bound to carbonyl compounds to form cyanohydrins. The formation of the latter compounds may explain the release of cyanide from cassava products in the absence of β-glucosidase, since cyanohydrins readily generate cyanide.

Although cyanide has been found in the free state in some plants, it generally arises from cyanogenic glucosides and cyanohydrins by the action of β-glucosidases and hydroxynitrilelyases. Cassava fermentation leads to a reduction of the cyanide content through the hydrolysis of the cyanogenic glycosides by β-glucosidases of the plant during chipping or pulping, and by microbial β-glucosidases during the fermentation. Oyenuga (1967) reports that "bruised or fermented cassava peel" may not be fed to sheep, goats and cattle, because the cyanide concentration in this feedstuff may be higher than that originally present in the peel.

IV. THE ORIGIN OF CYANIDE IN TROPICAL PLANTS

Cyanide has been detected in the free state in plants

Table IV Concentration of cyanide in cassava food products from Nigeria

Processed cassava	mg HCN/kg
Gari, Abeokuta Market	1300
Gari, Agege Market 1	1470
Gari, Agege Market 2	2400
Gari, Oshodi (F.I.I.R.)	2970
Gari, Ijebu Market	900
Gari, Mushin Market	930
Cassava Flour 1	1500
Cassava Flour 2	2600

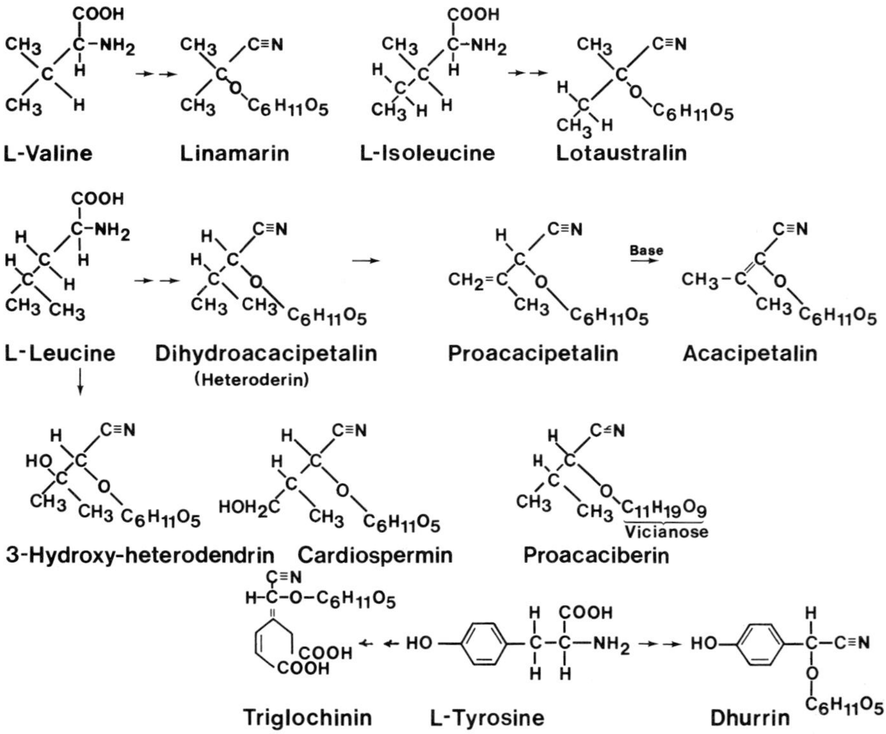

Fig. 1 Structural relations of some amino acids and cyanogenic glycosides

(Abrol, 1967), but generally, the precursors of cyanide in plants are relatively stable glycosidic derivatives of α-hydroxynitriles which on enzymic or non-enzymic hydrolysis yield HCN, sugars and carbonyl compounds. Fungal and bacterial cyanogenesis on the other hand yields unstable intermediates which readily break down, resulting in the accumulation of HCN in the growth medium or the atmosphere above it (Nartey, 1978).

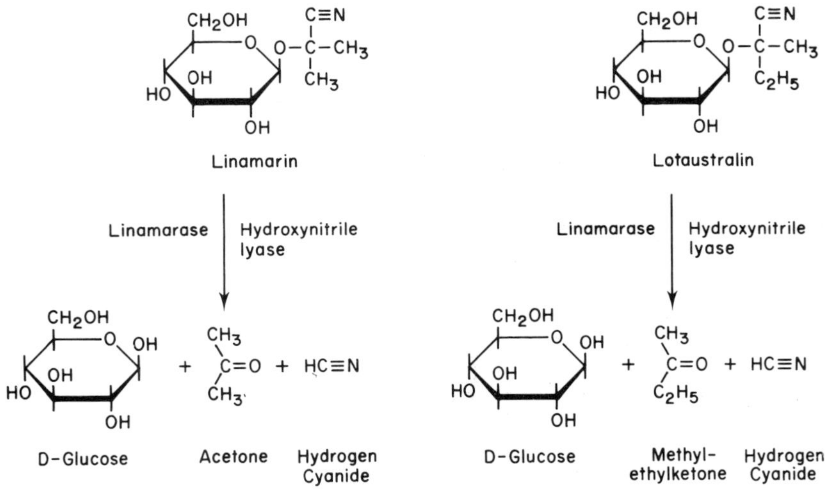

Fig. 2 Hydrolysis of linamarin and lotaustralin by cassava and microbial β-glucosidases

Plants utilized for foodstuffs and feed in the tropics include Cassava, Pulses, Sorghums and Millets, Cocoyams, Acacia, Cycads, Egyption and common vetch, several grasses and certain shrubs commonly referred to as "kill goats". As far as these plants are concerned, the most important precursors of cyanide are linamarin, lotaustralin, dhurrin, proacacipetalin, proacaciberin, vicianine, cyacasin and triglochinin (Fig. 1). Some of the less known cyanogenic glycosides in tropical plants are heterodendrin, 3-hydroxyheterodendrin and cardiospermin. Proacaciberin and 3-hydroxylheterodendrin have recently been isolated, together with several other cyanogenic compounds from *Acacia sieberiana* var. *woodii* (Tschierch, 1966; Ettlinger *et al.*, 1977; Seigler, 1977; Erb *et al.*, 1978; Nartey, 1978a; Zinsmeister, 1980). Some of the *Acacia* species of Australian origin contain sambunigrin, a cyanogenic glycoside with an aromatic aglucone. Hitherto, all cyanogenic glycosides identified in African *Acacia* species have been shown to possess aliphatic aglucones. This has been used as a taxonomic differentiation between African and Australian *Acacia* species (Rimington, 1935).

The biogenesis of HCN and cyanogenic glycosides has been extensively studied by Conn and his group at Davis (Conn and Buttler, 1969; Conn, 1973 and this volume) who have shown that the aglucone moieties of these compounds are derived from simple amino acids to which they bear structural relationships. Thus the aglucone moieties of linamarin and lotaustralin are derived from valine and isoleucine, respectively (Buttler and Buttler, 1960; Nartey, 1968), proacacipetalin, heterodendrin, cardiospermin and 3-hydroxyheterodendrin from leucine (Butterfield *et al.*, 1975; Seigler, 1976; Nartey, 1978a; Brimer *et al.*, 1980), dhurrin from tyrosine, and triglochinin from phenylalanine (Seigler, 1977).

With a few exceptions, cyanophoric plants synthesize cyanogens as well as their hydrolytic enzymes (Fig. 2). For example, certain species of the genera *Lotus* and *Trifolium* synthesize linamarin and lotaustralin but not the enzymes that hydrolyse them, or *vice versa* (Nartey, 1978a). All the cyanophoric tropical and subtropical plants that we have investigated do synthesize cyanogens and their hydrolytic enzymes. We have investigated species of *Manihot*, especially cultivars of *Manihot esculenta* from India, Africa, the West Indies, Asia, South America and most of the developing world because cassava forms one of the staple diets of most low-income populations of these areas. The utilization of cassava in the diet is known to give rise to several diseases such as cretinism, stunted growth in children and goitre. There is a mass of indirect evidence implicating cassava toxicity for lesions of the skin, mucous membrane, optic, auditory and peripheral nerves. The latter have been collectively termed Tropical Ataxic Neuropathy, and have been shown to be caused by prolonged exposure to varying levels of cyanide evolved in diets of cassava and cassava fermented products (Nartey, 1980a).

V. VARIATION OF CYANIDE IN CASSAVA

Cyanogenesis in cassava is continuous in that both low and high yielding cultivars exist (Cooke and Coursey, this volume). Although the synthesis and accumulation of cyanogenic materials in cassava tissue is genetically controlled, factors such as soil, humidity, rainfall and season have great influences on their accumulation. While these extrinsic factors play an important role, intrinsic factors such as valine and isoleucine levels, the activities of synthetic as well as hydrolytic enzymes, transport, storage and degradation of these secondary metabolites also influence the levels of cassava cyanogens a great deal (Nartey, 1973).

In spite of systematic screening to find cassava cultivars with zero cyanide levels, no such cultivars have yet been found. Cyanogenesis in cassava does not only vary with the age of individual plants, but it also varies with different clones and cultivars of the same species. Cassava exhibits intra- and inter-plant variation with respect to cyanogenesis. That is, cassava shows a genetic polymorphism in cyanogenesis which probably indicates that cyanogenesis in the plant is multigenic (Nartey, 1978).

Goats and sheep browse on cassava shrubs at specific times of the day without being poisoned by cyanide intoxication. However, the intake of the same amount of cassava leaf fodder at certain other times of the day by herbivores leads to poisoning and loss of stock (Ugochukwu, 1980), probably because the cyanogenic materials are at their highest levels at these times. This indicates a diurnal rhythm in cyanogenesis as has been shown for other plant secondary products, for example alkaloids (Fairbairn *et al.*, 1964).

Cassava leaves are incorporated into the diet in many developing countries, for example the Cameroons, Zaire and Guinea. Leaves have a very high protein content (Rogers, 1959; Omole, 1977), but also contain high levels of cyanide. Very young and unexpanded leaves contain higher levels of cyanide than do root tubers, and root tuber peel contains appreciably higher levels than root flesh (Ugochokwu *et al.*, 1980).

Whereas cyanogenesis in the cassava seed is negligible, unlike *Linum* (Smith *et al.*, 1980), it increases appreciably during germination, primarily in root tissue. As the primary leaves develop and become functional, cyanogenesis occurs predominantly in leaf tissues, and the cyanogens are thereafter transported basipetally to, and stored in, the roots, whose ability to synthesize cyanogens diminish (Fig. 3).

All parts of the cassava plant are capable of synthesizing cyanogens. Leaf, stem, stem-pith and root tissues maintained on agar medium, synthesize low levels of cyanide in the presence of added valine and isoleucine. Figures 3a and 3b are stem-pith and root tissue cultures. The tissue cultures were all found to form low levels of cyanide. Experiments are in progress to obtain root tissues in suspension cultures with the aim of genetically manipulating these cells so as to give progenies in which cyanogenesis does not occur, or is markedly reduced.

VI. FERMENTED FOODS

Yams, cassava, sorghum, millets and maize, apart from constituting a major fraction of diet in tropical countries directly, also form the carbohydrate-rich raw materials for indigenous fermentation processes for the production of alcoholic, non-alcoholic beverages and various foodstuffs. These fermentation processes improve the nutritive values of the low-protein and high-carbohydrate foods.

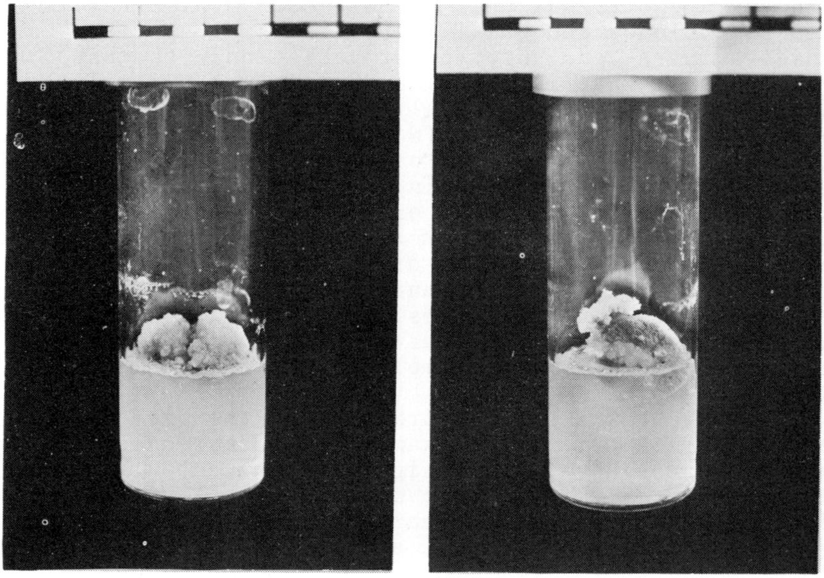

Fig. 3 Tissue cultures of stem-pith and tuber tissues of cassava grown on solid media incorporating valine, isoleucine, NAA (Kartha and Gamborg, 1975)

Sorghums and millets, varieties of which are cyanophoric, vigorously accumulate dhurrin and heterodendrin during germination, and traces of cyanide have been detected in the alcoholic beverage products of such fermentation. Cassava, maize and other cereal grains form substrages for a wide variety of non-alcoholic fermented foods in Africa, such as Gari, Purupuru, Eba, Akpo and Ogi. These food products contain cyanide, varying from traces to extremely high levels.

One of the most important raw materials for fermentation processes is cassava. The root crop forms an adjunct with sorghum in brewing alcoholic beverages such as Burukutu, but its major value resides in its use as substrate in the non-alcoholic fermented foods such as Gari and Akpo, variants of which are found all over the tropics (Jones, 1959).

A. MICROORGANISMS INVOLVED IN INDIGENOUS FERMENTATION

Indigenous fermentations are very complex, in that several microorganisms from the soil and the atmosphere infect the different substrates at different stages. For example, the sap of the palm tree, *Elaeis guineansis*, and the raphia palm, *Raphia hookeri*, are naturally infected by a host of organisms, including yeasts, *Lactobacilli*, *Bacilli*,

Aspergillus spp., *Penicillium spp.*, *Streptococcus spp.*, *Sarcina spp.* and *Leuconostoc spp.* in the brewing of palm wine. Similar organisms and *Mucor rouxii*, *Acetobacter spp.* and *Hansenula spp.* are also involved in the brewing of Buruktu and Kaffir beer (Ekundayo, 1980). The fermentation of maize and millets and soybeans to produce Ogi involves microorganisms such as yeast, *Aerobacter cloacae*, *Cephalosporium spp.*, *Fusarium spp.*, *Aspergillus spp.* and *Penecillium spp.* (Ekundayo, 1980).

Although some work has been done on the microbiology of indigenous fermentation, the organisms participating in the various indigenous fermentations, their physiology and their biosynthetic capabilities remain largely unknown. A major problem in all these fermentation processes is the contamination of fermented foods by undesirable microorganisms whose metabolic products constitute a serious health hazard to people incorporating such foods in the diet.

B. CASSAVA PSEUDOMONADS AND CYANIDE PRODUCTION

The fermentation of cassava to produce gari has been shown to occur by the aid of *Corynebacterium manihot* and *Geotrichum candidum* (Collard and Levi, 1959) in a two stage fermentation process in which *C. manihot* first breaks down cassava starch and produces various organic acids, including lactic acid, which lowers the pH of the mash and thus causes the hydrolysis of linamarin and lotaustralin with the concomitant release of hydrogen cyanide. The acid pH of the cassava mash then provides favourable growth conditions for a second organism, *G. candidum*, which produces various aldehydes and esters that impart the characteristic taste and aroma of gari (Akinrele, 1964). Further investigations have shown that *Lactobacillus spp.*, *Leuconostoc spp.* and *Alcaligenes spp.* are present in fermenting cassava mash at a later stage (Okafor, 1977). According to Ekundayo (1980) the low pH and the activity of cassava linamarase would appear to break down completely all the linamarin and lotaustralin present in the tuber mash (see Scheme 1).

Several reports appear to conflict with the suggestion that all or most of the cassava cyanogens are hydrolysed during grating, fermentation and roasting (see Table IV). Experiments designed to show that gari contains bound and free cyanide have demonstrated that both forms of cyanide exist in not only gari, but also cassava flour that has not undergone the process of "garification".

Recent investigations in our laboratory have shown that in addition to the microorganisms mentioned above, several other bacteria and fungi participate in the fermentation process. Through the kind collaboration of Dr Ayernor, International Institute of Tropical Agriculture, Ibadan, Nigeria, we have secured samples of juice from fermenting cassava meal from cassava-processing villages and from IITA in Nigeria, from which we have isolated these other

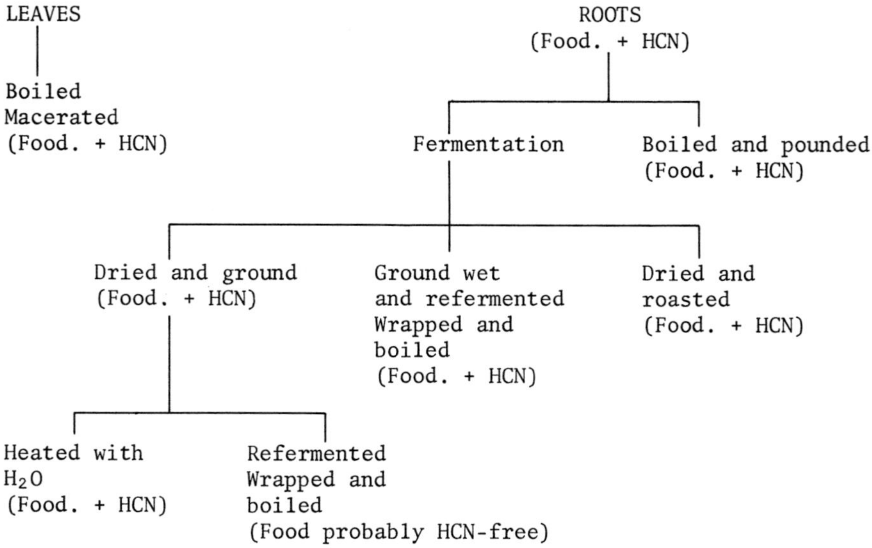

Scheme 1 Utilization of cassava as food in the tropics

organisms. In the early stages of cassava fermentation *Corynebacteria* and *Geotrichum spp.* were present, as well as several yeasts, including *Pichia*. Other microorganisms which were isolated in pure culture are *Aspergillus spp.*, *Penicillium spp.*, *Norcadia spp.*, *Streptomyces spp.*, *Pseudomonas spp.* and *Bacillus spp.*, including *B. cereus*, *B. subtillis* and *B. megaterium*, found to participate in the fermentation of cassava at a later stage.

Some of *Pseudomonads spp.* isolated from fermenting cassava have been studied in some detail in our laboratory primarily because they produce hydrogen cyanide during growth, and may account for the high levels of residual cyanide present in fermented cassava foodstuffs, probably in the form of cyanohydrins since sugars and various aldehydes have been found in gari (Akinrele, 1964).

Among the bacteria, *Pseudomonads* and *Chromobacterium violaceum* are known to be prolific producers of cyanide by oxidation of glycine (Wissing, 1968, 1974, 1978; Knowles, 1976; Castric, this volume).

A *Pseudomonas* species isolated from fermenting cassava was grown on several substrates, including cassava, maize, yam, and cocoyam extracts supplemented with inorganic salts. It was found that the organism grows well on these tropical food extracts and synthesizes *c.* 250 µM cyanide during the late logarithmic phase. Similar values for cyanide production were obtained when the organism was grown on inorganic salts supplemented with peptone, and on defined media consisting of inorganic salts, glycine, methionine and succinate (Nartey, 1980a). Figure 4 shows

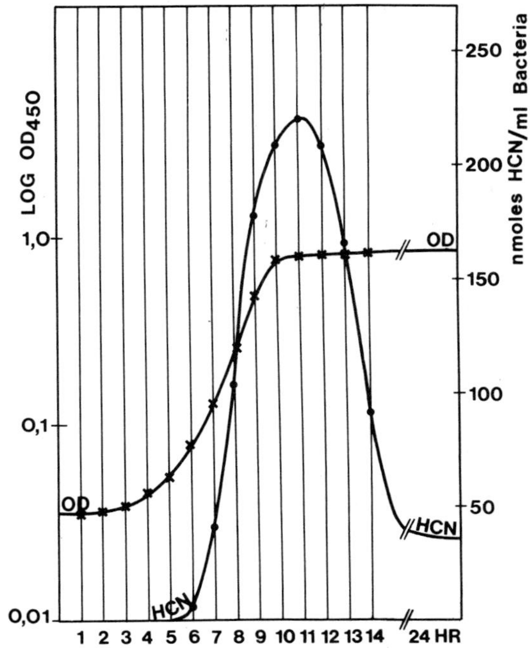

Fig. 4 Growth characteristics and cyanide production of a *Pseudomonad* isolated from a 3-day-old fermenting cassava meal. Substrate, glycine, methionine and succinate.

the growth characteristics and cyanide production of a *Pseudomonad* isolated from three-day old fermenting cassava.

Cassava cyanogens are hydrolysed by the plant enzyme linamarase, a β-glucosidase, during grating prior to fermentation. The question arises as to whether the major fraction of the cyanogens are thus detoxified by this enzyme, or whether microbial β-glucosidase activity also contributes to the hydrolysis of the cyanogens. This question has motivated investigations of the β-glucosidase activities of the microorganisms that ferment cassava. Most of the organisms involved in the fermentation of cassava form β-glucosidases which are able to hydrolyse proacacipetalin, proacaciberin, linamarin, lotaustralin, sambunigrin and amygdalin. The strain of *Pseudomonad* which produces cyanide was investigated with particular respect to the formation of β-glucosidases.

The organism does not form extracellular β-glucosidases capable of hydrolysing ρ-nitrophenyl-, β-galactoside and β-glucoside, but forms intracellular β-glucosidases that hydrolyse these substrates. The enzymes were partially purified by sonication of washed cells and precipitation of nucleic acids from the supernatant with streptomycin sulphate. Two protein fractions were obtained by precipitation with $(NH_4)_2SO_4$ at 40% (A) and 80% (B) saturation. After solubilizing the protein fractions in 0.07 M phosphate buffer pH 6.5 containing 0.3% Triton-X 100, dialysis and fractionation on a Sepharose-CL 6B column, two peaks with β-glucosidase activities could be separated, one in fraction 4 (10 ml) of A and the other in fractions 7 and 8 of B. Figures 5a,b and c show the separation and relative activities of β-glucosidases isolated from the organism. The fractions showing enzyme activities have been further separated into several peaks on DEAE-Sepharose CL 6B. The results of this separation will be published in a future communication elsewhere.

It is apparent that the *Pseudomonad* strain has at least two β-glucosidases with activities against linamarin and lotaustralin. Therefore, cassava linamarase and microbial β-glucosidases probably effect the hydrolysis of cassava cyanogens during grating and under fermentation of cassava meal.

Cassava itself contains the enzyme rhodanese which detoxifies cyanide by the formation of thiocyanate in the presence of sulphur amino acids (Nartey, 1973). It is capable of converting high levels of cyanide into asparagine and glutamate which are subsequently incorporated into protein, carbohydrates, lipids and other cellular components (Nartey, 1969). Thus the function of cyanogenesis in cassava plants may be the preservation of the cyanide group for metabolic activities. It has also been postulated that cyanogenesis in cassava may act as a detergent against ruminants, protect the plant against insects and exert some allellopathic influence against weeds (Swain, 1978).

C. DISEASES ENGENDERED BY CYANOGENESIS IN CASSAVA

Whatever the functions of cyanogenesis in cassava are, incorporation of the edible tuber and fermented tuber products into the diet has been associated with several diseases in the tropics, indicating that it constitutes a serious health hazard (Fig. 6). Cyanogenesis in cassava is known to lead to chronic and acute cyanide toxicities (Nestle, 1973), and the intoxication of cassava cyanogens is known to lead to the accumulation of the goitrogenic detoxification product thiocyanate (Ekpechi, 1973; De Lange, 1973). In the worst cases, the consumption of fermented products of cassava have been suspected of causing the deaths of entire families (Osuntokun, 1980).

Quite apart from the inhibitory activity of cyanide on most enzymes, particularly the terminal cytochrome oxidase of man, prolonged exposure to varying levels of cyanide has been shown to deplete the sulphane pool of the body, lead to vitamin B12 deficiency, cretinism and mental retardation (Dorozynski, 1978; Osuntokun, 1980). Throughout the tropics and subtropics, among island populations,

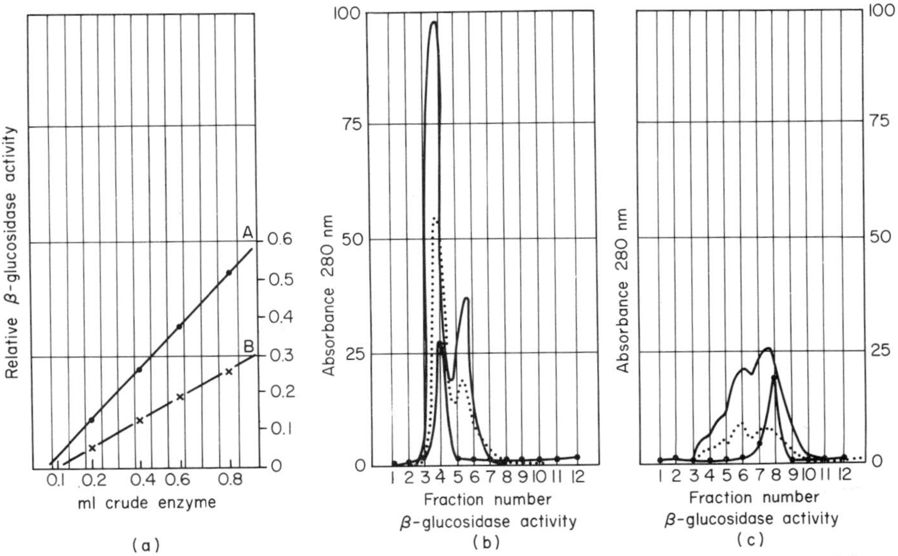

Fig. 5 Separation and activities of 2 β-glucosidases from a cyanide producing *Pseudomonad* isolated from 3-day-old fermenting cassava. (For explanation, see text).

and in parts of Europe and the Middle East, endemic goitre and cretinism have been shown to be due to high intake of cassava-based diets, and cruciferous plant foods which contain high levels of glucosinolate goitrogens (Goldsmith, 1963; Hoskins, 1978; Osuntokun, 1980). Apart from these syndromes, circumstantial evidence has been provided which implicates cassava cyanogens as the causative agents of tropical ataxic neuropathy (Osuntokun, 1980). In certain tropical countries, it appears that various neuropathies may be complicated by nutritional deficiencies as well as genetic predisposition.

The microbiology of indigenous fermentation is not well understood. Since fermented foodstuffs are of paramount importance in the tropics and subtropics, it is essential to identify the organisms that participate in these fermentations and to study their physiology and biochemistry as well as their potentials for synthesizing not only cyanide but other toxins that may occur as contaminants of tropical foodstuffs.

REFERENCES

Abrol, Y,P. (1967). *Ind. J. Exp. Biol.* 5, 191.
Akinrele, I.A. (1964). *J. Sci. Fd. Agric.* 15, 589-594.

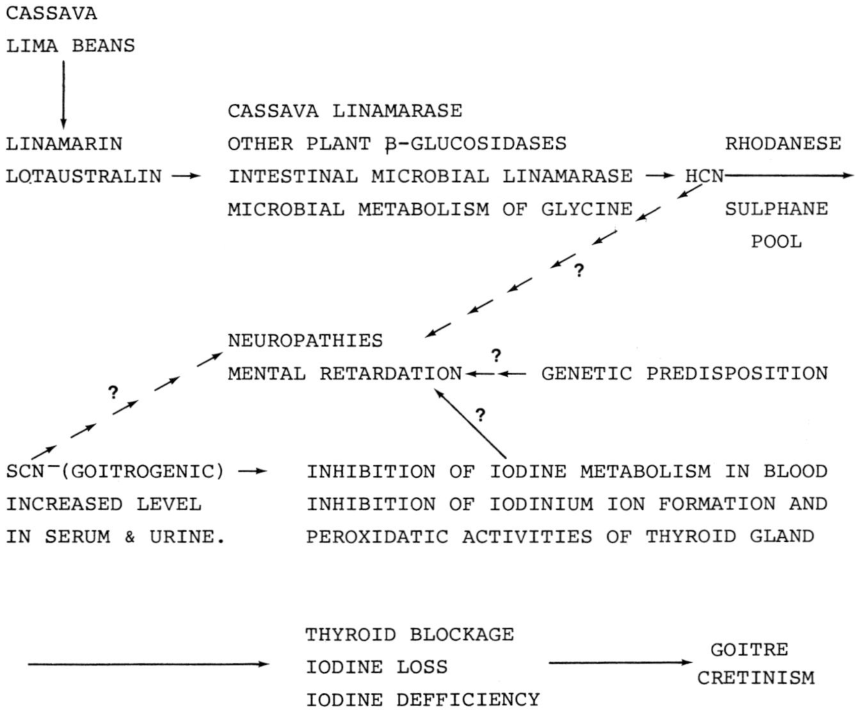

Fig. 6 Possible interrelations of cassava and lima beans linamarin and lotaustralin with goitre, cretinism, neuropathies and mental retardation, indicating areas for future research

Aplin, T.E.H. (1968). Bull. No. 3967. Western Austr. Dept. Agric.
Brimer, L., Nartey, F., Jaroszewski, J.W. and Christiansen, S.B. (1980). *Phytochemistry* (In press).
Butterfield, C., Conn, E.E. and Seigler, D.S. (1975). *Phytochemistry* 14, 993-997.
Butterworth, M.N. (1967). *Nutr. Abst. and Rev.* 37, 349-351.
Buttler, G.W. and Buttler, B.G. (1960). *Nature* 187, 780-781.
Collard, P. and Levi, S. (1959). *Nature* 183, 620-621.
Conn, E.E. and Buttler, G.W. (1969). *In* "Perspectives in Phytochemistry" (J.B. Harborne and T. Swain, eds). Academic Press, London.
Conn, E.E. (1973). *Bioch. Soc. Symp.* 38, 277-302.
Delange, F., Van der Velden, M. and Ermans, A.M. (1973). *In* "Chronic Cassava Toxicity" (B.L. Nestle and R. McIntyre, eds). I.D.R.C. Ottawa, Canada.
Dorozynski, A. (1978). *Nature* 272, 121.
Ekpechi, O.L. (1973). *In* "Chronic Cassava Toxicity" (B.L. Nestle and R. McIntyre, eds). I.D.R.C. Ottawa, Canada.
Ekundayo, J. (1980). *In* "Fungal Biotechnology" (J.E. Smith, D.R. Berry and B. Kristiansen, eds). Academic Press, London.
Epstein, J. (1947). *Anal. Chem.* 19, 272-274.

Erb, N., Zinsmeister, H.D., Lehman, G. and Nahrstedt, A. (1979). *Phytochemistry* 18, 1515-1518.
Ettlinger, M.G., Jaroszewski, J.W., Jensen, S.R., Nielsen, B.J. and Nartey, F. (1977). *J.C.S. Chem. Comm.* 24, 952-953.
Fairbairn, J.W. and Wassell, G. (1964). *Phytochemistry* 3, 253-258.
Gibbs, R.D. (1974). "Chemotaxonomy of Flowering Plants", Vols. I-IV. McGill - Wueen University Press, Montreal, Canada.
Goldsmith, E. (1963). "The Genetics of Migrant and Isolated Populations". Williams and Wilkins Co., Baltimore.
Göhl, B. (1975). "Tropical Feeds". FAO, Rome.
Hoskins, F.H. (1978). *In* "Chemical Toxicology of Food". Elsevier, North Holland, Amsterdam.
Hubel, W. and Nahrstedt, A. (1975). *Phytochemistry* 14, 2723-2725.
Irvine, F.R. (1961). "Woody Plants of Ghana". Oxford University Press, London.
Jones, W.O. (1959). "Manioc in Africa". Stanford University Press. California.
Jørgensen, K. (1955). *Acta Chem. Scand.* 9, 548.
Kartha, K.K. and Gamborg, O.L. (1975). *In* "Cassava Germ Plasma" (B. Nestel and R. McIntyre, eds). I.D.R.C. Ottawa, Canada and C.I.A.T., Colombia.
Kim, J.C. and de Ruiter, D. (1969). *Am. Ass. Cereal Chem.* 185-198.
Knowles, C. (1976). *Bacteriol. Rev.* 40, 652-680.
Montgomery (1969). *In* "Toxic Constituents in Plant Foodstuffs". (I.E. Liener, ed.). Academic Press, London.
Nartey, F. (1968). *Phytochemistry* 7, 1307-1312.
Nartey, F. (1969). *Physiol. Plant.* 22, 1085-1096.
Nartey, F. (1973). *In* "Chronic Cassava Toxicity". (B.L. Nestel and R. McIntyre, eds). I.D.R.C. Ottawa, Canada.
Nartey, F. (1978). "*Manihot esculenta* (Cassava): Cyanogenesis, Ultrastructure and Seed Germination". Munksgaard, Copenhagen.
Nartey, F. (1980a). *In* "Toxicology in the Tropics" (R.L. Smith and E.A. Bababunmi, eds). Taylor and Francis Ltd., London.
Nartey, F., Brimer, L. and Christiansen, S.B. (1981). *Phytochemistry* (In press).
Nestel, B.L. (1973). *In* "Chronic Cassava Toxicity" (B.L. Nestel and R. McIntyre, eds). I.D.R.C. Ottawa, Canada.
Nongoneirma, A. (1977). *Bull. de' I.F.A.N. T. 39 Ser. A. No. 1.*
Okafor, N. (1977). *J. Appl. Bact.* 42, 279-283.
Omole, T.A. (1977). *In* "Cassava as Animal Feed" (B.L. Nestel and M. Graham, eds). I.D.R.C. Ottawa, Canada.
Osuntokun, B.O. (1980). *In* "Toxicology in the Tropics" (C.R.L. Smith and E.A. Bababunmi, eds). Taylor and Francis Ltd., London.
Oyenuga, V.A. (1959). "Nigeria's Feeding-Stuffs: Their Composition and Nutritive Value". Ibadan University Press, Ibadan.
Rimington, C. (1935). *Onderspoort J. Vet. Anim. Ind.* 5, 445-464.
Rogers, D.J. (1959). *Econ. Bot.* 13, 261-263.
Seigler, D.S. (1977). *In* "Progress in Phytochemistry" (L. Reinhold, J.B. Harborne and T. Swain, eds). Vol. 4, pp. 83-120, Pergamon Press, Oxford.
Smith, C.R. Jn., Weileder, D., Miller, R.W., Palmer, I.S. and Olson, O.E. (1980). *J. Org. Chem.* 45, 507.
Standal, B.R. (1979). *In* "Tropical Foods: Chemistry and Nutrition"

(G.E. Inglett and G. Charalambus, eds). Academic Press, London.
Swain, T. (1977). *Ann. Rev. Plant. Phys.* 28, 479-501.
Tschiersch, B. (1966). *Flora* 157, 43-50.
Watt, J.M. and Breyer-Brandwijk, M.G. (1962). "The Medicinal and Poisonous Plants of Southern and Eastern Africa", 2nd edn. E. and S. Livingstone Ltd., Edinburgh and London.
Whiting, M.G. (1963). *Econ. Bot.* 17, 269-302.
Williams, R.J. and Langford, E.M. (1967). "Encyclopedia of Biochemistry", pp. 382-384. Reinhold Publishing Corp., New York.
Wissing, F. (1968). *Physiol. Plant.* 21, 589-593.
Wissing, F. (1974). *J. Bacteriol.* 21, 695-699.
Wissing, F. (1978). "Proc. Europ. Mol. Biol. Workshop on Cyanide Metabolism". University of Kent at Canterbury, England.
Ugochukwu, E.N. (1980). Personal communication.
Ugochukwu, E.N., Opoku, A.R. and Nartey, F. (1981). (To be published).
Zinsmeister, H.D., Erb, N. and Lehman (1980). *Z. Lebensm. Unters. Forsch.* (In press).

CYANOGENIC GLYCOSIDES AND LIPIDS: STRUCTURAL TYPES AND DISTRIBUTION

D.S. SEIGLER

Department of Botany, University of Illinois, Urbana, Illinois 61801, USA

I. INTRODUCTION

Many plants synthesize compounds which are capable of liberating hydrogen cyanide upon hydrolysis. This ability, known as cyanogenesis, has been recognized for centuries in such plants as apricots, peaches, almonds and other important food plants.

Two chemical types, cyanogenic glycosides and cyanolipids are responsible for this cyanophoric capability; both are derivatives of α-hydroxynitriles (cyanohydrins) and both liberate a carbonyl component and hydrogen cyanide when the sugar or the fatty acid moiety respectively is removed. The presence of hydrogen cyanide is readily detected by several simple and reasonably specific color tests (Tantisewie *et al*., 1969; Seigler 1975, 1977); these tests form the basis of most literature reports of cyanogenic plants. The isolation and characterization of cyanogens containing fatty acid moieties, which are much restricted in distribution has recently been reviewed (Mikolajczak, 1977).

Cyanogenic glycosides are known to occur in at least 2050 species of plants representing about 110 families (Gibbs, 1974; Hegnauer, 1977). They are known from ferns, gymnosperms, both monocotyledonous and dicotyledonous angiosperms, fungi, bacteria and several insects. In general, the highest concentrations are found in leaves but compounds of interest may be concentrated in the roots, seeds or other plant tissues. Despite the fact that many plants are known to be cyanogenic, the structures of only about 55 such compounds* have been reported, and the compounds responsible for activity have been studied in only about 200 species of plants. This is largely due to difficulties in isolation and purification, as well as the

---

* This figure excludes the pseudocyanogenic glycosides which are not treated in this review.

inherent instability of the aglycones of some upon hydrolysis. Enzymes within the plant decompose these compounds on damage to the tissues in which they occur. Furthermore, sugars and other glycosides with which they co-occur often make purification difficult. Only three cyanogenic compounds, amygdalin, prunasin and linamarin, are commercially available and reference standards of most others are difficult to obtain.

In the last few years interest in the chemistry and distribution of cyanogens has increased and it is the purpose of this work to review recent developments in the field subsequent to last major published reviews (Seigler, 1977, 1981; Tjon Sie Fat, 1979; Conn, 1979a, b, 1980a, b; Saupe, 1981). In many cases references are made to these reviews rather than to the original works. They should be consulted for background to this review.

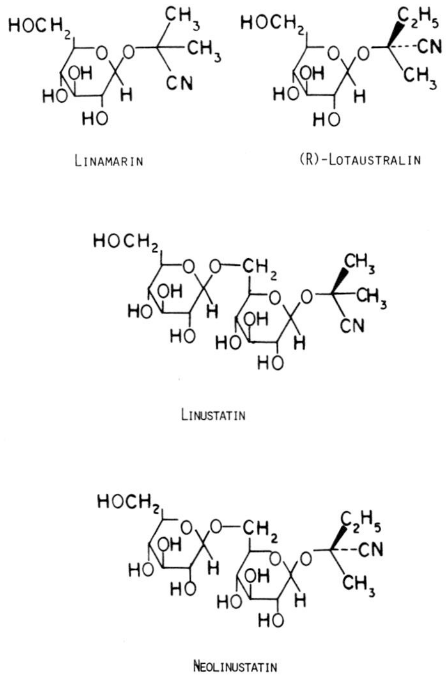

Fig. 1 Cyanogenic glycosides derived from valine and isoleucine

II. CYANOGENS DERIVED FROM VALINE AND ISOLEUCINE

Four cyanogenic glycosides appear to be derived from valine and isoleucine. These are linamarin and lotaustralin and the corresponding gentiobiosides, linustatin and neolinustatin (Fig. 1). The biosynthesis of linamarin and lotaustralin has been studied (Conn, 1979b), but that of linustatin and neolinustatin has not.

Linamarin and lotaustralin with few exceptions occur together although not necessarily in the same ratio. These glucosides occur in approximately 35 species from four families, the Asteraceae (Compositae), Fabaceae (Leguminosae), Euphorbiaceae and Linaceae. Linustatin and neolinustatin are only known from seed meal of flax, *Linum usitatissimum* L. (Smith, Jr. *et al.*, 1979).

The value of cyanogens derived from valine and isoleucine for systematic purposes is limited at the ordinal level but may be chemosystematically significant for understanding familial or infrafamilial (e.g. subfamily, tribe; genus) relationships (van Valen, 1979; Saupe, 1981).

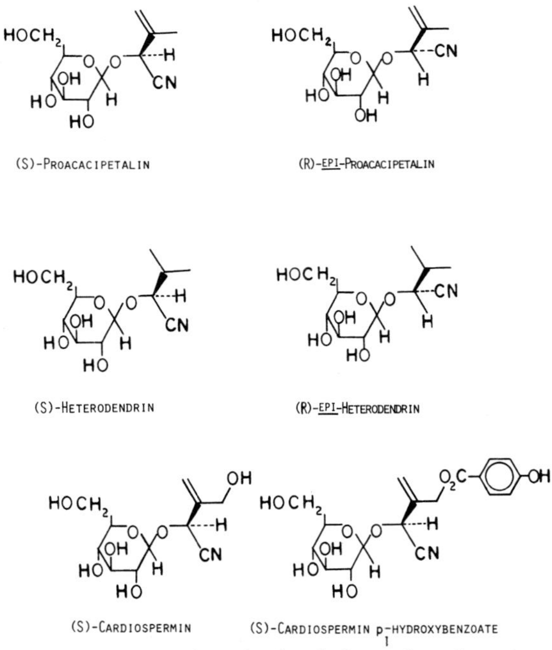

Fig. 2 Cyanogenic glycosides derived from leucine

III. CYANOGENS DERIVED FROM LEUCINE

All seven of the cyanogens derived from leucine are restricted in distribution (Figs. 2 and 3).

They are presently known to occur in the Rosaceae, Poaceae (Gramineae), Sapindaceae and Fabaceae (only in the genus *Acacia*). This pathway is especially prominent in the latter two groups. With the exception of the Poaceae, families synthesizing cyanogens from leucine are

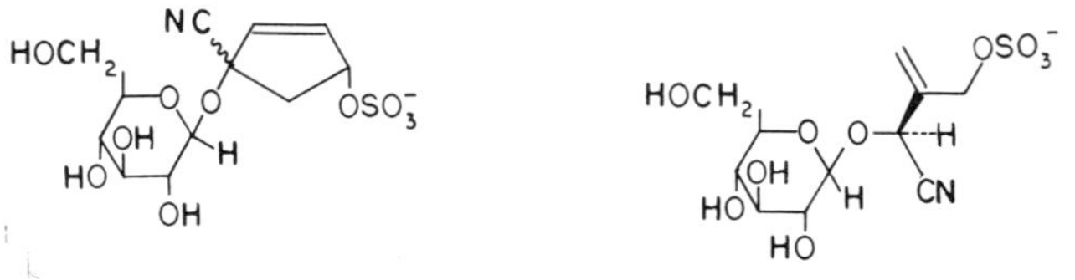

TETRAPHYLLIN B SULFATE

(S)-CARDIOSPERMIN SULFATE

Fig. 3 Sulfate containing cyanogens

generally considered to be closely related (Cronquist, 1968; Thorne, 1976; Saupe, 1981). The determination of structure and configuration of these compounds has been of much recent interest.

The most widespread member of the group, proacacipetalin, occurs in many species of section *Gummiferae* of the genus *Acacia* (Fabaceae: Mimosoideae) (Seigler, 1977, 1981). It has not been reported from other sources.

A related compound, acacipetalin, isolated from *Acacia sieberiana* DC var *woodii* (Burtt Davy) Keay and Brennan (*A. lasiopetala sensu* Steyn and Rimington not oliv.) and *A. hebeclada* DC (*A. stolonifera* Burch) (Steyn and Rimington, 1935; Rimington, 1935) is probably an artifact of isolation. The name acacipetalin has been inappropriately used for the naturally occurring cyanogen (proacacipetalin) (Ettlinger *et al.*, 1977).

Epiproacacipetalin has recently been isolated from *Acacia globulifera* Saff. (Seigler, Dunn, Conn and Pereira, unpublished data).

The saturated compounds corresponding to proacacipetalin and epiproacacipetalin have also been found in nature. (S)-Heterodendrin is known from *Acacia sieberiana* var *woodii* and *Heterodendron oleaefolium* Desf. (Sapindaceae) (Seigler, 1981) whereas (R)-epiheterodendrin is known only from barley (*Hordeum vulgard* L., Poaceae) (Erb *et al.*, 1979).

A series of compounds of this type in which a hydroxyl group occurs in the aglycone moiety is also known. Cardiospermin has been reported from two sapindaceous plants *Cardiospermum hirsutum* Willd. and *Heterodendron oleaefolium* (Seigler, 1981). The *p*-hydroxybenzoate (from *Sorbaria arborea* Schneid, Rosaceae) and the 5-sulfate from *Cardiospermum grandiflorum* Sw. are also known (Nahrstedt, 1976; Hübel and Nahrstedt, 1979).

IV. CYANOLIPIDS

Cyanolipids occur in the seed oils of many Sapindaceous plants. The chemistry and biology of this group of plants has recently been reviewed (Mikolajczak, 1977). The four known compounds of this type (Fig. 4) are all derived from leucine. They differ from cyanogenic glycosides in that the sugar is replaced by fatty acids. These fatty acids

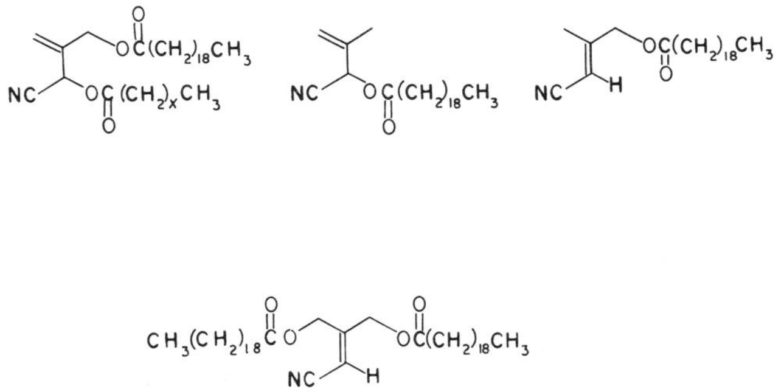

Fig. 4 Cyanolipids presently known from seed oils of the Sapindaceae

vary in chain length and degree of unsaturation. Although they often co-occur all four never are found in a single plant.

The simplest cyanolipid (which corresponds to proacacipetalin in structure) is known only from *Ungnadia speciosa*. A second which corresponds to cardiospermin in structure is more widespread and known from many sapindaceous plants. Two other cyanolipids (which appear to be related by an allylic rearrangement to the previously described compounds) are non-cyanogenic. They are also widespread among sapindaceous plants.

Cyanolipids have been reported from two genera, *Cordia* and *Heliotropium* of the Boraginaceae. Examination of voucher specimens of the *Cordia* collection indicated that the seed specimen was not *Cordia* and was probably a species of *Allophyllus* (Sapindaceae) (Seigler, 1976). The latter report (Ahmad *et al.*, 1979), which is the only reported occurrence of cyanolipids in non-sapindaceous plants, warrants confirmation.

V. CYANOGENS DERIVED FROM PHENYLALANINE

Five cyanogens are derived from phenylalanine (Fig. 5) and two others may possibly originate from this aromatic amino acid (Fig. 6).

These cyanogens occur in at least 44 species from 13 families. The Asteraceae, Fabaceae and Rosaceae are characterized by the production of phenylalanine derived cyanogens (Seigler, 1981; Saupe, 1981).

The disaccharide cyanogens amygdalin, vicianin, and lucumin (all of which have an R-configuration like that of prunasin) are each restricted to a single angiospermous family. Although only found in seeds of the Rosaceae, amygdalin is known from at least 17 species of that family (Saupe, 1980).

The production of cyanogens derived from the phenylalanine pathway is encountered among many families of the

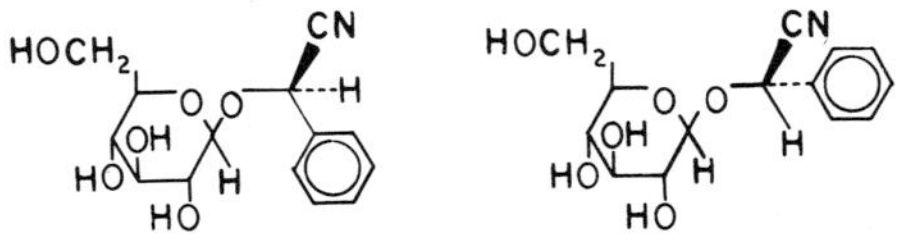

(R)-PRUNASIN (S)-SAMBUNIGRIN

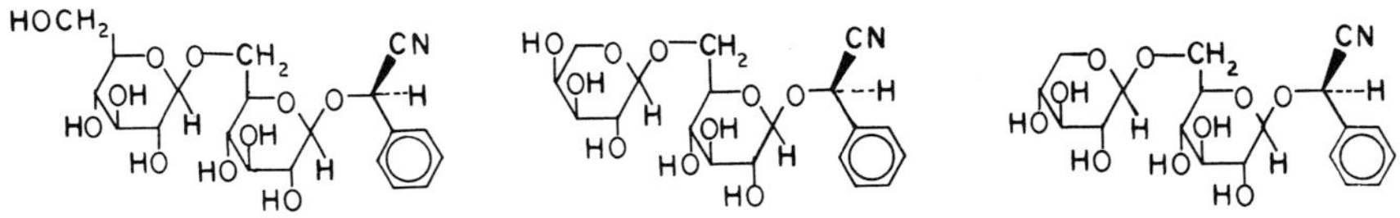

(R)-AMYGDALIN (R)-VICIANIN (R)-LUCUMIN

Fig. 5 Cyanogenic glycosides derived from phenylalanine

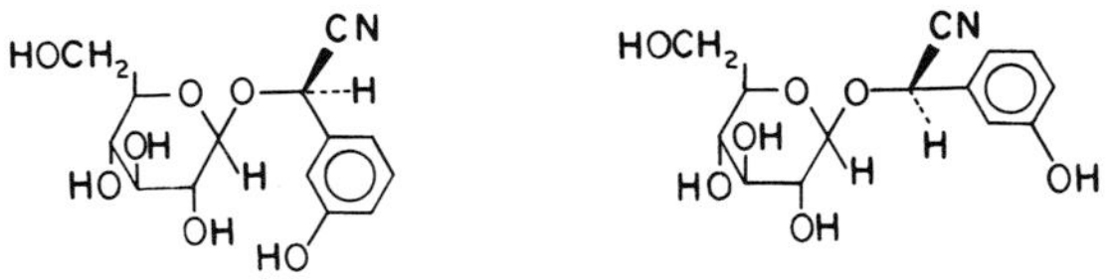

(R)-HOLOCALIN (S)-ZIERIN

Fig. 6 Cyanogenic glycosides probably derived from phenylalanine

Rosidae and Asteridae, the two most advanced subclasses of angiosperms (Cronquist, 1968; Saupe, 1981).

Pteridophytes are also characterized by the presence of cyanogens from this pathway (Hegnauer, 1977; Saupe, 1981).

The origin of holocalin and zierin (Fig. 6) is not clear. These compounds occur in the Fabaceae (*Holocalyx*), Rutaceae (*Zieria*) and Caprifolicaea (*Sambucus*) as well as the monocotyledonous genus *Chlorophytum* (van Valen, 1978a; Seigler, 1981). Hegnauer (1973) and van Valen (1978a) have suggested that holocalin may be synthesized via *m*-hydroxyphenylalanine (*m*-tyrosine). Seigler (1975) suggested that they are derived from phenylalanine, largely because they co-occur with prunasin and/or sambunigrin in *Holocalyx* and *Sambucus*. Clearly, biosynthetic studies are needed.

VI. CYANOGENS DERIVED FROM TYROSINE

Seven cyanogens have been reported that appear to be derived from tyrosine. These occur in at least 80 species belonging to 18 families (Figs. 7 and 8).

The simplest of these, (R)-taxiphyllin and (S)-dhurrin, occur widely in a number of monocotyledonous plants and

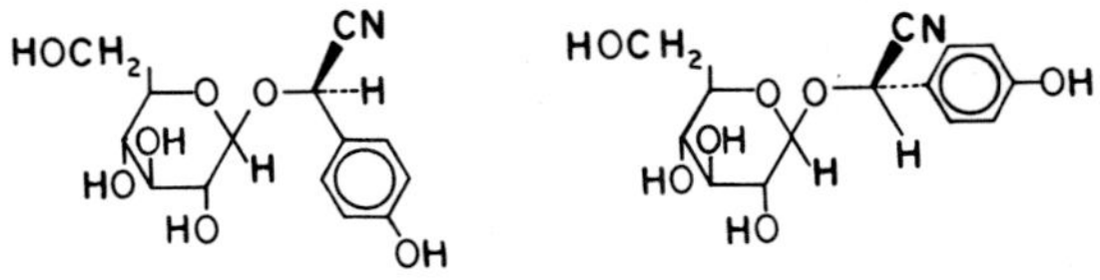

(R)-TAXIPHYLLIN (S)-DHURRIN

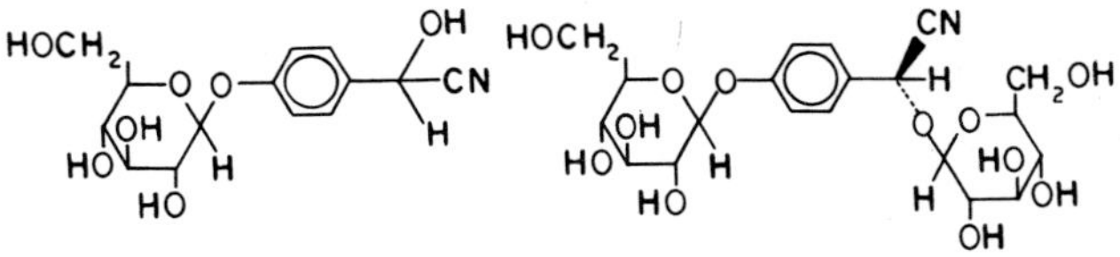

p-GLUCOSYLOXYMANDELONITRILE (S)-PROTEACIN

Fig. 7 Cyanogenic glycosides derived from tyrosine

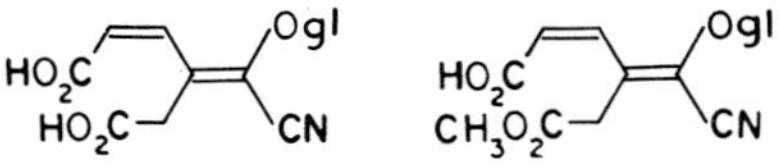

TRIGLOCHININ TRIGLOCHININ METHYL ESTER

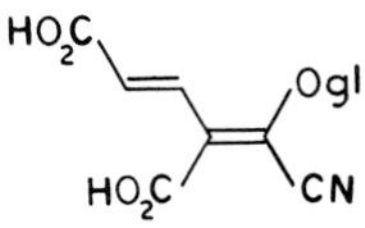

ISOTRIGLOCHININ

Fig. 8 Cyanogens derived from tyrosine which involve opening of the aromatic ring

in several dicotyledonous ones, especially members of the Magnoliidae.

An isomeric monoglycoside corresponding to dhurrin (or taxiphyllin), *p*-glucosyloxymandelonitrile, has been found in the Berberidaceae, (*Nandina domestica* Thunb.), Fabaceae (*Goodia lotifolia* Salisb.) and Ranunculaceae (*Thalictrum* spp.). A disaccharide corresponding to dhurrin, proteacin, occurs in the Proteaceae (*Macadamia* ssp.) and Ranunculaceae (*Thalictrum* spp.).

A second series of cyanogens derived from tyrosine possess structures which arise by opening of the aromatic ring (Fig. 8). Of these, isotriglochinin and trigochinin methyl ester may be artifacts of isolation (Hegnauer, 1977; Seigler, 1981).

The natural occurrence and chemosystematic significance of cyanogens derived from tyrosine is the most completely understood of any group. (Saupe, 1981). The Araceae,

Euphorbiaceae, Juncaginaceae, Magnoliaceae, Platanaceae, Poaceae, Papaveraceae, Berberidaceae, Calycanthaceae and Ranunculaceae are characterized by the production of tyrosine-derived cyanogens.

In dicots, tyrosine-derived cyanogens occur in the Magnoliidae, Hamamelidae, Rosidae, and Asteridae. Moreover, they have been isolated from all of Cronquist's (1968) subclasses of the Liliatae with the exception of the Liliidae (Saupe, 1981).

Monocotyledonous cyanogens are derived almost exclusively from tyrosine (Hegnauer, 1977). To date only two exceptions are known: epiheterodendrin from *Hordeum* (Erb *et al.*, 1979) and holocalin from *Chlorophytum* (Liliaceae, van Valen, 1978a).

The Magnoliidae, generally recognized as the most primitive group of Angiosperms (Cronquist, 1968; Thorne, 1978), is characterized by tyrosine-derived cyanogens (Hegnauer, 1977). All known tyrosine-derived cyanogens occur in this subclass.

The Hamamelidae, a relatively primitive group of woody dicots with highly reduced flowers (Cronquist, 1968) is also characterized by the production of tyrosine-derived cyanogens (Saupe, 1981). Dhurrin and triglochinin occur in the Trochodendraceae (van Valen, 1978b) and Platanaceae (Fikenscher and Ruijgrok, 1977), respectively.

This pathway also occurs sporadically in the Rosidae and Asteridae (Saupe, 1981).

It is generally agreed that the monocots were derived from ancestors resembling primitive dicots (Stebbins, 1974), but there is little agreement as to the ancestral group. The distribution of tyrosine-derived cyanogens strongly suggests that these taxa share a common ancestor (Hegnauer, 1973).

The tyrosine and phenyalanine pathways, which are the only routes of cyanogen formation in gymnosperms and ferns, respectively, probably represent the phylogenetically most ancient pathways of cyanogenesis in angiosperms (Hegnauer, 1977; van Valen, 1979b). The antiquity of the tyrosine pathway is further supported by its occurrence as the sole mechanism of cyanogen biosynthesis in primitive dicots and the predominant one in monocots. The absence of the cyclopentenoid and isoleucine/valine pathways in these taxa, suggest that these pathways are of more recent origin, perhaps arising after the divergence of the monocots (Saupe, 1981).

VII. CYANOGENS WHICH POSSESS A CYCLOPENTENOID NUCLEUS

Another area of current interest is the compounds which possess a cyclopentenoid nucleus (Fig. 9). The only compound with known configuration is gynocardin. This structure

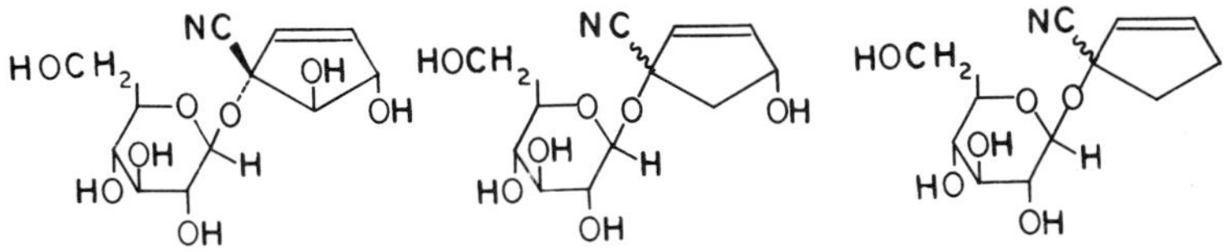

Fig. 9 Cyanogenic glycosides which possess a cyclopentenoid nucleus

has been determined by X-ray crystallography (Coburn and Long, 1966; Kim *et al.*, 1970). Two glucosides with cyclopentene rings, deidaclin and tetraphyllin A possess different NMR spectra and because they both contain glucose, must differ at the cyclopentene chiral center (Seigler, 1975, 1977). The configuration of both compounds is presently unknown. Epitetraphyllin B has recently been reported from an African plant *Adenia volkensii* (Passifloraceae), where it occurs admixed with tetraphyllin B (Gondwe *et al.*, 1978). Thus, at least five compounds are known in the series but configuration has been established for only one, gynocardin.

The cyclopentenoid nucleus is also found in fatty acids such as hydnocarpic acid from seed oils of members of the Flacourtiaceae (Mangold and Spener, 1977). These lipids are only known from this family.

Cyclopentenoid cyanogens, which are presently known only from the Flacourtiaceae, Turneraceae, and Passifloraceae, are extremely valuable phylogenetic markers (Hegnauer, 1977; Saupe, 1981). Gibbs (1965) and Tantisewie *et al.* (1969) have recently reviewed the cyanogens of these families, which are considered by most authorities to be closely related. The value of cyclopentenoid cyanogens at the tribal level has also been reviewed (Hegnauer, 1966).

VIII. FUNGAL CYANOGENS

The presence of cyanogens has been detected in approximately 30 species of fungi (all basidiomycetes) from five families, the Agaricaceae, Cortinariaceae, Polyporaceae, Rhodophyllaceae and the Tricholomataceae (Singer, 1975; Knowles, 1976). Most are found in the Tricholomataceae. To date the only cyanogens isolated from fungi (Fig. 10) are the cyanohydrins of pyruvic acid and glyoxylic acid which were isolated from an unidentified basidiomycete (snow mold) (Tapper and Macdonald, 1974).

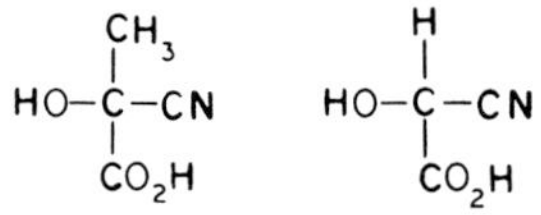

Fig. 10 Fungal cyanogens

ACKNOWLEDGEMENTS

I wish to thank E.E. Conn, A. Nahrstedt, W. Hübel, J.E. Dunn and S. Saupe for discussions. I further wish to acknowledge financial support by the National Science Foundation (NSF-PCM-7725767).

REFERENCES

Ahmad, I., Ansari, A.A. and Osman, S.M. (1978). *Chem and Ind.* 61-62.
Coburn, R.A. and Long, L. (1966). *J. Org. Chem.* 31, 4312-4315.
Conn, E.E. (1979). *In* "Herbivores" (G.A. Rosenthal and D.H. Janzen, eds). pp. 387-412. Academic Press, New York.
Conn, E.E. (1979b). *Naturwiss.* 66, 28-34.
Conn, E.E. (1980a). *In* "Secondary Plant Products" (Encyclopedia of Plant Physiology, Vol. 8) (E.A. Bell and B.V. Charlwood, eds). pp. 461-492. Springer Verlag, Berlin.
Conn, E.E. (1980b). *Ann. Rev. Physiol.* 31, 433-451.
Cronquist, A. (1968). "The Evolution and Classification of Flowering Plants". Houghton Mifflin, Boston.
Erb, N., Zinsmeister, H.D., Lehmann, G. and Nahrstedt, A. (1979). *Phytochemistry* 18, 1515-1517.
Ettlinger, M.G., Jaroszewski, J.W., Jensen, S.R., Nielsen, B.J. and Nartey, F. (1977). *Chem. Comm.* 952-953.
Fikenscher, L.H. and Ruijgrok, H.W.L. (1977). *Planta Medica* 31, 290-293.
Gibbs, R.D. (1965). *Lloydia* 28, 279-299.
Gibbs, R.D. (1974). "Chemotaxonomy of Flowering Plants" 4 Vols. McGill-Queen's University Press, Montreal.
Gondwe, A., Seigler, D.S. and Dunn, J.E. (1978). *Phytochemistry* 17, 271-274.
Hegnauer, R. (1973). *Biochem, Syst.* 1, 191-197.
Hegnauer, R. (1977). *Plant Syst. Evol., Suppl. 1*, 191-209.
Hübel, W. and Nahrstedt, A. (1979). *Tet. Lett.* 45, 4395-4396.
Kim, H.S., Jeffrey, G.A., Panke, D., Clapp, R.C., Coburn, R.A. and Long, L., Jr. (1970). *Chem. Comm.* 381-382.
Knowles, C.J. (1976). *Bacteriological Reviews* 40, 652-680.
Mangold, H.K. and Spener, F. (1977). *In* "Lipids and Lipid Polymers in Higher Plants" (M. Tevini and H.K. Lichtenthaler, eds). pp. 85-101. Springer Verlag, New York.
Mikolajczak, K.L. (1977). *Prog. Chem. Fats Other Lipids* 15, 97-130.
Nahrstedt, A. (1976). *Z. Naturforsch.* 31, 397-400.
Rimington, C. (1935). *Onderstepoort J. Vet. Sci. Anim. Ind.* 5, 445-465.

Saupe, S.G. (1981). *In* "Phytochemistry and Angiosperm Phylogeny" (D.A. Young and D.S. Seigler, eds). Praeger Press, New York.
Seigler, D.S. (1975). *Phytochemistry* 14, 9-29.
Seigler, D.S. (1977). *In* "Progress in Phytochemistry" (L. Reinhold, J.G. Harborne and T. Swain, eds). Vol. 4, pp. 83-120. Pergamon Press, Oxford.
Seigler, D.S. (1981). *Rev. Latinoam. Quim.* 12, 39-48.
Seigler, D.S. and Kawahara, W. (1976). *Biochem. Syst. Ecol.* 4, 263-265.
Singer, R. (1975). "The Agaricales in Modern Taxonomy", 3rd edn. J. Cramer, Vaduz.
Smith, C.R., Jr., Weisleder, D., Palmer, I.S. and Palmer, O.E. (1980). *J. Org. Chem.* 45, 507-510.
Stebbins, G.L. (1974). "Flowering Plants. Evolution Above the Species Level". Belknap Press of Harvard Univ. Press, Cambridge, Mass.
Steyn, D.B. and Remington, C. (1935). *Onderstepoort J. Vet. Sci. Anim. Ind.* 4, 51-63.
Tantisewie, B., Ruijgrok, H.W.L. and Hegnauer, R. (1969). *Pharm. Weekbl.* 104, 1341-1355.
Tapper, B.A. and Macdonald, M.A. (1974). *Can. J. Microbiol.* 20, 563-566.
Thorne, R.F. (1976). *In* "Evolutionary Biology" (M. Hecht, W. Steere and B. Wallace, eds) Vol. 9. Plenum Press, New York.
Tjon Sie Fat, L. (1979). Contribution to the Knowledge of Cyanogenesis in Angiosperms (Cyanogene Verbindingen buj Poaceae, Commelinaceae, Ranunculaceae en Companulaceae). Diss. R.U. Leiden.
van Valen, F. (1978a). *Proc. Koninkl. Nederl. Akad. Wetensch., Ser. C* 81, 132-140.
van Valen, F. (1978b). *Proc. Koninkl. Nederl. Akad. Wetensch., Ser. C* 81, 198-203.
van Valen, F. (1979a). *Planta Med.* 35, 141-145.
van Valen, F. (1979b). Contribution to the Knowledge of Cyanogenesis in Angiosperms. Diss. R.U. Leiden.

ISOLATION AND STRUCTURE ELUCIDATION OF CYANOGENIC GLYCOSIDES

ADOLF NAHRSTEDT

Institut für Pharmazeutische Biologie der Technischen Universität, D-3300 Braunschweig, West Germany

I. INTRODUCTION

In the last ten to twenty years the increased interest in cyanogenic compounds has led to better analytical procedures. Among these sample preparation, conditions of extraction, methods in gas chromatography (GLC), high pressure liquid chromatography (HPLC) and proton magnetic resonance (^{1}H-NMR) have been fully developed. Besides older summaries (Seifert, 1955; Dilleman, 1958) there are some excellent reviews in the last decade covering the cyanogenic glycosides (Eyjólfsson, 1970a; Seigler, 1975a,b) and cyanolipids (Mikolajczak, 1977) which contain much information on methods of isolation and structure elucidation. The present paper on cyanogenic glycosides reviews the literature through 1979 on the most useful of these methods together with our own experience in this field.

II. SAMPLE PREPARATION AND EXTRACTION

Structure elucidation involves the isolation of substances which are normally extracted from crude plant or animal material. Cyanogenic glycosides require special attention as most of them are not particularly stable, and isomerization and decomposition must be avoided during isolation. The normal way is to extract material which has been air dried carefully. However, one may have to accept loss in glycoside content because hydrolyzing enzymes (glucosidases) become active after damage to the plant material. In some plants (e.g. *Heterodendron oleaefolium*, Hübel, 1978) which contain high levels of tannins the activity of glucosidases is reduced. Some workers extract fresh plant material, which is sometimes frozen, and inactivate the hydrolyzing enzymes during extraction. In this case cold or hot methanol or ethanol (e.g. Gondwe *et al.*, 1978, for tetraphyllin; Gmelin *et al.*, 1973, for holocalin; Jensen and Nielsen,

1973, for sambunigrin; Butterfield *et al.*, 1975, for acacipetalin) have been used as extracting media. Sometimes formic or acetic acid (Reay, 1969, for dhurrin; Schwarzmaier, 1976, for taxiphyllin) have been combined with the alcohol. Aqueous perchloric acid (Bough and Gander, 1971, for dhurrin) and even hot water (e.g. Eyjólfsson, 1970b, for triglochinin) have also been used (Fig. 1). Extraction of fresh plant material is possible only if the plants are available near the laboratory. Since this cannot be realized in every case a suitable alternative method is to collect plants and place them directly in liquid nitrogen or dry ice, grind them under liquid nitrogen or dry ice in the lab and dry the resulting powder in a frozen condition by lyophilization (e.g. Nahrstedt, 1970, 1976a, b; Hübel and Nahrstedt, 1979). The material prepared in this manner is ready for extraction or can be stored for a long time at -18°C.

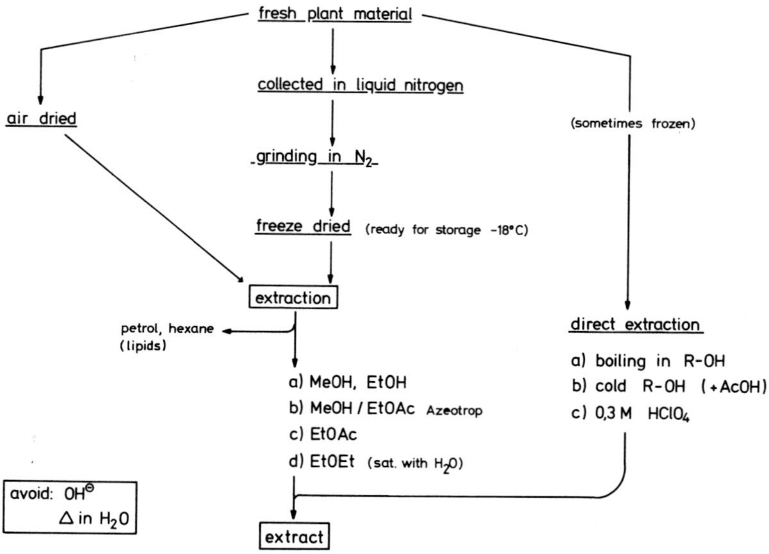

Fig. 1 Different ways of extracting fresh or dried plant material in order to obtain an extract containing cyanogenic glycosides

Dry material should be extracted first with petroleum ether to remove lipophilic compounds. Then, depending on the glycoside involved, different solvents are possible. Since all cyanogenic glycosides are rather polar substances, methanol or ethanol are excellent solvents. An azeotropic mixture of methanol and ethylacetate reduces the extraction temperature and avoids extraction of large amounts of polar substances such as sugars, some amino acids and peptides

(Nahrstedt, 1971). Cardiospermin-5-O-(4-hydroxy)-benzoate, for instance, is extractable with pure ethylacetate (Nahrstedt, 1976a), and prunasin with diethylether saturated with water. This latter method also allows the separation of prunasin from amygdalin, which is not soluble in this solvent (Trim, 1955). Even at this stage isolation has to be performed carefully to avoid decomposition, isomerization or derivatization of some cyanogenic glycosides.

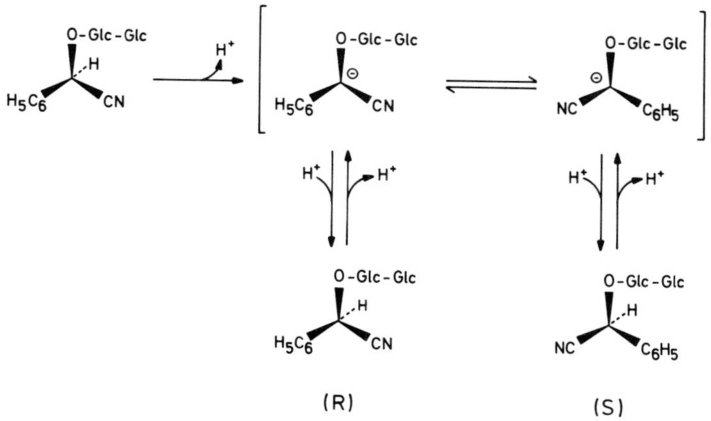

Fig. 2 Mechanism of epimerization of amygdalin (Nahrstedt, 1975c)

In the presence of small amounts of alkali epimerization occurs at the chiral centre of aglycones which have an acidic hydrogen attached at the cyanohydrin carbon (Nahrstedt, 1975c, for mandelonitrile glycosides; Ettlinger *et al.*, 1977, for proacacipetalin). The isomerization proceeds via a carbanion after elimination of the cyanohydrin proton (Fig. 2, Nahrstedt, 1975c; Turczan and Medwick, 1979). Reagents that cause epimerization are $Ba(OH)_2$-water, dilute concentrations of $Ca(OH)_2$ (resulting from an excess addition of $CaCO_3$ to aqueous extracts in order to neutralize plant acids), 0.005 N NH_4OH (Beilstein, 1938), and 0.7% triethylamine (Ettlinger *et al.*, 1977). Epimerization may even occur upon heating in aqueous solution (Nahrstedt, 1975c). Similarly epiheterodendrin was observed to epimerize upon standing in ethanol for several weeks (Erb *et al.*, 1979). This may be why epimeric pairs of glycosides are sometimes found in the same plant.

In the case of the *p*-hydroxymandelonitrile glucosides, decomposition occurs under alkaline conditions or simply upon heating in water and glucose, cyanide and *p*-hydroxybenzaldehyde are produced (Mao and Anderson, 1965; Schwarzmaier, 1976b). Another unstable cyanogenic glucoside is *p*-glucosyloxymandelonitrile (Abrol *et al.*, 1966; Sharples and Stoker, 1968) where the cyanohydrin group is not stabilized by glucosylation; these compounds are more stable in acidic solution. Triglochinin also decomposes in hot solvents and liberates cyanide.

Esterification of triglochinin, a strong dicarboxylic acid, may occur during extraction with boiling methanol. Hegnauer (pers. communication) could not isolate methyl-triglochinin from carefully prepared extracts of *Thalictrum aquilegifolium*, the original source of the methylester as reported by Sharples *et al*. (1972). Consequently, triglochinin-monomethylester is believed to be an artefact of the isolation procedure. There is evidence that isotriglochinin - often found in triglochinin preparations - is also an artificial product: cold isolated triglochinin-preparations did not show the typical signals of the trans protons in the ^{1}H-NMR-spectrum (Nahrstedt, 1975). Recently we have studied the stability of highly purified triglochinin in water at 40°C (Nahrstedt, 1979 unpublished). After about 20 h (Fig. 3), there are nearly 66% triglochinin, 30% iso-triglochinin and 4% of a third triglochinin isomer (see also Section VI.D.4). This indicates that triglochinin isomerizes under normal temperature conditions in water, and therefore small amounts of isotriglochinin may occur in the vacuole of the plant.

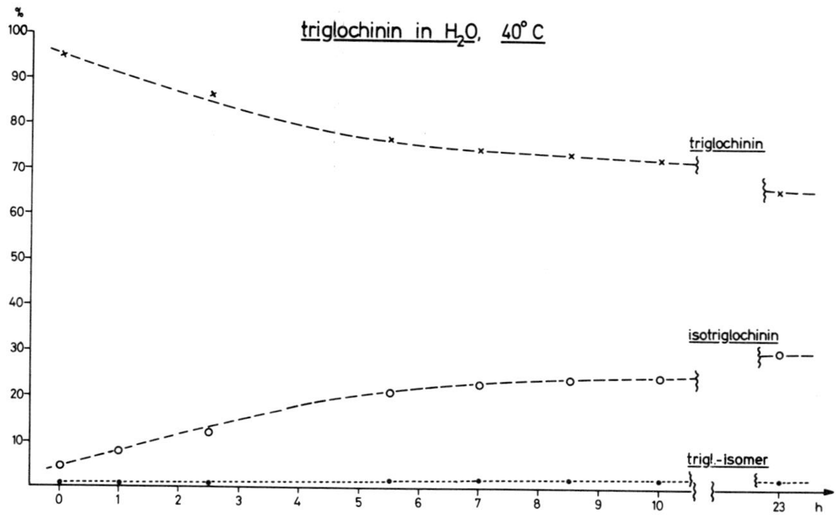

Fig. 3 Formation of isotriglochinin and a third triglochinin isomer from triglochinin dissolved in water (Nahrstedt, unpubl.).

III. PURIFICATION

During the purification of cyanogenic glycosides the main

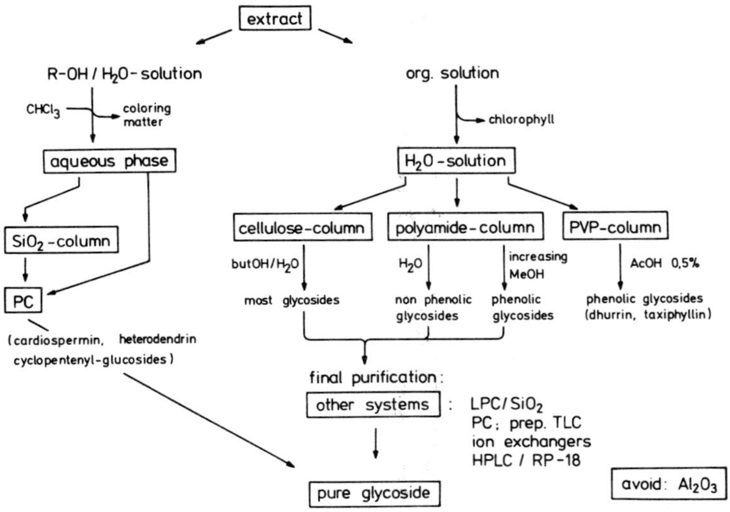

Fig. 4 Different ways of purifying cyanogenic glycosides from a crude extract

classes of compounds to be removed are sugars and glycosides of flavonoids, anthocyanins and related polar substances. There are several approaches that have been used successfully which can be summarized by the two general models shown (Fig. 4). The first starts from an extract obtained normally with water containing alcohols (Fig. 4, left side). Colouring matter is removed by chloroform treatment of the extract diluted with more water. These waste phases have to be controlled in every case for cyanogenesis. Chromatography by different systems, mainly paper chromatography sometimes combined with low pressure chromatography (LPC) on silica gel columns, often yields acceptably pure glycosides. In this manner cyclopentenyl glucosides (e.g. Gondwe *et al.*, 1978), cardiospermin (Seigler *et al.*, 1974) or heterodendrin (dihydroacacipetalin; Seigler *et al.*, 1975) were obtained in relatively pure forms.

Another approach (Fig. 4, right side) makes use of a change of solvent from an organic to an aqueous phase in order to remove most of the chlorophylls. In the next step the concentrated aqueous phase is chromatographed by LPC on different columns, such as cellulose, polyamide or polyvinylpyrrolidone (PVP). In the case of hydroxylated mandelonitrile glucosides such as dhurrin/taxiphyllin, pure substances are obtained by one step chromatography on a PVP column with weakly acidified water as the solvent (Reay, 1969). Also extracts of *Sorbaria spec.* which contain other cyanogenics as well as cardiospermin-5-O-(4-hydroxy)-benzoate can be purified using these systems (Nahrstedt and Scheid, 1981). Non-phenolic glycosides are eluted with water from polyamide in the solvent front. Phenolic substances such as flavonoids are retained on the column. This is a well proven way to get colourless fractions, but they still may contain sugars. By following this procedure with chromatographic systems, LPC on silica gel, paper chromatography (PC) or high pressure liquid chromatography (HPLC) on reversed phases (Section V,C) one normally can obtain pure substances. At this stage triglochinin can be purified by an anion exchange column with increasing concentration of acetic acid (Eyjólfsson, 1970b; Nahrstedt, 1975a).

The cardiospermin-5-O-(4-hydroxy)benzoate is also retaine on polyamide. By increasing the amounts of methanol in wate sugars are eluted first while phenolic material remains uneluted at the origin. The cyanogenic glucoside can be obtained in an intermediate fraction and then rechromatographed on silica gel (Nahrstedt, 1976a).

A useful but not very selective system is cellulose with butanol/water as a solvent. This system permits separation of nearly all cyanogenic glycosides from most of their contaminants. However, cardiospermin-5-O-sulphate (Hübel and Nahrstedt, 1979) is strongly retained on cellulose when there are high proportions of butanol in the solvent, as are flavonoid sulphates (Harborne and Williams, 1975). In every case a final purification with other chromatographic methods is necessary.

Systems that have found minor use in purification are the sephadexes (Pifferi, 1966; Gondwe *et al.*, 1978), charcoal (Towers *et al.*, 1964) and recently HPLC especially on reversed phases (see Section V.C). Aluminium oxide is probably not an appropriate stationary phase as it appears that isomerization of sambunigrin occurs during chromatography on this material (Schwarzmaier, 1975a). Preparative GLC of cyanogenic glycosides as their TMS-ethers is also an unsuitable method as the TMS-ethers produce strongly stabilized aerosols which are difficult to condense (Bissett *et al.*, 1969; Nahrstedt, 1971).

Column eluates are monitored by a wide spectrum of techniques. Of these detection of cyanogenesis within the collected fractions is the most useful since it is sensitive as well as specific and avoids masking of cyanogenics when large amounts of impurities are present. A suitable test involves the Feigl-Anger-test-paper (Tantisewie *et al.* 1969) for cyanide detection and crude enzyme preparations or emulsin as a hydrolysing agent in small test vials (see also Section V.A).

The relatively pure glycosides obtained by these methods of purification seldom crystallize and often are freeze-dried from a membrane-filtered, aqueous solution. As a precaution they should be stored under refrigeration. Fortunately, crystallization is not absolutely necessary in order to apply most of the modern physical methods for characterization and to degrade the glycosides. On the other hand, the melting point and optical rotation of the easily prepared peracetates, (for preparation see e.g. Davis and Nahrstedt, 1979), which usually crystallize readily, are useful constants as the crystals are generally very pure, the melting point is sharp and it is possible to distinguish (*R*)- and (*S*)-forms (Table I).

IV. DEGRADATION

Pure glycosides are normally degraded in order to recognize their subunits. The main methods of degradation involve hydrolysis by enzymes (e.g. Tantisewie *et al.*, 1969) or by dilute acids at elevated temperatures or in special cases by u.v.-irradiation (Takaishi *et al.*, 1977). Typical products are a carbonyl compound (aldehyde or ketone), a sugar and hydrogen cyanide (HCN) (Figs. 5A and C).

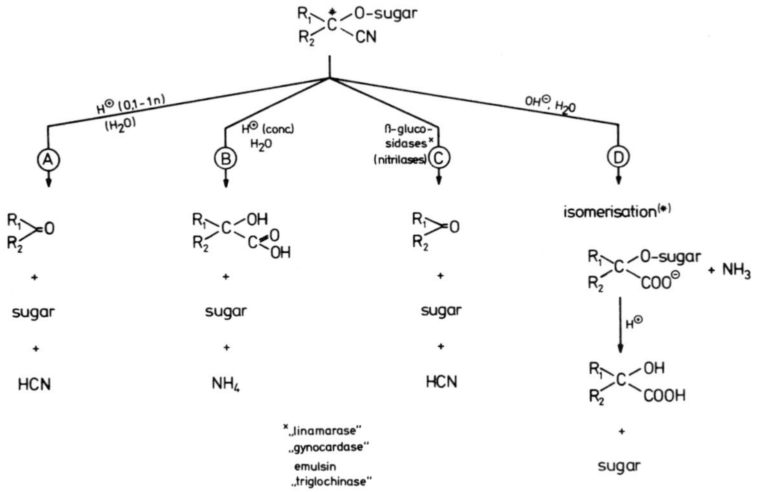

Fig. 5 Reactions for the degradation of cyanogenic glycosides useful for elucidation of their structure

A. HYDROGEN CYANIDE

The production of HCN is mainly used for qualitative detection of cyanogenic substances in plant material, on thin layer plates, or in column-eluates as well as for quantitative estimation of total cyanoglycoside content. There are several sensitive, and more or less specific, colour reactions for HCN that can be used both for rapid qualitative tests and quantitative estimation. The last review of these methods is that of Zitnak (1973). For the frequently used Guignard-Mirande-test (Mirande, 1909; technique see Seigler

Table I Melting points and optical rotation of cyanogenic glycosides and their peracetates. *, synthetic; **, partly isomerized (Nahrstedt, 1973c); ***, solvent not considered.

substance	underivatized: m.p. [°C]	$[\alpha]_D$***	t[°C]	as peracetate: m.p. [°C]	$[\alpha]_D$***	t[°C]	references
1. prunasin	15o-151	-3o.1	28	139-14o	-24	2o	Fischer and Bergmann (1917), Eyjolfsson (1968)
2. sambunigrin	151-152	-76.1	2o	125-126	-52.5	22	Fischer and Bergmann (1917), Karrer (1958)
3. amygdalin	215-22o	-42	18	171-172	-37.6		Beilstein (1938)
4. neoamygdalin	212	-59.2	26	174	-65.6		Beilstein (1938)
5. lucumin	184-185	-5o.5	2o	138-139			Eyjólfsson (1971)
6. vicianin	175-176	-2o.o	2o	17o-171	-29.6	2o	Eyjólfsson (1968)
7. p-glucosyloxy-mandelonitril	157-158 16o-164*			144-145			Mauthner (1912) Sharples and Stoker (1969)
8. proteacin	1o2-1o4			181-183 (2o8-2o9) remelted			from Seigler (1975)
9. taxiphyllin	168-169	-66.7	2o	144-144.8	-22.1	2o	Towers et al. (1964)
1o. dhurrin	163-165	-64	28	132-132.5	-5o.5	2o	Towers et al. (1964),Mao et al. (1965)
11. holocalin**	154-155	-59.1	2o				Gmelin et al. (1973)
12. zierin	153-156	-29.5	2o	115-118			Finnmore and Cooper (1936)

13. linamarin	143–144	-28.5	32	14o–141	-1o.8	14	Clapp et al. (1966); Fischer and Anger (1919)
14. lotaustralin	123.5–124.5	-19.15	25	116–116.5	- 2.88	28	Bissett et al. (1969)
15. epilotaustralin	117.5–118.5	-34.59	23	121–121.5	- 6.75	28	Bissett et al. (1969)
16. linustatin	123–123.5	-37	25	183.5–184.5			Smith et al. (198o)
17. neolinustatin	19o–192	-37	25	171.5–173			Smith et al. (198o)
18. proacacipetalin				112–113.5	-37	22	Ettlinger et al. (1977)
19. acacipetalin	176–177	-36.6	26	1o4	-16.2	26	Steyn and Rimington (1935)
2o. heterodendrin				1o6–1o8	-37.1	2o	Hübel (1978)
21. epiheterodendrin				144			Erb et al. (1979)
22. cardiospermin				1o1–1o2.5	-28.9	2o	Hübel (1978)
23. cardiospermin-5-O-(4-OH)-benzoate		-39.3	2o	137–138			Nahrstedt (1976)
24. tetraphyllin A	116–118	-14	25	1o8–1o9	- 2.o	25	Russell and Reay (1971)
25. deidaclin	127–128	-2o.4	27				Clapp et al. (197o)
26. tetraphyllin B	169–17o	-35.6	25	114–115	-25	25	Russell and Reay (1971)
27. barterin	157–158	-78					Paris et al. (1969)
28. gynocardin	165–166	+72.9	28	119–12o	+4o.2	25	Coburn and Long (1966)

et al., 1974), a critical survey is given by L.M. Larsen (1978) and L.M. Larsen and H. Sørensen (in prep.). Of all the tests available, that of Feigl and Anger (Feigl and Anger, 1966; technique see Tantisewie *et al.*, 1969) seems to be the most definite and sensitive of the quick tests although not absolutely specific. Methods of quantitative estimation of cyanide are referred to by Wissing and by Nahrstedt *et al.* in this volume.

B. SUGAR COMPONENTS

Detection of sugars normally is done by known TLC, PC or GLC methods. Some workers use the highly specific glucose oxidase method (Paris *et al.*, 1969) and glucose test strips (Gmelin *et al.*, 1973; Erb *et al.*, 1979). In the relatively rare cases of diglycosides, partial acidic hydrolysis to an intermediate monoglucoside was performed with lucumin (Eyjólfsson, 1971) and amygdalin (Takaishi *et al.*, 1977), and enzymatically with linustatin and neolinustatin (Smith *et al.*, 1980; Hegnauer, pers. comm.). In the latter case only the terminal glucose is split off by emulsin.

Since all known cyanogenic glycosides release only one molecule of cyanide, one obtains information about the length of the sugar side chain from a quantitative estimation of sugar/cyanide ratio.

C. CARBONYL COMPONENTS

Volatile carbonyl compounds obtained on hydrolysis of cyanogenic glycosides may be obtained by distillation as described by Butterfield *et al.* (1975), or by microdiffusion in a Conway chamber (technique see van Valen, 1979) as their 2,4-dinitrophenylhydrazones. In the case of non-volatile carbonyls, hydrolysis can be performed in the presence of the 2,4-dinitrophenylhydrazine reagent. The hydrazones are identifiable by different constants such as melting point, optical rotation, by TLC using differentiating spray reagents (Mehlitz *et al.*, 1963), GLC (Kallio, 1972, and lit. cited there), and ^{1}H-NMR-spectroscopy. However, some glycosides do not produce stable carbonyl compounds. These include cardiospermin and its derivatives, from which the theoretically expected 2-hydroxymethyl-propen-al was not detected (Seigler *et al.*, 1974; Nahrstedt, 1976a; Hübel and Nahrstedt, 1979). From the literature on cyanolipids type I, (for review see Mikolajczak, 1977), which have a nitrile-component identical to the aglycone of cardiospermin (see D.S. Seigler, this volume), one can assume that five membered methylhydroxylactones arise from complete hydrolysis of the aglycone. Another glycoside which does not yield a stable carbonyl on hydrolysis is triglochinin. Instead a ketene is produced which in turn yields a tricarboxylic acid, triglochinic acid, in aqueous solution (Eyjólfsson, 1970b,c). Acacipetalin yields α-keto isovaleric acid (Steyne and Rimington, 1935). The cyclopentenylglucosides seem to react differently, since tetraphyllin B (Russel and Reay, 1971) and deidaclin (Clapp *et al.*, 1970) result in the expected ketones whereas barterin (Paris *et al.*, 1969), gynocardin (Coburn and Long, 1966) and tetraphyllin A (Russel and Reay, 1971) do not.

D. β-GLUCOSIDASES

Some workers have used the more or less pronounced specificity of β-glucosidase-preparations which act on cyanogenic glycosides as a criterion for identification of the compound and even for its configuration at C-2. According to Hegnauer *et al.* emulsin is more active for mandelonitrile glycosides with the (*R*) configuration at C-2 than those with (*S*) configuration. The enzyme also is more reactive with aromatic glycosides than with the aliphatic ones and the cyclopentenylglucosides (Tjon Sie Fat, 1977). This technique has also been employed with TLC-plates (Fikenscher and Hegnauer, 1977). "Linamarase" prepared according to Coop (1940) hydrolysis linamarin three times faster than lotaustralin, whereas "gynocardase" (preparation according to Coop, 1940, from *Hydnocarpus*; see Tantisewie *et al.*, 1969) cleaves linamarin slightly faster than lotaustralin (van Valen, 1979). As expected "gynocardase" prefers cyclopentenylglucosides to mandelonitrile glycosides (Tantisewie *et al.*, 1969). A β-glucosidase with high selectivity for triglochinin has been isolated from *Alocasia* leaves (Hösel and Nahrstedt, 1975). This enzyme, sometimes called "triglochininase", was successfully employed in characterizing triglochinin in several plants (e.g. Fikenscher and Ruijgrok, 1977; van Valen, 1978a, c; Tjon Sie Fat, 1979). A survey on crude enzymes used for hydrolysis of cyanogenic glycosides is given by Seigler (1975a). W. Hösel reviews this subject in detail in this volume.

E. α-HYDROXY ACIDS

Hydrolysis of glycosides in concentrated acids (e.g. 36% hydrochloric acid) yields α-hydroxy acids with retention of configuration at the chiral centre at C-2 of the aglycone (Fig. 5B). This is an important reaction since one is able to establish the configuration of the aglycone by correlation or by measurement of the optical rotation of the resulting acid. This procedure has been employed with some mandelonitrile glycosides (Kofod and Eyjólfsson, 1969). and lotaustralin (Bisset *et al.*, 1969). For these reactions normally 20-25 mg of substance are necessary. The (*S*) configuration for heterodendrin and proacacipetalin was determined with 5-10 mg of material (Nahrstedt and Hübel, 1978; Hübel and Nahrstedt, 1978) by hydrolysing the glucosides to the corresponding α-hydroxyl-3-methyl-butyric acid. Proacacipetalin was previously hydrogenated to "dihydroproacacipetalin". The acids were esterified with (-)

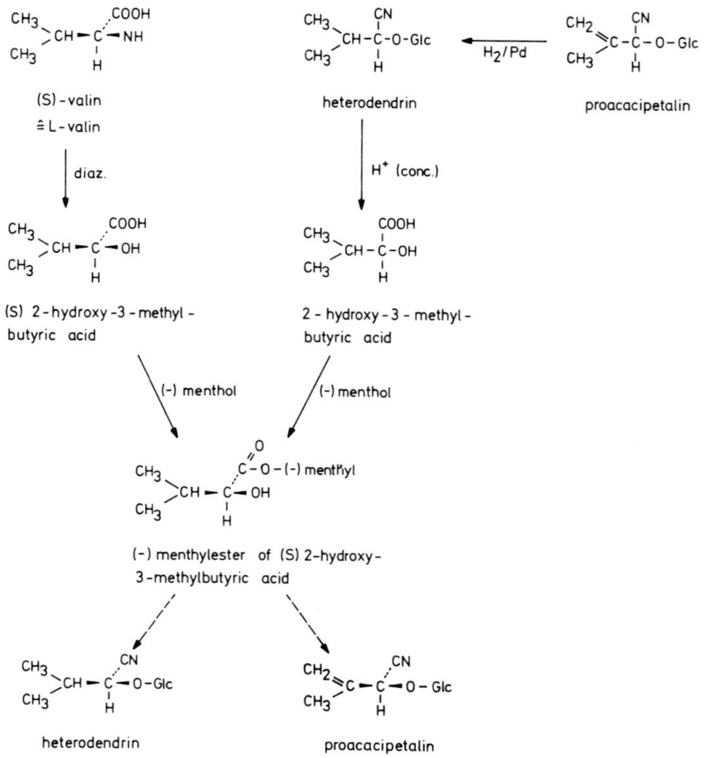

Fig. 6 Degradation of heterodendrin and proacacipetalin to the corresponding α-hydroxy acids whose configurations were established by correlation GLC

menthol and the resulting ester had an identical retention time in GLC analysis with that of the known (*S*)α-hydroxy-3-methyl-butyric acid prepared from valine (Fig. 6). In this way the (*S*) configuration was established for this series of glucosides.

Another reaction (Fig. 5D) using strong bases is less important and seldom used for structure elucidation. It yields the corresponding glycosidic acid but produces razemisation at the α-C. This is then followed by acidic hydrolysis resulting in a racemic α-hydroxy acid.

Although all of these reactions are helpful it is not absolutely necessary to degrade pure glycosides. There do exist several chromatographic correlation methods that allow recognition of known cyanogenic glycosides. However, for these methods one needs a collection of reference substances for comparison.

In addition, modern spectroscopic methods give data that allow the structure to be deduced. Nevertheless, good analytical procedures are often required in order to determine the structure unambiguously.

V. CHROMATOGRAPHIC CORRELATION METHODS

A. TLC- AND PC-SYSTEMS

There is no cyanogenic glycoside which has not been chromatographed by TLC or PC. Consequently, many chromatographic systems exist, for which a tabulated overview is given by Seigler (1975a). Since all cyanogenic glycosides are rather polar substances, all of the solvent systems employed are polar containing methanol, ethanol, propanol, *n*-butanol, acetone, methylethylketone, butanone, ethylacetate, chloroform, pyridine (isomerization possible) or water. It is advantageous for phenolic glucosides (e.g. dhurrin) and the triglochinins to add small amounts of organic acids such as formic or acetic to reduce dissociation during chromatography. Since diglycosides, the triglochinins and cardiospermin-5-O-sulphate are the most polar compounds of this group, they exhibit relatively low R_f-values. Heterodendrin/epiheterodendrin, deidaclin, prunasin/sambunigrin, lotaustralin and linamarin lacking hydroxyl function(s) in their aglycones are relatively apolar and therefore show relatively high R_f-values. However, in every case co-chromatography with known glycosides in different solvents is necessary. The work with mandelonitrile glycosides (van Valen, 1978b; Tjon Sie Fat, 1979), linamarin and lotaustralin (van Valen, 1979) or amygdalin, prunasin, linamarin, lotaustralin and gynocardin (Tantisewie *et al.*, 1969) serve as informative examples.

Although several cyanogenic glycosides fluoresce upon the use of a fluorescence indicator on TLC-plates (mandelonitril glycosides, the triglochins, the ester of aromatic acids with cardiospermin) these compounds can often be detected on chromatograms by different spray reagents. One class of reagents acts on the sugar moiety before or after hydrolysis on the chromatogram (see Seigler (1975a) for a tabulated overview). However, these reagents of course are not specific and detect other glycosides as well as several non-glycosidic substances. A more specific method is the detection of cyanogenesis upon the chromatogram after hydrolysis by β-glucosidases. This technique, normally employed as a sandwich technique, is described by Tantisewie *et al.* (1969) using picrate-paper or Feigl/Anger-paper for detection of cyanide in those areas of the chromatogram where a cyanogenic substance liberates cyanide under the conditions chosen. This method is applicable to silica gel plates as well as to cellulose systems. The detection of liberated cyanide directly on the plate or paper sheet using *p*-nitrobenzaldehyde and *o*-dinitrobenzene as reagents (Bennet and Tapper, 1968) only works on cellulose systems. By changing the sequence of the spray reagents (Nahrstedt, 1970) the method was made more certain. The limit of detection using these techniques is about 5-15 μg of glycoside. However, as indicated above not all cyanogenic glycosides are hydrolysed sufficiently by the same enzyme preparation. The enzymes used are emulsin (commercially available), "linamarase", "triglochininase" and "gynocardase" (see Section IV.D). In the case of unknown glycosides, Eyjólfsson (1970a) advises additional treatment of the chromatograms with an aqueous extract of the fresh parent plant.

There are some special colour reactions which occur during detection which indicate distinct cyanogenic glycosides or groups of such glycosides. Hegnauer and Ruijgrok (1971) observed that *p*-hydroxybenzaldehyde arising from hydrolytic cleavage of *p*-hydroxymandelonitrile glycosides produces a yellow-coloured spot after spraying with benzidine (carcinogenic!)/trichloroacetic acid which is distinguishable by its tint from that of *m*-hydroxybenzaldehyde arising from holocalin/zierin. Fikenscher and Ruijgrok (1977) observed a characteristic pink spot for triglochinin after spraying with β-glucosidase. During the detection of *p*-hydroxymandelonitrile glucosides, Bennett and Tapper (1968) noticed a brown zone within the purple spot normally caused by cyanide.

Schwarzmaier (1975b) has used 2,3,5-triphenyltetrazolium-hydroxide to detect mandelonitrile glycosides specifically with a limit of 2-5 μg. Recently Zitnak *et al.* (1977) reported a method for detecting linamarin on paper chromatograms using its reaction with p-anisaldehyde at 85°C; linamarin, but not lotaustralin, produces a pink colour which is brightly fluorescent at 366 nm. Another 25 substances, apart from sinigrin, were found to react more weakly than linamarin.

Epimeric pairs of cyanogenic glycosides normally are not separable by the common TLC or PC systems; recently the separation of heterodendrin and its epimer on silica gel was observed using EtOAc/MeOH/H_2O as a solvent (Erb *et al.*, 1979). However, epimeric forms of mandelonitrile glycosides are distinguishable on silica gel plates by a colour reaction developed by Schwarzmaier (1975a) and modified by van Valen (1978b). This method uses the different acidity of the (*R*) and (*S*) forms which, after spraying with a hydroxylamine/iron-III-chloride reagent, form blue spots in the case of the compound with the (*R*) configuration and red brown ones in the case of the (*S*) configuration, after one hour.

Some of these methods of detection allow a semi-quantitative evaluation against pure substances (see, for example, Zitnak, 1977). Quantitative estimation of taxiphyllin and triglochinin was accomplished by enzymatically liberating cyanide after separating the compounds on silica gel by

Table II Stationary phases used in GLC separation of epimeric pairs of cyanogenic glycosides. -, no separation; +, 3σ-separation; ++, 4σ-separation; +++. 6σ-separation. * Nahrstedt (unpubl.).

(R) / (S)-mixture	derivate	stationary GLC-phase:						references
		SE-3o	OV-1	OV-17	OV-225	ECNSS-M	others	
1. amygdalin/ neoamygdalin	TMS	–	++	+	+++*	decomp		Nahrstedt, 1973
2. prunasin sambunigrin	TMS	–	+	++	+++*	++ (decomp)		Nahrstedt, 1973
3. (S)-/(R)-lucumin	TMS	–	+	+				Nahrstedt, 1973
4. (S)-/(R)-vicianin	TMS	–	(+)	+				Nahrstedt, 1973
5. taxiphyllin/ dhurrin	TMS	 –*	 –*		 +++		QF-1 	Reay and Conn, 1974 Nahrstedt et al., 1978
6. holocalin/ zierin	TMS		–*	–*	++			Nahrstedt, 1973
7. epiproacacipetalin/ proacacipetalin	TMS						OV-25; 1,4-butanediol-succinate	Ettlinger et al., 1977
8. epiheterodendrin/ heterodendrin	TMS		+				UCCW: +	Erb et al., 1979
9. lotaustralin/ epilotaustralin	TMS acetate		–* 	–* 	–* 	 ++		Nahrstedt and Davis (1981)

TLC (Nahrstedt *et al.*, 1979). Studies of the *in situ* determination on TLC-plates of prunasin and amygdalin have been performed by Wingertszahn (1978).

B. GLC-SYSTEMS

The stationary phase first used in GLC of cyanogenic glycosides was methylsilicone SE-30 (Furuya, 1965; Bissett *et al.*, 1969). However, its selectivity was poor as epimeric pairs of cyanogenic glycosides were not separated. This situation was improved by introducing more selective methyl silicone phases (OV-1, OV-101), weakly polar phenyl-methyl-silicones such as OV-17 and OV-25 and the more polar phenyl-cyanopropyl-methyl-silicone (OV-225) and QF-1-fluorsilicone (see Table II). In every case the non volatile glycosides were chromatographed as their per-trimethylsilyl-ethers (TMS-ethers) prepared by several methods (Sweeley *et al.*, 1963; Donike *et al.*, 1973; Klebe *et al.*, 1966; Donike, 1969). A new reagent allows silylation even in wet samples (Weiss and Tambawala, 1972).

From the results listed in Table II one can assume that selectivity of epimeric pairs increases with polarity of the stationary phase. On the other hand increasing the polarity is limited by instability of the polar phases and the temperatures necessary (between 160°C and 250°C) for separation as well as instability of TMS-ethers with strong polar phases such as ECNSS-M (Table II) or polyethylene-glycol succinate (PEG-S). Thus weak and medium polar silicon phases seem to be the most suitable for separation of TMS-ethers of epimeric cyanogenic glycosides.

All GLC-systems listed in Table II separate epimeric TMS-ethers in the same order: glycosides of (*R*) configuration at C-2 of the aglycone are eluted after those with the(*S*) configuration. The pairs 1-6 in Table II show that this may be a general rule for mandelonitrile glycosides. Recently epimeric pairs of glucosides possessing an aliphatic aglycone have been separated in the same order (pairs 7 and 8 in Table II), suggesting that this rule may be true for all cyanogenic glycosides which possess a proton at the chiral centre at C-2 of the aglycone. Furthermore, (*R*) lotaustralin and (*S*) epilotaustralin, which are not separable in our experience as their TMS-ethers, have been successfully separated on ECNSS-M as their peracetates and have the same order of elution as do the TMS-ethers (pair 9 in Table II); this system, which also works with crude methanolic extracts after acetylation, now provides the means for determining the configuration of the numerous substances reported to be lotaustralin. In contrast to these observations Cairns *et al.* (1978) separated the trifluoracetic acid esters of (*R*)/(*S*) amygdalin on GE-versilube-F-50 (trichlorphenyl-methylsilicon) in the reverse order, (*R*) - before (*S*) - form.

As far as we know, no GLC-systems for the cyclopentenylglucosides are available. This is unfortunate since they might be helpful in elucidating the unsolved question of identity of tetraphyllin A with deidaclin and tetraphyllin B with barterin (Seigler, 1975). GLC of triglochinin is not possible because of its thermal instability (Nahrstedt, unpublished). Hübel (unpublished) was unable to silylate cardiospermin-5-O-sulphate in view of its insolubility in silylating solvent systems.

In general poorer results have been obtained from crude extracts of plant material than from those of insect material, as the latter contains fewer substances that cause interference (Davis and Nahrstedt, 1979; Nahrstedt and Davis, 1981). Plant extracts need purification by PC (e.g. Zilg and Conn, 1974, for linamarin and lotaustralin), TLC or by LPC using small columns (Nahrstedt, 1972) before derivatization for qualitative or quantitative GLC estimation (Nahrstedt, 1970, 1972, 1973a, for prunasin and amygdalin; Hübel, 1978, for cardiospermin).

C. HPLC-SYSTEMS

In the last few years high pressure liquid chromatography (HPLC) has been applied to cyanogenic glycosides. HPLC possesses the following advantages compared to GLC: strongly polar substances do not need to be derivatized, the system works at room temperature and the substances can be trapped after passing the detector. All these properties make HPLC a most suitable method for purification and subsequent isolation of cyanogenic glycosides even as distinct epimers. However, detection is more difficult than in GLC, as unspecific and sensitive detectors are lacking. Detectors used in HPLC of cyanogenic glycosides are the u.v. detector for u.v. absorbing glycosides and the refraction index detector for non absorbing glycosides. Only the former possesses the sensitivity of the flame ionization detector used in GLC, and this only in a few cases, depending on the specific extinction of glycosides to be analysed.

Table III shows the systems applied to cyanogenic glycosides. Separation of epimeric mixtures was successful on silica gel (2, 3, 4, 5, 8 in Table III), but also on reversed phases (6, 7 in Table III). In the case of amygdalin/neoamygdalin (6a) the separation was not very efficient. Epimeric mixtures of the mandelonitrile glycosides as well as heterodendrin and its epimer are eluted from a silica gel column in the same order as by GLC. These observations allow the application of the elution order from GLC to HPLC (the thermodynamic reason of course is different).

As expected the order of elution of epimeric pairs on reversed phases is also reversed: glycosides with (*R*) con-

Table III HPLC-systems used for cyanogenic glycosides

substance	stationary phase	mobile phase	detector	references
1. prunasin dhurrin holocalin amygdalin	RP-18	H_2O/AcCN/AcOH 94:5:1	UV, 265 nm	Nahrstedt (1978)
2. prunasin sambunigrin 3. taxiphyllin dhurrin 4. holocalin zierin 5. amygdalin neoamygdalin	silica gel	EtOAc/MeOH 97:3	UV, 265 nm	Nahrstedt (1978)
6. amygdalin neoamygdalin	RP-18	a) H_2O/AcCN 99.8:o.2 b) KH_2PO_4 o.1 M	UV, 254 nm UV	Cairns et al. (1978) Culcasi et al. (1978)
7. taxiphyllin dhurrin triglochinin isomers tyrosin 3-OH benzoic acid (standard)	RP-18	H_2O/AcCN/AcOH 95:4,5:o,5 (flow program)	UV, 232 nm	Nahrstedt (1979)
8. epiheteroden-drin	silica gel	EtOAc/MeOH 95:5	RI	Erb et al. (1979)
9. linamarin lotaustralin	RP-18	H_2O/AcCN 95:5	RI	Davis and Nahrstedt (1979)
1o. linustatin neolinustatin	RP-18	a) H_2O/MeOH 85:15 (preparative) b) H_2O/AcCN 96:4	 RI	Smith et al. (198o) Nahrstedt (unpubl.)
11. cardiospermin cardiospermin-5-O-sulfate	RP-18	H_2O/MeOH 9o:1o containing tetra-methylammonium phosphate o.o2 M, pH 7.2	RI	Hübel (1981)
12. cardiospermin-5-O-ester	RP-18	H_2O/AcCN/iProp/AcOH 77,4:15:7,5.o1	UV, 27o nm	Nahrstedt and Scheid (1981)

figuration appear earlier than those of (*S*) configuration (6, 7 in Table III).

Chromatographic experiments performed by Hübel with cardiospermin-5-O-sulphate showed that this substance was not retained on RP-phases and therefore was not separable from other substances eluted in the front. The problem was successfully solved by using ion-pair-chromatography with tetramethylammonium as the cation; this method allows determination of cardiospermin and its 5-O-sulphate within one run (Hübel, 1981).

All systems mentioned in Table III are useful for semi-preparative or preparative work. Even from columns of analytical dimensions enough glycosides are available from several runs for modern spectroscopic analysis. This has been demonstrated for epiheterodendrin (Erb *et al.*, 1979), linamarin and lotaustralin (Davis and Nahrstedt, 1979) and some cardiosperm esters (Nahrstedt and Scheid, 1981). A 2.5 g sample containing linustatin and neolinustatin was separated in one run only by using a 5.7 x 30 cm RP-18 column (Smith *et al.*, 1980).

Besides normal analytical and preparative application of GLC and HPLC systems, these methods allow additional determination of the configuration at C-2 of the aglycone of the cyanogenic glycosides by the use of the observed elution rule. Most glycosides are isomerizable in alkaline solution (see Section II), and therefore chromatography of a pure substance compared to its isomerization product gives a clear result (e.g. Nahrstedt, 1973c; Nahrstedt, 1975c; Ettlinger *et al.*, 1977; Erb *et al.*, 1979).

VI. SPECTROSCOPY

A. U.V.- AND I.R.-SPECTROSCOPY

Cyanogenic glycosides containing chromophores exhibit u.v. absorptions in solvents such as water, methanol or acetonitrile. A rather low specific absorption is observed for the unsubstituted mandelonitrile glycosides with λ_{max} at 262 nm (1, 2 Table IV). Aromatic glycosides with auxochromic gourps such as a hydroxyl group exhibit stronger signals with a molar extinction between 10^3 and 10^4 as found for dhurrin (3, Table IV) with its major absorption at about 230 nm and holocalin at 222 nm.

Presence of a phenolic hydroxyl is indicated by a bathochromic shift after adding small amounts of alkali (NaOMe, NaOH) as shown for dhurrin, holocalin and cardiospermin-5-O-(4-hydroxy)benzoate. Of course this shift is not observed in those glycosides in which the phenolic hydroxyl is glucosylated as in proteacin and the p-glucosyloxylmandelonitrile (6, 7 in Table IV).

Non-aromatic glycosides normally possess absorption below 220 nm with two exceptions; these are the triglochinins, which have a system of conjugated double bonds including a carboxyl and a nitrile group, and cardiospermin-5-O-(4-hydroxy)benzoate and related compounds which are esters of aromatic acids. The difference between the molar extinction of triglochinin (8, Table IV) and isotriglochinin (9, Table

Table IV u.v.-maxima and molar absorptivity of some cyanogenic glycosides (solvent: MeOH or H_2O).

substance	neutral solution		OH^- added			references
	λ_{max} [nm]	ϵ	λ_{max} [nm]	ϵ	shift	
1. prunasin	262	low				Zechner, 1966
2. amygdalin	262	o.35 x 1o^{3}				Nahrstedt, unpubl.
3. dhurrin	23o 228	1.o7 x 1o^{4} 1.3 x 1o^{4}	255	1.51 x 1o^{4}	+ 25	Mao et al., 1965 Towers et al., 1964
4. taxiphyllin	228 232	9.87 x 1o^{3} 1.12 x 1o^{4}				Towers et al., 1964 Schwarzmaier, 1976
5. holocalin	222 28o	3.3 x 1o^{3} 2.2 x 1o^{3}	246 3o4	3.5 x 1o^{3} 2.6 x 1o^{3}	+ 24 + 24	Gmelin et al., 1973
6. p-glucosyloxymandelo-nitrile	27o		27o			Sharples and Stoker, 1969 Abrol et al., 1966
7. proteacin	27o					Sharples and Stoker, 1969
8. triglochinin	275	1.1 x 1o^{4}				Ettlinger and Eyjólfsson, 1972
9. isotriglochinin	283	2.2 x 1o^{4}				Ettlinger and Eyjólfsson, 1972
1o. acacipetalin	22o	1o^{4}				Ettlinger et al., 1977
11. cardiospermin-5-O-(4-OH)benzoate	257	1.75 x 1o^{4}	298	2.15 x 1o^{4}	+ 41	Nahrstedt, 1976

IV) might indicate a *s-cis* conformation of the double bond system of triglochinin and a *s-trans* conformation for isotriglochinin.

I.r. spectra give specific information about the degree of saturation in 2,3-position of the aglycone. The absorption of a nitrile group with an oxygen in α-position is quenched (Bellamy, 1956). Most α,β-saturated nitrile glycosides such as prunasin or amygdalin exhibit only a weak or no nitrile absorption in the range of 2240-2260 cm^{-1} whereas the cyclopenten derivates tetraphyllin A and B show a clear absorption at 2290 cm^{-1} (Russell and Reay, 1971). On the other hand α,β-unsaturated nitriles (e.g. triglochinin) although containing oxygen in the α-position show a pronounced absorption and a hyposochromic shift down to 2220 cm^{-1} (Fig. 7). Some descriptive information on i.r.-spectra is given by Ettlinger *et al.* (1977; acacipetalin, proacacipetalin), Seigler *et al.* (1974; cardiospermin), Eyjólfsson (1970b; triglochinin), Gmelin *et al.* (1973: holocalin), Nahrstedt (1976a; cardiospermin-5-O-(4-OH) benzoate), Hübel and Nahrstedt (1975; heterodendrin), Bissett *et al.* (1969; linamarin and lotaustralin), and Smith *et al.* (1980; linustatin and neolinustatin).

B. MASS SPECTROMETRY

Since all cyanogenic glycosides are polar and non-volatile substances they normally need derivatisation before introduction into a mass spectrometer. Derivatives used are the TMS-ethers (Bissett *et al.*, 1969, for linamarin and lotaustralin), peracetates (Sharples *et al.*, 1972, for triglochinin) and trifluoracetates (Cairns *et al.*, 1978, for amygdalin). In the case of cyanogenic cyclopentenyl-glucosides, underivatized samples were used, normally resulting in M-49 as the highest peak, but in case of tetraphyllin B even a M^+ signal was obtained (Clapp *et al.*, 1970; Russell and Reay, 1971). Although M^+ signals are often not observed, other products of fragmentation sometimes give useful information on the aglycone as well as the sugar portion. The TMS-derivatives produce a M^+-15(-CH_3)-ion, as is observed for many TMS-flavonoid glycosides (Schels *et al.*, 1977, 1978). Cairns *et al.* (1978) point out that both epimers, (*R*) amygdalin and (*S*) neoamygdalin are identical in their mass spectra as TFA-derivatives.

Since a M^+ signal is seldom obtainable by the normal MS methods, field desorption MS (FD-MS) has been used in several cases for estimation of molecular weight (e.g. Seigler *et al.*, 1975, for heterodendrin; Butterfield *et al.*, 1975, for proacacipetalin; Nahrstedt, 1976a, for cardiospermin-5-O-(4-hydroxy)benzoate; Hübel and Nahrstedt, 1979, for cardiospermin-5-O-sulphate). Very recently Dreifuss *et al.* (1980) investigated principles of fragmentation by FD-MS using 6 cyanogenic glycosides.

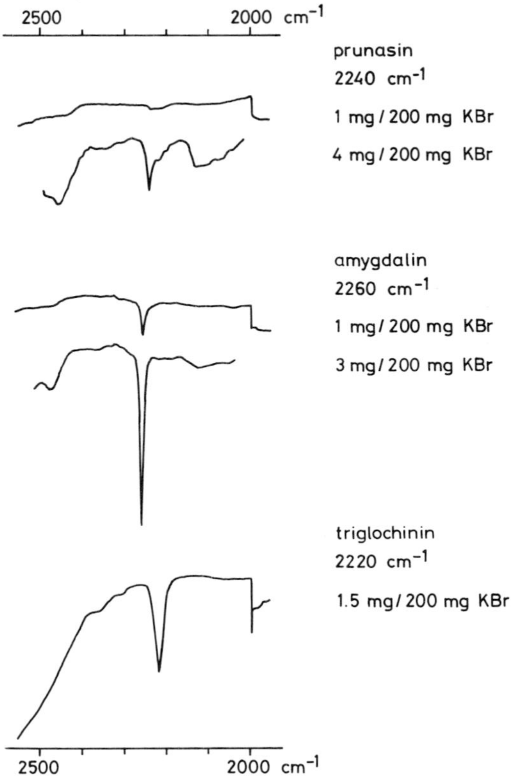

Fig. 7 I.r.-nitrile absorption of some cyanogenic glycosides

C. ^{1}H-NMR

Proton resonance spectroscopy has been very useful and spectra for every known glycoside have been recorded in the last 12-15 years. Most spectra have been run as trimethylsilylethers in CCl_4. However, TMS-ethers are derivatives and need to be prepared as well as destroyed if the compound is needed for other reactions (for techniques of preparation and destruction, see Seigler, 1975a). Therefore, more polar solvents such as dimethylsulphoxide-d_6, deuterium oxide, methanol-d_4, acetone-d_6 or acetonitrile-d_3 are useful for measurement of spectra of underivatized glycosides. Since a lot of cyanogenic glycosides do not exhibit signals to higher field of 3 p.p.m. DMSO-d_6, acetone-d_6 and acetonitrile-d_3, with their own signals at c. 2.5, 2 and 1.9 p.p.m. resp., are especially suitable solvents. In those cases where protic solvents are necessary, the hydroxyl protons of the solvents as well as of the sample can be shifted to lower field by adding a small amount of DCl or TFA-d_1.

It is advisable to record a substance, derivatized as well as underivatized, in several solvents. For example: TMS-heterodendrin in CCl_4 shows a pseudotriplet for the anomeric proton at C-1' and the C-2-proton which coincide in the region $\delta = 4.3$ p.p.m. (6 in Fig. 10). Since the C-2-H-doublet of the underivatized glucoside in MeOH-d_4 is near the solvent signal, this spectrum again is not unambiguous (2 in Fig. 10). Although the spectrum recorded in DMSO-d_6 shows broader signals, two well resolved doublets for the C-1' proton and the C-2 proton are observed (Hübel and Nahrstedt, 1975; Erb *et al.*, 1979).

Quantitative information about the number of different protons is available from integration of a well recorded spectrum; this is especially valuable for the determination of the aglycone:sugar ratio. After acetylation the number of hydroxyl groups can be estimated by integration of the methyl-signals resulting from the acetyl groups. Furthermore, acetylated alcoholic and phenolic hydroxyl groups are distinguishable by location of the methyl resonances in the spectrum (e.g. Towers *et al.*, 1973; Nahrstedt, 1976a). The position of a C-2 proton is detectable by isomerization of the compound in D_2O; in this case the C-2 proton signal disappears as shown for amygdalin (Nahrstedt, 1975c). Finally, in the case of amygdalin quantitative estimation was performed by Turczan and Medwick (1977) using trinitrobenzene as an internal standard.

TMS-ethers of several of the cyanogenic glycosides are discussed by Seigler (1975a). Therefore, in the following discussion only similarities and common features of these compounds are pointed out. Using schematic idealized 60 or 100 MHz "stick spectra" the glycosides are compiled into groups characterized by their chemical and spectroscopic properties. Spectra taken from the literature are marked by their reference; all other spectra were recorded by the author's group.

1. 2-Alkyl-propionitrile glucosides (Fig. 8)

In contrast to most other glycosides, these glucosides do not possess methine protons at C-2. Thus, we only find the doublet(s) of the anomeric proton(s) in the downfield region at about $\delta = 4.4$ p.p.m. In the case of the two gentiobiosides (4 and 5, Fig. 8) the doublets at higher field are correlated with the proton attached to C-1' (for discussion see Turczan *et al.*, 1978). These doublets all exhibit an axial coupling constant of 7-8 Hz indicating a β-configuration at the glycosidic bond; the remaining sugar protons all resonate in the range between 2.8 to 4.3 p.p.m. Both observations are of value for all other known cyanogenic glycosides. The two methyl groups of linamarin (1, Fig. 8) and linustatin (4, Fig. 8) fall together at 1.6 and 1.7 p.p.m. respectively. Glycosides with an ethyl side chain (2, 3, 5 in Fig. 8) exhibit a quartet centred at about 1.9 p.p.m. and a triplet at 1.05 p.p.m. produced

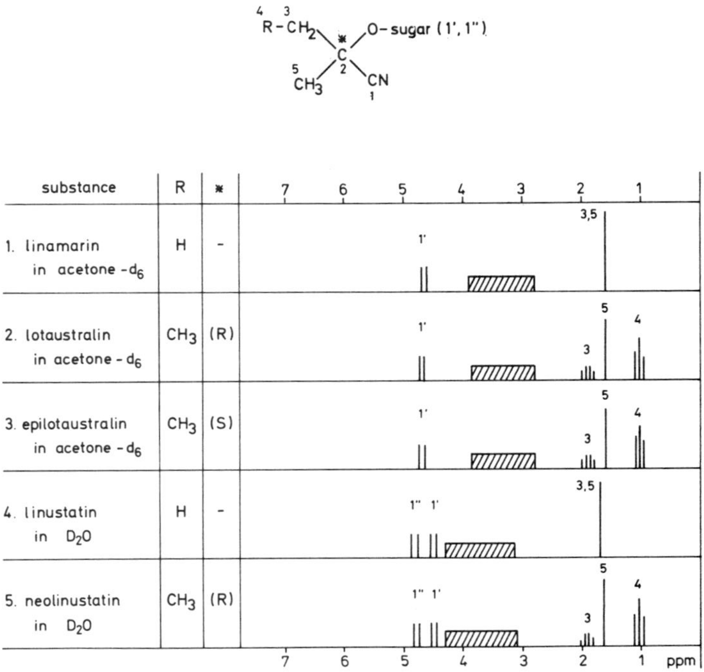

Fig. 8 Schematic ^{1}H-NMR spectra of derivatives of 2-alkylpropionitrile glycosides; δ-scale in p.p.m.

by the methylene and the methyl group respectively. Epilotaustralin (3, Fig. 8), presently only known as a synthetic compound (Bissett *et al.*, 1969), is nearly identical with the spectrum of its epimer lotaustralin. According to Bissett *et al.* (1969), there are slight differences in the position of the resonance of the methyl groups in the spectra of the peracetylated compounds; the signal of the methyl group of (*S*)epilotaustralin is shifted downfield by 0.09 p.p.m. in comparison to (*R*)lotaus-ralin. However, these two epimers are better distinguished by GLC of their peracetates (see Section V.B).

2. Mandelonitrile glycosides (Fig. 9)

Many cyanogenic glycosides possess an aromatic aglycone. Without any ring substitution the aromatic protons appear at about 7.3 p.p.m. as indicated for TMS-prunasin, TMS-sambunigrin, TMS-amygdalin and TMS lucumin (1, 2, 3, 4 in Fig. 9). p-Substituted mandelonitrile glycosides show the typical symmetric AA'-BB'-system as indicated for TMS-taxiphyllin and TMS-dhurrin (5, 6 in Fig. 9); TMS-holocalin with a meta-disubstituted benzene-ring shows a complex pattern of resonance lines in this region.

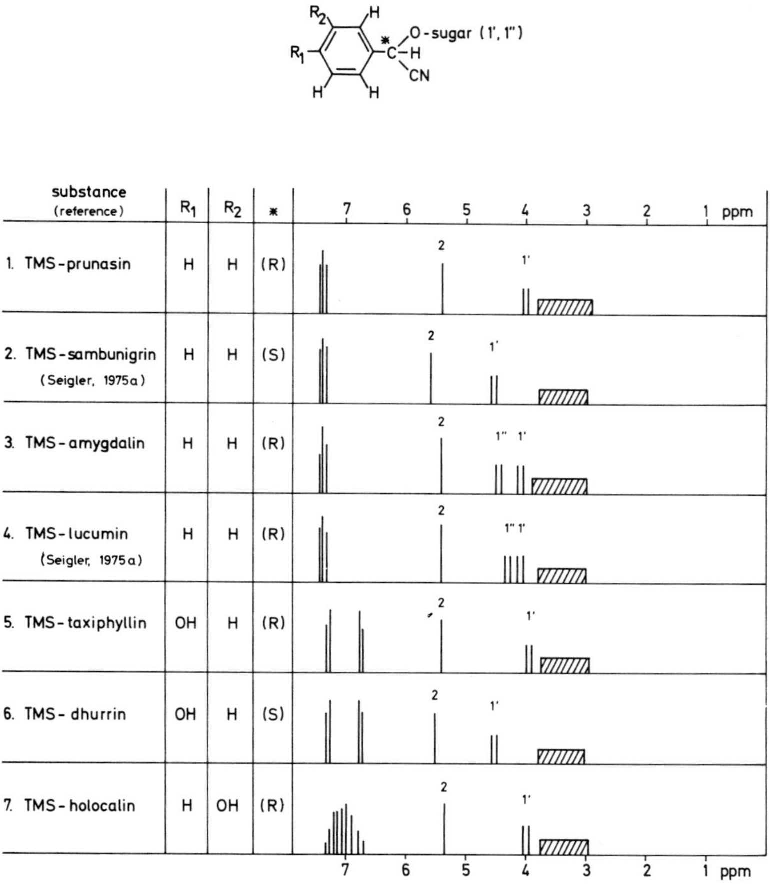

Fig. 9 Schematic H-NMR spectra of some mandelonitrile glycosides; δ-scale in p.p.m. TMS: pertrimethylsilylethers in CCl_4

The position of the cyanohydrin proton at C-2 of the TMS-ether can be observed in two areas of the spectrum, one downfield from 5.5 p.p.m., the other upfield. These differences allow distinction between epimeric forms of aromatic cyanogenic glycosides. The C-2 proton of compounds with an (*S*) configuration resonates downfield from 5.5, whereas those with an (*R*) configuration appear upfield from 5.5 p.p.m. Towers *et al.* (1964) explain these differences as a long range effect on the methine hydrogen of the aromatic ring system by hindered free rotation of the aryl moiety in case of dhurrin, whereas (*R*) taxiphyllin does not exhibit this anisotropic effect.

Although the configuration at C-2 may be determined by the position of the methine proton absorption, it is more clearly indicated by the position of the doublet of the anomeric proton of the first sugar attached to the aglycone. Again Towers *et al.* (1964) show that the nitrile group and the anomeric hydrogen may be almost eclipsed in case of (*S*) dhurrin, whereas in (*R*) taxiphyllin the methine proton is eclipsed with the anomeric hydrogen resulting in different long-range effects on the resonance position of the anomeric hydrogen doublet of (*R*)- and (*S*) forms. In TMS-monoglucosides with an (*R*) configuration at C-2, such as prunasin, taxiphyllin and holocalin, this doublet resonates at about 4 p.p.m., whereas in compounds with an (*S*) configuration, such as sambunigrin and dhurrin, those doublets are shifted about 0.5 p.p.m. downfield to 4.5 p.p.m. A similar difference is also observed in the spectra of peracetates from dhurrin (δ = 5.02), taxiphyllin (δ = 4.62) (Towers *et al.*, 1964) and prunasin (δ = 4.55; Nahrstedt, unpubl.). The corresponding anomeric proton of proteacin octaacetate resonates at 5.03 and its C-2 hydrogen is also shifted by 0.35 p.p.m. to lower field compared to taxiphyllin pentaacetate suggesting that proteacin also possesses a (*S*) configuration at C-2 (R.L. Young, pers. comm. to E.E. Conn). Using underivatized mandelonitrile glycosides in D_2O the differences between (*R*)- and (*S*)-form resonances for the anomeric proton are about 0.2 p.p.m. and, for the methine proton at C-2, nearly 0.15 p.p.m. (Schwarzmaier, 1976a).

3. *Butyronitrile glucosides*

In this class of cyanogenic glucosides we encounter a series of structurally related compounds (including the cyanolipids which are not discussed here; for ^{1}H-NMR spectra see Mikolajzak, 1977) starting with a glucoside possessing a saturated aglycone (heterodendrin and its epimer, 1,2 in Fig. 10) and terminating in esters of the desaturated and hydroxylated analogues. The electron withdrawing effect of the substituents increases in this order and is reflected by the ^{1}H-NMR-spectra:

The two methyl groups of heterodendrin and its epimer exhibit two doublets arising from the diastereotopic effect of the chiral centre at C-2 (Hübel and Nahrstedt, 1975). Inspection of the TMS-ethers (6-10 in Fig. 10) indicates that the methyl absorption at C-5 undergoes a downfield shift upon introduction of a double bond (7, 8 in Fig. 10), the addition of a hydroxyl group (9 in Fig. 10) and their subsequent esterification with an aromatic acid (10 in Fig. 10). The same trend in this order is observed for the C-4 protons, the C-2 proton and less clearly for the anomeric glucose proton. The C-3 proton of the saturated compound appearing as an octet near 2.1 p.p.m. disappears upon introduction of the 3, 4 double bond, and consequently a single signal is observed for the C-2 proton of butyronitrile-3-ene derivatives. As observed by Ettlinger *et al.* (1977), the C-2 proton of TMS-epipro-

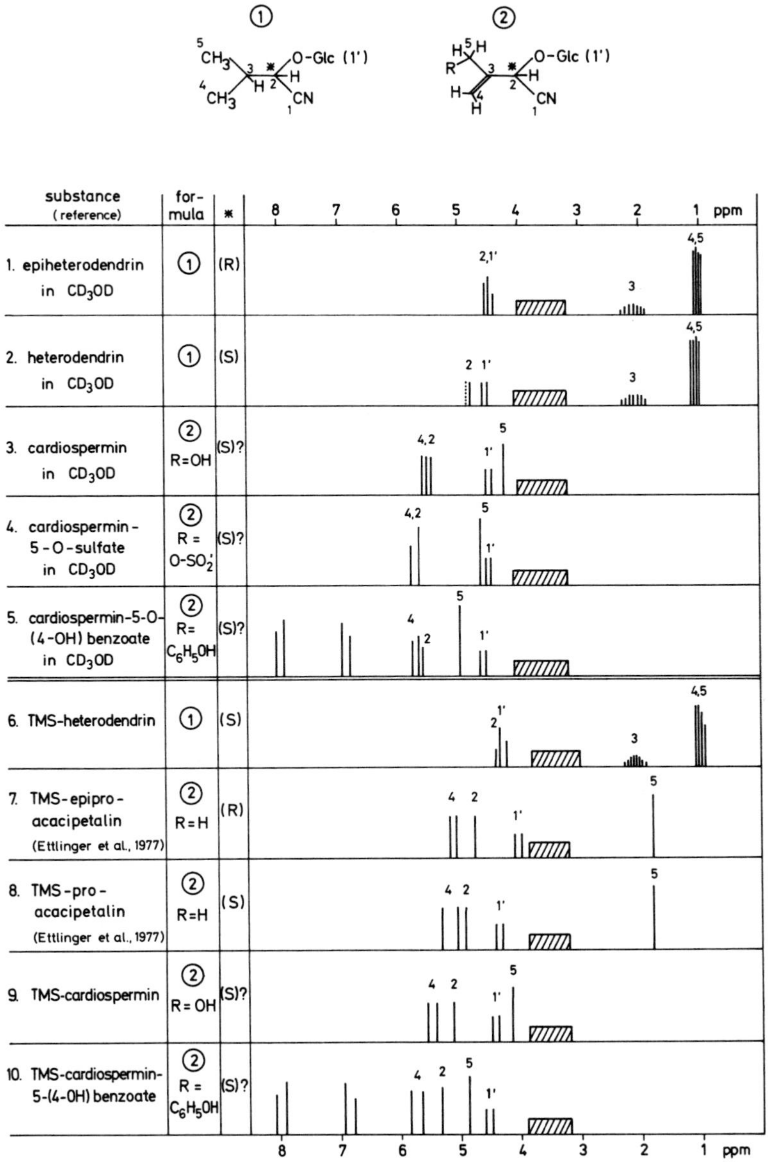

Fig. 10. Schematic ^{1}H-NMR spectra of butyronitrile glucosides; δ-scale in p.p.m. TMS: pertrimethylsilylethers in CCl_4

acacipetalin is shifted by about 0.15 p.p.m. and the anomeric proton of the same compound by about 0.3 p.p.m. to higher field compared to TMS-proacacipetalin (7, 8 in Fig. 10). Again, in the case of heterodendrin and epiheterodendrin, the same trend was observed for both protons (Erb *et al.*, 1979). This is in a good agreement with the corresponding protons of epimeric pairs of mandelonitrile glycosides indicating the (*R*) configuration for epiheterodendrin and epiproacacipetalin.

In the spectrum of cardiospermin-5-O-sulphate recorded in MeOH-d_4, one of the vinyl protons at C-4 overlaps the methine proton at C-2. This coincidence can be resolved by changing the solvent. Recording the substance in D_2O (with trace amounts of TFA-d_1) Hübel and Nahrstedt (1979) observed well resolved signals of all three protons. Cardiospermin shows the same effect; recorded in DMSO-d_6 or acetone-d_6, these three protons exhibit two broad signals whereas the spectrum in MeOH-d_4, and that of the TMS-ether in CCl_4, is well resolved. The coincidence of the two doublets of the C-2 and the anomeric proton of TMS-heterodendrin is discussed above. Although these two doublets of heterodendrin are well resolved in the CD_3OD-spectrum of the underivatized compound (2 in Fig. 10), the same protons of epiheterodendrin in CD_3OD again exhibit a pseudo triplet. However, both heterodendrin and its epimer show well resolved doublets when recorded in DMSO-d_6 (Hübel and Nahrstedt, 1975; Erb *et al.*, 1979).

The configuration of cardiospermin and its esters at C-2 is not yet established. As shown by the TMS-ethers the anomeric proton of the (*S*) butyronitrile glucosides (6, 8 in Fig. 10) resonate to lower field of 4.2 p.p.m. whereas those of the (*R*) epimeric TMS-epiproacacipetalin (7, Fig. 10) appear at 4.03 p.p.m. From these observations as well as from biogenetic reasons which are not discussed here the (*S*) configuration of cardiospermin and its derivatives, all of which exhibit an anomeric proton signal lower than 4.4 p.p.m., seems likely (see also resonance position of glc-C_1 of compound 1 in Table Vc compared to compounds 2-6 in Table Vc).

4. *Triglochinins (Fig. 11)*

With the exception of acacipetalin, which is probably an artifactual product and whose spectrum is additionally shown in Fig. 11 (1), the triglochinins are the only group of α,β-unsaturated cyanogenic glucosides. Because of their two double bonds, four isomers are possible: 2,3(E)-4,5(Z)triglochinin and 2,3(Z)-4,5(Z)triglochinin, called triglochinin A and B by Jaroszewski (1978), and 2,3(E)-4,5(E)triglochinin and 2,3(Z)-4,5(E)triglochinin called isotriglochinin A and B by the same author. The data published in the literature only show clear evidence of the configuration of the 4,5 double bond from ^{1}H-NMR data. TMS-ethers of triglochinin preparations (2 in Fig. 11) exhibit a strong signal within the range of sugar absorption corresponding to the C-6 protons, the anomeric proton doublet at about 4.9 p.p.m and an AB pattern arising from the C-4 and C-5 proton centred at 5.9

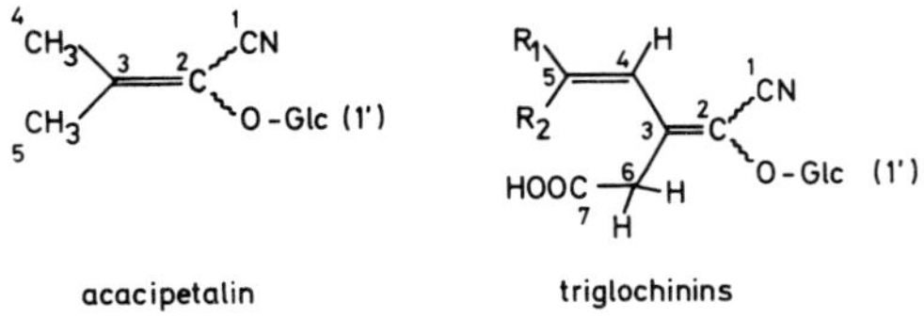

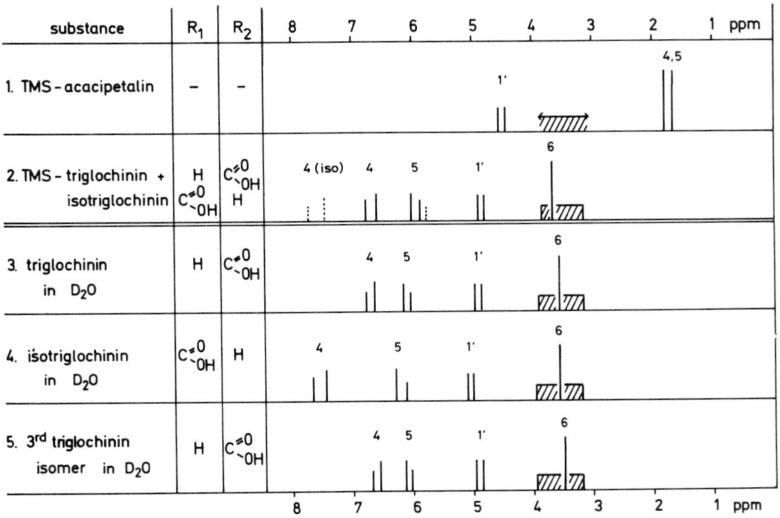

Fig. 11 Schematic ^{1}H-NMR spectra of acacipetalin and triglochinin and isomers; δ-scale in p.p.m. TMS: pertrimethylsilylethers in CCl_4

and 6.7 p.p.m. with a coupling constant of 12.5 Hz (Eyjólfsson, 1970b). Sometimes additional signals of a vinyl group centered at 7.0 and 7.65 p.p.m. with J_{AB} = 16 Hz are observed (Nahrstedt, 1975a, b). The position and coupling constants associated with these signals indicate the presence of a 4,5(Z) - together with a 4,5 (E)triglochinin, the latter being called isotriglochinin in the literature (Ettlinger and Eyjólfsson, 1972).

Recently a crude triglochinin preparation was separated by HPLC (see Section V.C) and three fractions were found to be cyanogenic (Nahrstedt, unpubl.). The compound eluted last from the RP-18 column was the main component and exhibited the spectrum of triglochinin (3 in Fig. 11). The second minor compound showed the spectrum of isotriglochinin (4 in Fig. 11), and the first eluted compound present in traces exhibited a spectrum identical to that of triglochinin together with a small upfield shift of the C-6 protons of 0.06 p.p.m. (5 in Fig. 11). The third compound of course must be a 2,3-isomer of triglochinin, but the data at present do not allow determination of the configuration by ^{1}H-NMR. Furthermore, the situation becomes more complex since several conformations of the diene system are possible (see Section VI.A).

5. *Cyclopentenone-cyanohydrin glucosides (Fig. 12)*

A group of cyanogenic glucosides which is closely distributed in the plant kingdom contain a cyclopentenyl moiety. These are all β-glucosides as indicated by a 7 Hz coupling constant of the anomeric proton resonating at 4.4 - 4.5 p.p.m. in case of the TMS-ethers and at 4.8-5 p.p.m. in case of underivatized compounds in D_2O. The olefinic protons of all these glucosides except TMS-gynocardin (4, Fig. 12) appear as two doublets, with evidence for allylic coupling in the range of 6 p.p.m. Underivatized gynocardin shows a complex pattern of signals for these protons as they are part of a complex ABXY spin system.

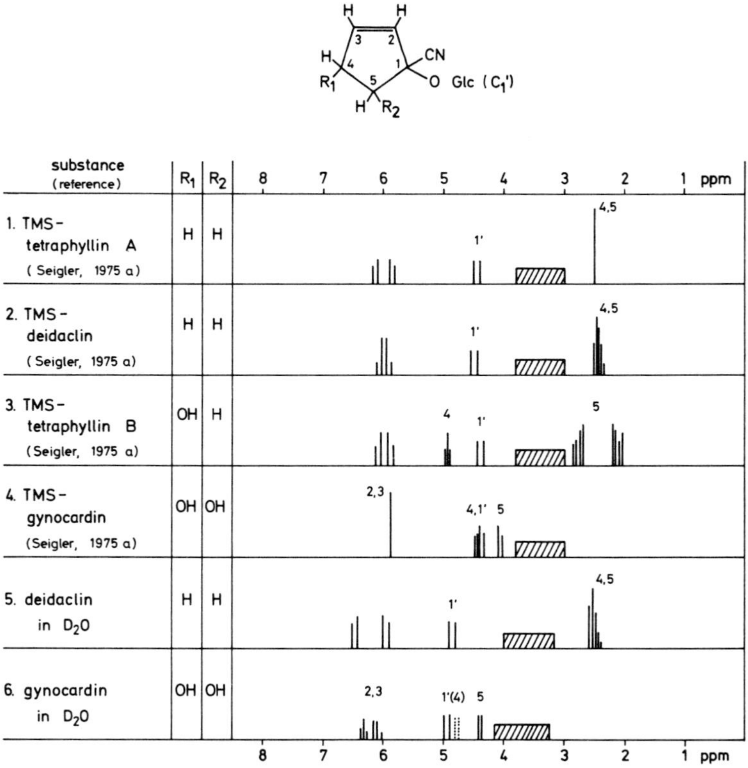

Fig. 12 Schematic ^{1}H-NMR spectra of some cyclopentenone-cyanohydrin glucosides; δ-scale in p.p.m.; TMS: pertrimethylsilylethers in CCl_4

Both cyclic methylene groups of TMS-tetraphyllin A (1, Fig. 12) and TMS-deidaclin (2, Fig. 12) appear as a broad singlet and multiplet respectively centred at 2.5 p.p.m. These differences including a slight variation in the position of the anomeric and the vinyl protons, which are also observed for these compounds recorded underivatized in D_2O (Clapp *et al.*, 1970; Russell and Reay, 1971), prove that both compounds are not identical and perhaps are epimeric at C-1.

Introduction of a hydroxyl group (3, Fig. 12) at C-4 results in a strong shift of the remaining C-4 proton down to 4.9 p.p.m. with the appearance of a triplet from an overlapping double doublet (Seigler, 1975a; Gondwe *et al.*, 1978). Additionally, the non-equivalent geminal C-5 protons (Russell and Reay, 1971) appear as the AB part of an ABX system with centres at 2.15 and 2.83 p.p.m. Recently Gondwe *et al.* (1978) isolated a mixture of 4-hydroxylated cyclopenten-cyanhydrin glucosides which were suggested, from ^{1}H-NMR data, to be tetraphyllin B and its C-1-epimer. Two sets of quartets for the C-5 protons and a triplet resulting from two overlapping doublets of two species of anomeric protons led to this interpretation.

TMS-gynocardin, as the 4,5-dihydroxy compound, exhibits two doublets for the methine protons attached at C-4 and C-5, the former one overlapping the anomeric proton doublet (4, Fig. 12). The singlet produced by both olefinic hydrogens is surprising as the protons are expected to be non-equivalent. However a complex pattern of the expected ABXY system is visible in the spectrum of underivatized gynocardin in D_2O (6, Fig. 12, see also Coburn and Long, 1966).

Although ^{1}H-NMR spectra of this group of glucosides contain much information they are difficult to interpret because of the complex spin systems from the cyclopentenyl moiety. It is expected that ^{13}C-NMR and high-field (400 MHz) ^{1}H-NMR spectroscopy will be of particular importance in structural elucidation of these compounds.

D. ^{13}C-NMR

In the last few years ^{13}C-NMR spectroscopy has been applied to the structural elucidation of some of the cyanogenic glycosides (linustatin and neolinustatin: Smith *et al.*, 1980; acacipetalin: Ettlinger *et al.*, 1977; amygdalin: Cairns *et al.*, 1978; cardiospermin-5-O-sulphate: Hübel and Nahrstedt, 1979). Although Jaroszewski (1978) demonstrated the usefulness of ^{13}C-NMR in the investigation of cyanogenic glycosides, a systematic examination of different groups of these compounds still has not been published. Recently Hübel *et al.* (1981) have recorded data for a series of cyanogenic glycosides and this is shown in Table V, a-d.

Table V ^{13}C-assignments from proton decoupled ^{13}C-NMR spectra referenced to TMS, recorded in D_2O (*Va*) 2-alkyl-propionitrile glycosides (for structure see Fig. 8); (*Vb*) mandelonitrile glycosides (for structure see Fig. 9); (*Vc*) butyronitrile glucosides (for structure see Fig. 10); (*Vd*) cyclopentenone-cyanohydrin glucosides (for structure see Fig. 12).

Va:	substance	nitrile C	C-2	C-3	C-5	C-4	glc C-1'	glc C-6'	glc C-1"	glc C-6"	glc C-2'(") - C-5'(")
1.	linamarin	122.32	72.92	27.05;	27.67	-	99.79	61.48	-	-	76.96; 76.38; 73.72; 70.37
2.	linustatin	122.29	72.72	27.73;	26.78	-	99.58	69.11	103.44	61.58	76.67; 76.40; 76.19; 75,89; 73.94; 73.59; 70.48; 70.04;
3.	lotaustralin	121.97	76.73	33.86	24.08	8.69	99.49	61.48	-	-	77.00; 76.49; 73.74; 70.40
4.	neolinustatin	121.92	76.39	33.93	23.81	8.66	99.28	69.02	103.43	61.60	76.68; 76.39; 76.30; 76.03; 74.01; 73.60; 70.53; 70.10;

Vb:	substance	nitrile C	C-2	aromatic carbons 1	2	3	4	5	6	glc C-1	glc C-6	glc C-2 - C-5
1.	prunasin	119.36	69.65	133.23	130.25	128.78	131.42	128.78	130.25	101.91	61.40	77.08; 76.40; 73.64; 70.24
2.	sambunigrin	118.69	69.48	133.17	130.21	128.80	131.35	128.80	130.21	101.23	61.44	77.14; 76.45; 73.58; 70.26
3.	taxiphyllin	119.48	69.21	124.97	130.86	116.91	158.33	116.91	130.86	101.35	61.41	77.50; 76.41; 73.60; 70.26
4.	dhurrin	118.71	68.88	124.76	130.63	116.70	158.02	116.70	130.63	100.89	61.35	76.92; 76.34; 73.44; 70.13
5.	holocalin	119.28	69.32	134.83	115.43	157.16	120.62	131.68	118.34	101.93	61.40	77.07; 76.40; 73.64; 70.24
6.	zierin	118.61	69.18	134.77	115.56	157.14	120.53	131.64	118.29	101.24	61.43	77.13; 76.46; 73.57; 70.25

Vc: substance	nitrile C	C-2	C-3	C-4	C-5	glc C-1	glc C-6	glc C-2 - C-5	4(OH)benzoyl
1. epiheterodendrin	119.98	74.79	32.20	17.65;	17.26	104.21	61.35	76.18; 76.31; 73.76; 70.23	-
2. heterodendrin	119.01	73.54	32.07	18.03;	17.44	101.54	61.45	77.09; 76.42; 73.54; 70.38	-
3. proacapipetalin	118.18	71.01	137.84	118.70	18.43	101.02	61.45	76.44; 76.07; 73.51; 70.28	-
4. cardiospermin	118.01	68.04	140.82	119.36	61.95	101.02	61.46	77.10; 76.46; 73.52; 70.31	-
5. cardiospermin-5-O-(4-OH)benzoate	117.49	67.83	136.39	121.85	64.57	101.15	61.43	76.04; 75.40; 72.50; 69.25	carboxyl: 168.12; 121.35(1); 132.83(2) 116.12(3); 161.72(4)
6. cardiospermin-5-O-sulfate	116.76	66.67	135.32	121.97	67.36	100.22	60.47	76.96; 76.34; 73.45; 70.18	-

Vd: structure	nitrile C	C-1	C-2	C-3	C-4	C-5	glc C-1	glc C-6	glc C-2 - C-5
1. deidaclin	120.92	84.98	143.14	128.73	31.43	37.67	100.26	61.47	77.08; 76.42; 73.78; 70.34
2. gynocardin	116.67	85.65	140.91	128.39	78.59	87.36	100.13	61.70	77.01; 76.43; 73.69; 70.61

E. OTHER METHODS

Several other methods that have not been frequently used in structure elucidation of cyanogenic glycosides are mentioned here. Using Klyne's rule (Klyne, 1950) the terminal sugar and configuration of its glycosidic bond in lucumin was established by molecular rotation (Eyjólfsson, 1971). Correlation of the ORD curves of linustatin and neolinustatin with those of linamarin, lotaustralin and amygdalin allowed all the chiral centres of these new gentiobiosides to be defined (Smith *et al.*, 1980). X-ray crystallographic structure determination was used to determine absolute configurations at C-1, C-2 and C-3 of the cyclopentenring of gynocardin (Kim *et al.*, 1970).

ACKNOWLEDGEMENTS

I am most thankful to Dr V. Wray and Dr D.S. Seigler for their linguistic advice during preparation of the whole manuscript as well as parts of it. Dr V. Wray determined most of the NMR spectra. Samples of cyanogenic glycosides have been graciously provided by Drs R.C. Clapp, E.E. Conn, R. Gmelin, R. Hegnauer and L. Fikenscher. I would like to thank Drs W. Hübel, V. Wray and H.D. Zinsmeister for information regarding past results and for discussion of numerous problems arising from our common work.

REFERENCES

Abrol, Y.P., Conn, E.E. and Stoker, J.R. (1966). *Phytochemistry* 5, 1021.

Beilsteins Handbuch der organischen Chemie (1938), 4th edn. Vol 31, pp. 399-400. J. Springer, Berlin.

Bellamy, L.J. (1956). "The Infrared Spectra of Complex Molecules", p. 225. John Wiley, New York.

Bennet, W.D. and Tapper, B.A. (1968). *J. Chromatogr.* 34, 428.

Bissett, F.H., Clapp, R.C., Coburn, R.A., Ettlinger, M.G. and Long, L. Jr. (1969). *Phytochemistry* 8, 2235-2247.

Bough, W.A. and Gander, J.E. (1971). *Phytochemistry* 10, 67-77.

Butterfield, C.S., Conn, E.E. and Seigler, D.S. (1975). *Phytochemistry* 14, 993-997.

Cairns, Th., Froberg, J.E., Gonzales, S., Langham, W.S. and Stamp, J.J. (1978). *Anal. Chemistry* 50, 317-322.

Clapp, R.C., Ettlinger, M.G. and Long, L. Jr. (1970). *J. Amer. Chem. Soc.* 92, 6378-6379.

Coburn, R.A. and Long, L. (1966). *J. Org. Chem.* 31, 4312.

Coop, I.E. (1940). *New Zealand J. Sci. Technol.* 22, 71 B.

Culcasi, M., Cheung, A., Singai, E., Jee, J. and Lim, P. (1978). *J. Pharm. Sci.* 67, 1190-1192.

Davis, R.H. and Nahrstedt, A. (1979). *Comp. Biochem. Physiol.* 64B, 395-397.

Dilleman, G. (1958). *In* "Handbuch der Pflanzenphysiologie" (W. Ruhland,

ed.), Vol. VIII, p. 1050. Springer, Berlin.
Donike, M. (1969). *J. Chromatogr.* 42, 103-104.
Donike, M., Zuzberg, H. and Jaenicke, L. (1973). *J. Chromatogr.* 85, 9-17.
Dreifuss, P.A., Wood, G.E., Roach, J.A.G., Brumley, W.G., Andrzewski, D. and Sphon, J.A. (1980). *Biomed. Mass Spectrom.* 7, 201-204.
Erb, N., Zinsmeister, H.D., Lehmann, G. and Nahrstedt, A. (1979). *Phytochemistry* 18, 1515-1517.
Ettlinger, M. and Eyjólfsson, R. (1972). *J.C.S. Chem. Comm.* 572-573.
Ettlinger, M., Jaroszewski, J.W., Jensen, S.R., Nielsen, B.J. and Nartey, F. (1977). *J.C.S. Chem. Comm.* 952-953.
Eyjólfsson, R. (1970a). *In* "Fortschritte der Chemie organischer Naturstoffe" (W. Herz, H. Grisebach and A.I. Scott, eds), Vol. 28, p. 74. Springer, Wien, New York.
Eyjólfsson, R. (1970b). *Phytochemistry* 9, 845-851
Eyjólfsson, R. (1970c). *Acta Chem. Scand.* 24, 3075.
Eyjólfsson, R. (1971). *Acta Chem. Scand.* 25, 1898-1900.
Feigl, F. and Anger, V. (1966). *Analyst* 91, 282.
Fikenscher, L.H. and Hegnauer, R. (1977). *Planta Med.* 31, 266-269.
Fikenscher, L.H. and Ruijgrok, H.W.L. (1977). *Planta Med.* 31, 290-293.
Finnmore, H. and Cooper, J.M. (1938). *J. Soc. Chem. Ind. (London)* 57, 166.
Fischer, E. and Anger, G. (1919). *Chem. Ber.* 52, 854.
Fischer, E. and Bergmann, M. (1917). *Chem. Ber.* 50, 1047.
Furuya, T. (1965). *J. Chromatogr.* 18, 152-156.
Gmelin, R., Schüler, M. and Bordas, E. (1973). *Phytochemistry* 12, 457-461.
Gondwe, A.T.D., Seigler, D.S. and Dunn, J.E. (1978). *Phytochemistry* 17, 271-274.
Harborne, J.B. and Williams, C.A. (1975). *In* "The Flavonoids" (J.B. Harborne, T.J. Mabry and H. Mabry, eds), p. 403. Chapman and Hall, London.
Hegnauer, R. and Ruijgrok, H.W.L. (1971). *Pharm. Weekblad* 106, 263-270.
Hösel, W. and Nahrstedt, A. (1975). *Hoppe-Seylers. Z. physiol. Chem.* 356, 1265-1275.
Hübel, W. (1978). Dissertation, Universität Freiburg, FRG.
Hübel, W. (1981). *Planta Med.* 42, 128.
Hübel, W. and Nahrstedt, A. (1975). *Phytochemistry* 14, 2723-2725.
Hübel, W. and Nahrstedt, A. (1978). *Planta Med.* 33, 283.
Hübel, W. and Nahrstedt, A. (1979). *Tetrahedron Letters* (45), 4395-4396.
Hübel, W., Nahrstedt, A. and Wray, V. (1981). *Arch. Pharm.* 314, 609.
Jaroszewski, J.W. (1978). Glucosides of Ketene Cyanohydrins. Symposium paper (Embo Workshop on Cyanide Metabolism), Canterbury.
Jensen, S.R. and Nielsen, B.J. (1973). *Acta Chem Scand.* 27, 2661-2662.
Kallio, H. (1972). *J. Chromatogr.* 65, 355.
Karrer, W. (1958). "Konstitution und Vorkommen der organischen Pflanzenstoffe", p. 947. Birkhäuser, Basel, Stuttgart.
Kim, S.H., Jeffrey, G.A., Pauke, D., Clapp, R.C., Coburn, R.A. and Long, L. Jr. (1970). *J.C.S. Chem. Comm.* 381-382.
Klebe, J.F., Finkbeiner, H. and White, D.M. (1966). *J. Amer. Chem. Soc.* 88, 3390-3395.

Klyne, W. (1950). *Biochem. J.* 47, xli-xlii.
Kofod, H. and Eyjólfsson, R. (1969). *Phytochemistry* 8, 1509-1511.
Larsen, L.M. (1978). Paper presented at the EMBO Workshop on Cyanide Metabolism, Canterbury, 14-18 August.
Mao, C.-H. and Anderson, L. (1965). *J. Org. Chem.* 30, 603-607.
Mao, C.-H., Blocher, J.P., Anderson, L. and Smith, D.G. (1965). *Phytochemistry* 4, 297-303.
Mauthner, F. (1912). *J. Prakt. Chem.* 85, 564.
Mehlitz, A., Gierschner, K. and Minas, T. (1963). *Chem. Ztg., Chem. App.* 87, 573-576.
Mikolajczak, K.L. (1977). *In* "Progress in the Chemistry of Fats and other Lipids" (R.T. Holman, ed.), Vol. 15, pp. 97-130. Pergamon Press, Oxford.
Mirande, M. (1909). *Compt. Rend.* 149, 140.
Nahrstedt, A. (1970). *Phytochemistry* 9, 2085-2089.
Nahrstedt, A. (1971). Dissertation, Universität Freiburg, FRG.
Nahrstedt, A. (1972). *Phytochemistry* 11, 3121-3126.
Nahrstedt, A. (1973a). *Phytochemistry* 12, 1539-1542.
Nahrstedt, A. (1973b). *Planta Med.* 24, 83-89.
Nahrstedt, A. (1973c). *Phytochemistry* 12, 2799-2800.
Nahrstedt, A. (1975a). *Phytochemistry* 14, 1339-1340.
Nahrstedt, A. (1975b). *Phytochemistry* 14, 2627-2628.
Nahrstedt, A. (1975c). *Arch. Pharm.* 308, 903-910.
Nahrstedt, A. (1976a). *Z. Naturforsch.* 31c, 397-400.
Nahrstedt, A. (1976b). *Phytochemistry* 15, 1983-1984
Nahrstedt, A. (1978). *J. Chromatogr.* 152, 265-268.
Nahrstedt, A. (1979). *J. Chromatogr.* 177, 157-161.
Nahrstedt, A. and Davis, R.H. (1981). *Comp. Biochem. Physiol.* 68B, 575-577.
Nahrstedt, A. and Hübel, W. (1978). *Phytochemistry* 17, 314-315.
Nahrstedt, A., Hösel, W. and Walther, A. (1979). *Phytochemistry* 18, 1137-1141.
Nahrstedt, A. and Scheid, H. (1981). *Phytochemistry* 20, 1309-1310.
Paris, M., Bouquet, A. and Paris, R. (1969). *C.R. Acad. Sci. Paris* 268, 2804.
Pifferi, P.G. (1966). *Bull. Sci. Fac. Chim. Ind. Bologna* 24, 215.
Reay, P.F. (1969). *Phytochemistry* 8, 2259-2260.
Reay, P.F. and Conn, E.E. (1974). *J. Biol. Chem.* 249, 5826-5830.
Russell, G.B. and Reay, P.F. (1971). *Phytochemistry* 10, 1373-1377.
Schels, H., Zinsmeister, H.D. and Pfleger, K. (1977). *Phytochemistry* 16, 1019-1023.
Schels, H., Zinsmeister, H.D. and Pfleger, K. (1978). *Phytochemistry* 17, 523-526.
Schwarzmaier, U. (1975a). *J. Chromatogr.* 111, 430-433.
Schwarzmaier, U. (1975b). *J. Chromatogr.* 114, 235-236.
Schwarzmaier, U. (1976a). *Chem. Ber.* 109, 3250-3251.
Schwarzmaier, U. (1976b). *Chem. Ber.* 109, 3379-3389.
Seifert, P. (1955). *In* "Moderne Methoden der Pflanzenanalyse". (K. Paech and M.V. Tracey, eds), Vol. IV, p. 680. Springer, Berlin.
Seigler, D.S. (1975a). *Phytochemistry* 14, 9-29.
Seigler, D.S. (1975b). *Phytochemical Bulletin* 8 (1).
Seigler, D.S., Eggerding, C. and Butterfield, C. (1974). *Phytochemistry* 13, 2330-2332.

Seigler, D.S., Butterfield, C.S., Dunn, J.E. and Conn, E.E. (1975). *Phytochemistry* 14, 1419-1420.
Sharples, D. and Stoker, J.R. (1969). *Phytochemistry* 8, 597-601.
Sharples, D., Spring, M.S. and Stoker, J.R. (1972). *Phytochemistry* 11, 3069-3071.
Smith, C.R. Jr., Weisleder, D., Miller, R.W., Palmer, I.S. and Olsen, O.E. (1980). *J. Org. Chem.* 45, 507-510.
Steyn, D.G. and Rimington, C. (1935). *Onderstepoort J. Vet. Sci. Anim. Ind.* 4, 51.
Sweeley, C.C., Bentley, R., Makita, M. and Wells, W.W. (1963). *J. Amer. Chem. Soc.* 85, 2497.
Takaishi, K., Kuwajima, H., Hatano, H. and Go, H. (1977). *Chem. Pharm. Bull.* 25, 3075-3077.
Tantisewie, B., Ruijgrok, H.W.L. and Hegnauer, R. (1969). *Pharm. Weekblad* 104, 1341-1355.
Tjon Sie Fat, L. (1977). *Proc. Koninkl. Nederl. Akad. Wetensch.* 80C, 227-237.
Tjon Sie Fat, L. (1979). *Proc. Koninkl. Nederl. Akad. Wetensch.* 82C, 165-170.
Towers, G.H.N., McInnes, A.G. and Neish, A.G. (1964). *Tetrahedron* 20, 71-77.
Trim, A.R. (1955). *In* "Moderne Methoden der Pflanzenanalyse" (K. Paech and M.W. Tracey, eds), Vol. II, p. 304. Springer, Berlin.
Turczan, J.W. and Medwick, Th. (1977). *Anal. Letters* 10, 581-590.
Turczan, J.W. and Medwick, Th. (1979). *J. Ass. Off. Anal. Chem.* 62, 190-196.
Valen, F. van (1978a). *Planta Med.* 34, 408-413.
Valen, F. van (1978b). *Proc. Koninkl. Akad. Wetensch.* 81C, 132-140.
Valen, F. van (1978c). *Proc. Koninkl. Akad. Wetensch.* 81C, 492-499
Valen, F. van (1979). *Planta Med.* 35, 141-149.
Weiss, A.H. and Tambawala, H. (1972). *J. Chromatogr. Sci.* 10, 120.
Wingertszahn, U. (1978). Staatsarbeit, Universität des Saarlandes, Saarbrücken.
Zechner, L. (1966). *In* "Die Rohstoffe des Pflanzenreichs" (J.V. Weisner, ed.), 5th edn., Lieferung 5, p. 66. J. Cramer, Weinheim.
Zilg, H. and Conn, E.E. (1974). *J. Biol. Chem.* 249, 3112-3115.
Zitnak, A. (1973). *In* "Chronic Cassava Toxicity" (B. Nestel and R. McIntyre, eds) pp. 89-96. Intern. Development Research Centre, Ottawa.
Zitnak, A., Hill, D.C. and Alexander, J.C. (1977). *Anal. Biochemistry* 77, 310-314.

BIOSYNTHESIS OF CYANOGENIC GLYCOSIDES

ERIC E. CONN

Department of Biochemistry and Biophysics, University of California, Davis, California 95616, USA

I. INTRODUCTION

The ability of living organisms to produce hydrogen cyanide (HCN) is known as cyanogenesis. Such ability is exhibited by many (approximately 2000 species) higher plants, numerous microorganisms (fungi and bacteria) and a few animals. The sources of HCN in higher plants are two, cyanogenic glycosides and lipids. Their structure, distribution, isolation and characterization are described in chapters by Seigler and Nahrstedt (this volume). This chapter is restricted to a discussion of the general features of biosynthesis of the cyanogenic glycosides, a subject which has been reviewed in greater detail elsewhere (Conn, 1973, 1979, 1980a).

II. THE BIOSYNTHETIC PATHWAY

A. PRECURSOR-PRODUCT RELATIONSHIPS

The aglycones of a majority (23) of the 28 known cyanogenic glycosides are derived from five proteinaceous amino acids, L-valine, L-isoleucine, L-leucine, L-phenylalanine and L-tyrosine. The precursor-product relationship for four such cyanogenic glycosides is shown in Fig. 1.

The specific relationships shown in Fig. 1 were selected because there is extensive experimental evidence, to be reviewed below, showing that dhurrin (or more precisely its aglycone) for example is indeed produced from L-tyrosine. Examination of the structures of the known cyanogenic glycosides (Seigler, this volume) will suggest that taxiphyllin, triglochinin, *p*-glucosyloxymandelonitrile and proteacin should also be derived from L-tyrosine and there is supporting evidence in these cases also. Older studies involving the use of ^{14}C-labelled L-tyrosine have shown this amino acid to be efficiently converted to taxiphyllin (Bleichert *et al.*, 1966), *p*-glucosyloxymandelonitrile

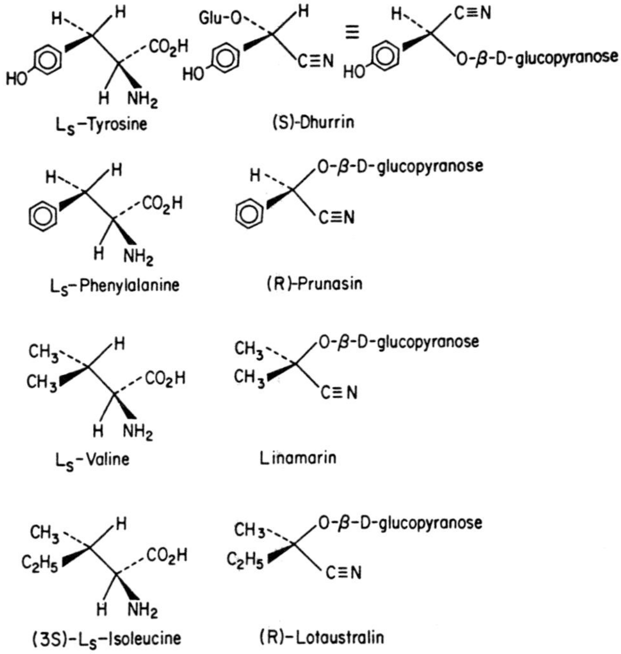

Fig. 1 The precursor product relationships for four cyanogenic glycosides. Reprinted with permission from Conn (1979).

(Abrol *et al.*, 1966; Sharples and Stoker, 1966) and proteacin (Sharples and Stoker, 1966). More recent enzymatic work (Hösel and Nahrstedt, 1980) has demonstrated that L-tyrosine is a precursor of taxiphyllin (and probably triglochinin).

A detailed investigation by Tapper and Butler (1971) established that L-phenylalanine is converted to prunasin in cherry laurel and peach tissue. This was predicted in earlier experiments which showed that ^{14}C-labelled phenylalanine is a precursor of prunasin (Mentzer and Favre-Bonvin, 1961; Ben-Yehoshua and Conn, 1964). Studies by Abrol (1967) also showed conversion of ^{14}C-labelled phenlyalanine to amygdalin in bitter almonds. While (*R*)-holocalin and (*S*)-zierin presumably ultimately arise from phenylalanine, there is no experimental evidence indicating when the *meta*-hydroxyl group is introduced into the aromatic ring. It obviously could be introduced either at the amino acid level, possibly by conversion of phenylalanine to *m*-hydroxyphenylalanine (*m*-tyrosine) or by *meta*-hydroxylation of (*R*)-prunasin and (*S*)-sambunigrin respectively.

Extensive studies, to be discussed below, also have shown that valine and isoleucine are the precursors of linamarin and lotaustralin. Again, such a precursor-product relationship was predicted by early radiochemical studies showing the conversion of ^{14}C-labelled valine and isoleucine to linamarin and lotaustralin (Butler and Butler, 1960). Undoubtedly, the recently described (Smith *et al.*, 1980) disaccharides linustatin and neolinustatin are derived from valine and isoleucine. While seven structurally related cyanogens (proacacipetalin, *epi*-proacacipetalin, heterodendrin, *epi*-heterodendrin, cardiospermin and its *p*-hydroxybenzoate and sulfate esters) presumably derive their aglycone from L-leucine, only one limited radiochemical study supports this relationship (Butterfield *et al.*, 1975).

In this connection it is important to note that not all radiochemical studies on the biosynthesis of cyanogenic glycosides have been without errors. In 1966, Abrol concluded that *Papaver nudicaule* seedlings contained linamarin and lotaustralin based on the apparent ability of seedlings of this species to convert [U-^{14}C]-valine and [U-^{14}C]-isoleucine into $H^{14}CN$ (Abrol, 1966). The $H^{14}CN$ was not rigorously identified or distinguished from $^{14}CO_2$ which could be produced from the labelled amino acids. While chromatographic evidence for linamarin and lotaustralin was provided, there was no evidence given for these compounds being labelled when the ^{14}C-labelled amino acids were administered. Ideally, the glycosides, if labelled, should have been isolated, purified and then degraded to yield $H^{14}CN$. Recently van Valen (1978) has isolated and identified dhurrin and triglochinin from leaves of flowering plants of *P. nudicaule*.

The five cyanogenic glycosides (Seigler, this volume) having a cyclopentenoid aglycone may well be derived from the non-protein amino acid cyclopentenyl glycine, whose biosynthesis in *Caloncoba echinata* (Flacourtiaceae) has recently been described (Cramer *et al.*, 1980). This precursor-product relationship seems especially possible in the case of tetraphyllin A and its presumed epimer deidaclin which have an unsubstituted cyclopentenoid aglycone. The other three glycosides in this group have one or two hydroxyl groups on the cyclopentene ring which could be introduced by hydroxylation of tetraphyllin A or deidaclin. Alternatively, a hydroxylated isomer of cyclopentene glycine might be the immediate precursor of these glycosides.

In the radiochemical studies just described, the use of amino acids specifically labelled with ^{14}C unequivocally established that the C-2 and C-3 carbons respectively were converted to the nitrile carbon atom and the carbon atom of the aglycone to which the sugar moiety is attached (Fig. 2). However, experiments involving amino acids labelled with ^{15}N and ^{14}C in the C-2 position were particularly informative regarding the biosynthetic pathway for cyanogenic glycosides (Butler and Conn, 1964; Uribe and Conn, 1966; Bleichert *et al.*, 1966). Such experiments showed that the amino acids were converted to their related cyanogenic glycoside with little change in the ratio of

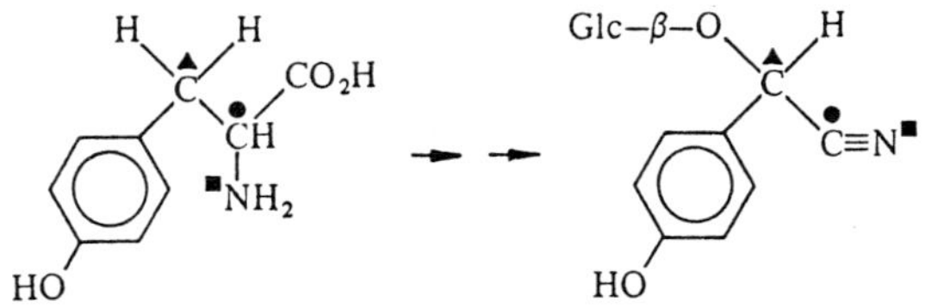

Fig. 2 Precursor-product relationship between certain atoms in L-tyrosine and the aglycone of dhurrin. Reprinted with permission from Conn (1980a).

^{15}N to ^{14}C. Such data obviously indicated that the nitrogen-carbon bond in the amino acid was not broken as biosynthesis occurs and therefore dictated that all intermediates contained nitrogen.

Another experiment involving L-tyrosine doubly labelled in the C-2 and C-3 position indicated that this carbon-carbon bond was maintained intact as L-tyrosine was converted to dhurrin (Koukol *et al.*, 1962) in sorghum. This experiment was conducted to examine whether the nitrile moiety of the cyanogenic glycoside in sorghum might arise directly from HCN addition plus glycosylation of the corresponding cyanohydrin, *p*-hydroxy-(*S*)-mandelonitrile. In retrospect, such experiments seem unnecessary since there was no evidence for a pool of *p*-hydroxybenzaldehyde required for synthesis of the cyanohydrin. Moreover, studies involving the administration of $H^{14}CN$ to sorghum seedlings (and several other cyanogenic species) showed that this compound was converted almost exclusively to ^{14}C-asparagine (Conn and Butler, 1969; Conn, 1980a). However, the capacity of sorghum seedlings to convert ^{14}C-labelled L-tyrosine to dhurrin with the remarkable yields of 25-35 per cent (Rosen *et al.*, 1975) sharply contrasted with our inability to demonstrate any labelled biosynthetic intermediates.

Similar large conversions (25% or more) of ^{14}C-labelled valine to linamarin in flax seedlings (Butler and Conn, 1964; Tapper and Butler, 1971) also predicted that ^{14}C-labelled intermediates should be detectable in such experiments. However, it was only when DL-*O*-methylthreonine, an inhibitor of linamarin biosynthesis in flax seedlings, was administered simultaneously with ^{14}C-valine that radioactive compounds which might be related to the biosynthesis of linamarin were detected in flax seedlings (Tapper and Butler, 1972). When these compounds were tentatively identified as isobutyraldoxime and its *O*-β-glucoside (Tapper, 1968) and that information was generously communicated prior to publication (Tapper and Butler, 1972) to others working in the field, efforts were concentrated on the possible role of oximes as intermediates in the biosynthesis of cyanogenic glycosides. Experiments soon established that ^{14}C-labelled isobutyraldoxime (Tapper *et al.*, 1967) and phenylacetaldoxime (Tapper, 1968) were converted either equally or more efficiently into linamarin and prunasin, respectively. Simultaneously and independently, oximes were recognized as intermediates in the biosynthesis of glucosinolates (Underhill, 1967) and it appeared that the biosynthesis of these two groups of natural products might be related.

B. EXPERIMENTS WITH LABELLED PRECURSORS AND INTERMEDIATES

A possible pathway for biosynthesis of a cyanogenic glycoside from an amino acid was proposed in 1968 after oximes and the related nitriles were shown to serve as precursors of linamarin and prunasin (Hahlbrock *et al.*, 1968). That pathway, which was subsequently revised in 1979 (Conn, 1979) to include an *N*-hydroxyamino acid as an additional intermediate (Fig. 3), was then tested in a large number of experiments.

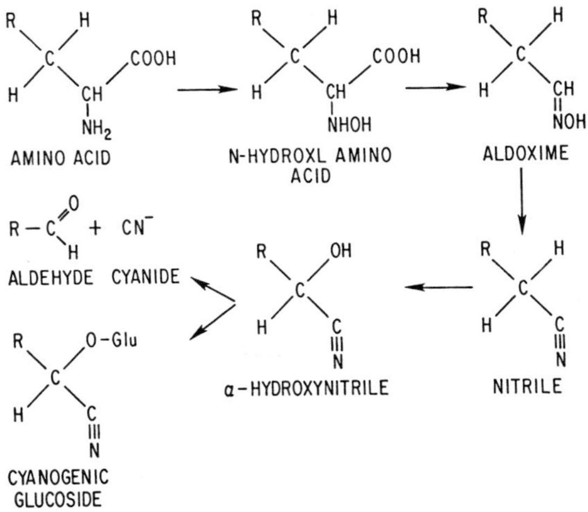

Fig. 3 The biosynthetic pathway for cyanogenic glucosides. Reprinted with permission from Conn (1979).

Three types of experiments were designed to ascertain the biosynthetic role of the aldroxime, nitrile and α-hydroxynitrile (cyanohydrin). The first involved the synthesis of ^{14}C or ^{3}H labelled compounds, their administration to cyanogenic plant tissues (i.e. sorghum, flax, cherry laurel and peach) and comparison of their incorporation with that of the known amino acid precursor. In a second type of experiment, the ^{14}C-labelled amino acid was administered simultaneously with unlabelled aldoximes or nitriles to increase the metabolic pools of these intermediates. After a period of metabolism, the aldoxime or nitrile was reisolated from the plant and examined to see whether any radioactive aldoxime or nitrile, produced from the labelled amino acid, had been "trapped" in the pool of added intermediate. These studies, which have been evaluated in recent reviews (Conn, 1973, 1980a) supported the proposed biosynthetic pathway (Fig. 3).

The third type of experiment involved the detection, partial purification and characterization of enzymes which catalyzed the last step in biosynthesis, i.e. the glucosylation of the α-hydroxynitrile to form the product cyanogenic glycoside. Such studies demonstrated the presence of enzymes in flax (Hahlbrock and Conn, 1970) and in sorghum (Reay and Conn, 1974) which catalyzed the reasonably specific synthesis of the cyanogenic glycosides characteristic of those species. Interesting differences in the stereospecificity of these two enzymes do exist, however, and these have been reviewed elsewhere (Conn, 1980a).

Although many experiments with labelled precursors, intermediates and metabolic traps were carried out, these did not settle all questions regarding the pathway postulated in Fig. 3. As an example, there are two possible routes (Fig. 4) for the conversion of aldoximes to α-hydroxynitriles (Shimada and Conn, 1977). The route that is utilized in the biosynthetic pathway is shown in Fig. 3. It involves the dehydration of the aldoxime to form a nitrile which then is subsequently oxidized to an α-hydroxynitrile. The other possibility is the oxidation of the aldoxime to an α-hydroxyaldoxime which subsequently is dehydrated to yield the α-hydroxynitrile (Fig. 4). Because of the lability of α-hydroxyaldoximes, we could not anticipate meaningful results being obtained in an experiment in which a labelled sample of α-hydroxyaldoxime would be administered to a plant. Similarly, it seemed unlikely that a trapping experiment involving unlabelled α-hydroxyisobutyraldoxime and intact plants would be informative. It was only after a cell-free enzyme system in sorghum microsomes was obtained and partially characterized that

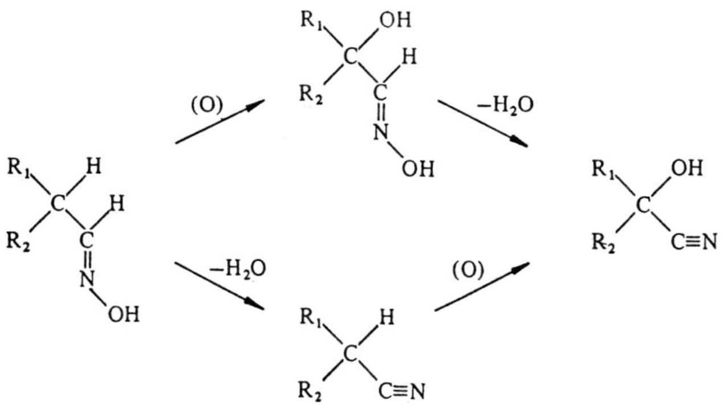

Fig. 4 Two alternative routes for the conversion of an aldoxime to an α-hydroxynitrile. Reprinted with permission from Conn (1980a).

this matter could be examined. As described in Section III, the results obtained (Shimada and Conn, 1977) appeared to rule out a role for an α-hydroxyaldoxime in the pathway.

Another unanswered question in these earlier studies concerned the nature of the intermediate, if any, between the parent amino acid and the aldoxime. The conversion of an amino acid to the homologous aldoxime represents a 4-electron oxidative decarboxylation. This is a process unlikely to proceed without at least one intermediate although the oxidative decarboxylation of amino acids to their homologous amides, which are isoatomic with aldoximes, is known to occur (Ohnishi *et al.*, 1976). Moreover, Kindl and Underhill (1968) had suggested that *N*-hydroxyphenylalanine might be an intermediate in the conversion of phenylalanine to phenylacetaldoxime in certain crucifers. Progress in sorting out the early steps in the pathway was delayed until the cell-free enzyme system, to be described now, was available and could be characterized.

III. STUDIES WITH MEMBRANE-BOUND ENZYME PREPARATIONS

The formation of the α-hydroxynitrile (Fig. 3) received substantial attention in the earlier studies in our laboratory. Zilg *et al.* (1972) demonstrated that $^{18}O_2$ was extensively incorporated into the glucosidic-linkage oxygen of linamarin and lotaustralin in flax seedlings. Thus, a direct oxygenation of the secondary carbon atom of isobutyronitrile was indicated even though dehydrogenation and hydration between that carbon atom and one of the branch methyl carbons could also serve to introduce the hydroxyl group. In the case of dhurrin biosynthesis, however, oxygenation of the methylene carbon atom in the side chain of *p*-hydroxyphenylacetonitrile would be the only alternative. For these reasons, it appeared likely that a mixed function oxidase (monooxygenase) might well be involved in the conversion of nitrile to α-hydroxynitrile. Efforts were therefore made to detect such an enzyme in the high-speed particle (microsomal) fraction from dark-grown sorghum seedlings, and Dr I.J. McFarlane was almost immediately successful in this effort.

In 1975 McFarlane *et al.* reported that microsomal fractions from sorghum seedlings could catalyze the conversion of *p*-hydroxyphenylacetonitrile to *p*-hydroxymandelonitrile in the presence of NADPH. Even more important, however, such preparations also oxidized L-tyrosine to the α-hydroxynitrile and did so more rapidly than they oxidized the nitrile. The multi-step conversion required only O_2 and NADPH (or a NADPH generating system) in addition to L-tyrosine, and the reaction was followed by measuring the HCN or *p*-hydroxybenzaldehyde formed on dissociation of the *p*-hydroxymandelonitrile. Typical data, shown in Table I, demonstrated that NADH was only about one-third

Table I Conversion of L-[U-^{14}C]-tyrosine to *p*-hydroxybenzaldehyde*

Conditions	nmols *p*-hydroxybenzaldehyde/ h/mg protein
Complete	193
minus NADPH generating system	2
minus NADPH generating system + NADPH (0.75 μmoles)	111
minus NADPH generating system + NADH (0.75 μmoles)	63
Complete, pellet fraction boiled	5
Complete, anaerobic	12
Complete, after O_2 flush	202
Complete	50[a]
Complete	0.2[b]

[a] The product measured here was *p*-hydroxyphenylacetaldoxime
[b] The product measured here was *p*-hydroxypenylacetonitrile
* Reprinted from McFarlane *et al.* (1975) with permission of the copyright owner, the American Society of Biological Chemists, Inc.

as effective as a NADPH generation system. There was an absolute requirement for O_2 and the enzyme(s) involved were saturated at the O_2 concentration (20%) in air. Significant quantities of *p*-hydroxyphenylacetaldoxime could be detected in the incubation mixture; this constitutes probably the best evidence for an aldoxime intermediate in the biosynthetic pathway (Fig. 3). Only trace amounts of *p*-hydroxyphenylacetonitrile were ever observed, however, and this is consistent also with data acquired later during studies on metabolic channelling.

As noted above, the particulate system in sorghum has been indispensible in obtaining information which could not be obtained with intact plants. The participation of the corresponding α-hydroxyaldoxime (i.e. 2-hydroxy-(4-hydroxyphenyl)-acetaldoxime) in the biosynthesis of dhurrin (Fig. 4) was examined by performing trapping experiments using either *p*-hydroxyphenylacetonitrile or the α-hydroxyaldoxime as traps (Shimada and Conn, 1977). While the nitrile did serve as a trap, the 2-hydroxyaldoxime did not and this latter compound has not been further considered as a biosynthetic intermediate.

The sorghum microsomal enzyme system was also invaluable in examining the initial steps in the biosynthetic pathway. Several lines of evidence indirectly suggested that an *N*-hydroxyamino acid might be an early intermediate in the pathway. Thus, Kindl and Underhill (1968) had proposed that *N*-hydroxyphenylalanine might be an intermediate in the formation of phenylacetaldoxime from L-phenylalanine in crucifers. These authors had also described the enzymatic conversion of *N*-hydroxyphenylalanine to phenylacetaldoxime in extracts of *Nasturtium officinale, Sinapis alba* and *Tropaeolum majus* although they did not show the formation of *N*-hydroxyphenylalanine in their plants. While the reported lability of *N*-hydroxyamino acids (Spenser and Ahmad, 1961) did little to encourage work with these compounds, it seemed essential that *N*-hydroxytyrosine be synthesized and examined as a possible first intermediate in the biosynthesis of dhurrin.

Møller *et al.* (1977) therefore developed a method for synthesis of ^{14}C-labelled (and unlabelled) *N*-hydroxytyrosine as well as a method for detecting *N*-hydroxytyrosine and separating it (Møller, 1977) from the other intermediates (and L-tyrosine) in dhurrin biosynthesis. Using these methods, Møller and Conn (1979) have shown that *N*-hydroxytyrosine is indeed formed from L-tyrosine by the sorghum particles and that *N*-hydroxytyrosine, in turn, may be enzymatically converted to the homologous aldoxime, nitrile and α-hydroxynitrile (Fig. 3) by the particles.

While the sorghum particulate enzyme system has been extremely useful in studying the biosynthesis of dhurrin, we do not yet understand all the results obtained with this system. For example, the conversion of the aldoxime to the nitrile may be formally represented as a dehydration reaction. However, this reaction when carried out as described (McFarlane *et al.*, 1975; Møller and Conn, 1979) requires NADPH for full activity. It has also not been possible to clearly establish cofactor requirements for the oxidation of *N*-hydroxytyrosine by the particles. Møller has pointed out (this volume) that there is a lack of information on the enzymatic oxidation of *N*-hydroxyamino acids and has proposed, as did Møller and Conn (1979) that 3-(4-hydroxyphenyl)-2-nitroso propionic might be an intermediate in the oxidative decarboxylation of -hydroxytyrosine to *p*-hydroxyphenylacetaldoxime. Such nitroso acids are extremely labile and the specific one required for testing in the sorghum system has not been examined.

The usefulness of the sorghum microsomal enzyme system in clarifying several aspects of dhurrin biosynthesis led to numerous attempts in the author's laboratory to obtain a particulate system with similar enzymatic capacities from another cyanogenic plant. Discouragingly negative results obtained in California were balanced by Hösel and Nahrstedt (1980) in Germany who obtained active particles from young seedlings of *Triglochin maritima*. Their particles catalyzed the formation of *p*-hydroxymandelonitrile (presumably the (*R*)-epimer) from L-tyrosine in the presence of NADPH. When a soluble protein fraction from the plant was combined with particles, tyrosine, NADPH and UDP-glucose, these authors demonstrated the synthesis of (*R*)-taxiphyllin.

Taking a clue from this work, Cutler and Sternberg

(unpubl.) in the author's laboratory have now isolated an active microsomal preparation from linen flax seedlings that catalyze the oxidation of L-valine and L-isoleucine to HCN and, presumably, acetone and 2-butanone, respectively. The clue to a successful experiment was the need to remove all traces of flax seed coat adhering to the young seedlings. If this was not done with the *T. maritima* seedlings, particles with little or no activity were obtained (Hösel and Nahrstedt, 1980). Apparently, some material in the seed coat of these two species is strongly inhibitory to the oxidation of the amino acid described.

IV. CHANNELLING OF BIOSYNTHETIC INTERMEDIATES

In the course of using the sorghum microsomal enzyme preparation to sort out the biosynthetic pathway, certain observations on the catalytic activity of the particles appeared inconsistent with the sequence of intermediates as given in the biosynthetic pathway (Fig. 3). For example, McFarlane *et al.* (1975) observed that L-tyrosine and *p*-hydroxyphenylacetaldoxime were oxidized at higher rates than *p*-hydroxyphenylacetonitrile. Later Shimada and Conn (1977) confirmed that *p*-hydroxyphenylacetaldoxime was oxidized to *p*-hydroxybenzaldehyde and HCN about three times more rapidly by the same particle preparation than was *p*-hydroxyphenylacetonitrile. Still later, Møller and Conn (1979) observed that L-tyrosine and *p*-hydroxyphenylacetaldoxime were oxidized to HCN three and eight times as rapidly, respectively, as was *p*-hydroxyphenylacetonitrile. While the rate of oxidation of the nitrile was usually more variable than the other two compounds, it was always the least rapidly oxidized.

These differences in rate appeared to conflict with the order in which these compounds occur in the biosynthetic sequence. Specifically, if the oxidation of *p*-hydroxyphenylacetonitrile is the last reaction in the formation of the α-hydroxynitrile, then neither the prior intermediates nor tyrosine itself should be oxidized more rapidly. Such a statement of course assumes that the intermediates, when added to the particles, have unrestricted access to the catalytic site(s) and that the intermediates when produced *in situ* from tyrosine readily dissociate from the membrane-associated enzymes.

The kinetic data just described resemble those of Gaertner *et al.* (1970) who have studied the conversion of 3-deoxy-D-*arabino*-heptulosonate-7-phosphate to 3 enolpyruvylshikimate-3-phosphate in *Neurospora crassa*. This sequence of five reactions was originally attributed to a multienzyme complex and is now assigned to a single polypeptide enzyme cluster (Gaertner and Cole, 1977) which exhibits the phenomenon of "catalytic facilitation". Such complexes or clusters may display an apparent increase in catalytic efficiency as they direct the flow of carbon atoms through a series of tightly bound intermediates. Such a collection of enzyme proteins (or catalytic sites in a single protein) can also account for the existence of separate metabolic pools and channelling that is observed. Gaertner (1978) has recently discussed the expected properties of such enzyme complexes or clusters.

Using two different approaches, Møller and Conn (1980) have obtained data demonstrating that the conversion of L-tyrosine to *p*-hydroxymandelonitrile in sorghum microsomes is a metabolically channelled process. The first approach, which patterned earlier studies by Kindl and coworkers (1979), involved the simultaneous addition of two differently labelled substrates, e.g. [^{3}H]-tyrosine and [^{14}C]-*p*-hydroxyphenylacetonitrile, to the sorghum microsomes, together with NADPH and buffer. After a period of metabolism, the *p*-hydroxyphenylacetonitrile was reisolated from the reaction mixture and its content of [^{3}H] and [^{14}C] compared with that in the *p*-hydroxymandelonitrile (actually *p*-hydroxybenzaldehyde). The latter of course would contain [^{3}H] obtained from [^{3}H]-tyrosine and [^{14}C] from [^{14}C]-*p*-hydroxyphenlyacetonitrile. To the extent that [^{3}H]-nitrile was more efficiently converted to the end product than was the [^{14}C]-nitrile added, this represented a preferential conversion of the [^{3}H]-nitrile produced *in situ*. Such experiments produced a channelling ratio of 112 which means that not more than one molecule of *p*-hydroxyphenylacetonitrile (^{3}H-labelled) exchanged with the pool of externally added [^{14}C]-nitrile when 112 molecules of [^{3}H]-tyrosine were converted to [^{3}H]-*p*-hydroxymandelonitrile via [^{3}H]-*p*-hydroxyphenylacetonitrile.

The second approach resembled that of Gaertner *et al.* (1970) in that two different labelled substrates were added sequentially to the sorghum microsomes. In this way one could monitor the ability of one substrate to displace the other substrate involved from a catalytic site on the sorghum microsomes. Specifically, when [^{14}C]-aldoxime was added to sorghum particles, it was not displaced by [^{3}H]-labelled aldoxime produced from [^{3}H]-tyrosine. In the reciprocal experiment, however, [^{3}H]-aldoxime produced from [^{3}H]-tyrosine was readily displaced by [^{14}C]-aldoxime added after the experiment was initiated. In a comparison experiment, *p*-hydroxyphenylacetonitrile added to particles which were actively metabolizing [^{3}H]-tyrosine could not displace the low concentration of [^{3}H]-nitrile produced *in situ* from [^{3}H]-tyrosine. However, when [^{3}H]-tyrosine was added to particles already metabolizing [^{14}C]-nitrile, the [^{3}H]-nitrile produced *in situ* nearly completely stopped the metabolism of [^{14}C]-nitrile, even though the latter compound was present at a much higher concentration.

The results from the two different types of experiments (Møller and Conn, 1980) were in excellent agreement in that they indicated that *p*-hydroxyphenylacetonitrile and

N-hydroxytyrosine are effectively channelled in sorghum microsomes which convert L-tyrosine to *p*-hydroxyphenylacetonitrile while *p*-hydroxyphenylacetaldoxime is not. This technique needs now to be applied to the microsomal preparations from *T. maritima* and flax to examine the degree and nature of channelling, if any, in these membrane-bound enzyme systems.

The channelling of metabolites observed with the sorghum particles presumably is an important factor in the tyrosine metabolism of young sorghum seedlings. As noted earlier, three-day-old seedlings contain 3-4% (dry weight) of dhurrin while the ungerminated seed contains no detectable cyanogenic glycoside. Therefore, there is a remarkable conversion of tyrosine to this secondary metabolite at a time when tyrosine is also being converted to protein, lignin and several phenolic compounds. The plant presumably requires an efficient mechanism for channelling the flow of carbon atoms from its tyrosine pool(s) into dhurrin. Such a channelled process could also be a mechanism for stabilizing labile intermediates (i.e. *N*-hydroxytyrosine) which, if allowed to dissociate from the protection of membrane-bound enzymes, might be lost in side reactions. The channelling phenomenon can even account for the fact, referred to in Section II.A, that it was never possible to detect biosynthetic intermediates either during dhurrin synthesis in sorghum seedlings or linamarin biosynthesis in flax seedlings.

V. CONCLUSION

While the available experimental evidence supports the biosynthetic pathway for cyanogenic glycosides presented in Fig. 3, much work remains to clarify the details of the reactions involved. Solubilization and characterization of the individual membrane-localized enzymes would appear to be an essential approach in this objective. Unfortunately, efforts made to date in this direction in the author's laboratory have not been successful.

There are other questions which can be asked regarding the biosynthesis of these interesting compounds (Conn, 1980b). Why, for example, do only five protein amino acids (and one non-protein amino acid) serve as precursors of these compounds? Is there something unique about the favoured five that is not shared by alanine, methionine and tryptophan which are similarly nonpolar or hydrophobic in character? Amino acids such as lysine, histidine, tryptophan, ornithine and aspartic acid are precursors of other secondary compounds (e.g. alkaloids) in plants. While the property is shared by phenylalanine and tyrosine, the branch chain amino acids haven't been noted in this regard. But leaving aside the matter of biosynthetic origin, there remain other questions regarding the sites of synthesis, their storage place in the plant cell, and ultimately their role. Fortunately, information on some of these matters is becoming available (Conn, 1980b).

REFERENCES

Abrol, Y.P. (1966). *Indian J. Chem.* 4, 251-252.
Abrol, Y.P. (1967). *Indian J. Biochem.* 4, 54-55.
Abrol, Y.P., Conn, E.E., Stoker, J.R. (1966). *Phytochemistry* 5, 1021-1027.
Ben-Yehoshua, S. and Conn, E.E. (1964). *Plant Physiol.* 39, 331-333.
Bleichert, E.F., Neish, A.C., Towers, G.H.N. and Billek, G. (eds) (1966). Vol. 3, Proc. 2nd Meet. Fed. Eur. Biochem. Soc., Pergamon Press, Oxford.
Butler, G.W. and Butler, B.G. (1960). *Nature* 187, 780-781.
Butler, G.W. and Conn, E.E. (1964). *J. Biol. Chem.* 239, 1674-1679.
Butterfield, C.S., Conn, E.E. and Seigler, D.S. (1975). *Phytochem.* 14, 993-997.
Conn, E.E. (1973). *Biochem. Soc. Symp.* 38, 277-302.
Conn, E.E. (1979). *Naturwissenschaften* 66, 28-34.
Conn, E.E. (1980a). *Encycl. Plant Physiol. New Series* 8, 461-492.
Conn, E.E. (1980b). *Ann. Rev. Plant Physiol.* 31, 433-451.
Conn, E.E. and Butler, G.W. (1969). *In* "Perspectives in Phytochemistry" (J.B. Harborne and T. Swain, eds) pp. 47-74. Academic Press, London.
Cramer, U., Rehfeldt, A.G. and Spener, F. (1980). *Biochemistry* 19, 3074-3080.
Gaertner, F.H. (1978). *Trends in Biochem. Sci.* 3, 63-65.
Gaertner, F.H. and Cole, K.W. (1977). *Biochem. Biophys. Res. Commun.* 75, 259-264.
Gaertner, F.H., Ericson, M.C. and DeMoss, J.A. (1970). *J. Biol. Chem.* 245, 595-600.
Hahlbrock, K. and Conn, E.E. (1970). *J. Biol. Chem.* 245, 917-922.
Hahlbrock, K., Tapper, B.A., Butler, G.W. and Conn, E.E. (1968). *Arch Biochem. Biophys.* 125, 1013-1016.
Hösel, W. and Nahrstedt, A. (1980). *Arch. Biochem. Biophys.* 203, 753-757.
Kindl, H. (1979). *Fed. Eur. Biochem. Soc.* 55, 49-61.
Kindl, H. and Underhill, E.W. (1968). *Phytochem.* 7, 745-756.
Koukol, J., Miljanich, P. and Conn, E.E. (1962). *J. Biol. Chem.* 237, 3223-3228.
McFarlane, I.J., Lees, E.M. and Conn, E.E. (1975). *J. Biol. Chem.* 250, 4708-4713.
Mentzer, C. and Favre-Bonvin, J. (1961). *C.R. Acad. Sci.* 253, 1072-1074.
Møller, B.L. (1977). *Anal. Biochem.* 81, 292-304.
Møller, B.L. and Conn, E.E. (1979). *J. Biol. Chem.* 254, 8575-8583.
Møller, B.L. and Conn, E.E. (1980). *J. Biol. Chem.* 255, 3049-3056.
Møller, B.L., McFarlane, I.J. and Conn, E.E. (1977). *Acta Chem. Scand. B.* 31, 343-344.
Ohnishi, T., Yamamoto, S., Hayaishi, O., Izumi, T. and Shiba, T. (1976). *Arch. Biochem. Biophys.* 176, 358-365.
Reay, P.F. and Conn, E.E. (1974). *J. Biol. Chem.* 249, 5826-5830.

Rosen, M.A., Farnden, K.J.F., Conn, E.E. and Hanson, K.P. (1975). *J. Biol. Chem.* 250, 8302- 8308.
Sharples, D. and Stoker, J.R. (1969). *Phytochem.* 8, 597-601.
Shimada, M. and Conn, E.E. (1977). *Arch. Biochem. Biophys.* 180, 199-207.
Smith, C.R. Jr., Weisleder, D., Miller, R.W., Palmer, I.S. and Olson, O.E. (1980). *J. Org. Chem.* 45, 507-510.
Spenser, I.E. and Ahmad, A. (1961). *Proc. Chem. Soc. Lond.* 375.
Tapper, B.A. (1968). PhD Thesis, Massey University, Palmerston North, New Zealand.
Tapper, B.A. and Butler, G.W. (1971). *Biochem. J.* 124, 935-941.
Tapper, B.A. and Butler, G.W. (1972). *Phytochem.* 11, 1041-1046.
Tapper, B.A., Conn, E.E. and Butler, G.W. (1967). *Arch. Biochem. Biophys.* 119, 593-595.
Underhill, E.W. (1967). *Eur. J. Biochem.* 2, 61-63.
Uribe, E. and Conn, E.E. (1966). *J. Biol. Chem.* 241, 92-94.
van Valen, F. (1978). *Proc. Konink. Nederl. Akad. Wetensch.* 81C, 492-498.
Zilg, H., Tapper, B.A. and Conn, E.E. (1972). *J. Biol. Chem.* 247, 2384-2386.

THE INVOLVEMENT OF *N*-HYDROXYAMINO ACIDS AS INTERMEDIATES IN METABOLIC TRANSFORMATIONS

BIRGER LINDBERG MØLLER

Department of Physiology, Carlsberg Laboratory,
10 Gamle Carlsberg Vej,
DK-2500 Copenhagen Valby, Denmark

I. INTRODUCTION

N-Hydroxylation constitutes an important mechanism for the mammalian metabolism of xenobiotics. Both aromatic and aliphatic amino drugs can be *N*-hydroxylated and the pharmacological importance of this process is under extensive investigation (Weisburger and Weisburger, 1973; Gorrod, 1978). *N*-Hydroxylation of naturally occurring compounds has been reported in only a few cases, most of which involve the *N*-hydroxylation of amino acids. However, the demonstration of *N*-hydroxyamino acids as intermediates in metabolic pathways has been strongly impeded by the chemical instability of these compounds, by the lack of proper analytical techniques and by their occurrence in only minute quantities in biological material. So far, *N*-hydroxyamino acids have only been implicated as intermediates in the biosynthesis of cyanogenic glucosides (Møller and Conn, 1979), glucosinolates (Kindl and Underhill, 1968), and hydroxamic acids (Stevens and Emery, 1966). In this review, the present knowledge on the involvement of *N*-hydroxyamino acids as intermediates in biological pathways is summarized with emphasis on the nature of the eyzymatic transformations responsible for their production and utilization within each pathway. The possible involvement of *N*-hydroxyamino acids in additional biosynthetic pathways is discussed. The experimental difficulties encountered in studying the metabolism of *N*-hydroxyamino acids justifies an initial presentation of analytical methods.

II. ANALYSIS OF *N*-HYDROXYAMINO ACIDS

A frequently used criterion to establish a compound as an intermediate in a biosynthetic pathway is demonstration of its occurrence. Direct isolation of an underivatized free *N*-hydroxyamino acid from biological material has not yet been achieved. As a consequence, the formation of *N*-hydroxyamino acids in biological systems has only been inferred using more or less indirect assays (Emery, 1963; Murray *et al.*, 1977; Møller, 1977). To understand the nature of such assays, the chemical properties of *N*-hydroxyamino acids need to be considered.

N-Hydroxyamino acids are colourless crystalline compounds. They are stable when kept as solids and moderately stable for periods up to several weeks when dissolved in concentrated or dilute hydrochloric or sulphuric acids (Tomlinson and Viswanatha, 1973; Møller, 1978). When the pH of solutions containing *N*-hydroxyamino acids is increased above pH 3, the rate of decomposition is greatly accelerated. For α-*N*-hydroxyamino acids, this decomposition primarily involves oxidative decarboxylation and results in the formation of the corresponding aldoxime. When no other oxidants are present, molecular oxygen serves as the oxidant (Møller, 1978) and the rate of decomposition can be diminished by flushing the solutions with nitrogen gas. Other oxidants, i.e. ferric ions, will also smoothly effect this conversion. This becomes particularly important in experiments dealing with very small amounts of α-*N*-hydroxyamino acids, i.e. during synthesis of material of high specific radioactivity for biosynthetic studies, where trace amounts of oxidants present in solvents or on glassware can cause complete decomposition of the α-*N*-hydroxyamino acid into an aldoxime. The pH dependence of the rate of decomposition reflects the more facile oxidation of an unprotonized hydroxylamine group. The dissociation constants for an α-*N*-hydroxyamino acid are:

$$\mathrm{p}K_1\ 2.0\ \text{to}\ 2.5\ \left(\mathrm{R{-}CH(NH_2^{\oplus}{-}OH){-}COOH} \rightleftarrows \mathrm{R{-}CH(NH_2^{\oplus}{-}OH){-}COO^{\ominus}} + \mathrm{H}^{\oplus}\right)$$

and

$$\mathrm{p}K_2\ 5.2\ \text{to}\ 6.0\ \left(\mathrm{R{-}CH(NH_2^{\oplus}{-}OH){-}COO^{\ominus}} \rightleftarrows \mathrm{R{-}CH(NH{-}OH){-}COO^{\ominus}} + \mathrm{H}\right)^{\oplus}$$

(Ahmad, 1974; Møller *et al.*, 1977b). Other *N*-hydroxyamino acids are also converted oxidatively into aldoximes. However, above pH 7, the decomposition appears more complex (Emery, 1966; Tomlinson and Viswanatha, 1973).

α-*N*-Hydroxyamino acids disproportionate into the parent amino acids and the corresponding aldoximes when refluxed under nitrogen (Møller *et al.*, 1977b). The earlier reported formation of the corresponding ketoxime as a product of this reaction (Spenser and Ahmad, 1961) seems questionable. Both the oxidative decarboxylation reactions of *N*-hydroxyamino acids into aldoximes and the disproportionation reaction may involve α-nitroso acids as intermediates. These are extremely unstable and give rise to aldoximes upon decarboxylation (Pritzkow and Rosler, 1967).

The labile nature of *N*-hydroxyamino acids greatly reduces the number of analytical methods applicable for their determination. The most direct analytical method reported for the identification and quantitation of an *N*-hydroxyamino acid in biological material is based on trimethylsilylation. The complex mixture of trimethylsilyl derivatives obtained including the stable trimethylsilyl derivative of the *N*-hydroxyamino acid is then analyzed by gas liquid chromatography (Møller, 1977). Coupling of the gas chromatograph to a gas proportional counter and use of radioactively labelled substrates allows determination of accumulated intermediates without interference from any other trimethylsilyl derivatives formed from the biological material (Møller and Conn, 1979). Coupling the gas chromatograph to a mass spectrometer and the use of stable isotope labelled precursors allows identification of the intermediates even in the presence of unlabelled carrier material (Møller *et al.*, 1977a, 1979). The procedure described (Møller, 1977; Møller and Conn, 1979) should be of general applicability and has been used to identify and quantitate intermediates including *N*-hydroxytyrosine involved in the synthesis of the cyanogenic glucosides dhurrin and taxiphyllin by microsomal preparations from *Sorghum bicolor* and *Triglochinin maritima* , respectively (Møller 1979; Hösel and Nahrstedt, 1980).

Analysis of *N*-hydroxyamino acids by either thin-layer or paper chromatography, or by high-voltage electrophoresis has proven to be difficult. Thus the radioactivity patterns obtained upon thin-layer chromatography of [U-^{14}C]-*N*-hydroxytyrosine on cellulose plates by use of a variety of solvent systems are greatly altered when the separations are carried out in a nitrogen atmosphere (Møller, 1978), indicating a high degree of oxidative decomposition of the *N*-hydroxyamino acid in the presence of oxygen.

Paper chromatographic analysis of *N*-hydroxyamino acids (Spenser and Ahmad, 1961; Emery, 1963; Cooper and Griffith, 1979) also seems to be accompanied by decomposition reactions. When six different α-*N*-hydroxyamino acids were analysed by paper chromatography, ninhydrin spots which correspond to those of the parent amino acids were observed (Spenser and Ahmad, 1961). This observation was explained by disproportionation of the α-*N*-hydroxyamino acid during chromatography. *N*-Hydroxyamino acids have also been studied by high voltage electrophoresis. *N*-hydroxyaspartic acid was analysed at pH 5 in a pyridine-acetate buffer, but the use of either a higher or lower pH results in decomposition of the *N*-hydroxyamino acid (Emery, 1963). Unfortunately, the electrophoretic mobilities of *N*-hydroxyaspartic acid and aspartic acid are identical at pH 5. Under the same conditions, δ-*N*-hydroxyornithine can be separated from its parent amino acid ornithine and from its oxidation product, glutamic acid-γ-semialdehyde oxime, with only negligible decomposition (Emery, 1966).

N-hydroxyamino acids may be visualized on chromatograms or electropherograms by use of spray reagents. Due to the reducing capacity of *N*-hydroxyamino acids, a red colour is obtained with triphenyltetrazolium chloride (Snow, 1954; Emery, 1963; Nagasawa *et al.*, 1972) and a black colour with silver nitrate (Spenser and Ahmad, 1961). Depending on the compound and conditions, ninhydrin has been reported to give no colour (Snow, 1954; Ahmad and Spenser, 1961), brown to purple colour (Emery, 1963), blue colour (Emery and Neilands, 1961) and orange colour (Møller, 1978). The latter colour obtained after thin layer chromatography of *N*-hydroxytyrosine under a nitrogen atmosphere could originate from an oxidation product of *N*-hydroxytyrosine formed on the thin layer plate when this was exposed to the atmosphere after termination of the chromatographic separation. Use of acid ninhydrin results in no colour formation (Tomlinson and Viswanatha, 1973). When analysed under standard conditions in the amino acid analyser the ninhydrin colour yield of *N*-hydroxyamino acids relative to that of norleucine varied between 4 and 26% (Cooper and Griffith, 1979). However, *N*-hydroxyamino acids are unstable under this analytical procedure giving rise to skewed evanescent peaks (Tomlinson and Viswanatha, 1973).

Other methods to detect *N*-hydroxyamino acids involve their reduction to the parent amino acids either by catalytic hydrogenation (Neelakantan and Hartung, 1958; Emery and Neilands, 1961; Emery, 1963; Tomlinson and Viswanatha, 1973) or by extended reflux in 6 *N*-hydrochloric acid (Tomlinson and Viswanatha, 1973). With these methods, the presence of the parent amino acid in the material to be analysed poses additional requirements with respect to preliminary separations or additional assays.

An analytical procedure used to quantitate *N*-hydroxyamino acids is based on colorimetric determination of hydroxylamine (Tomlinson *et al.*, 1971; Parniak *et al.*, 1979). The *N*-hydroxyamino acid is converted by iodine treatment into the corresponding oxime. The hydroxylamine liberated upon hydrolysis of the aldoxime is oxidized to nitrite by iodine and the nitrite is estimated colorimetrically by diazotization of sulphanilic acid and coupling with α-naphthylamine. However, the recovery of nitrate from most *N*-hydroxyamino acids is low (Tomlinson *et al.*, 1971) and the procedure has therefore to be calibrated for individual *N*-hydroxyamino acids and seems unsuitable for their mixtures.

Several experimental approaches have been developed to achieve the synthesis of both α- and ω-*N*-hydroxyamino acids. These procedures include:

(1) reaction of hydroxylamine with the appropriate α-halogenocarboxylic acid (Hantszch and Wild, 1896; Cook and Slater, 1956; Lancini *et al.*, 1966; Kamiński and Sokołowska, 1973) or with α,β-unsaturated carboxylic

acids (Posner, 1912; Emery, 1963)

(2) partial reduction of oximes with diborane or sodium cyanoborohydride (Feuer *et al.*, 1965; Borch *et al.*, 1971; Ahmad, 1974; Møller *et al.*, 1977b; Cooper and Griffith, 1979)

(3) synthesis and hydrolysis of appropriate nitrone derivatives (Buehler and Brown, 1967)

(4) synthesis via cyclization of the hydroxamate of the corresponding ω-halogenocarboxylic acid (Smrt *et al.*, 1959)

(5) partial reduction of the corresponding nitro derivative (Bamberger, 1884; Beckmann, 1909; Marvel and Kamm, 1919; Leeds and Smith, 1951; Neilands and Azari, 1963; Rogers and Neilands, 1963; Tomlinson and Viswanatha, 1973).

(6) reaction of nitrogen oxide with alkylated derivatives of acetoacetic ester (Traube, 1894, 1895) or malonic ester (Neelakantan and Hartung, 1958) followed by hydrolysis

(7) addition of hydrogen cyanide to oximes and subsequent hydrolysis (Miller and Plöchl, 1893; Porter and Hellerman, 1944; Neelakantan and Hartung, 1958; Duynstee *et al.*, 1965)

(8) partial oxidation of the corresponding amines with hydrogen peroxide (Rogers, 1955)

(9) synthesis of cyclic *N*-hydroxyamino acids by oxidation of the corresponding cyanoethylated amino acid (Nagasawa *et al.*, 1972)

(10) synthesis using enzymatic transformations (Emery, 1963; Møller, 1978).

The easiest route of most *N*-hydroxyamino acids seems to be the one based on partial reduction of the corresponding ketoxime to the *N*-hydroxyamino acid (Borch *et al.*, 1971). This route presumably results in the production of a mixture of D- and L-stereoisomers. D- and L-amino acid oxidases have recently been shown to catalyse a stereo-specific conversion of D- and L-*N*-hydroxyamino acids, respectively into their corresponding ketoximes (Cooper and Griffith, 1979); this transformation will be useful in resolving *N*-hydroxyamino acids. Several of the synthetic routes for *N*-hydroxyamino acids are believed to produce mainly one stereoisomer (Cook and Slater, 1956; Liberek and Palacz, 1971; Nagasawa *et al.*, 1972). However, the use of these methods are restricted and the yields generally low. It should be noted that many *N*-hydroxyamino acids can be obtained easily by hydrolysis of hydroxamic acids produced in gram quantities by microorganisms (Rogers and Neilands, 1963; Emery, 1966; Stevens and Emery, 1966). The difficulties encountered in obtaining *N*-hydroxyamino acids free of impurities derived either from their synthesis or by decomposition is clearly reflected in the variation of the melting points reported for the same *N*-hydroxyamino acid (McKinney *et al.*, 1950; Cook and Slater, 1956; Neelakantan and Hartung, 1958; Liberek and Palacz,

1971; Nagasawa *et al.*, 1972; Kamińsky and Sokołowska, 1973; Ahmad, 1974; Møller *et al.*, 1977b; Cooper and Griffith, 1979).

III. *N*-HYDROXYAMINO ACIDS AS INTERMEDIATES IN BIOSYNTHETIC REACTIONS

A. BIOSYNTHESIS OF CYANOGENIC GLUCOSIDES

The five protein amino acids valine, leucine, isoleucine, phenylalanine, and tyrosine, are the primary precursors of cyanogenic glucosides (Seigler, 1975). A pathway for the biosynthesis of cyanogenic glucosides involving aldoximes, nitriles, and cyanohydrins as intermediates was proposed by Conn (1969). Biosynthetic studies with microsomal membranes isolated from etiolated sorghum seedlings lend support to the proposed pathway (McFarlane *et al.*, 1975; Shimada and Conn, 1977). Additional studies on the involvement of *N*-hydroxyamino acids in the biosynthesis of cyanogenic glucosides have been carried out using this same microsomal preparation and are discussed below.

The first intermediate which could be readily identified in earlier studies was the aldoxime (Fig. 1). Aldox-

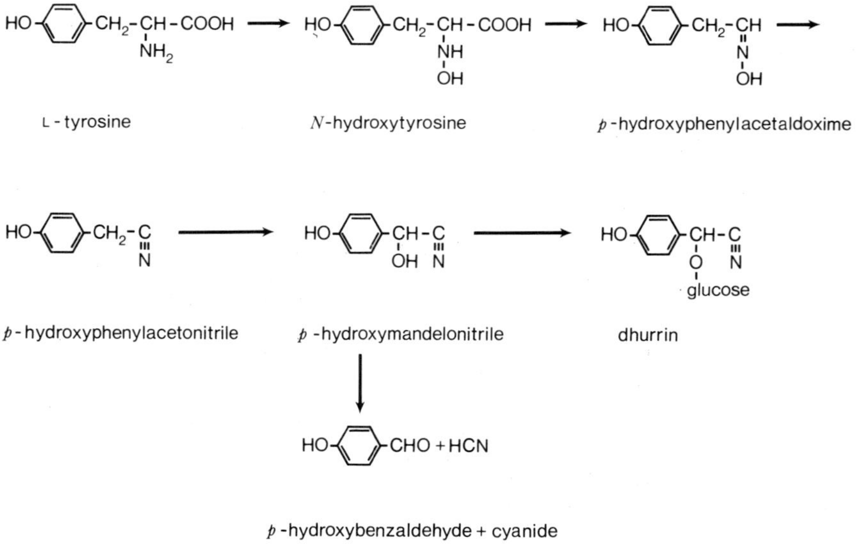

Fig. 1. Biosynthetic pathway for the cyanogenic glucoside dhurrin.

imes can formally be obtained from their parent amino acids by a four electron oxidative decarboxylation. Various reaction mechanisms for this transformation were tested by addition of the suspected intermediate compounds to the microsomal preparation with NADPH added as a cofactor. Under such conditions the particles oxidize tyrosine to *p*-hydroxymandelonitrile which dissociates into *p*-hydroxybenzaldehyde and cyanide. The amount of cyanide produced is therefore a convenient measure of metabolic activity. Of the compounds tested (Møller and Conn, 1979), only *N*-hydroxytyrosine gives rise to cyanide formation suggesting *N*-hydroxytyrosine as an intermediate in the conversion of tyrosine to *p*-hydroxyphenylacetaldoxime. However, the disproportionation of *N*-hydroxytyrosine into tyrosine and *p*-hydroxyphenylacetaldoxime had earlier been demonstrated (Møller *et al.*, 1977b). Furthermore, *N*-hydroxytyrosine is slowly converted to *p*-hydroxyphenylacetaldoxime by oxidizing agents. The decomposition products thus formed are known precursors of dhurrin, and therefore the cyanide formation observed upon administration of *N*-hydroxytyrosine to the microsomal membranes could reflect metabolism of the decomposition products rather than conversion of *N*-hydroxytyrosine itself. This was tested in the following ways: First, the microsomal membranes were preincubated with *N*-hydroxytyrosine in the absence of NADPH. After addition of NADPH the rate of cyanide production observed was not enhanced compared to experiments where no preincubation was made. Secondly, when *N*-hydroxytyrosine was used as substrate the rate of cyanide formation was not changed upon addition of tyrosine decarboxylase. Thus, the observed metabolism of *N*-hydroxytyrosine is neither due to initial non-enzymatic disproportionation or to oxidative decarboxylation reactions, nor to an initial reduction of *N*-hydroxytyrosine to tyrosine by the microsomal membranes.

Additional evidence for *N*-hydroxytyrosine as an intermediate in the pathway is the demonstration of its formation by the microsomal membranes (Møller and Conn, 1979). When carbon-14 labelled L-tyrosine is administered to the microsomal preparation in the presence of NADPH the radiochemically labelled products generally observed are small amounts of *p*-hydroxyphenylacetaldoxime and large amounts of *p*-hydroxybenzaldehyde (or its enzymatic oxidation product *p*-hydroxybenzoic acid) formed by dissociation of *p*-hydroxymandelonitrile. The production of radioactively labelled *N*-hydroxytyrosine is observed only when large amounts of unlabelled *N*-hydroxytyrosine are added as a trap. The [^{14}C]-*N*-hydroxytyrosine which accumulates was identified by the use of a gas chromatograph coupled to a gas proportional counter after trimethylsilylation of the lyophilized reaction mixtures (Møller, 1977).

The production of *N*-hydroxytyrosine from tyrosine seems to be catalyzed by a mixed function oxidase. The reaction is strongly dependent on NADPH and molecular oxygen and stable isotope experiments with $^{18}O_2$ have shown the quantitative incorporation of ^{18}O into the hydroxylamine and oxime oxygen atoms of *N*-hydroxytyrosine and *p*-hydroxyphenylacetaldoxime, respectively (Møller *et al.*, 1977a). The use of α-d_1-L-tyrosine as substrate showed that the α-hydrogen atom of tyrosine is retained in *N*-hydroxytyrosine and *p*-hydroxyphenylacetaldoxime. The mass spectrometric analysis of these stable isotope experiments provides independent, unambiguous demonstration of *N*-hydroxytyrosine formation by the microsomal membranes. The enzyme system catalyzing the *N*-hydroxylation reaction has a high degree of substrate specificity. Thus neither D- and L-phenylalanine, D- and L-histidine, L-valine, nor D-tyrosine were metabolized. This suggests that the biosynthesis of other cyanogenic glucosides is catalysed by enzyme systems each specific for the corresponding parent amino acid (Møller and Conn, 1979).

Compared to the formation of *N*-hydroxytyrosine, the mechanism of its enzymatic utilization is less well understood. The results of biosynthetic experiments point towards *p*-hydroxyphenylacetaldoxime as an intermediate in the biosynthesis of dhurrin since this compound is a good substrate for the microsomal preparation and is formed as the major product when L-tyrosine is used as a substrate for microsomes prepared in the absence of β-mercaptoethanol (Shimada and Conn, 1977; Møller and Conn, 1979, 1980). Conversion of *N*-hydroxytyrosine into *p*-hydroxyphenylacetaldoxime is a two electron oxidative decarboxylation and should be dependent on an oxidized cofactor such as NAD^+, $NADP^+$, FAD, or FMN. No absolute requirement for any of these cofactors has been demonstrated although the addition of strong reducing agents which convert these cofactors into their reduced forms inhibited *N*-hydroxytyrosine utilization. No accumulation of *N*-hydroxytyrosine was observed under these conditions when tyrosine was used as a substrate. Recent studies where differently labelled intermediates were administered to the microsomal membranes point towards the catalysis of the biosynthetic pathway by either a multienzyme complex or by a multifunctional enzyme exhibiting the phenomenon of metabolic channeling (Møller and Conn, 1980), although other interpretations of the results can be proposed (Gaertner, 1978). It is possible, that the $NADP^+$ formed upon the oxygenation of tyrosine is regenerated to NADPH in the following oxidative decarboxylation reaction without the possibility for an exchange with externally added $NADP^+$.

The next putative step in the biosynthetic pathway for dhurrin is the conversion of *p*-hydroxyphenylacetaldoxime into *p*-hydroxyphenylacetonitrile (Fig. 1). This reaction can be formulated as a simple dehydration reaction supposedly catalysed by a hydro-lyase. The transformation is strongly dependent upon NADPH as a cofactor for the hydrolyase whereas the typical cofactor for soluble hydrolyases is pyridoxal-phosphate (IUPAC, 1972). The only hydro-lyases reported to be dependent upon pyridine nucleotides are those involved in the biosynthesis of deoxysugars (Elbein and Heath, 1965; Hey and Elbein, 1966: Matsuhashi *et al.*, 1966; Wang and Gabriel, 1969). These hydro-lyases are soluble and the dehydration reaction seems to occur by a two-step procedure involving a 4-keto-6-deoxyhexose nucleotide as an intermediate (Matsuhashi *et al.*, 1966, Melo *et al.*, 1968). The overall dehydration reaction is therefore composed of an oxidation and a reduction process which makes the requirement for pyridine nucleotides understandable. The direct conversion of an aldoxime into a nitrile by a similar mechanism involving redox processes seems difficult to formulate. A soluble hydro-lyase from the fungus *Gibberella fujikuroi* is known specifically to catalyse the conversion of indoleacetaldoxime into indoleacetonitrile (Shukla and Mahadevan, 1968). The properties of this anzyme differ from those of the membrane bound enzyme converting *p*-hydroxyphenylacetaldoxime into *p*-hydroxyphenylacetonitrile.

The last biosynthetic step catalysed by the microsomal membranes is the hydroxylation of *p*-hydroxyphenylacetonitrile into *p*-hydroxymandelonitrile (Shimada and Conn, 1977). The latter is then converted by a soluble UDPG-glucosyltransferase into dhurrin (Reay and Conn, 1974).

B. BIOSYNTHESIS OF GLUCOSINOLATES

More than 80 different glucosinolates are known and are presumably derived from amino acids (Larsen, 1981). Seven of the known glucosinolates can be formulated as derivatives of the protein amino acids alanine, valine, leucine, isoleucine, phenylalanine, tyrosine, and tryptophan. The remaining glucosinolates are supposedly formed either from non-protein amino acids produced from protein amino acids by a chain lengthening process or by modifications of the side chains at the glucosinolate level. As yet, no cell free system catalysing several of the reactions involved in the biosynthesis of glucosinolates has been obtained which has made detailed studies of the biosynthetic pathway difficult. The biosynthetic pathway for glucosinolates is considered to proceed from an amino acid via a *N*-hydroxyamino acid, an aldoxime, a thiohydroximic acid, and finally a desulphoglucosinolate. The evidence available for the involvement of these intermediates is discussed below.

Amino acids have been established as precursors of glucosinolates (Ettlinger and Kjaer, 1968; Mahadevan, 1973; Larsen, 1981) (Fig. 2). The next intermediate in the pathway is believed to be an *N*-hydroxyamino acid. Incorporation of radioactively labelled DL-*N*-hydroxyphenylalanine into glucotropaeolin has been reported (Kindl and Underhill, 1968). As discussed above for the biosynthesis of cyanogenic glucosides, the interpretation of this result is ambiguous because of the easy decomposition of *N*-hydroxyamino acids into aldoximes which by themselves are intermediates (Møller *et al.*, 1977; Møller, 1979). The formation of *N*-hydroxyphenylalanine in the preparation studied was not demonstrated.

Evidence for aldoximes as intermediates in the biosynthesis of glucosinolates has been obtained by demonstrating that aldoximes are natural constituents of glucosinolate-producing plants (Underhill, 1967) and by incorporating labelled aldoximes into glucosinolates (Tapper and

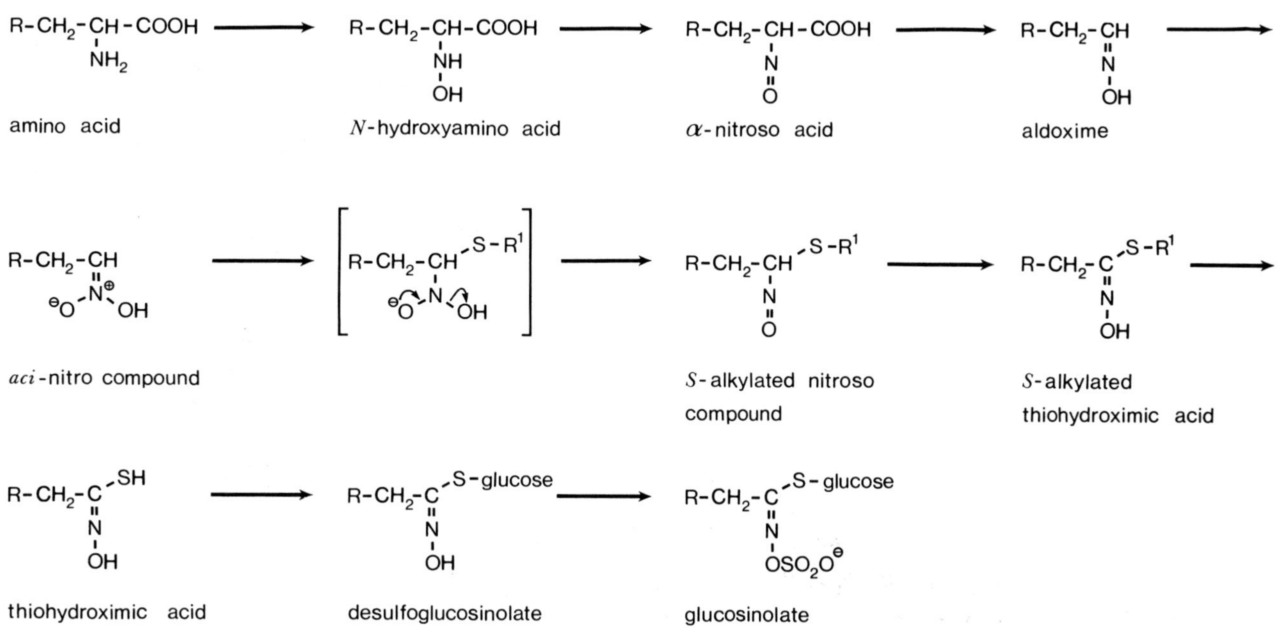

Fig. 2. Proposed biosynthetic pathway for glucosinolates.

Butler, 1967; Underhill, 1967). Conversion of an *N*-hydroxyamino acid into an aldoxime has been reported with partially purified enzyme preparations (Kindl and Underhill, 1968). In contrast to the analogous enzyme transformation described in sorghum seedlings (Møller and Conn, 1979), the enzyme activity associated with this reaction in Tropaeolum leaves was soluble. A marked increase in total and specific activity, obtained by heat treatment, was interpreted to indicate the removal of an inhibitor. A similar stimulation of the conversion of *N*-hydroxytyrosine to *p*-hydroxyphenylacetaldoxime was observed upon heating of the microsomal parti cles from sorghum. This was explained by perturbation of the membrane structure resulting in increased accessibility of the *N*-hydroxyamino acid to compounds in the membranes which then chemically oxidize *N*-hydroxyamino acids (Møller, unpubl.).

Aldoximes are transformed into glucosinolates with thiohydroximic acids and desulphoglucosinolates as known intermediates (Matsuo and Underhill, 1969; Underhill and Wetter, 1969) Fig. 2). Intermediates in the conversion of aldoximes into thiohydroximic acids have not been identified with certainty. The *aci* tautomers of nitro compounds have been implicated in this transformation (Ettlinger and Kjær, 1968) and it was subsequently demonstrated that phenylacetaldoxime is enzymatically converted into 1-nitro-2-phenylethane in *Tropaeolum majus* (Matsuo *et al.*, 1972). The nitro compound was also shown to be a natural constituent of this plant and to be incorporated into benzylglucosinolate (Matsuo *et al.*, 1972). The sulphur atom of the thiohydroximic acids seems to derive from cysteine (Wetter and Chisholm, 1968) and one possible route to the formation of the thiohydroximic acid involves the addition of cysteine to the *aci* form of the nitro compound (Ettlinger and Kjær, 1968) (Fig. 2). The *S*-alkylated nitroso compound thus formed is tautomeric to an *S*-alkylated thiohydroximic acid. The thiohydroximic acid can be obtained by enzymatic dealkylation probably involving a C-S lyase of similar nature to those already described (Binkley, 1950; Schwimmer and Kjær, 1960; Moore and Thompson, 1967) and can subsequently be converted into a desulphoglucosinolate (Matsuo and Underhill, 1969; Matsuo and Underhill, 1971) and the glucosinolate itself (Underhill *et al.*, 1973).

C. BIOSYNTHESIS OF HYDROXAMATES

A substantial number of hydroxamates are found in nature, originating mainly from microbial sources (Neilands, 1967; Emery, 1971; Neilands, 1973). Hydroxamates are formed from the amino acids glycine, alanine, leucine, isoleucine, tyrosine, lysine, and ornithine, and may contain one, two, or three -CON(OH)- groups. The biosynthesis of the hydroxamates hadacidin (Stevens and Emery, 1966), ferrichrome (Emery, 1966), rhodotorulic acid (Akers and Neilands, 1973), and aerobactin (Parniak *et al.*, 1979) seems to proceed from

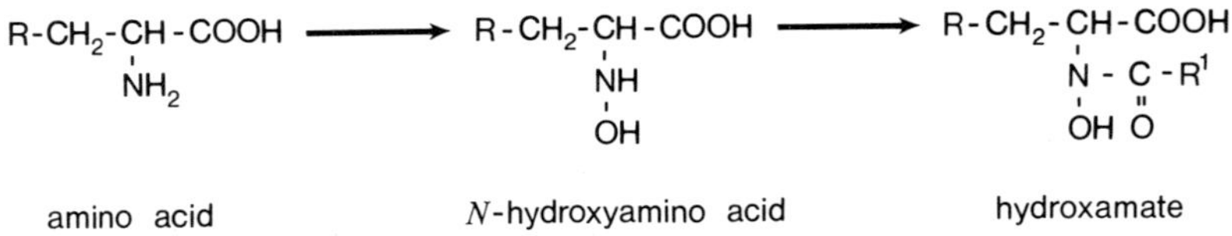

Fig. 3. Biosynthetic pathway for hydroxamates.

the parent amino acid with an *N*-hydroxyamino acid as the first intermediate followed by an acylation reaction and the final production of the hydroxamate (Fig. 3). Although *N*-hydroxyamino acids have not yet been isolated from any hydroxamate producing microorganism, strong evidence for their involvement has been obtained by use of cell-free extracts from *Aerobacter aerogenes* (Murray *et al.*, 1977; Parniak *et al.*, 1979). Upon incubation of these extracts with L-lysine, a product was obtained which by iodine and performic acid oxidation and by paper chromatography behaved similarly to ε-*N*-hydroxylysine. In earlier studies, *N*-hydroxyglycine (Stevens and Emergy, 1966) and δ-*N*-hydroxyornithine (Emery, 1966) were administered to cultures of *Penicillium aurantio-violaceum* and *Ustilago sphaerogena* and were shown to be incorporated into hadacidin and ferrichrome, respectively. In contrast to the situation with cyanogenic glucosides and glucosinolates, oxidative decomposition products of *N*-hydroxyamino acids cannot serve as precursors for hydroxamic acids and the presence of a metabolic pathway interrelating the *N*-hydroxyamino acid and the hydroxamate is therefore unambiguously demonstrated. The oxygen atom of the hydroxamate group is derived from molecular oxygen (Stevens and Emery, 1966; Akers and Meilands, 1978). This is also true for the oxygen atom of hydroxamates produced by an alternative biosynthetic pathway in which the acylation step precedes that of the *N*-hydroxylation (Micetich and MacDonald, 1964; MacDonald, 1965). Free *N*-hydroxyamino acids are not intermediates in this pathway. It should be noted that the biosynthesis of 2,4-dihydroxy-7-methoxy-1,4-benzoxazin-3-one (DIMBOA), a cyclic hydroxamate produced by plants, involves such a hydroxylation of an amide structure (Reimann and Byerrum, 1964; Tipton *et al.*, 1967).

Cell-free systems capable of synthesizing siderophores of the ferrichrome-type have recently been obtained from *Aspergillus fumigatus* and *A. quadricinctus* (Müller and Diekmann, 1977). This should greatly facilitate more detailed studies on the biosynthesis of hydroxamates.

D. BIOSYNTHESIS OF NITRO COMPOUNDS

The occurrence of nitro groups in compounds of biological origin is rare (Larsen, 1968). Two nitro compounds, 3-nitropropionic acid and 1-nitro-2-phenylethane, and their glucosides are known from higher plants. These compounds were early postulated to arise through oxidation of the amino acids aspartic acid and phenylalanine, respectively, with α-nitrocarboxylic acids as intermediates (Gottlieb *et al.*, 1961). α-Nitrocarboxylic acids have never been isolated from natural sources and decarboxylate easily (Pedersen, 1934). In agreement with the above speculation it has been shown in fungi that both the amino group and the carbon skeleton of aspartic acid are incorporated directly into 3-nitropropionic acid (Shaw and McCloskey, 1969) and that the nitro group is not derived from oxidation of inorganic nitrogen compounds such as the ammonium ion (Shaw and DeAngelo, 1969). 3-Nitroacrylate is converted in cell-free extracts of *Penicillium atrovenetum* into 3-nitropropionic acid and an enzyme with a high degree of substrate specificity has been partially purified from these extracts (Shaw, 1967). No data on intermediates having the nitrogen atom in oxidation states between that of aspartic acid and 3-nitropropionic acid were provided.

1-Nitro-2-phenylethane has been shown to be a constituent of the shoots of *Tropaeolum majus* and its formation from phenylacetaldoxime was demonstrated in a trapping experiment (Matsuo *et al.*, 1972). Thus the final step in the biosynthesis of 1-nitro-2-phenylethane seems to be *N*-hydroxylation of phenylacetaldoxime to form the tautomeric *aci*-nitro compound. In analogy with the biosynthetic pathway for cyanogenic glucosides and glucosinolates, this result indicates that those nitro compounds which can be derived easily from amino acids may be formed with *N*-hydroxyamino acids, aldoximes and *aci*-nitro compounds as intermediates.

IV. CONCLUDING REMARKS: A UNIFYING PRINCIPLE

It is apparent from the preceeding discussions that the biosynthetic routes to cyanogenic glucosides, glucosinolates, hydroxamates and nitro compounds all share common intermediates. It is therefore tempting to speculate that these four classes of secondary plant products may be derived from a common pathway with various branchpoints determining which class of compounds is finally produced (Fig. 4). Amino acids would be listed as precursors for all four classes of compounds in such a scheme and *N*-hydroxyamino acids would be the first intermediate. A side-branch would then involve acylation of the *N*-hydroxyamino acid resulting in the formation of hydroxamates. The main route would involve oxidative decarboxylation of the *N*-hydroxyamino acid to produce an aldoxime most likely with an α-nitroso acid as an intermediate.

The biosynthesis of cyanogenic glucosides and glucosinolates probably diverges at the aldoxime level (Mahadevan, 1973) (Fig. 4). To form cyanogenic glucosides, the aldoxime is dehydrated into a nitrile which then by hydroxylation is transformed into a cyanohydrin yielding the cyanogenic glucoside upon glucosylation. The formation of gluc-

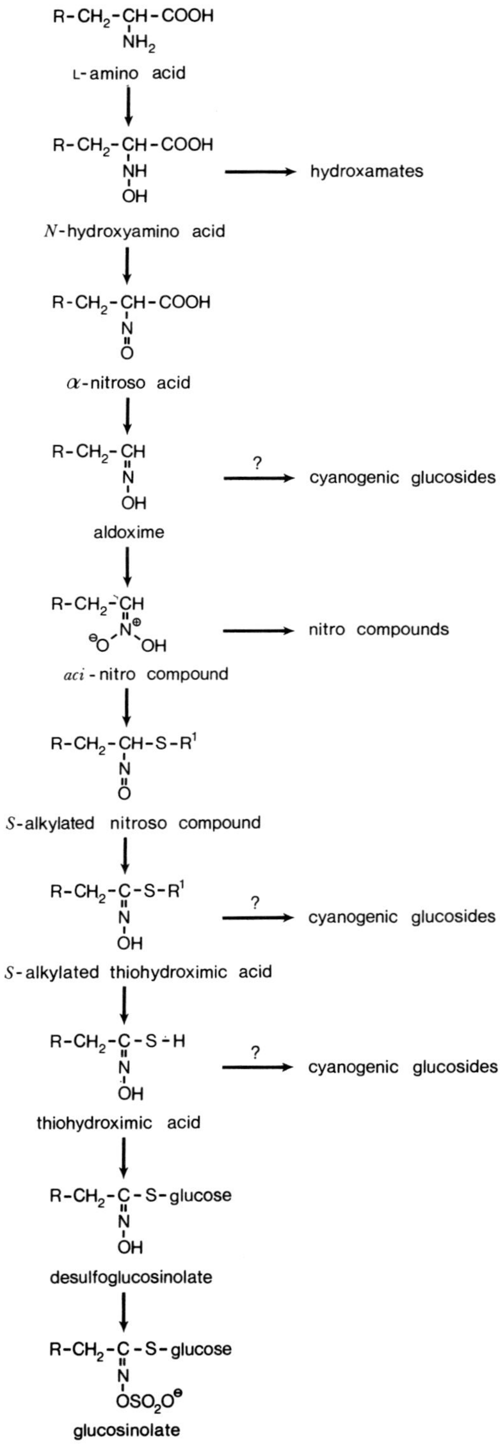

L-amino acid
hydroxamates
N-hydroxyamino acid
α-nitroso acid
?
cyanogenic glucosides
aldoxime
nitro compounds
aci-nitro compound
S-alkylated nitroso compound
?
cyanogenic glucosides
S-alkylated thiohydroximic acid
?
cyanogenic glucosides
thiohydroximic acid
desulfoglucosinolate
glucosinolate

osinolates most likely involves an additional *N*-hydroxylation step to form an *aci*-nitro compound. The *aci*-nitro compound may give rise to nitro compounds by tautomerization or may be metabolized into glucosinolates by addition of cysteine to form an *S*-alkyl thiohydroximic acid. Enzymatic dealkylation produces a thiohydroximic acid which by glucosylation is converted into a desulphoglucosinolate. Finally the glucosinolate is formed by enzymatic sulphurylation. A number of additional possibilities exist for the metabolism of aldoximes. These are discussed elsewhere (Mahadevan, 1973).

The most detailed studies on the biosynthesis of cyanogenic glucosides have been carried out by the use of microsomes from etiolated sorghum seedlings catalysing all except the last step in the biosynthesis of dhurrin (McFarlane *et al.*, 1975). The intermediates expected according to the general pathway outlined above (Fig. 1) have all been unambiguously identified in the microsomal reaction mixtures. However, the cofactor requirements observed for the conversion of *N*-hydroxytyrosine into *p*-hydroxyphenylacetonitrile were surprising. This may be related to the catalysis of the biosynthetic pathway by a highly organized multi-enzyme complex or by a multifunctional protein of poorly understood nature (Møller and Conn, 1980). However, it may also indicate that our knowledge of the nature of the intermediates involved in the pathway is not so complete as generally believed. One possibility is that the biosynthesis of cyanogenic glucosides and glucosinolates do not diverge at the aldoxime level but also have a nitro compound and an *S*-alkylated thiohydroximate or a thiohydroximate as common intermediates (Fig. 4). This speculation is supported by the notion that 1-nitro-2-*p*-hydroxy-phenylethane is produced by the sorghum microsomes (Møller, unpubl.). Such a biosynthetic pathway would also explain the earlier observed peculiar requirement for NADPH and thiols in the conversion of aldoximes into nitriles (Møller and Conn, 1976; Shimada and Conn, 1977). NADPH would be required in the reductive cleavage of the α-C-S bond in the alkylated thiohydroximate resulting in the formation of the nitrile. The suggested cleavage of the α-C-S bond is analogous to the well-known cleavage of acyl derivatives of coenzyme A (Lynen and Reichert, 1951) except that the carbonyl group is replaced by the oxime function. The cleavage may also occur at the opposite side of the sulphur atom producing a free thiohydroximate as observed in the biosynthesis of glucosinolates (Binkley, 1950; Schwimmer and Kjær, 1960; Moore and Thompson, 1967). Thiohydroximates are chemically labile and decompose into nitriles and free sulphur (Ettlinger and Lundeen, 1957).

Fig. 4 Possible branching points in the biosynthesis of cyanogenic glucosides, glucosinolates, hydroxamates, and nitro compounds.

NADPH could then be involved in a corresponding enzymatic reduction of the thiohydroximate into the nitrile.

Several other possibilities can be formulated for the transformation of the nitro compound. 1-Nitro-2-phenylethane can be converted chemically into benzaldehyde and cyanide by treatment with alkali (Gottlieb *et al.*, 1962). Considering the mechanism proposed for this conversion it seems an unlikely route for cyanohydrin formation in the biosynthetic pathways. The involvement of a nitrile oxide (Edward and Tremaine, 1971) as an intermediate between the *aci*-nitro compound and the nitrile is an alternative possibility which has not been investigated.

The evidence for the involvement of *N*-hydroxyamino acids in the biosynthesis of four classes of natural products have been presented and the similarities between the enzymatic transformations necessary to produce each class of compounds have been indicated. It is possible that *N*-hydroxyamino acids are also involved in the biosynthesis of other natural products such as alkaloids. Epidithiodioxopiperazines are derived from amino acids and contain a sulphur atom bound to the α-carbon atom of the parent amino acid (Kirby, 1979). The biosynthesis of a few representatives within this family of more than thirty toxic fungal metabolites has been studied (Neuss *et al.*, 1968; Johns and Kirby, 1971; Kirby, 1974). *cyclo*-(L-Phenylalanyl-L-seryl) was identified as an intermediate in the biosynthesis of gliotoxin (Kirby *et al.*, 1978). Unpublished data also suggests the involvement of the di(methylthio) derivative (Kirby, 1979). No additional data are available on the mechanism by which the sulphur atoms are inserted.

The *N*-hydroxylation of amino acids is not limited to plants and microorganisms. Thus the biochemical basis for cyanide production by millipedes are cyanogenic glucosides most likely synthesized by a pathway identical to the one known from plants (Duffey and Towers, 1978). The presence of *N*-hydroxylated polypeptides have also been reported in tumours of the human brain (Neunhoeffer, 1970; Nagasawa *et al.*, 1972) and future studies may reveal the involvement of *N*-hydroxyamino acids in additional metabolic pathways.

REFERENCES

Ahmad, A. (1974). *Bull. Chem. Soc. Japan* 47, 1819-1820.

Akers, H.A. and Neilands, J.B. (1973). *Biochemistry* 12, 1006-1010.

Akers, H.A. and Neilands, J.B. (1978). "Biological Oxidation of Nitrogen" (J.W. Gorrod, ed.) pp. 429-436. Elsevier/North-Holland Biomedical Press, Amsterdam.

Bamberger, E. (1894). *Ber. Dtsch. Chem. Ges.* 27, 1548-1557.

Beckmann, E. (1909). *Justus Liebigs Ann. Chem.* 365, 201-214.

Binkley, F. (1950). *J. Biol. Chem.* 186, 287-296.

Borch, R.F., Bernstein, M.D. and Durst, H.D. (1971). *J. Am. Chem. Soc.* 93, 2897-2904.

Buehler, E. and Brown, G.B. (1967). *J. Org. Chem.* 32, 265-267.

Conn, E.E. (1969). *J. Agri. Food Chem.* 17, 519-526.

Cook. A.H. and Slater, C.A. (1956). *J. Chem. Soc.* 4130-4133.

Cooper, A.J.L. and Griffith, O.W. (1979). *J. Biol. Chem.* 254, 2748-2753.

Copenhaver, J.W. (1957). U.S. Patent 2,786,865.

Duffey, S.S. and Towers, G.H.N. (1978). *Can. J. Zoo.* 56, 7-16.

Duynstee, E.F.J., Hennekens, J.P. and Mevis, M.E.A.H. (1965). *Recl. Trav. Chim. Pays-Bas* 84, 1442-1451.

Edward, J.T. and Tremaine, P.H. (1971). *Can. J. Chem.* 49, 3489-3492.

Elbein, A.D. and Heath, E.C. (1965). *J. Biol. Chem.* 240, 1926-1931.

Emery, T.F. (1963). *Biochemistry* 2, 1041-1045.

Emery, T.F. (1966). *Biochemistry*, 5, 3694-3701.

Emery, T.F. (1971). *Adv. Enzymol. Relat. Areas Mol. Biol.* 35, 135-185.

Emery, T.F. and Neilands, J.B. (1961). *J. Am. Chem. Soc.* 83, 1626-1628.

Ettlinger, M.G. and Kjær , A. (1968). *Recent Adv. Phytochem.* 1, 59-144.

Ettlinger, M.G. and Lundeen, A.J. (1957). *J. Am. Chem. Soc.* 79, 1764-1765.

Feuer, H., Vincent, B.F. Jr. and Bartlett, R.S. (1965). *J. Org. Chem.* 30, 2877-2882.

Gaertner, F.H. (1978). *TIBS* 3, 63-65.

Gorrod, J.W. (1978). "Biological Oxidation of Nitrogen". Elsevier/North-Holland, Biomedical Press, Amsterdam.

Gottlieb, O.R., Magalhães, M.T. and Mors, W.B. (1961). *Ann. Acad. Bras. Cienc.* 33, 301-303.

Gottlieb, O.R., Souza, I.S. de and M.T. Magalhães (1962). *Tetrahedron* 18, 1137-1141.

Hantzsch, A. and Wild, W. (1896). *Justus Liebigs Ann. Chem.* 289, 285-309.

Hey, A.E. and Elbein, A.D. (1966). *J. Biol. Chem.* 241, 5473-5478.

Hösel, W. and Nahrstedt, A. (1980). *Arch. Biochem. Biophys.* 203, (In press).

IUPAC (1973). Enzyme Nomenclature 1972, pp. 286-298. Elsevier Scientific Publishing Company, Amsterdam.

Johns, N. and Kirby, G.W. (1971). *J. Chem. Soc., Chem. Commun.* pp.163-164.

Kamiński, K. and Sokołowska, T. (1973). *Ann. Soc. Chim. Pol.* 47, 653-656.

Kindl, H. and Underhill, E.W. (1968). *Phytochemistry* 7, 756-7

Kirby, G.W. (1974). *J. Chem. Soc., Chem. Commun.*, pp. 833-834.

Kirby, G.W. (1979). *Pure and Appl. Chem.* 51, 705-708.

Kirby, G.W., Patrick, G.L. and Robins, D.J. (1978). *J. Chem. Soc. Perkin Trans.* 1, pp. 1336-1338.

Lancini, G.C., Diena, A. and Lazzari, E. (1966). *Tetrahedron Lett.* 1769-1772.

Larsen, L.M. (1968). *Dansk Tidsskr. Farm.* 42, 272-283.

Larsen, P.O. (1981). "The Biochemistry of Plants, A Comprehensive Treatise" (P.K. Stumpf, and E.E. Conn, eds). Vol. 7 (In press).

Leeds, M.W. and Smith, G.B.L. (1951). *J. Electrochem. Soc.* 98, 129-133.

Liberek, B. and Palacz, Z. (1971). *Ann. Soc. Chim. Pol.* 45, 1173-1177.

Lynen, F. and Reichert, E. (1951). *Angew. Chem.* 63, 47-48.

MacDonald, J.C. (1965). *Biochem. J.* 96, 533-538.
Mahadevan, S. (1973). *Ann. Rev. Plant Physiol.* 24, 69-88.
Marvel, C.S. and Kamm, O. (1919). *J. Am. Chem. Soc.* 41, 276-282.
Matsuhashi, S., Matsuhashi, M., Brown, J.G. and Strominger, J.L. (1966). *J. Biol. Chem.* 241, 4283-4287.
Matsuo, M., Kirkland, D.F. and Underhill, E.W. (1972). *Phytochemistry* 11, 697-701.
Matsuo, M. and Underhill, E.W. (1969). *Biochem. Biophys. Res. Commun.* 36, 18-23.
Matsuo, M. and Underhill, E.W. (1971). *Phytochemistry* 10, 2279-2286.
McFarlane, I.J., Lees, E.M. and Conn, E.E. (1975). *J. Biol. Chem.* 250, 4708-4713.
McKinney, L.L., Uhing, E.H., Setzkorn, E.A. and Cowan, J.C. (1950). *J. Am. Chem. Soc.* 72, 2599-2603.
Melo, A., Elliott, W.H. and Glaser, L. (1968). *J. Biol. Chem.* 243, 1467-1474.
Micetich, R.G. and MacDonald, J.C. (1964). *J. Chem. Soc.* 1507-1510.
Miller, W. and Plöchl, J. (1893). *Ber. Dtsch. Chem. Ges.* 26, 1545-1548.
Møller, B.L. (1977). *Anal. Biochem.* 81, 292-304.
Møller, B.L. (1978). *J. Label. Compd. Radiopharm.* 14, 663-671.
Møller, B.L. and Conn, E.E. (1976). 16th Symposium and Annual Meeting of the Phytochemical Society of North America, Vancouver, British Columbia, August 8-11, 1976; p.14. Phytochemical Society of North America.
Møller, B.L. and Conn, E.E. (1979). *J. Biol. Chem.* 254, 8575-8583.
Møller, B.L. and Conn, E.E. (1980). *J. Biol. Chem.* 255, 3049-3056.
Møller, B.L., Conn, E.E., Martin, R. and Sweeley, C.C. (1977a). 11th FEBS Meeting, August 14-19, 1977, Copenhagen Abstract LB400.
Møller, B.L., McFarlane, I.J. and Conn, E.E. (1977b). *Acta Chem. Scand. Ser.* B 31, 343-344.
Møller, B.L., Conn, E.E. and Sweeley, C.C. (1979). *Carlsberg Res. Commun.* 44, 367-379.
Moore, D.P. and Thompson, J.F. (1967). *Biochem. Biophys. Res. Commun.* 28, 474-479.
Müller, H.-G. and Diekmann, H. (1977). 113, 243-246.
Murray, G.J., Clark, G.E.D., Parniak, M.A. and Viswanatha, T. (1977). *Can. J. Biochem.* 55, 625-629.
Nagasawa, H.T., Kohlhoff, J.G., Fraser, P.S. and Mikhail, A.A. (1972). *J. Med. Chem.* 15, 483-486.
Neelakantan, L. and Hartung, W.H. (1958). *J. Org. Chem.* 23, 964-967.
Neilands, J.B. (1967). *Science* 156, 1443-1447.
Neilands, J.B. (1973). "Inorganic Biochemistry", (G.L. Eichhorn, Ed.) Vol. I, pp. 167-202. Elsevier, Amsterdam.
Neilands, J.B. and Azari, P. (1963). *Acta Chem. Scand.* 17, 190-
Neunhoeffer, O. (1970). *Z. Naturforsch. B.* 25, 299-301.
Neuss, N., Boeck, L.D., Brannon, D.R., Chue, J.C., Delong, D.C., Gorman, M., Huckstep, L.L., Lively, D.H., Mabe, J., Marsh, M.M., Molloy, B.B., Nagarajan, R., Nelson, J.D. and Stark, W.M. (1968). *Antimicrob. Agents Chemother*, pp. 213-219.
Parniak, M.A., Jackson, G.E.D., Murray, G.J. and Viswanatha, T. (1979). *Biochim. Biophys. Acta* 569, 99-108.
Pedersen, K.J. (1934). *J. Phys. Chem.* 38, 559-571.
Porter, C.C. and Hellerman, L. (1944). *J. Am. Chem. Soc.* 66, 1652.

Posner, T. (1912). *Justus Liebigs Ann. Chem.* 389, 1-120.
Pritzkow, W., and Rosler, W. (1967). *Justus Liebigs Ann. Chem.* 703, 66-76.
Reay, P.F. and Conn, E.E. (1974). *J. Biol. Chem.* 249, 5826-5830.
Reimann, J.E. and Byerrum, R.U. (1964). *Biochemistry* 3, 847-851.
Rogers, M.A.T. (1955). *J. Chem. Soc.* 769-772.
Rogers, S. and Neilands, J.B. (1963). *Biochemistry*, 2, 6-9.
Schwimmer, S. and Kjær, A. (1960). *Biochim. Biophys. Acta* 42, 316-324.
Siegler, D.S. (1975). *Phytochemistry* 14, 9-29.
Shaw, P.D. (1967). *Biochemistry* 6, 2253-2260.
Shaw, P.D. and DeAngelo, A.B. (1969). *J. Bacteriol.* 99, 463-468.
Shaw, P.D. and McCloskey, J.A. (1967). *Biochemistry* 6, 2247-2253.
Shimada, M. and Conn, E.E. (1977). *Arch. Biochem. Biophys.* 180, 199-207.
Shukla, P.S. and Mahadevan, S. (1968). *Arch. Biochem. Biophys.* 125, 873-883.
Smrt, J., Beránek, J. and Horák, M. (1959). *Collect. Czech. Chem. Commun.* 24, 1672-1676.
Snow G.A. (1954). *J. Chem. Soc.*, 2588-2596.
Spenser, I.D. and Ahmad, A. (1961). *Proc. Chem. Soc.* 375-376.
Stevens, R.L. and Emery, T.F. (1966). *Biochemistry* 5, 74-81.
Tapper, B.A. and Butler, G.W. (1967). *Arch. Biochem. Biophys.* 120, 719-721.
Tipton, C.L., Klun, J.A., Husted, R.R. and Pierson, M.D. (1967). *Biochemistry* 6, 2866-2870.
Tomlinson, G., Cruickshank, W.H. and Viswanatha, T. (1971). *Anal. Biochem.* 44, 670-679.
Tomlinson, G. and Viswanatha, T. (1973). *Can. J. Biochem.* 51, 754-763.
Traube, W. (1894). *Ber. Dtsch. Chem. Ges.* 27, 1507-1510.
Traube, W. (1895). *Ber. Dtsch. Chem. Ges.* 28, 1785-1797, 2297-2302.
Underhill, E.W. (1967). *Eur. J. Biochem.* 2, 61-63.
Underhill, E.W. and Wetter, L.R. (1969). *Plant Physiol.* 44, 584-590.
Underhill, E.W., Wetter, L.R. and Chisholm, M.D. (1973). "Nitrogen Metabolism in Plants" (T.W. Goodwin and R.M.S. Smillie, eds). pp. 303-326, Biochemical Society Symposium No.38. The Biochemical Society, London.
Wang, S.-F. and Gabriel, O. (1969). *J. Biol. Chem.* 244, 3430-3437.
Weisburger, J.H. and Weisburger, E.K. (1973). *Pharmacol. Rev.* 25, 1-66.
Wetter, L.R. and Chisholm, M.D. (1968). *Can. J. Biochem.* 46, 931-935.

THE ENZYMATIC HYDROLYSIS OF CYANOGENIC GLUCOSIDES

WOLFGANG HÖSEL

Lehrstuhl für Biochemie der Planzen
der Westfälischen Wilhelms-Universität
Hindenburgplatz 55, D-4400 Münster, Germany

I. INTRODUCTION

The production of hydrocyanic acid (HCN) upon injury of plant tissue containing a cyanogenic glucoside is a well known phenomenon. It was first investigated by Liebig and Wöhler (1837). They prepared an extract from bitter almonds which they called emulsin and which was capable of bringing about the release of HCN from the particular cyanogenic glucoside of that plant, amygdalin. It has become obvious over the next hundred years that this liberation of HCN is due to the sequential action of two types of enzymes, a β-glucosidase and a α-hydroxynitrile lyase, as outlined schematically in Fig. 1.

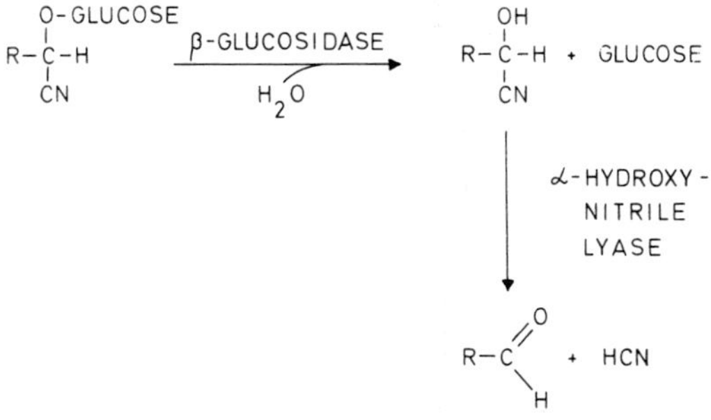

Fig. 1 General scheme of the enzymatic hydrolysis of cyanogenic glucosides.

The general scheme depicted in Fig. 1 holds for the hydrolysis of most cyanogenic glucosides (for the structures of the individual cyanogenic glucosides, refer to Chapters 1 and 2).

The amygdalin-emulsin system in bitter almonds is an exception to the general pattern in so far as the glucoside contains two glucose units. This gave rise earlier to the question whether the two glucose moieties are hydrolysed by the same β-glucosidase or by two different ones, a question which is dealt with in more detail in a later section.

It also became obvious at an early point that the β-glucosidases responsible for the hydrolysis of the cyanogenic glucosides display some degree of specificity for the type of compound with which they co-occur (Armstrong *et al.*, 1908; cf. Robinson, 1930). This fact has not always been appreciated in the past, and many investigations concentrated only on the specificity for the sugar unit (cf. Robinson, 1930; Helferich, 1948). This occurred primarily because of the availability and wide use of synthetic glycosidic substrates (mostly phenolic glycosides) but also because the crude glycosidase preparations ("emulsin") studied nearly always contained a mixture of different glycosidases. It is the aim of this chapter to give a state of the art summary on the β-glucosidases responsible for the hydrolysis of cyanogenic glucosides. The main emphasis has been placed on the well-characterized enzymes rather than trying to give a comprehensive account of all β-glucosidases reported so far which act on cyanogenic glucosides. A considerable part of the emphasis is directed towards the aglycone specificity of the β-glucosidases, since it is from that part of the cyanogenic glucoside molecule that the HCN originates. It should therefore be of special interest from a physiological point of view.

II. β-GLUCOSIDASES FOR LINAMARIN/LOTAUSTRALIN

Unfortunately no β-glucosidase responsible for the hydrolysis of linamarin/lotaustralin has so far been purified to homogeneity from any plant. Nevertheless it can be stated that plants which contain these cyanogenic glucosides also possess β-glucosidases which display preferential specificity for these substances. This is clearly demonstrated by the results given in Table I which lists the plant extracts known to hydrolyse linamarin or lotaustralin.

In spite of the fact that all plants investigated show high β-glucosidase activity (measured with a synthetic β-glucoside), only those which contain linamarin/lotaustralin are able to hydrolyse these substances effectively. It does not matter whether the plants which yield ineffective extracts contain other cyanogenic glucosides. Thus even high activities of bitter almond β-glucosidase catalyse only a slow hydrolysis of linamarin (Butler *et al.*, 1965). That linamarin/lotaustralin are the preferred substrates for one or several β-glucosidases of linseed, white clover, birdsfoot trefoil and cassava has been further substantiated by partial purification and characterization of the respective enzymes (Butler *et al.*, 1965; Hughes and Maher, 1973; Rissler and Millar, 1977; Cooke *et al.*, 1978; Wilkinson and Millar, 1979). The relative rates of hydrolysis and K_m values determined with the partially purified

Table I Comparison of the hydrolysis of linamarin/lotaustralin and other glucosidic substrates by various plant extracts (data taken from the references listed)

Plant	linamarin lotaustralin	salicin arbutin amygdalin cellobiose	
(+)Trifolium repens (leaves)	+	+	Butler *et al.*, (1965).
(+)Linum usitatissimum (shoots)	+	+	"
Sambucus nigra (leaves)	-	+	"
Trifolium pratense (leaves)	-	+	"
Triticum vulgare (sprouted wheat)	-	+	"
Vicia faba (sprouted broad beans)	-	+	"
Conium maculatum (leaves)	-	+	"
Populus alba (shoots)	-	+	"
Photinea serrulata (leaves)	-	+	"
(+)Dimorphotheca cuneata	+		Marais and Rimington (1934)
(+)Manihot utilissima (peel)	+		Wood (1966)
(seedlings)	+		Nartey (1968)
(parenchymal tissue)	+		Cooke *et al.*, (1978)
(+)Lotus corniculatus (leaves)	+		Millar and Higgins (1970)

(+)Plants that contain linamarin/lotaustralin.

Table II Relative hydrolytic velocities of different substrates and K_m values of linamarin for linamarase from different origin.

Substrate	% hydrolysis by linseed linamarase(1)	% hydrolysis by cassava leaves linamarase(2)	K_m (mM) cassava(3)	K_m (mM) white clover(4)
Linamarin	76.2	81.5	1.45	0.7
Lotaustralin		79.1		
Prunasin	51.6			
Amygdalin	0	0.2		
Phloridzin	30.0			
Arbutin	34.2			
Salicin	32.7	11.4		0.5
β-Methylglucoside	1.1	1.4		

(1)Butler *et al.*, (1965). (2)Nartey (1968). (3)Cooke *et al.*, (1978). (4)Hughes and Maher (1973).

linamarases from these plants are given in Table II.

In no case has linamarase from the plant species listed in Table II been unequivocally shown to be a single enzyme. Butler *et al.* (1965) were clearly dealing with several different β-glycosidases in linseed. Hughes and Maher (1973), on the other hand, has some indication by mixed substrate experiments and by immunological studies that the β-glucosidase activity of white clover plants consists of only one type of β-glucosidase ("linamarase"). The same seems to hold for *Lotus corniculatus* (Rissler and Millar, 1977). A thorough purification with a subsequent conclusive proof of a single β-glucosidase activity will be necessary, however, before a final evaluation of the exact substrate specificity of linamarase can be made.

III. β-GLUCOSIDASES WITH SPECIFICITY FOR AROMATIC CYANOGENIC GLUCOSIDES

A. AMYGDALIN AND PRUNASIN

As was mentioned earlier, the β-glucosidases from almonds have been under investigation for a long time; indeed, they are among the very first enzymes ever described (Liebig and Wöhler, 1837). Nevertheless only a few papers have been published where the presumed physiological substrates, i.e. amygdalin and prunasin, of these β-glucosidases have been used. The work of Haisman and Knight (1967), Haisman *et al.* (1967) and Lalégérie (1974) confirmed earlier results (e.g. Armstrong *et al.*, 1912) that amygdalin is hydrolysed in a consecutive fashion by two different β-glucosidases in bitter almonds.

As depicted in Fig. 2, a first β-glucosidase is responsible for the removal of one glucose molecule; the prunasin thus produced is subsequently hydrolysed by another β-glucosidase yielding mandelonitrile and a second molecule of glucose. The intact disaccharide unit, gentiobiose, has never been detected in any assay. That two different β-glucosidases are indeed involved in the hydrolysis of amygdalin has been concluded from competition experiments using amygdalin and prunasin (Haisman and Knight, 1967) and by complete separation of both enzymes using continuous flow electrophoresis (Haisman *et al.*, 1967). Later Lalégérie (1974) also purified a β-glucosidase from almonds which displayed better activity towards amygdalin than prunasin. The crude extract ("emulsin") on the other hand, hydrolysed both substrates equally. Figure 2 includes the K_m values for the two substrates determined by Haisman and Knight (1967) and Lalégérie (1974). There is good agreement as far as the K_m for the prunasin is concerned, but the amygdalin values differ considerably.

Synthetic glycosidic substrates have often been used both in the past and in recent studies of the almond β-glucosidases. Much of this work was done by Helferich and co-workers (e.g. Helferich, 1933; 1948) who succeeded in

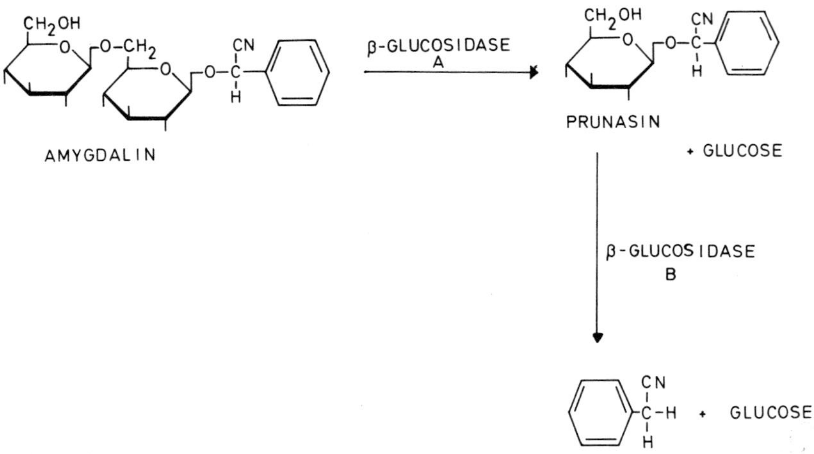

Fig. 2 Hydrolysis of amygdalin and prunasin by the almond β-glucosidases. Following K_m and V_{max} data have been determined for the almond β-glucosidases:

	Amygdalin			Prunasin		
	K_m (mM)	V_{max}	V_{max}/K_m	K_m (mM)	V_{max}	V_{max}/K_m
β-Glucosidases mixture A+B[(1)]	1.5	35	23	1.7	40	24
β-Glucosidase A[(2)]	7.5	53	7	5.5	6.3	1.1

[(1)] Haisman and Knight (1967)

[(2)] Lalégérie (1974)

isolating β-glucosidases with different molecular weights (e.g. Kleinschmidt *et al.*, 1970) and different catalytic activities (e.g. Helferich and Kleinschmidt, 1967). These investigations with artificial substrates have had considerable impact on the development of our understanding of enzyme catalysis, especially on the mechanism of glycosidase action (for reviews see Veibel, 1951; Jermyn, 1961; Nisizawa and Hashimoto, 1970).

One of the most controversial points over a long period of time has been whether glycosidic substrates with different sugar units (e.g. β-glucosides and β-galactosides) are hydrolysed by the same almond enzyme or by different ones. Most data appeared to favour the hydrolysis of both sugars by one β-glucosidase (e.g. Heyworth and Walker, 1962). However, the existence of a bifunctional enzyme with independent glucosidase and galactosidase sites has recently been postulated again (Grover *et al.*, 1977; Grover and Cushley, 1977). This claim, however, was questioned a short time later by Walker and Axelrod (1978), who, using a β-glucosidase purified to exactly the same extent as Grover *et al.*, (1977), came up with fairly convincing evidence for one catalytic site. Legler and Harder (1978) have recently managed to identify a short amino acid sequence at the catalytic site of bitter almond β-glucosidase. For this purpose they used a covalent binding of the β-glucosidase inhibitor, 6-bromo-6-deoxy conduritol B epoxide, to an aspartic acid residue in the catalytic site.

Despite these interesting and valuable results concerning the catalytic properties of almond β-glucosidase, it can only again be deplored that most investigations have used inappropriate synthetic substrates. This lack of interest in the nature of the aglycone originated obviously from the fact that the almond β-glucosidases, which are by far the most extensively studied glycosidases from plant sources, do not show as distinct an aglycone specificity as do other β-glucosidases described below.

B. DHURRIN AND TAXIPHYLLIN

A β-glucosidase with a fairly prominent aglycone specificity became known only very recently when Eklund and Conn (1980) reinvestigated the β-glucosidases from *Sorghum bicolor* seedlings. Mao and Anderson (1967) had purified the β-glucosidases from sorghum seedlings to some extent, but they had not obtained a β-glucosidase with preferential specificity towards dhurrin, the cyanogenic glucoside in sorghum. In contrast Eklund and Conn have been able to purify two β-glucosidases by molecular sieve and anion exchange chromatography. Their very pronounced specificity for dhurrin can be seen from Table III.

This example demonstrates again that the determination of glycosidase specificity is likely to be meaningful only after a thorough separation which results in a single enzyme.

A β-glucosidase which effectively hydrolyses taxiphyllin, the epimer of dhurrin, has been isolated from *Triglochin maritima* seedlings, a plant known to contain this cyanogenic glucoside (Nahrstedt *et al.*, 1979). This plant also contains another cyanogenic glucoside, triglochinin (Eyjólfsson and Ettlinger, 1972), which is hydrolyzed by β-glucosidase(s) present in this species. A separation of the β-glucosidase activities of *T. maritima* seedlings by anion exchange chromatography is shown in Fig. 3.

The seedlings obviously possess β-glucosidases with different specificities towards the two cyanogenic glucosides. Thus β-glucosidase B displays a high specificity

Table III Substrate specificities of the β-glucosidases purified from *Sorghum bicolor* (Eklund and Conn, 1980) and *Triglochin maritima* (Nahrstedt *et al.*, 1979).

Substrate	β-glucosidase from *Sorghum bicolor*			β-glucosidase (enzyme C in Fig. 3) from *Triglochin maritima*	
	Concentration (mM)	Enzyme A	Enzyme B	K_m (mM)	V_{max} (Mol/min·mg)
Dhurrin	0.9	100 (K_m=0.1 mM)	100	0.4	0.7
p-Nitrophenylglucoside	4	33	0.4	0.13	4
Coniferin	1	4	0.1	-	-
Syringin	1	5	0.2	-	-
Salicin	0.86	0	0	-	-
6-Bromo-2-naphthol-glucoside	0.5	0	0.5	-	-
Taxiphyllin	1.4	1.4	0.1	0.4	3.5
Sambunigrin	0.7	70 (K_m=0.3 mM)	60	-	-
Prunasin	1	2	0	-	-
Benzyl glucoside	0.75	1	0.4	-	-
Triglochinin	0.26	5	2.5	2	20
Linamarin	1	0.1	0.04	-	-
4-Methylumbelliferyl-β-glucoside	-	-	-	0.1	6

(-)Not determined.

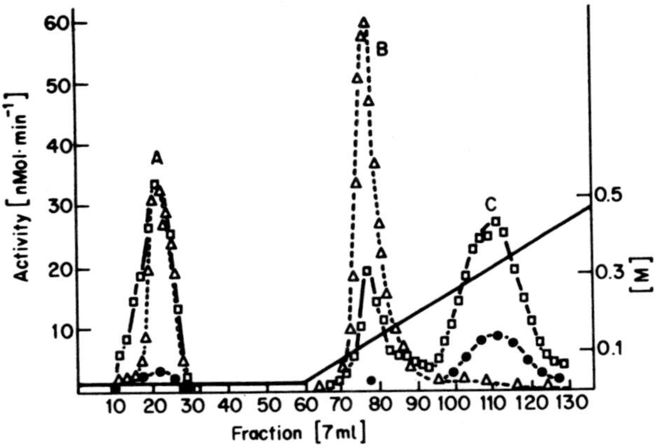

Fig. 3 Separation of *Triglochin maritima* β-glucosidases by DEAE anion exchange column chromatography. Δ-----Δ Hydrolysis of triglochinin; O———O Hydrolysis of taxiphyllin; □———□ Hydrolysis of 4-nitrophenyl-β-glucoside; ——— Buffer gradient Tris-HCl, pH 7. (Data taken from Nahrstedt *et al.*, 1979, by courtesy of Pergamon Press.)

for triglochinin (see next section) whereas only β-glucosidase C hydrolyses taxiphyllin to a notable extent. Although the specificity of this latter enzyme for taxiphyllin has not been found to be as strict as that of the sorghum β-glucosidase for dhurrin (see Table III), it also has not yet been demonstrated that β-glucosidase C (see Fig. 3) is a pure β-glucosidase. It may still be contaminated by another glucosidase activity.

IV. TRIGLOCHININ SPECIFIC β-GLUCOSIDASES

As was mentioned briefly in the previous section, a β-glucosidase with high specificity for triglochinin is present in *Triglochin maritima* seedlings (see Fig. 3). Such a β-glucosidase was first described from *Alocasia macrorrhiza* (Hösel and Nahrstedt, 1975), a plant which contains triglochinin as its only cyanogenic glucoside. Nearly all of the β-glucosidase activity extracted from *Alocasia* leaves showed specificity for triglochinin. This was clearly demonstrated by the fact that the crude protein extract and the highly purified β-glucosidase displayed identical relative hydrolysis rates on various glycosidic substrates (Hösel and Klewitz, 1977). After a comparatively low enrichment (11-fold), the purification procedure produced a homogenous protein as judged by alkaline disc electrophoresis in the presence and absence of sodium dodecylsulphate. The molecular weight of the monomeric form was estimated at 55,000-60,000. A hexamer with a molecular weight of 310,000 is probably the β-glucosidase form present *in vivo*. A dimeric form (MW 110,000) was also found in course of the purification. It obviously originates *in vitro* by dissociation from the hexamer without any loss of activi-

Table IV Substrate specificity of the β-glucosidases from *Alocasia macrorrhiza* (Hösel and Nahrstedt, 1975) and *Triglochin maritima* (Nahrstedt *et al.*, 1979).

	Alocasia β-glucosidase				*Triglochin* β-glucosidase (enzyme B in Fig. 3)		
	Relative activity (2 mM substrate concentration)	K_m (mM)	V (μMol/min·mg)	V/K_m	K_m (mM)	V_{max}	V_{max}/K_m
4-Nitrophenyl-β-glucoside	100	3	40	13.3	2	1.1	0.55
4-Nitrophenyl-β-galactoside	10	10	6.6	0.66			
4-Nitrophenyl-α-glucoside	0	-	-	-			
Triglochinin	1000	0.3	400	1333	0.6	43	72
Dhurrin (S)	14	-	-	-	2	1	0.5
Taxiphyllin (R)	<1	-	-	-	-	-	-
Sambunigrin (S̄)	5	-	-	-	-	-	-
Prunasin (R)	<1	-	-	-	-	-	-
Amygdalin (R)	<1	-	-	-	-	-	-
Linamarin	<1	-	-	-	-	-	-
Epilotaustralin (S)	<1	-	-	-	-	-	-
Lotaustralin (S)	<1	-	-	-	-	-	-
4-Methylumbelliferyl-β-glucoside	20	1.5	25	16.6	2	1.4	0.7
Salicin	1	-	-	-	-	-	-
Cellobiose	0	-	-	-	-	-	-

ty. The protein properties of the two triglochinin-specific β-glucosidases from *Alocasia macrorrhiza* and *Triglochin maritima* are very similar. The substrate specificities of the enzymes are nearly identical (see Table IV).

Triglochinin is by far the best substrate for the two β-glucosidases and the only other cyanogenic glucosides which can be hydrolysed are those with an aromatic aglycone and *S*-configuration (e.g. dhurrin and sambunigrin). These, however, are hydrolysed only very slowly.

The β-glucosidase from *Alocasia macrorrhiza* has been further characterized with respect to several properties, especially the influence of a variety of known inhibitors of β-glucosidases (Hösel and Nahrstedt, 1975; Hösel and Klewitz, 1977).

V. GENERAL PROPERTIES OF β-GLUCOSIDASES SPECIFIC FOR CYANOGENIC GLUCOSIDES

The enzymes described in the previous sections share certain common properties among themselves and with other β-glucosidases. They all show maximal activity at a slightly acidic pH (pH 4-6) and several are competitively inhibited by glucono-1,5-lactone (e.g. Heyworth and Walker, 1962; Hösel and Nahrstedt, 1975; Eklund and Conn, 1980). However, not enough information based on work with pure enzymes is presently available for a detailed evaluation of other possible common properties.

On the other hand it is also clear that significant differences exist both among β-glucosidases specific for the various cyanogenic glucosides and between these and other β-glucosidases. Thus it has been found that the triglochinin-specific β-glucosidase from *Alocasia macrorrhiza* responds differently to active site-directed inhibitors like conduritol B epoxide or bromoconduritol (Hösel and Klewitz, 1977) than other β-glycosidases (Legler, 1973). Even the triglochinin-specific β-glucosidase from *Triglochin* seems to be different in its catalytic properties from that of *Alocasia* since the former is not inhibited by sulphhydryl blocking reagents whereas that of *Alocasia* is (Nahrstedt *et al.*, 1979).

VI. PHYSIOLOGICAL ASPECTS OF CYANOGENIC GLUCOSIDE HYDROLYSIS

The concept that cyanogenic glucosides and their respective hydrolysing enzymes (β-glucosidase and α-hydroxynitrile lyase) are only brought into contact when the plant tissue is disrupted was suggested several decades ago (Czapek, 1921; Robinson, 1930). HCN would then be released and could exert its toxic effect on living organisms, perhaps acting as a protective agent for the plant (see the chapters of D. Jones and W. Fry in this volume; Conn, 1980). It was not until recently, however, that it was shown for the first time that a cyanogenic glucoside and

Table V The distribution of dhurrin and enzymes involved in its metabolism in different fractions from six-day-old sorghum leaf blades (data taken from Kojima *et al.*, 1979, by courtesy of Plant Physiology).

Component	Epidermal protoplasts		Mesophyll protoplasts			Bundle sheat strands	
	per 10^6 protoplasts	per mg protein	per 10^6 protoplasts	per mg protein	per mg chlorophyll	per mg protein	per mg chlorophyll
Dhurrin (μmol)	5.3	26.5	0.47	1.27	10.4	0.006	0.054
Dhurrin β-glucosidase (μmol/h)	0.55	2.75	8.5	23	191	1.65	11.6
Hydroxynitrile lyase (μmol/h)	0.99	4.95	19.7	53	441	2.23	13.4

its hydrolysing enzymes are indeed physically separated within intact plant tissue (Kojima *et al.*, 1979). Table V shows the distribution of dhurrin, the dhurrin-specific β-glucosidase and the α-hydroxynitrile lyase activity in the leaves of young *Sorghum bicolor* plants.

It can clearly be seen that the cyanogenic glucoside is contained in the epidermal layer whereas both hydrolysing enzymes are nearly exclusively present in the mesophyll cells. This distribution provides a clear intercellular separation of substrate and enzyme within the leaves.

A more detailed investigation on the intracellular localisation of the dhurrin-specific β-glucosidase has revealed that a significant fraction of this activity seems to be present within the plastids of the mesophyll cells (Thayer and Conn, 1981).

In a study on linamarin specific β-glucosidase in *Lotus corniculatus* Rissler and Millar (1977) found that the activity *in situ* was localized in the phloem, epidermis and mesophyll in healthy and in infected (by *Stemphylium loti*) leaves. These results, however, were obtained using a coupling azo-dye technique and the synthetic substrate bromonaphthyl glucoside and should therefore be confirmed by another, more specific, method. There has been a great deal of work on plants which contained cyanogenic glucosides but lack β-glucosidases for these substrates. Since there is a separate chapter by M. Hughes in this volume dealing with that phenomenon the reader is referred to that.

VII. CONCLUSIONS

The currently available data clearly support the concept that cyanogenic glucosides are accompanied by β-glucosidases which frequently display a very pronounced specificity for these substrates. Indeed, in every case where a thorough purification has been performed, a β-glucosidase with a preferential specificity towards the cyanogenic glucoside present in the same plant has been found. The aglycone as well as the sugar part of the substrate obviously plays a role in this specificity; in some cases, in fact, the aglycone is the main determinant (e.g. Hösel and Nahrstedt, 1975; Eklund and Conn, 1980). This is similar to the behaviour of the β-glycosidases which show specificity for phenolic, and especially flavonoid, glycosides (for review see Hösel, 1981). In my view, this can be regarded as a general property of all β-glycosidases which show specificity for any secondary plant glycoside. It seems reasonable to predict that β-glucosidases also exist which will display preferential specificity for those cyanogenic glucosides for which specific β-glucosidases have yet to be found (vicianin, acacipetalin, cardiospermin, holocalin, zierin, cyclopentene derived glucosides, sulphated cyanogenic glucosides and others). Indeed, reports on vicianin hydrolysis (Bertrand and Rivkid, 1907; Courtois *et al.*, 1964) and preliminary results on cardiospermin in *Cardiospermum grandiflorum* (Hübel and Nahrstedt, unpublished) seem to support this hypothesis. Another reasonable assumption seems to be that the cyanogenic glucosides and their hydrolysing enzymes are located in separate compartments and are likely to come in contact only after disruption of the plant tissue. As a consequence, the system cyanogenic glucoside – β-glucosidase seems to be optimized for a rapid release of HCN after disruption of the plant tissue, thus providing a protective mechanism against HCN-sensitive organisms which attack the plant. However, it is also possible that the hydrolysing enzymes are also involved in the endogenous turnover of the cyanogenic glucosides which has been described several times (Abrol and Conn, 1966; Tschiersch, 1966; Bough and Gander, 1971; Jones, 1972).

Finally, it may be stated that most of the points which have been made in this chapter regarding β-glucosidases presumably also hold for the α-hydroxynitrile lyases. The few investigations carried out so far on substrate specificity (Bové and Conn, 1961; Becker *et al.*, 1963; Seely *et al.*, 1966) or localization (Kojima *et al.*, 1979) of the latter enzymes show the same pattern of results as has been reported for the β-glucosidases.

ACKNOWLEDGEMENT

The author's research described in this chapter has been supported by the Deutsche Forschungsgemeinschaft. He thanks Professor Dr Brian E. Ellis, University of Ontario, Guelph, Canada, for linguistic revision of the manuscript.

REFERENCES

Abrol, Y.P. and Conn, E.E. (1966). *Phytochemistry* 5, 237-242.
Armstrong, Armstrong and Horton (1908). *Proc. Roy. Soc. B*, 80, 321.
Armstrong, Armstrong and Horton (1912). *Proc. Roy. Soc. B*, 85, 359.
Becker, W., Benthin, U., Eschenhof, E. and Pfeil, E. (1963). *Biochemische Zeitschrift* 337, 156-166.
Bertrand, G. and Rivkid, L. (1907). *Bull. Soc. Chim. Biol.* 4, 497.
Bough, W.A. and Gander, J.E. (1971). *Phytochemistry* 10, 67-77.
Bové, C. and Conn, E.E. (1961). *J. Biol. Chem.* 236, 207-210.
Butler, G.W., Bailey, R.W. and Kennedy, L.D. (1965). *Phytochemistry* 4, 369-381.
Conn, E.E. (1980). *In* "Herbivores: Their Interaction with Secondary Plant Metabolites" (G.A. Rosenthal and D.H. Janzen, eds), Academic Press, New York.
Cooke, R.D., Blake, G.G. and Battershill, J.M. (1978). *Phytochemistry* 17, 381-383.
Courtois, J.E., Percheron, F. and Quang, H.N. (1964). *Bull. Soc. Chim. Biol.* 46, 984-986.
Czapek, F. (1921). "Biochemie der Pflanzen", 2nd edn., Vol. III, pp. 205-220, Gustav Fischer Verlag, Jena.
Eklund, S. and Conn, E.E. (1980). Personal communication.

Eyjólfsson, R. and Ettlinger, M. (1972). *J. Chem. Soc. Chem. Commun.* 572.
Grover, A.K. and Cushley, R.J. (1977). *Biochim. Biophys. Acta* 482, 109-124.
Grover, A.K., Macmurchie, D.D. and Cushley, R.J. (1977). *Biochim. Biophys. Acta* 482, 98-108.
Haisman, D.R. and Knight, D.J. (1967). *Biochem. J.* 103, 528-534.
Haisman, D.R., Knight, D.J. and Ellis, M.J. (1967). *Phytochemistry* 6, 1501-1505.
Helferich, B. (1933). *Ergeb. Enzymforschg.* 2, 74-89.
Helferich, B. (1948). FIAT Rev. German. Sci. 1939-46, Biochem. Pt. III, 125-138.
Helferich, B. and Kleinschmidt, T. (1967). *Hoppe-Seyler's Z. Physiol. Chem.* 348, 753-758.
Heyworth, R. and Walker, P.G. (1962). *Biochem. J.* 83, 331-335.
Hösel, W. (1981). *In* "The Biochemistry of Plants - A comprehensive treatise" (E.E. Conn and P.K. Stumpf, eds), Vol. VII, Academic Press, New York.
Hösel, W. and Nahrstedt, A. (1975). *Hoppe-Seyler's Z. Physiol. Chem.* 356, 1265-1275.
Hösel, W. and Klewitz, O. (1977). *Hoppe-Seyler's Z. Physiol. Chem.* 358, 959-966.
Hughes, M.A. and Maher, E.B. (1973). *Biochemical Genetics* 8, 1-12.
Jermyn, M.A. (1961). *Rev. Pure Appl. Chem.* 11, 92.
Jones, D.A. (1972). *In* "Phytochemical Ecology" (J.B. Harborne, ed.) Ch. 7, Academic Press, New York.
Kleinschmidt, T., Glossmann, H. and Horst, J. (1970). *Hoppe-Seyler's Z. Physiol. Chem.* 351, 349-358.
Kojima, M., Poulton, J.E., Thayer, S.S. and Conn, E.E. (1979). *Plant Physiol.* 63, 1022-1028.
Lalégérie, P. (1974). *Biochimie* 56, 1163-1172.
Legler, G. (1973). *Molec. & Cellul. Biochem.* 2, 31-38.
Legler, G. and Harder, A. (1978). *Biochim. Biophys. Acta* 524, 102-108.
Liebig, J. and Wöhler, F. (1837). *Annalen* 22, 11.
Mao, C.-H. and Anderson, L. (1967). *Phytochemistry* 6, 473-483.
Marais, J.S.C. and Rimington, C. (1934). *Onderstepoort J. Vet. Sci.* 3, 111-117.
Millar, R.L. and Higgins, V.J. (1970). *Phytopathology* 60, 104-110.
Nahrstedt, A., Hösel, W. and Walther, A. (1979). *Phytochemistry* 18, 1137-1141.
Nartey, F. (1968). *Phytochemistry* 7, 1307-1312.
Nisizawa, K. and Hashimoto, Y. (1970). *In* "The Carbohydrates" (W. Pigman and D. Horton, eds) Vol. IIA, Ch. 33, pp. 241-299, Academic Press, New York.
Rissler, J.F. and Millar, R.L. (1977). *Protoplasma* 92, 57-70.
Robinson, M.E. (1930). *Biolog. Rev.* 5, 126-141.
Seely, M.K., Criddle, R.S. and Conn, E.E. (1966). *J. Biol. Chem.* 241, 4457-4462.
Thayer, S.S. and Conn, E.E. (1981). *Plant Physiol.* 67, 617-622.
Tschiersch, B. (1966). *Flora* 157, 43-50.
Veibel, S. (1951). *In* "The Enzymes" (J.B. Summer and K. Myrbäck, eds), Vol.I, pp. 584-634, Academic Press, New York.
Walker, D.E. and Axelrod, B. (1978). *Arch. Biochem. Biophys.* 178,

102-107.
Wilkinson, H.T. and Millar, R.L. (1979). *Can. J. Bot.* 57, 69-73.
Wood, T. (1966). *J. Sci. Fd. Agric.* 17, 85-90.

THE METABOLISM OF HYDROGEN CYANIDE BY BACTERIA

PETER A. CASTRIC

Department of Biological Sciences, Duquesne University, Pittsburgh, Pennsylvania 15219, USA

Hydrogen cyanide is a highly potent metabolic inhibitor, and so would not seem to be a very practicable metabolite. However, the contributions to this book indicate that this is not necessarily the case. The ability to produce, assimilate, or detoxify HCN spans the spectrum of nature from animals and higher plants to microbes. Within the microbes representatives among the fungi, true algae and bacteria are able to metabolize HCN. This chapter will focus on cyanide metabolism by bacteria and will exclude algal cyanogenesis and fungal cyanide metabolism, topics covered in other sections of this book (Vennesland and Pistorius; Solomonson; Fry; Bunch and Knowles). Emphasis is primarily on work done since this subject was last examined (Knowles, 1976). Since research efforts in bacterial cyanide metabolism during this time have been directed mostly towards the study of cyanogenesis, this topic will receive a disproportionate emphasis in this review.

I. BACTERIAL HCN BIOSYNTHESIS

Questions arising during a criminal trial concerning the possible liberation of cyanide from decomposing protein led to the first observation of bacterial cyanide production (Emerson *et al*, 1913). The organisms isolated and others found to be cyanogenic were examined further in subsequent papers (Clawson and Young, 1913; Patty, 1921). The apparent taxonomic distribution of the cyanogenic bacteria is well recorded by Clawson and Young (1913) where *Bacillus pyocyaneus (Pseudomonas aeruginosa)*, *Bacillus fluorescens (Pseudomonas fluorescens)*, *Bacillus violaceus* (possibly *Chromobacterium violaceum)*, and a bacterial strain resembling *Pseudomonas aureofaciens* are described as being cyanogenic. Subsequent evidence has indicated that bacterial cyanogenesis is confined to *Chromobacterium violaceum* (Sneath, 1956; Sneath, 1960; Sneath, 1966; Michaels and Corpe, 1965; Rodgers and Knowles, 1978) and to members of a closely related group of *Pseudomonas* species characterized by their ability to produce fluorescent pigments (Doudoroff and Palleroni, 1974). Within this group *P. aeruginosa* (Lorck, 1948; Castric, 1975), *P. fluorescens* (Freeman *et al*, 1975, 1976; Castric, 1975), *P. aureofaciens* (Michaels and Corpe, 1965) and *Pseudomonas chlororaphis* (Michaels and Corpe, 1965) have been shown to be cyanogenic. Other members of the fluorescent pseudomonad group seem to be cyanide negative, *Pseudomonas putida* (Freeman *et al*, 1975, 1976; Castric, 1975) and *Pseudomonas cichorii* (Castric, 1975), or have not been tested, e.g. *Pseudomonas syringae*. *Pseudomonas* strains that are cyanogenic but which have not been identified as to species have been described (Bugel and Muller, 1963; Wissing, 1968). The taxonomic distribution of this trait is however, far from clear. For example, cyanogenesis occurs in *P. aeruginosa* at a frequency of about 70% (Castric, 1975) indicating that a number of strains of each species must be tested to provide meaningful results. Such a study might be of interest in clarifying the taxonomic relationship between *C.violaceum* and the fluorescent pseudomonads.

A. METABOLIC PATHWAY OF BACTERIAL CYANOGENESIS

The metabolic precursor of cyanide in bacteria is glycine. Glycine-enhanced cyanide production was first indicated by Lorck (1948) with *P. aeruginosa* and later by Michaels and Corpe (1965) with *C. violaceum*. Collins *et al* (1980) noted a stimulation of HCN production when *C. violaceum* was grown on a glutamate-salts medium containing L-threonine. This organism presumably has an enzyme capable of converting L-threonine to glycine. This was found to be the case in *P. aeruginosa* where threonine also enhanced cyanogenesis, and where extracts were able to convert L-U-^{14}C-threonine to ^{14}C glycine (Castric, 1977). This is further suggested by the evidence that while U^{14}-C threonine is a good radioactive precursor of H^{14}CN in *P. aeruginosa*, the addition of unlabelled glycine greatly diminishes the incorporation of label. L-phenylalanine also stimulated cyanide production in *P. aeruginosa*. Whereas carbon-labelled glycine and threonine were good precursors of radioactive cyanide, L-U-^{14}C-phenylalanine was only slightly converted to H^{14}CN (Castric, 1977). These results possibly point to a regulatory role with phenylalanine, or a metabolite of phenylalanine, causing a diversion of carbon to glycine and hence to HCN.

The origin of cyanide carbon in *C. violaceum* is the methylene group of glycine. Washed cells are able to convert 2-^{14}C-glycine to H^{14}CN efficiently with a dilution factor of 0.94 (Michaels *et al*, 1965). 1-^{14}C-glycine was a poor precursor of labelled cyanide. Here the dilution factor was less than 0.01, with the label being apparently converted primarily to $^{14}CO_2$. The origin of cyanide nitrogen in *C. violaceum* is the amino nitrogen of glycine. $H^{14}C^{15}N$ produced by this organism growing on a glutamate-salts medium supplemented with 2-^{14}C,^{15}N-glycine had the same $^{15}N/^{14}C$ ratio as the precursor glycine (Brysk *et al*, 1969a). In *P. aeruginosa* the methylene carbon of glycine is a good precursor of cyanide (Castric, 1977) with a dilution of label of 0.63. However, unlike the glycine feeding pattern described above, 1-^{14}C glycine is also incorporated into cyanide, albeit with the lower dilution factor of 0.36. The apparent utilization of the carboxyl group as an HCN precursor here may reflect either (1) a fundamental difference in the mode of conversion of glycine to cyanide by this organism as compared to *C. violaceum* or, (2) intermediary metabolism of glycine in *P. aeruginosa* which results in a partial randomization of label prior to the conversion of glycine to cyanide. The latter possibility might occur if glycine was metabolized to a purine which then might be degraded to glyoxylate (Vogels and Van der Drift, 1976). The carboxyl group of glyoxylate could be derived from the methylene carbon while the aldehyde group would come from the carboxyl group of glycine. Transamination of the glyoxylate (Campbell, 1956) would yield glycine. When 1-^{14}C glycine and 2-^{14}C-glycine were fed together to *P. aeruginosa* the average dilution was 0.92, indicating that nearly all the cyanide carbon is coming from exogenous glycine.

Fungal cyanogenesis is metabolically similar in many respects to HCN production by bacteria (Fry, this volume). The metabolic precursor of HCN in the snow mold basidiomycete is glycine where the methylene carbon and amino nitrogen are converted to cyanide carbon and nitrogen (Ward *et al*, 1977). This organism is, under certain cultural conditions, also able to produce labelled cyanide when fed 1-^{14}C-glycine (Bunch and Knowles, this volume). Here it is suggested that the reversible conversion of glycine to oxalate, via glyoxylate and glycollate, could allow a randomization of carbons 1 and 2 prior to the oxidation of this amino acid to CO_2 and HCN.

Although the precursor of HCN is well established in bacteria the metabolic pathway involved is far from clear. The minimal reaction in the conversion of glycine to HCN and CO_2 requires a decarboxylation and removal of four electrons. Three proposed schemes which could account for this conversion are depicted in Fig. 1. The path represented by steps (a), (b) and (c) has been suggested by Conn (1973) in analogy to the initial steps of plant cyanogenic glycoside biosynthesis (Conn, 1979, this volume). Alternatively, the decarboxylation step of this

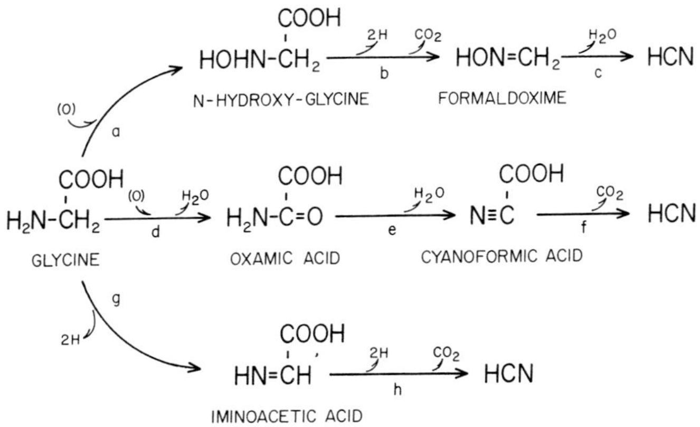

Fig. 1 Proposed pathways for the biosynthesis of HCN by bacteria.

proposed pathway might occur after the oxidation of N-hydroxyglycine in which case glyoxylate oxime, a probable intermediate in algal cyanide formation (Solomonson, 1978; Solomonson and Spehar, 1979) would be produced. Steps (d), (e) and (f) represent the major components of a pathway suggested by Michaels *et al* (1965). These authors also suggest the further conversion of cyanoformic acid to cyanuric acid and HCN as a possible branch. More recently Wissing (1974) has suggested a path, steps (g) and (h), in which an imine would serve as an intermediate. This type of intermediate is inviting since it is known to be involved in other microbial enzymes catalyzing amino acid oxidation, i.e., L-glutamate dehydrogenase (Smith *et al*, 1975), D or L amino acid oxidases (Hafner and Wellner, 1971). Inhibition studies by Wissing (1974) on cyanide biosynthesis by an unidentified pseudomonas species implicates a flavoprotein in the oxidation of glycine to cyanide and carbon dioxide, a further similarity to the amino acid oxidases. Wissing, however, indicates that due to the apparent Km of the cyanogenic enzyme system, as measured in whole cells, and the lack of inhibition by benzoic acid, a D-amino acid oxidase was unlikely to be involved in cyanogenesis here.

These paths must remain speculative until more definitive work is done, especially on the nature of the cyanogenic enzyme system. This enzyme system, HCN synthase, has been demonstrated in homogenates of an unidentified cyanogenic pseudomonad (Wissing, 1975) and more recently, in extracts of *P. aeruginosa* (Castric *et al*, 1979). Aspects of the bacterial cyanogenic enzyme system are discussed elsewhere in this book (Castric *et al*; Wissing).

B. PHYSIOLOGICAL FACTORS OF BACTERIAL CYANOGENESIS

1. *Nutritional Factors*

a. Glycine Whereas glycine is required for maximal cyanogenesis (Fig. 2), cyanide is produced in small amounts in the absence of added glycine by *C. violaceum* (Michaels and Corpe, 1965; Rodgers and Knowles, 1978), by a *Pseudomonas* species (Wissing, 1968) and by *P. aeruginosa* (Castric, 1977). In all of these cases the only carbon available is the medium carbon source, thus the low levels of HCN produced represent a diversion of materials from primary metabolism.

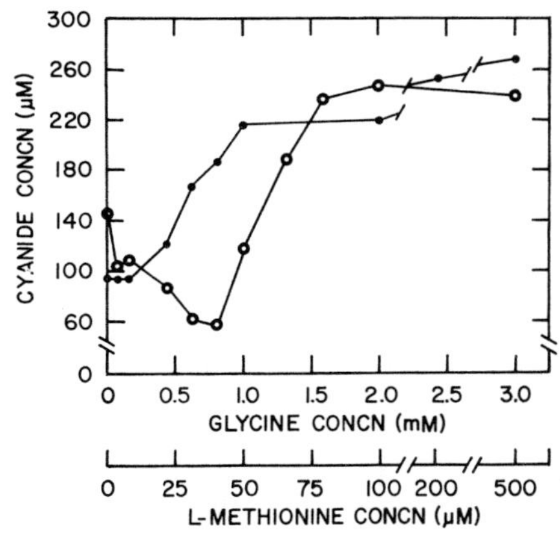

Fig. 2 The effect of initial cultural glycine and methionine levels on cyanogenesis by *Chrombacterium violaceum*. Growth was in a synthetic medium initially containing 0.5 mM methionine and glycine at various concentrations (○), or in the presence of 2 mM glycine with methionine at various concentrations (●). From Collins *et al* (1980); figure reproduced by the courtesy of the *Journal of General Microbiology*.

In neither *P. aeruginosa* (Castric, 1977) nor *C. violaceum* (Collins *et al*, 1980) does glycine serve as a good carbon and energy source. Glycine supported very slow growth, with a generation time of about 72 hours, for *P. aeruginosa* (Castric, 1977). Thus in a situation where this amino acid is synthesized faster than required for biosynthesis, pools of glycine would be available for cyanogenesis. *P. aeruginosa*, if continually subcultured in a glycine-salts medium, becomes "trained" to use this amino acid as a sole carbon and energy source (Castric, K.F., and P.A. Castric, unpub. obsv.). This organism produces no detectable HCN when grown in this manner, but produces normal amounts of cyanide when grown on a glutamate-glycine-salts medium. These results may indicate that cyanogenesis functions to regulate glycine levels when the bacterium cannot utilize this amino acid in another way. This point will be re-examined in a later section.

Whereas the role of glycine as substrate for bacterial cyanide production is clear, its role in the regulation of synthesis of the HCN synthase is not. Although glycine might be expected to be an inducer, the omission of this amino acid from a synthetic *P. aeruginosa* growth medium results in a slight increase in specific activity of HCN synthase rather than a decline (Castric *et al*, 1979). Even so, intracellular glycine increases under these conditions and accounts for over one-third of the non-carbon source amino acid pool (Castric *et al*, this volume). These levels may be high enough to cause induction. In *C. violaceum* the addition of small amounts of glycine to a glutamate-methionine salts medium actually suppress HCN production partially, although higher amounts enhance cyanogenesis (Collins *et al*, 1980). Altogether these results suggest caution in the interpretation of the role of glycine in the regulation of HCN synthase biosynthesis.

Another role for glycine may be in the maintenance of stability of this enzyme during cyanogenesis. The HCN synthase of *P. aeruginosa* is extremely sensitive to aerobic conditions and is only present in significant amounts when cultural oxygen levels are low (Castric *et al*, this volume). Glycine protects against this oxygen-mediated inactivation *in vitro*, and may also have this function *in vivo*.

b. Methionine In all cases examined methionine has an important influence on bacterial cyanide production (Michaels and Corpe, 1965; Wissing, 1968; Castric, 1977; Collins *et al*, 1980). Whereas methionine cannot replace glycine in the stimulation of cyanogenesis it significantly enhances the amounts of cyanide produced. This is demonstrated in Fig. 2 where 0.2 to 0.5 mM methionine is required for the maximal activity by *C. violaceum* in the presence of 2 mM glycine. Methionine does not act as a metabolic precursor since neither methyl labelled methionine in *C. violaceum* (Michaels *et al*, 1965) nor uniformly labelled methionine in *P. aeruginosa* (Castric, 1977) are converted, to a significant extent, to labelled cyanide.

The role of methionine in cyanogenesis is enigmatic. Michaels and Corpe (1965) have suggested that it functions as a methyl group donor and so indirectly influences HCN biosynthesis. This is based on the findings that methyl carriers such as betaine and choline will substitute for methionine in enhancing cyanogenesis in *C. violaceum*. Collins *et al* (1980) were unable to substantiate these findings, but did find that structurally related compounds such as D-methionine, cystathionine, and S-adenosyl-L-homocysteine were able to substitute for L-methionine in this organism. These authors suggest that HCN could be produced to reduce glycine levels which would allow the continued production, from serine by serine transhydroxymethylase, of vital one-carbon units as well as glycine. Methionine would reduce the one carbon demand, hence altering the flow of glycine and thus enhance cyanogenesis.

These results warrant a closer examination of the physiologically significant routes of glycine biosynthesis in the cyanogenic organisms and the patterns of regulation of these paths. For example, is the serine transhydroxymethylase regulated in these organisms as it is in *Salmonella typhimurium* (Stauffer and Brenchley, 1977)? If this is so, then the presence of methionine might repress the synthesis of this enzyme resulting in lowered glycine production. Of equal interest, is glycine produced from serine via the serine transhydroxymethylase? Can transaminases such as serine: glyoxylate aminotransferase or glutamate: glyoxylate amino transferase, enzymes which have been shown to occur in *Pseudomonas* species (Campbell, 1956; Quayle, 1972), serve this function? Can the conversion of threonine to glycine serve as a source of glycine as it can under certain conditions in *Escherichia coli* (Newman *et al*, 1976; Potter *et al*, 1977)? Finally, one can question the influence of HCN production on methionine biosynthesis. With some strains of *E. coli* growth inhibition by 5 mM azide or 25 μM cyanide is accompanied by a drop in intracellular methionine (Nazar and Wong, 1973). This interference with cell growth, which is reversed by the addition of methionine, is interpreted by the authors as being due to cyanide inhibition of the B_{12}-dependent homocysteine transmethylase, one of the two *E. coli* enzymes capable of catalyzing this last step in methionine biosynthesis (Taylor and Weissbach, 1973). Could the HCN produced by the cyanogenic bacteria partially inhibit methionine biosynthesis, thus requiring the addition of this amino acid for normal metabolism and cyanogenesis?

Alternately methionine may influence apparent cyanide levels by inhibiting assimilation, but not production, of HCN. Rodgers (this volume) presents evidence that this is the case with *C. violaceum*, a bacterium which is able actively to convert HCN to β-cyanoalanine. The influence of both glycine and methionine on cyanogenesis by *C. violaceum* is further examined elsewhere in this book (Nazly *et al*).

Finally methionine may act as either an inducer of synthesis of the HCN synthase or a positive effector of this enzyme. Induction of cyanogenesis by methionine in *C. violaceum* has been suggested (Michaels and Corpe, 1965; Rodgers and Knowles, 1978). In *P. aeruginosa* this is probably not the case since, as indicated above, exogenous methionine is not required for maximal HCN synthase activity. Further, in the absence of added methionine the intracellular levels of methionine never rise above a basal level (Castric, P.A., unpub. obsv.) during the culture cycle while the cyanogenic enzyme system is synthesized mainly during the latter part of the log phase (Castric *et al*, 1979). An influence by methionine on the activity of the HCN synthase, as suggested by Collins *et al* (1980) may well occur, but elucidation of this must await further work on the enzyme system.

c. Carbon source L-Glutamate has been the usual carbon and energy source in studies with the cyanogenic bacteria. Substituting glucose for this amino acid with *C.violaceum* (Collins *et al*, 1980) resulted in a slight increase in total cyanide produced, while substituting glucose for succinate as carbon and energy source for an unidentified pseudomonad (Wissing, 1968) resulted in a decline in HCN production. Such a carbon source effect is quite pronounced with *P. aeruginosa* (Ebert, R.F., and P.A. Castric, unpub. obsv.) where using either a glucose-urea or a glucose-ammonia medium results in a little cyanide production and very low levels of HCN synthase. It is inviting to think that these results imply carbon catabolite repression (Drew and Demain, 1974; Demain *et al*, 1979). With *P. aeruginosa*, it is probably not so, since the intermediates of the tricarboxylic acid cycle are preferred carbon sources over glucose (Ng and Dawes, 1973). It is particularly interesting to note that cyclic AMP reduces cyanogenesis in *C. violaceum* grown on glucose (Collins *et al*, 1980) which may indicate a carbon source mediated regulation in this organism. The addition of cyclic AMP has no influence on the glucose effect seen with *P. aeruginosa*. This is not really surprising since this organism, while containing significant levels of cyclic AMP, does not appear to be subject to regulation by this nucleotide (Seigel *et al*, 1977).

2. *Aeration*

Some of the earliest reports on bacterial cyanogenesis (Clawson and Young, 1913; Patty, 1921) note the relationship between aerobic conditions and cyanide production. More recently it has been shown that aerobic stationary *P. aeruginosa* cultures produced significantly less HCN as compared to shake cultures (Castric, 1975). This organism, grown anaerobically using nitrate respiration, produced very low amounts of HCN (Castric, 1975). These conditions influence both growth and cyanogenesis, thus the role of oxygen is not apparent.

The influence of oxygen was examined more closely on an unidentified cyanogenic pseudomonad (Wissing, 1974) where resting cells produced HCN at only a low rate under anaerobic conditions as seen in Fig. 3. The addition of O_2 under these conditions results in a significant and immediate increase in cyanide production. Artificial electron acceptors substitute for oxygen with an order of reactivity of: O_2 >phenazine methosulfate >methylene blue >2,6-dichlorophenolindophenol >potassium ferricyanide. There is no apparent relationship between redox potential of these electron acceptors and their ability to support anaerobic cyanogenesis. Although these results indicate that oxygen acts as an electron acceptor several problems remain. If oxygen is a physiological electron acceptor in the oxidation of glycine to cyanide and CO_2, it has to be established whether this molecule acts directly on the cyanogenic enzyme system or whether a series of electron carriers lie between the oxidation of glycine and the reduction of oxygen. In this regard, it has been noted recently that the HCN synthase in extracts of *P. aeruginosa*, while producing no cyanide under anaerobic conditions, carries out the oxidation of glycine to cyanide in the presence of oxygen (Castric *et al*, this volume). Phenazine methosulfate supported anaerobic cyanide production by these extracts, but unlike the whole cells mentioned above, at several times the oxygen-mediated rate. These results indicate that oxygen may not be the direct physiological electron acceptor and might require intact electron transport components to act in this manner. Finally, one can question whether oxygen is an obligatory physiological electron acceptor in cyanogenesis. The work by Nazly *et al* (this volume) strongly indicates not. Here cyanide is produced by *C. violaceum* growing anaerobically using glucose as carbon and energy source and fumarate as electron acceptor.

Oxygen also appears to influence regulation of bacterial cyanogenesis. Aerobic conditions result in the inactivation of the cyanogenic enzyme system and may play a physiological role in the termination of cyanogenesis during the *P. aeruginosa* culture cycle (Castric *et al*, this volume). This point is discussed elsewhere in this chapter.

Two physiological predicaments become apparent from the above discussion. In the first, good aeration favors cyanogenesis but aerobic conditions inactivate the HCN synthase. This may be explained by good aeration favoring vigorous growth and metabolism by these aerobic organisms, and hence cyanogenesis. Vigorous growth and metabolism require a high respiratory rate which could result in a reduced oxygen tension within the cell which, in turn, could protect the HCN synthase. This, along with high

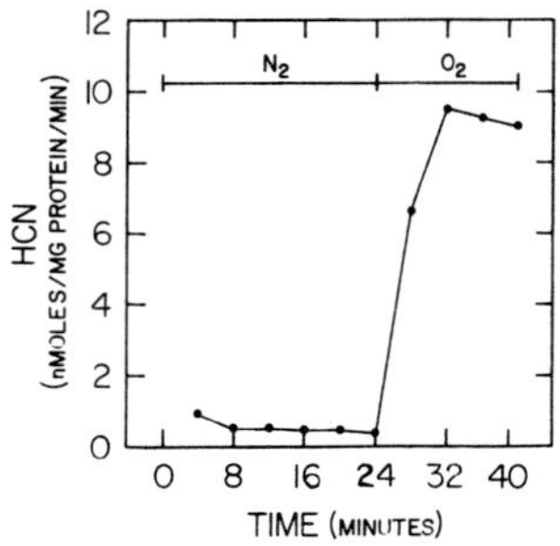

Fig. 3 Response of cyanide production by whole cells of a *Pseudomonas* species to oxygen. From Wissing (1974); figure reproduced by the courtesy of the *Journal of Bacteriology*.

internal glycine levels, could result in significant enzyme protection. In the second predicament, aerobic conditions favor cyanogenesis, yet also favor respiration for which cyanide is a classic inhibitor. To avoid this, cyanogenic organisms may (1) metabolically detoxify cyanide as with *C. violaceum* (Rodgers and Knowles, 1978), or (2) selectively turn to cyanide resistant respiration during cyanogenesis as is the case with both *C. violaceum* (Niven *et al*, 1975) and *P. aeruginosa* (Kralik and Castric, 1979). These above mentioned methods of microbial cyanide resistance are discussed later in this article and elsewhere in this book (Rodgers; Bunch and Knowles; Fry; Henry).

3. *Growth Phase*

A characteristic of bacterial cyanogenesis in batch cultures is the temporal relationship between HCN production and growth phase (Michaels and Corpe, 1965; Wissing, 1968; Castric, 1975; Rodger and Knowles, 1978). Cyanide is produced mainly during a discrete portion of the culture cycle corresponding to the transition between log and stationary phases. This is represented in Fig. 4 with the time-course of cumulative HCN production and cell growth of *P. aeruginosa* growing on a glutamate-glycine-methionine-salts medium. Cyanogenesis does not occur exclusively during this period however. With *C. violaceum* (Rodgers and Knowles, 1978) as well as the pseudomonads examined (Wissing, 1968; Castric *et al*, 1979) it can be seen that very low levels of cyanide are produced during log growth. The massive production of HCN at the end of log growth represents an amplification of this low rate. This amplification can be prevented by inhibitors of protein synthesis (Castric, 1975; Rodgers and Knowles, 1978). Thus synthesis of the cyanogenic enzyme system must occur during the latter part of the culture cycle, a conclusion which is supported by the

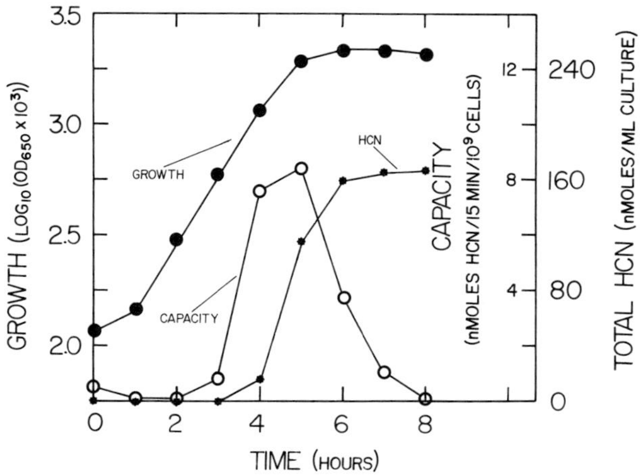

Fig. 4 The change in cyanide production (*) and cyanogenic capacity (○) as compared to growth (●) of *Pseudomonas aeruginosa*. From Castric *et al* (1979); figure reproduced by the courtesy of *Current Microbiology*.

dramatic increase in specific activity of the HCN synthase as the culture cycle progresses (Castric *et al*, this volume).

4. Mineral Influences

a. Iron. The production of HCN by *C. violaceum* (Rodgers and Knowles, 1978) or *P. aeruginosa* (Castric, 1975) is significantly influenced by iron. Figure 5 demonstrates that iron concentrations which allow complete cell growth, added as ferric chloride with *P. aeruginosa* or ferrous sulfate with *C. violaceum*, limit cyanogenesis by these organisms. It can also be seen that the concentration response to this metal ion is different with these two organisms. With *P. aeruginosa* the influence is specific to iron; cobalt, copper, manganese or zinc cannot act as substitute (Castric, 1975).

b. Inorganic phosphate. Bacterial cyanogenesis responds dramatically to cultural phosphate levels. This occurs in both *C. violaceum* (Rodgers and Knowles, 1978) and *P. aeruginosa* (Castric, 1975; Meganathan and Castric, 1977) as represented by Fig. 5. HCN production is dramatically influenced by concentrations of phosphate which permit optimal culture growth. As with the iron effect, there are significant differences in the response of these two organisms to inorganic phosphate. With *P. aeruginosa* maximum HCN production occurs within a narrow range of

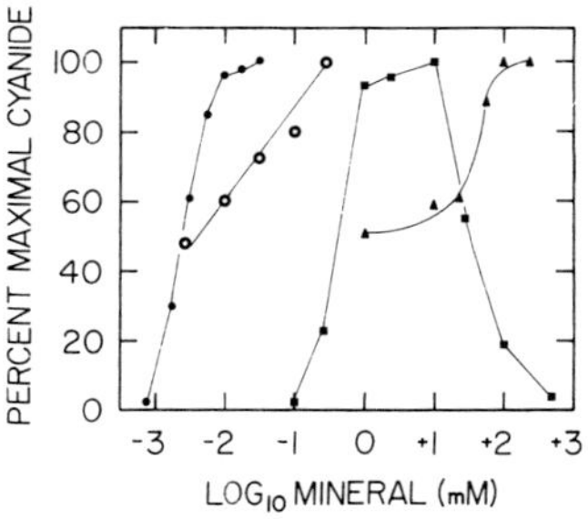

Fig. 5 The influence of cultural iron and inorganic phosphate levels on cyanide production by *Chromobacterium violaceum* (○, iron; ▲, inorganic phosphate) and *Pseudomonas aeruginosa* (●, iron; ■, inorganic phosphate). From Castric (1975), Meganathan and Castric (1977), Rodgers and Knowles (1978); composite figure produced by the permission of the *Canadian Journal of Microbiology*, *Archives of Microbiology*, and the *Journal of General Microbiology*.

phosphate concentrations which are sufficient to cause only minimal HCN production by *C. violaceum*.

Optimal levels of phosphate in *P. aeruginosa* are needed at the time cyanogenesis is occuring (Meganathan and Castric, 1977). Shifting phosphate at this time of the culture cycle from lower non-permissive (0.1 mM) to permissive (10.0 mM) levels is quickly followed by HCN production. This sort of response occurs with shift-ups of iron levels, 0.5 to 20 μM, also during the period of cyanogenesis (Meganathan R., McDevitt, D., and P.A. Castric, unpub. obsv.). These shift-ups are accompanied by synthesis of the HCN synthase which is preventable by protein synthesis inhibitors. Shifting phosphate from permissive (10.0 mM) to upper non-permissive (200 mM) levels results in prematurely shutting down cyanogenesis.

The mode of action of these minerals is not clear. While mineral influences of this nature have been seen with other metabolites (Weinberg, 1977; Weinberg, 1978) we must seek explanations which are specific for cyanogenesis. Since the HCN synthase system is an oxido-reductase it might contain iron which could act as a cofactor. Iron limitation might then result in the production of an inactive apo-enzyme resulting in no HCN production. On the other hand, the mode of action of phosphate may involve regulation of enzymatic activity as might be indicated by the phosphate shift experiment (10 mM to 200 mM) described above. In addition, cultures grown with non-permissive phosphate levels (250 mM) produce significant levels of HCN synthase but are not particularly cyanogenic (Castric *et al*, 1979).

The iron and phosphate influence may be of a much more general nature, and control cyanogenesis only indirectly. One possibility might be energy metabolism where the influence of iron may be primarily on respiration. This would be expected to alter the levels of a variety of metabolites. Cultural phosphate levels might result in altered adenine nucleotide content and adenylate charge of these cells (Chapman and Atkinson, 1977; Tsai *et al*, 1979). Such compounds might then be the intracellular factors regulating cyanogenesis.

C. POSSIBLE PHYSIOLOGICAL FUNCTIONS OF BACTERIAL CYANOGENESIS

The physiological function of cyanogenesis in certain organisms may be idscussed with some confidence. For example, with algal cyanogenesis there is evidence that this process is involved in the regulation of the assimilatory nitrate reduction system of these organisms (Solomonson, 1978; Solomonson and Spehar, 1979; Solomonson, this volume). However the role of cyanogenesis in bacteria is not apparent. This is further complicated by the evidence that this process is not required for cell growth, or, if required, is necessary at very low levels. For example, many *P. aeruginosa* isolates are not cyanogenic (Castric, 1975). Cyanide-negative mutants of *P. aeruginosa* have been obtained (Kralik and Castric, 1979) which seem to grow normally. Strains of *P. aeruginosa* "trained" to use glycine as a carbon and energy source, as described in a previous section, are not cyanogenic under these conditions but do produce cyanide when grown on a glutamate-glycine-methionine-salts medium. Finally the environmental factors discussed previously result in low or undetectable levels of HCN, without disturbing cell growth, in both *C. violaceum* (Rodger and Knowles, 1978) and *P. aeruginosa* (Castric, 1975).

While the above might imply a minor role for cyanogenesis in these bacteria the magnitude of the HCN produced would indicate otherwise. In *C. violaceum*, where cyanide can be produced to levels of 2-3 millimoles per liter (Brysk *et al*, 1969; Rodgers and Knowles, 1978), the amounts of glycine converted to cyanide must easily rival the amounts of this amino acid used for biosynthesis.

Some of the physiological factors described in the previous section which influence cyanogenesis, environmental factors and growth phase dependence, have been considered to be characteristics of microbial secondary metabolism (Weinberg, 1970, 1971). The characteristics for cyanogenesis described in this section, lack of apparent function and the non-requirement for cell growth, are also considered to be attributes of secondary metabolites (Demain, 1979). Whereas being a secondary metabolite does not ascribe a function to bacterial cyanogenesis it does provide a series of approaches which may prove useful in establishing the physiological relevance of this process.

1. *Ecological Significance*

The production of HCN could be beneficial to the producer organisms in a number of ways. As pointed out by Knowles (1976), this process could (1) increase the competitiveness of the cyanogenic organism; (2) decrease its chances of predation by other microbes; (3) enhance any parasitic nature of the cyanogenic organism. Given the natural environment, soil and water, of the cyanogenic bacteria there could be many competitive and predatory microbes present.

It has recently been proposed (Hassan and Fridovitch, 1980) that another secondary metabolite of *P. aeruginosa*, the blue pigment pyocyanine, is produced by this organism as an anti-microbial agent. Pyocyanine could enter neighboring cells and divert electron flow to production of highly toxic superoxide which could overwhelm the superoxide dismutase present, resulting in cell death. It is possible that cyanide produced by *P. aeruginosa* might act in concert with pyocyanine by inhibiting electron transport and thus causing an increase in intracellular oxygen. Electrons diverted via pyocyanine would produce the superoxide and, subsequently, hydrogen peroxide.

C. violaceum can be a human pathogen (Sneath *et al*, 1953), and *P. aeruginosa* is well known both as a plant and human pathogen (Elrod and Braun, 1941; Sands *et al*, 1970; Lowbury, 1975). It is interesting to note that the fluorescent pseudomonads produce a number of secondary metabolites other than HCN (Leisinger and Margraff, 1979). Some of these are phytotoxins and play a specific role in plant pathogenesis (Strobel, 1977). Whether or not cyanogenesis plays a role in some plant or animal diseases cannot, at present be established.

The same arguments may be made against this type of role for cyanogenesis as are made against such a role for secondary metabolites in general (Weinberg, 1970; Demain, 1974). The narrow range of conditions necessary for cyanogenesis might be an unusual set of circumstances for these organisms in their soil or water environment. Thus amounts of HCN produced might be insignificant. This coupled with the ability of many organisms to carry out cyanide resistant respiration (Knowles, 1976; Jones, 1979) might make this an ineffective ecological mechanism. These possibilities are nevertheless intriguing and certainly warrant further examination.

2. *Regulatory Significance*

Although HCN is an extremely toxic compound its production may have nothing to do with its biological activity. This is simply restating a concept which proposes that the process of secondary metabolism relieves some negative influence brought on by a metabolic crisis, such as a nutrient deficiency, while the product is of no value (Weinberg, 1971). Evidence in favor of this idea shows that cultural conditions which favor secondary metabolism enhance long-term viability whereas cultural conditions unfavorable to secondary metabolism result in reduced long-term viability (Weinberg and Goodnight, 1970; Gentry *et al*, 1971). This idea may be applied to cyanogenesis (Castric, 1975) since glycine, while a central molecule in the metabolism of these bacteria (being a precursor to other amino acids, protein, purines and hemes), is capable of major inhibitory effects. High concentrations of glycine interrupt bacterial cell wall biosynthesis (Schleifer *et al*, 1976). Glycine also acts as a negative effector of the glutamine synthetase of *P. fluorescens* (Hubbard and Stadtman, 1967).

Conditions which might result in metabolic stress and thus cause cyanogenesis could be the presence of high exogenous glycine concentrations or the inability of the cell to regulate synthesized glycine levels under certain particular situations in the absence of added glycine. The latter conditions would give rise to overflow metabolism as described by Tempest and Neijssel (1978), a conditions which, in times of metabolic stress, results in the diversion of normal metabolites to excretion products. More specific suggestions are proposed by Rodgers and Knowles (1978) with regards to cyanogenesis in *C. violaceum* where cyanide production may be related to the ability of these cells to maintain one-carbon metabolism as indicated previously. These authors suggest also that cyanogenesis could be involved in the removal of nitrogen by the cells in a form other than ammonia.

The above discussion proposes several intriguing but somewhat speculative explanations for the physiological role of bacterial cyanogenesis. This role might well be more easily explained. It is possible that cyanogenesis in bacteria plays some role in regulating metabolism in these organisms as it does in the algae (Solomonson, 1978; Solomonson, this volume). This might function by inactivating cyanide sensitive components such as particular terminal oxidases of the branched electron transport system. Such possibilities, although currently without support, deserve further examination.

III. HCN ASSIMILATION BY BACTERIA

Whereas certain bacteria are able to produce HCN, others in turn are able to assimilate and detoxify this compound. HCN assimilation, unlike HCN formation by bacteria, is not restricted to closely related organisms and involves a number of different pathways.

A. PATHWAYS OF ASSIMILATION

1. β-*Cyanoalanine Formation*

The condensation of HCN with a three-carbon molecule to form β-cyanoalanine, as indicated in step (a) of Fig. 6, has been demonstrated in extracts or whole cells of several bacterial species. These include *Escherichia coli* (Dunnill and Fowden, 1965), *Bacillus megaterium* (Castric and Strobel, 1969), and *C. violaceum* (Brysk *et al*, 1969b). β-cyanoalanine formation also occurs in the alga *Chlorella pyrenoidosa* (Fowden and Bell, 1965) as well as in higher plants where the reaction was first discovered (Blumenthal-Goldschmidt *et al*, 1963; Blumenthal *et al*, 1968). With both *C. violaceum* (Brysk *et al*, 1969a, b) and *B. megaterium* (Castric and Strobel, 1969) cyanide carbon is incorporated only in the C-4 position of β-cyanolanine and the carbon-nitrogen bond of cyanide is retained in the cyano portion of this amino acid. With *C. violaceum* the isotope ration was maintained on conversion of [2-$^{14}C^{15}N$] glycine to $H^{14}C^{15}N$ and, subsequently, to the cyano group of β-cyanoalanine. Likewise the non-cyanogenic *B. megaterium* converted $K^{13}C^{15}N$ to the cyano portion of β-cyanoalanine with no change of ratio. While L-serine is a precursor for the three-carbon fragment in bacteria (Castric and Strobel, 1969; Brysk *et al*, 1969b) the immediate precursor may be either L-cysteine or O-acetyl-L-serine (Castric and Conn, 1971).

The nature of the enzyme which catalyzes the formation of β-cyanoalanine in bacteria is not clear. In the plant blue lupine (*Lupinus angustifolia*) two enzymes are present which can produce β-cyanoalanine (Hendrickson and Conn, 1969). One is cysteine synthase [EC 4.2.99.8] referred to in several of the references cited as O-acetyl-L-serine sulfhydrylase, which produces L-cysteine from O-acetyl-L-serine and H_2S, but also, with a 90% reduction in specific activity, converts O-acetyl-L-serine and HCN to β-cyanoalanine. The other is termed β-cyanoalanine synthase [EC 4.4.1.9] which condenses L-cysteine and HCN to β-cyanoalanine, and also produces cysteine from O-acetyl-L-serine and H_2S (the latter having only 4% the specific activity of the former). *B. megaterium* extracts were able to synthesize β-cyanoalanine from L-cysteine and HCN but only at 0.05% of the rate of synthesis of cysteine from O-acetyl-L-serine and H_2S (Castric and Conn, 1971). These activities were coordinately repressed by L-cysteine, but were induced by sulfate or L-djenkolic acid. This manner of regulation is seen with the cysteine synthase (O-acetyl serine sulfhydrylase) of *Salmonella typhimurium* (Kredich and Tomkins, 1966). Furthermore, the β-cyanoalanine forming activity of

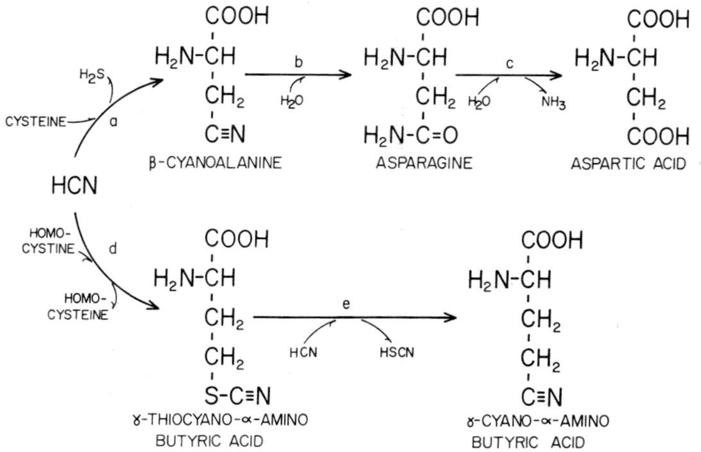

Fig. 6 The β-cyanoalanine and γ-cyano-α-aminobutyric acid pathways of cyanide assimilation.

extracts of *B. megaterium* was copurified with cysteine synthase through a 30-fold purification and was co-eluted by ion-exchange chromatography and gel filtration. It appears that this organism produces β-cyanoalanine using its cysteine synthase (Castric and Conn, 1971). But what about the cyanogenic bacteria? Cell free production of β-cyanoalanine in extracts of *C. violaceum* has been demonstrated (Rodgers and Knowles, 1978). It would be most interesting to know whether this activity is due to a cysteine synthase, a true β-cyanoalanine synthase, or whether this organism, like the blue lupine, has two distinct β-cyanoalanine synthesizing enzymes. Other aspects of β-cyanoalanine formation are examined elsewhere in this book (Rodgers).

The β-cyanoalanine formed by these bacteria can be hydrolyzed further to asparagine as indicated by step (b) of Fig. 6. This reaction also may be catalyzed as a secondary reaction of another enzyme. For example, the L-asparaginases [EC 3.5.1.1.] of guinea pig serum and *E. coli* can carry out this reaction (step (c) of Fig. 6) (Lauinger and Ressler, 1970). With the *E. coli* asparaginase, nitrilase maximum velocity is 30% of the asparaginase rate; the Km for asparagine is 0.011 mM while that for β-cyanoalanine is 12 mM. In contrast, the blue lupine has a β-cyanoalanine nitrilase [EC 4.2.1.65], (Castric *et al*, 1972) which will not hydrolyze L-asparagine. As with the nitrile-synthesizing enzymes, the role of nitrilases in bacterial β-cyanoalanine metabolism provides an interesting area for study.

2. *γ-Cyano-α-aminobutyric Acid Production*

HCN is metabolized in another manner in *C. violaceum* as described by Brysk and Ressler (1970). Here γ-cyano-α-aminobutyric acid, a compound never previously described as a natural product, is produced from γ-thiocyanobutyric acid (step (e) of Fig. 6). This step is enzymatically catalyzed by γ-cyanoaminobutyric acid synthase (Ressler *et al*, 1973). The γ-thiocyanobutyric acid is produced non-enzymatically from homocystine and HCN (step (d) of Fig. 6).

The γ-cyanoaminobutyric acid synthase has been purified and characterized (Ressler *et al*, 1973). This enzyme has a molecular weight of 130,000, as estimated by gel filtration, and an iso-electric point at pH 4.2-4.4. The optimal pH varied with substrate concentration but was in the range of 8.3-10.5. The Km for cyanide was 30 mM while the Km for γ-thiocyanobutyric acid was 29 mM. Thiocyanate, the other end product of this reaction, inhibited the enzyme 40% at 0.01 M and 90% at 0.10 M while γ-cyano-α-aminobutyric acid had no negative influence at 0.01 M. The γ-cyanoaminobutyric acid synthase required pyridoxal phosphate for activity as did the plant β-cyanoalanine synthase (Akopyan *et al*, 1975). Complete loss of activity followed the destruction of the enzyme-bound pyridoxal with hydroxylamine. Nearly complete recovery of activity accompanied the readdition of this co-enzyme. It is of interest that the same reaction as that catalyzed by this enzyme, replacement of the thiocyano group with a cyano group, is catalyzed by plant β-cyanoalanine synthase (Akopyan *et al*,1975) using as substrate the structural homologue β-thiocyanoalanine.

As with the β-cyanoalanine pathway the physiological significance is not absolutely clear. The γ-cyanoaminobutyric acid synthase has a non-enzymatically produced precursor and quite high Km's for its substrates which might indicate that it has another, primary, catalytic function. However, this enzyme was shown not to be γ-cystathionase, homocysteine desulfhydrase, rhodanese, or β-mercaptopyruvate sulfurtransferase (Ressler *et al*, 1973). Further, a relation to the presence of HCN was established when Rodgers and Knowles (1978) showed an increase in γ-cyanoaminobutyric acid synthase during the portion of the culture cycle when cyanogenesis occurs most actively. This was interpreted by these authors to mean that cyanide may have been acting as an inducer. γ-Cyano-α-aminobutyric acid is not further metabolized by *C. violaceum* indicating a possible detoxification role (Brysk and Ressler, 1970).

3. *Thiocyanate Production*

While thiocyanate is one of the products of cyanide

assimilation via the γ-cyano-α-aminobutyric acid pathway, it is the sole product in the two steps depicted in Fig. 7. Reaction (a), catalyzed by the enzyme rhodanese [EC 2.8.1.1.] occurs in plants and animals, as well as in microbes (Westly, 1973; Sörbo, 1975). This enzyme is found in a variety of bacteria including *C. violaceum* and *P. aeruginosa* (Vandenbergh *et al*, 1979). Regulation of rhodanese in *C. violaceum* was examined by Rodgers and Knowles (1978) who found that this enzyme increased during the part of the culture cycle where HCN was produced. Enhancement of rhodanese levels by the addition of HCN has been noted in *Thiobacillus denitrificans* (Bowen *et al*, 1965) and *Rhodospirillum palustris* (Yoch and Lindstrom, 1971). The evidence cited above suggests a detoxification role for this enzyme in bacteria, but this may not be the case. Westley (1973) suggested several possible functions including (1) HCN detoxification; (2) H_2S detoxification; (3) thiol biosynthesis, and (4) thiosulfate oxidation. Sulfur oxidation by chemolithotrophic bacteria (Suzuki, 1974) would be an example of the last function. It is interesting to note that rhodanese has also been implicated in sulfur metabolism in the cyanogenic bacterium *P. aeruginosa* (Hall and Berk, 1968; Shook and Berk, 1978). This enzyme may serve as a general sulfur transferase and so carry out all or a number of the above functions as the metabolic situation requires (Westley, 1973). A further discussion of rhodanese by Westley may be found in this book.

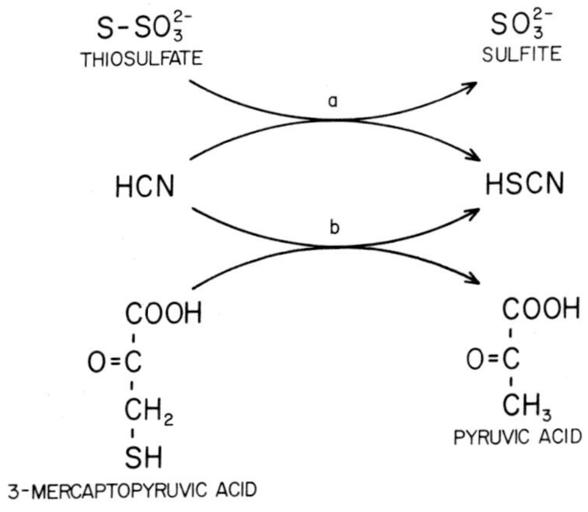

Fig. 7 The conversion of hydrogen cyanide to hydrogen thiocyanate.

Step (b) of Fig. 7 shows the reaction catalyzed by mercaptopyruvate sulfurtransferase [EC 2.8.1.2], an enzyme demonstrated in *E. coli* (Vaschek and Wood, 1972) as well as in animal sources (Sörbo, 1975). Westley (1973) compares this enzyme to rhodanese, indicating a role of sulfur transfer. In a non-microbial system this enzyme is involved in sulfur transfer to an iron-sulfur protein, adrenodoxin (Toniguchi and Kimura, 1974). Likewise rhodanese, again from an animal source, is implicated in sulfur transfer to succinic dehydrogenase (Bonomi *et al*, 1977). Whether such a role is involved in microbial systems is not clear.

B. CYANIDE ASSIMILATION BY CYANOGENIC BACTERIA

The two general facets of bacterial cyanide metabolism are reflected in the organisms which can assimilate as well as produce cyanide. The bacterium *C. violaceum* is an example. As indicated previously the methylene carbon and amino nitrogen of glycine serve as precursors for cyanide which, in turn, serves as a precursor for the cyano group of β-cyanoalanine (Brysk *et al*, 1969b). In addition, glycine is a one-carbon donor which, with the aid of serine transhydroxymethylase, condenses with another molecule of glycine to form serine. Serine is, in turn, the direct or indirect three carbon precursor of β-cyanoalanine. This intertwining of cyanide formation and assimilation was demonstrated by Brysk *et al* (1969a). Whereas $H^{14}CN$ was incorporated by whole cells into carbon 4 of β-cyanoalanine, [^{14}C]-formaldehyde, a precursor to one carbon metabolism, was incorporated into carbons 2 or 3. Furthermore, incubation of whole cells with [2-^{14}C] glycine resulted in the incorporation of label in carbons 2 or 3 in addition to incorporation in the carbon 4 position of β-cyanoalanine. Thus glycine is capable of serving as the complete precursor for β-cyanoalanine which can then be hydrolysed by the cell to the protein amino acids asparagine and aspartic acid. The effect of this conversion of glycine to aspartic acid on the metabolism of these amino acids has not been studied.

The β-cyanoalanine synthase, rhodanese and γ-cyanoaminobutyric acid synthase of *C. violaceum* have been studied with regard to their relationship to cyanogenesis (Rodgers and Knowles, 1978). As mentioned above, the synthesis of these enzymes is stimulated during the portion of the culture cycle where maximal cyanogenesis occurs. This stimulation is followed by a sharp decrease in HCN, indicating a degradation of the cyanide produced. The addition of chloramphenical, which prevents further synthesis of these enzymes, prevents the decline in cyanide levels. These results indicate a physiological relation between cyanide biosynthesis and cyanide degradation in *C. violaceum*. The formation of β-cyanoalanine is examined further by Rodgers (this volume).

Cyanide uptake by the cyanogenic pseudomonads has not been studied in detail. Where it has been examined it would appear that these organisms do not have the extensive ability to metabolize HCN demonstrated by *C. violaceum*. Wissing (1974) demonstrated a nearly 1:1 ratio between glycine utilized and HCN produced by resting cells of an unidentified pseudomonad, indicating no further metabolism of HCN under these conditions. HCN levels of *P. aeruginosa* cultures do not decline in the manner described for *C. violaceum* (Castric, unpub. obsv.). However the pseudomonads do contain rhodanese (Shook and Berk, 1978; Vandenbergh *et al*, 1979), and the proper conditions for demonstrating HCN assimilation or detoxification in these organisms may not have been achieved.

C. NUTRITIONAL UTILIZATION OF HCN

Very little work has been done in specifically examining the utilization of cyanide as carbon, nitrogen or energy sources. This is unusual considering the number of indications that microbes, and particularly bacteria, are able to use this compound for such purposes. The biochemistry of such a process could be straightforward; enzymatic hydrolysis of cyanide would yield formamide or formic acid and ammonia, from which a bacterium might satisfy many of its nutritional needs. The ammonia would be a ready source of nitrogen; the utilization of formate as a carbon source or as an energy source by a variety of bacteria is well documented (Colby *et al*, 1979).

The metabolism of nitriles by bacteria would be analogous to such a process. The hydrolysis of the nitrile ricinine by a *Pseudonomas* species allows this organism to use this compound as a carbon and energy source (Robinson and Hook, 1964). Presumably the production of ammonia by the ricinine nitrilase [EC 3.5.5.2] would also allow this organism to use ricinine as a nitrogen source (Hook and Robinson, 1964). Acetonitrile can serve as sole carbon and energy source (and, presumably, nitrogen source) for *Corynebacterium nitrilophilus* (Mimura *et al*, 1969) and an unidentified *Pseudomonas* species (Firmin and Gray, 1976). The necessary nitrilase (Arnaud *et al*, 1977) has been isolated and characterized from a species belonging to the genus *Brevibacterium* which is able to use acetonitrile as the sole source of nitrogen. *Nocardia rhodochrous* can use acetonitrile, propionitrile, hydroacrylonitrile, and succinonitrile as both carbon and nitrogen source, and can use acrylonitrile and butenenitrile as nitrogen source but is unable to utilize benzonitrile (DiGeronimo and Antoine, 1976). The enzymatic hydrolysis of acetonitrile and propionitrile by extracts of this organism was demonstrated. A bacterium identified as belonging to the genus *Nocardia* is able to use benzonitrile as sole carbon, energy and nitrogen source (Harper, 1977). The enzyme catalyzing this hydrolysis of benzonitrile was purified and characterized by this author.

The breakdown of HCN to formamide, which occurs in fungi, is catalyzed by the enzyme formamide hydro-lyase [EC 4.2.1.66],(Fry and Millar, 1972). Formamide hydrolyzing enzymes are not uncommon (Clark and Ornston, 1975), and would produce formate and ammonia. Formamide hydrolyase has been demonstrated in the fungi *Stemphylium loti* (Fry and Millar, 1972) and *Gloeocercospora sorghi* (Fry and Munch, 1975). The ability of the unidentified psycrophilic basidiomycete termed snow mold to convert HCN to CO_2 may indicate the presence of this enzyme (Bunch and Knowles, 1980). Formamide hydro-lyase appears to be involved in cyanide detoxification in these fungi. Therefore, it or a similar enzyme, could play a nutritional role in other organisms, including bacteria (see also Fry and Myers, this volume).

A number of bacteria seem to use HCN for nutrition (Knowles, 1976). In the earliest reports a cyanide utilizing bacterium, apparently an actinomycete (Pettet and Ware, 1955; Ware and Painter, 1955), was described. Skowronski and Strobel (1969) isolated an HCN utilizing strain of *Bacillus pumilus* from soil which had supported growth of cyanogenic flax plants for 73 consecutive years. This organism, in addition to being extremely cyanide resistant, was able to reduce the HCN content of a culture medium, initially 0.1 M, indicating metabolism of this compound. The feeding of $K^{14}C^{15}N$ to this organism resulted in the production of $^{14}CO_2$ and $^{15}NH_3$. Further, a cyanide utilizing bacterium has been isolated from soil polluted with electroplating waste water (Furuki *et al*, 1972).

III. ECOLOGICAL ASPECTS OF BACTERIAL CYANIDE METABOLISM

A. HCN IN NATURAL ENVIRONMENTS

While many aspects of bacterial HCN metabolism are understood some are not. One of these is the role in nature for the assimilation and production of HCN by bacteria and other microbes. The ability of the natural microflora of soil samples to utilize HCN has been clearly demonstrated by Strobel (1967) who showed that $K^{14}CN$ was converted to $^{14}CO_2$ by a variety of soil types. The feeding of doubly labelled cyanide, $K^{14}C^{15}N$, showed a greater retention of the cyanide nitrogen by the soil, possibly indicating its use as a microbial nitrogen source.

On the other hand cyanide production in natural environments has been demonstrated by Krutz (1979; this volume). The cyanide content in rural German watersheds were shown to be significant (0.7-2.1 μg/liter), and, most importantly, were not associated with industrial pollution.

In addition, a seasonal change in HCN levels was observed. High HCN concentrations in the fall and the winter were interpreted as arising from seasonal decomposition of plant material by microbes.

As pointed out by Krutz (1979) another source of the HCN found in soil and water could be the cyanogenic plants. Rangaswami and Balasubramanian (1963a, b) analyzed the HCN contents of sorghum roots and found them to be high. However, a definite relationship between the microbes of the rhizosphere and the cyanide content of the roots was not established. Even so, the sorghum rhizosphere microbes increased 5-fold when given a 24 hour treatment with a volatile extract of sorghum which contained HCN.

Allen and Strobel (1966) have used such information to propose a "Cyanide Microcycle" in which cyanogenic members of a soil ecosystem including bacteria produce HCN which could then be assimilated by cyanide metabolizing members, again including bacteria. The magnitude of HCN fixation and release would depend on the flora as well as the abiotic components present. Thatcher and Weaver (1976) proposed the presence of a specific ecological relationship involving elements of the "Cyanide Microcycle". These investigators isolated a methylotrophic bacterium designated BL-4, from a lesion on the leaf of a species of *Sorghum* plant. This plant was infected with the pathogen *Gloeocercospora sorghi*, a fungus described before as being able to detoxify cyanide. In this situation the phytopathogenic fungus might cause the cyanogenic plant to release HCN as a breakdown product of its cyanogenic glycosides. In response, the fungus would be able to convert HCN to formamide using its formamide hydrolyase which would then serve as carbon, energy and nitrogen source for the methylotroph. CO_2 and NH_3, produced during this process, could serve as carbon and nitrogen sources for other organisms, including plants.

The above discussion assumes specific roles for HCN metabolism in a specific ecosystem; i.e. the *Sorghum* plant produces HCN as a defense mechanism and the fungus hydrolyzes HCN to detoxify it. While various aspects of bacterial cyanide metabolism in nature have been examined in this chapter, specific roles remain elusive.

B. HCN AS AN INDUSTRIAL POLLUTANT

The use of cyanide utilizing organisms in the control of industrial cyanide wastes have long been considered possible (see discussion in Knowles, 1976). By enrichment, Ilyalemdinov *et al* (1977), produced a mixed population of HCN utilizing microbes and established conditions in which treatment ponds seeded with these organisms might be used. Raef *et al* (1977a, b) indicated that in an HCN treatment system four mechanisms are important in cyanide removal: (a) chemical reactions, i.e. hydrolysis, polymerization, cyanohydrin formation; (b) adsorption to solids; (c) stripping; (d) metabolism. These authors showed that sewage cultures grown with aeration were capable of converting $K^{14}CN$ to $^{14}CO_2$ to a significant extent, and they concluded that under the conditions described, stripping and metabolism accounted for most of the HCN removal. Further, pretreating cyanide and glucose with high levels of base resulted in cyanohydrin production which, in turn, was a good substrate for these sewage microbes. This indicates the possibility of mixing cyanides and aldose wastes prior to a base treatment and biodegradation.

While the above mentioned organisms show promise in controlling HCN wastes, the enzymes of cyanide assimilation and detoxification present methods for detecting this compound. β-Cyanoalanine synthase can be immobilized by attachment to glass, agarose, or polyacrylamide and used to detect cyanide by liberation of H_2S upon incubation in the presence of cysteine (Gutknecht and Guilbault, 1971; Svenson and Andersson, 1977). This product may be measured colorimetrically (Svenson and Andersson, 1977) or potentiometrically (Gutknecht and Guilbault, 1971). Cyanide also can be accurately measured using both β-cyanoalanine synthase and rhodanese immobilized on glass beads (Mattiasson *et al*, 1977). Here thermistors measure the heat change produced by these reactions. These techniques offer the possibility of continuous, on-line monitoring of effluents of industries producing HCN as a by product.

IV. PROSPECTS

It can be seen that there are many facets to bacterial HCN metabolism. These range from topics, such as industrial cyanide waste treatment, which have direct application, to topics of a more basic nature. While some of these are currently under study others are presently in a relative state of neglect, i.e. bacterial HCN degradation. A topic of particular promise would be the study of the ecological significance of HCN metabolism. In soil, for example, which organisms are responsible for HCN release? What is the magnitude of the HCN produced? What is the influence of the cyanide produced on the flora and fauna present? What is the role of cyanide assimilation and the detoxification pathways?

Other aspects of bacterial HCN metabolism are fascinating in nature but difficult to study. Cyanide a component of interstellar gases, is implicated as both precursor and intermediate in prebiotic evolution (Fox and Dose, 1977). The first living cells probably grew heterotrophically, indicating at least the possibility of HCN metabolism under these primitive conditions. Could any such ability have been retained as these primitive cells and their environments evolved? Can remnants of this trait be seen today as HCN assimilation and detoxification? Can such remnants be seen as nitrogenase, an enzyme which can, as a secondary function, reduce cyanide to methane and ammonia? Could the ability to oxidize glycine to cyanide and CO_2 have evolved into the ability to reduce N_2 to the level of ammonia? Or, as suggested by Meganathan (1979) could cyanogenic bacteria avoid assimilation of the plasmid-borne nitrogenase trait since this new enzyme would result in an energetically wasteful futile cycle? Bacterial cyanogenesis impinges on many areas of biological and biochemical research, ranging from the basic to the applied, and thereby offers significant potential for future research.

ACKNOWLEDGEMENTS

I would like to thank K.F. Castric, R. Meganathan, D. McDevitt, and J. Kuchta for helpful discussions. My own research in this area was supported by grants BMS 74-16398 and PCM 77-24144 from the National Science Foundation.

REFERENCES

Akopyan, T.N., Braunstein, A.E. and Goryachenkova, E.V. (1975). *Proc. Natl. Acad. Sci. U.S.A.* 72, 1617-1621.
Allen, J. and Strobel, G.A. (1966). *Can. J. Microbiol.* 12, 414-416.
Arnaud, A., Galzy, P. and Jallageas, J.C. (1977). *Agric. Biol. Chem.* 41. 2183-2191.
Blumenthal, S.G., Hendrickson, H.R., Abrol, Y.P. and Conn, E.E. (1968) *J. Biol. Chem.* 243, 5302-5307.
Blumenthal-Goldschmidt, S., Butler, G.W. and Conn, E.E. (1963). *Nature* 197, 718-719.
Bonomi, F., Pagani, S., Cerletti, P. and Canella, C. (1977). *Eur. J. Biochem.* 72, 17-24.
Bowen, T.J., Butler, P.J. and Happold, F.C. (1965). *Biochem. J.* 97, 651-657.
Brysk, M.M., Lauinger, C. and Ressler, C. (1969a). *Biochem. Biophys. Acta.* 184, 583-588.
Brysk, M.M., Corpe, W.A. and Hankes, L.V. (1969b). *J. Bacteriol.* 97, 322-327.
Brysk, M.M. and Ressler, C. (1970). *J. Biol. Chem.* 245, 1156-1160.
Bunch, A.W. and Knowles, C.J. (1980). *J. Gen. Microbiol.* 116, 9-16.
Bugel, P. and Muller, D. (1963). *Protoplasma.* 57, 158-159.
Campbell, L.L. (1956). *J. Bacteriol.* 71, 81-83.
Castric, P.A. (1975). *Can. J. Microbiol.* 21, 613-618.
Castric, P.A. (1977). *J. Bacteriol.* 130, 826-831.
Castric, P.A. and Conn, E.E. (1971). *J. Bacteriol.* 108, 132-136.

Castric, P.A., Ebert, R.F. and Castric, K.F. (1979). *Current Microbiol.* 2, 287-292.
Castric, P.A., Farnden, K.J.F. and Conn, E.E. (1972). *Arch. Biochem. Biophys.* 152, 62-69.
Castric, P.A. and Strobel, G.A. (1969). *J. Biol. Chem.* 244, 4089-4094.
Chapman, A.G. and Atkinson, D.E. (1977). *In* "Advances in Microbial Physiology" (A.H. Rose and D.W. Tempest, eds) Vol. 15, pp. 254-306. Academic Press, London.
Clarke, P.H. and Ornston, L.N. (1975). *In* "Genetics and Biochemistry of Pseudomonas" (P.H. Clarke and M.H. Richmond, eds) pp. 263-340. John Wiley and Sons, London.
Clawson, B.J. and Young, C.C. (1913). *J. Biol. Chem.* 15, 419-422.
Colby, J., Dalton, H. and Whittenbury, R. (1979). *Ann. Rev. Microbiol.* 33, 481-517.
Collins, P.A., Rodgers, P.B. and Knowles, C.J. (1980). *J. Gen. Microbiol.* 117, 73-80.
Conn, E.E. (1973). *In* "Nitrogen Metabolism In Plants" (T.N. Goodwin and R.M.S. Smellie, eds) Vol. 38, Biochemical Society Symposium, pp. 277-302. The Biochemical Society, London.
Conn, E.E. (1979). *Naturwissenschaften* 66, 28-34.
Demain, A.L. (1974). *Ann. New York Acad. Sci.* 235, 601-612.
Demain, A.L., Kennel, Y.M. and Aharonowitz, Y. (1979). *In* "Microbial Technology: Current State, Future Prospects" (A.T. Bull, D.C. Ellwood and C. Ratledge, eds) Twenty-Ninth Symposium of the Society for General Microbiology, pp. 163-185. Cambridge University Press, Cambridge.
DiGeronimo, M.J. and Antoine, A.D. (1976). *Appl. Microbiol.* 31, 900-906.
Doudoroff, M. and Palleroni, N.J. (1974). *In* "Bergey's Manual of Determinative Bacteriology" (R.E. Buchanan and N.E. Gibbons, eds) 8th Edition, pp. 217-243. The Williams and Wilkins Company, Baltimore.
Drew, S.W. and Demain, A.L. (1977). *Ann. Rev. Microbiol.* 31, 343-356.
Dunnill, P.M. and Fowden, L. (1965). *Nature* 208, 1206-1207.
Elrod, R.P. and Braun, A.C. (1941). *Science* 94, 520-521.
Emerson, H.W., Cady, H.P. and Bailey, E.H.S. (1913). *J. Biol. Chem.* 15, 415-417.
Firmin, J.L. and Gray, D.O. (1976). *Biochem. J.* 158, 223-229.
Fowden, L. and Bell, E.A. (1965). *Nature* 206, 110-112.
Fox, S.W. and Dose, K. (1977). "Molecular Evolution and the Origin of Life," M. Dekker Inc., New York and Basel.
Freeman, L.R., Angelini, P., Silverman, G.F. and Merritt, C. (1975). *Appl. Microbiol.* 29, 560-561.
Freeman, L.R., Silverman, G.J., Angelini, P., Merritt, C. and Esselen, W.B. (1976). *Appl. Microbiol.* 32, 222-231.
Fry, W.E. and Millar, R.L. (1972). *Arch. Biochem. Biophys.* 151, 468-474.
Fry, W.E. and Munch, D.C. (1975). *Physiol. Plant. Pathol.* 7, 23-33.
Furuki, M., Yamamoto, T., Shimura, T. and Tachibana, S. (1972). *J. Ferment. Technol.* 50, 298-304.
Gentry, M.J., Smith, D.K., Schnute, S.F., Werber, S.L. and Weinberg, E.D. (1971). *Microbios.* 4, 205-215.
Gutknecht, W.F. and Guilbault, G.G. (1971). *Environ. Lett.* 2, 51-57.

Halfner, E.W. and Wellner, D. (1971). *Proc. Natl. Acad. Sci. USA* 68, 987-991.
Hall, M.R. and Berk, R.S. (1968). *Can. J. Microbiol.* 14, 515-523.
Harper, D.B. (1977). *Biochem. J.* 167, 685-692.
Hassan, H.M. and Fridovich, I. (1980). *J. Bacteriol.* 141, 156-163.
Hendrickson, H.R. and Conn, E.E. (1969). *J. Biol. Chem.* 244, 2632-2640.
Hook, R.H. and Robinson, W.G. (1964). *J. Biol. Chem.* 239, 4263-4267.
Hubbard, J.S. and Stadtman, E.R. (1967). *J. Bacteriol.* 93, 1045-1055.
Ilyalemdinov, A.N., Enker, P.B. and Vlasova, Z.G. (1977). *Mikrobiologiya* 46, 358-362.
Jones, C.W. (1979). *In* "Microbial Biochemistry" (J.R. Quayle, ed.) Vol. 21 of International Review of Biochemistry, pp. 49-84. University Park Press, Baltimore.
Knowles, C.J. (1976). *Bacteriol. Rev.* 40, 652-680.
Kralik, C.A. and Castric, P.A. (1979). *Current Microbiol.* 3, 71-74.
Kredich, N.M. and Tomkins, G.M. (1966). *J. Biol. Chem.* 241, 4953-4965.
Krutz, H. (1979). Veroffentlichurgen des Instituts fur Wasserforschung Gmbh Dortmund und der Hydrologischen Abteilung der Dortmunder Stadtwerke AG. Nr 28.
Lauinger, C. and Ressler, C. (1970). *Biochim. Biophys. Acta.* 198, 316-323.
Leisinger, T. and Margraff, R. (1979). *Microbiol. Rev.* 43, 422-442.
Lorck, H. (1948). *Physiol. Plant.* 1, 142-146.
Lowbury, E.J.L. (1975). *In* "Genetics and Biochemistry of Pseudomonas" (P.H. Clarke and M.H. Richmond, eds) pp. 37-65. John Wiley and Sons, London.
Mattiasson, B., Mosbach, K. and Svenson, A. (1977). *Biotechnol. Bioeng.* 19, 1643-1651.
Meganathan, R. (1979). *J. Theor. Biol.* 80, 301-304.
Meganathan, R. and Castric, P.A. (1977). *Arch. Microbiol.* 114, 51-54.
Michaels, R. and Corpe, W.A. (1965). *J. Bacteriol.* 89, 106-112.
Michaels, R., Hankes, L.V. and Corpe, W.A. (1965). *Arch. Biochem. Biophys.* 111, 121-125.
Mimura, A., Kawano, T. and Yamaga, K. (1969). *J. Ferment. Technol.* 47, 631-638.
Nazar, R.N. and Wong, J.T.-F. (1973). *Biochim. Biophys. Acta.* 324, 218-225.
Newman, E.B., Kapoor, V. and Potter, R. (1976). *J. Bacteriol.* 126, 1245-1249.
Ng, F.M.-W. and Dawes, E.A. (1973). *Biochem. J.* 132, 129-140.
Niven, D.F., Collins, P.A. and Knowles, C.J. (1975). *J. Gen. Microbiol.* 90, 271-285.
Patty, A.F. (1921). *J. Infect. Dis.* 29, 73-77.
Pettet, A.E.J. and Ware, G.C. (1955). *Chem. Ind.* 1955, 1232-1238.
Potter, R., Kapoor, V. and Newman, E.R. (1977). *J. Bacteriol.* 132, 385-391.
Quayle, J.R. (1972). *In* "Advances in Microbial Physiology" (A.H. Rose and D.W. Tempest, eds) Vol. 7, pp. 119-203. Academic Press, London.
Raef, S.F., Characklis, W.G., Kessick, M.A. and Ward, C.H. (1977a). *Water Res.* 11, 477-483.

Raef, S.F., Characklis, W.G., Kessick, M.A. and Ward, C.H. (1977b). *Water Res.* 11, 485-492.
Rangaswami, G. and Balasubramanian, A. (1963a). *Can. J. Microbiol.* 9, 719-725.
Rangaswami, G. and Balasubramanian, A. (1963b). *Indian J. Exptl. Biol.* 1, 215-217.
Ressler, C., Abe, O., Kondo, Y., Cottrell, B. and Abe, K. (1973). *Biochemistry* 12, 5369-5377.
Robinson, W.G. and Hook, R.H. (1964). *J. Biol. Chem.* 239, 4257-4262.
Rodgers, P.B. and Knowles, C.J. (1978). *J. Gen. Microbiol.* 108, 261-267.
Sands, D.C., Schroth, M.N. and Hildebrand, D.C. (1970). *J. Bacteriol.* 101, 9-23.
Schliefer, K.H., Hammes, W.P. and Kandler, O. (1976). *In* "Advances in Microbial Physiology" (A.H. Rose and D.W. Tempest, eds) Vol. 13, pp. 245-292. Academic Press, London.
Schook, L.B. and Berk, R.S. (1978). *J. Bacteriol.* 133, 1377-1382.
Siegel, L.S., Hylemon, P.B. and Phibbs, P.V. (1977). *J. Bacteriol.* 129, 87-96.
Skowronski, B. and Strobel, G.A. (1969). *Can. J. Microbiol.* 15, 93-98.
Smith, E.L., Austen, B.M., Blumenthal, K.M. and Nyc, J.F. (1975). *In* "The Enzymes" (P. Boyer, ed.) Vol. XI, pp. 293-367. Academic Press, New York.
Sneath, P.H.A. (1956). *J. Gen. Microbiol.* 15, 70-98.
Sneath, P.H.A. (1960). *Iowa State J. Sci.* 34, 243-410.
Sneath, P.H.A., Whelan, J.P.F., Singh, R.B. and Edwards, D. (1953). *Lancet* 265, 276-277.
Sneath, P.H.A. (1966). *In* "Identification Methods for Microbiologists" (B.M. Gibbs and F.A. Skinner, eds), pp. 15-20. Academic Press, London.
Solomonson, L.P. (1978). *In* "Microbiology-1978" (D. Schlessinger, ed.) pp. 315-319. American Society for Microbiology, Washington.
Solomonson, L.P. and Spehar, A.M. (1979). *J. Biol Chem.* 254, 2176-2179.
Sörbo, B. (1975). *In* "Metabolism of Sulfur Compounds" (D.M. Greenberg, ed.) Vol. VII, 3rd edition of Metabolic Pathways, pp. 433-456. Academic Press, New York.
Stauffer, G.V. and Brenchley, J.E. (1977). *J. Bacteriol.* 129, 740-749.
Strobel, G.A. (1967). *Soil Science.* 103, 299-302.
Strobel, G.A. (1977). *Ann. Rev. Microbiol.* 31, 205-224.
Suzuki, I. (1974). *Ann. Rev. Microbiol.* 28, 85-101.
Svenson, A. and Andersson, B. (1977). *Anal. Biochem.* 83, 739-745.
Taniguchi, T. and Kimura, T. (1974). *Biochim. Biophys. Acta.* 364, 284-295.
Taylor, R.T. and Weissbach, H. (1973). *In* "The Enzymes" (P.D. Boyer, ed.) Vol. IX, pp. 121-165. Academic Press, New York.
Tempest, D.W. and Neijssel, O.M. (1978). *In* "Advances in Microbiol Ecology" (M. Alexander, ed.) Vol. 2, pp. 105-153. Plenum Press, New York.
Thatcher, R.C. and Weaver, T.L. (1976). *Science* 192, 1234-1235.
Tsai, J.C., Aladegbami, S.L. and Vela, G.R. (1979). *J. Bacteriol.* 139, 639-645.

Vachek, H. and Wood, J.L. (1972). *Biochim. Biophys. Acta.* 258, 133-146.
Vandenbergh, P.A., Bawdon, R.E. and Berk, R.S. (1979). *Intl. J. Syst. Bacteriol.* 29, 339-344.
Vogels, G.D. and Van der Drift, C. (1976). *Bact. Rev.* 40, 403-468.
Ward, E.W.B., Starratt, A.N. and Robinson, J.R. (1977). *Can. J. Bot.* 55, 2065-2069.
Ware, G.C. and Painter, H.A. (1955). *Nature* 175, 900.
Weinberg, E.D. (1970). *In* "Advances in Microbiol Physiology" (A.H. Rose and J.F. Wilkinson, eds) Vol. 4, pp. 1-44. Academic Press, London and New York.
Weinberg, E.D. (1971). *Perspect. Biol. Med.* 14, 565-577.
Weinberg, E.D. (1977). *In* "Microorganisms and Minerals" (E.D. Weinberg, ed.) pp. 289-315. M. Dekker, Inc, New York and Basel.
Weinberg, E.D. (1978). *Folia Microbiol.* 23, 496-504.
Weinberg, E.D. and Goodnight, S.A. (1970). *Antonie van Leeuwenhoek J. Microbiol. Serol.* 36, 73-80.
Westley, J. (1973). *In* "Advances in Enzymology" (A. Meister ed.) Vol. 39, pp. 327-368. John Wiley and Sons, New York.
Wissing, F. (1968). *Physiol. Plant.* 21, 589-593.
Wissing, F. (1974). *J. Bacteriol.* 117, 1289-1294.
Wissing, F. (1975). *J. Bacteriol.* 121, 695-699.
Yoch, D.C. and Lindstrom, E.S. (1971). *J. Bacteriol.* 106, 700-701.

FACTORS INFLUENCING THE TERMINATION OF CYANOGENESIS IN *PSEUDOMONAS AERUGINOSA*

PETER A. CASTRIC*, KATHLEEN F. CASTRIC and R. MEGANATHAN**

Department of Biological Sciences,
Duquesne University,
Pittsburgh, Pennsylvania, 15219, U.S.A.

I. SUMMARY

Pseudomonas aeruginosa produces hydrogen cyanide from glycine by an enzyme system which is herein referred to as HCN synthase. In batch cultures this production halted when stationary phase was reached. The loss of the capacity of the culture to produce HCN, which was accompanied by a decline in HCN synthase activity, was not prevented by inhibitors ofprotein synthesis. This loss of cyanogenic capacity was prevented by imposing anaerobic conditions on the culture. The HCN synthase activity of cell extracts was quickly lost under aerobic conditions in the absence of glycine. Significant protection of this enzyme system was afforded by anaerobic conditions or by the inclusion of either glycine or dithiothreitol under aerobic conditions. Desalting by gel filtration did not protect the enzyme system. Extracts from post-cyanogenic cells did not inhibit cyanide production by extracts of cyanogenic cells.

II. INTRODUCTION

The production of hydrogen cyanide has been noted in a variety of microbes, but only in a few bacterial species found in the genera *Chromobacterium* and *Pseudomonas* (Knowles, 1976). Microbial secondary metabolism may be defined by a number of characteristics which apply to bacterial cyanide production (Wissing, 1968; Castric, 1975; Meganathan and Castric, 1977; Rodgers and Knowles, 1978; Collins *et al.*, 1980). One characteristic is that the pro-

*To whom offprint requests should be sent.

**Present address: Department of Biological Sciences, University of Pittsburgh, Pittsburgh, Pennsylvania 15260, U.S.A.

duct is apparently not required for cell growth (Demain *et al.*, 1979). Another involves the selective effects of certain environmental factors on secondary metabolite production (Weinberg, 1978). Yet another characteristic is the temporal relationship between metabolite formation and the culture cycle (Weinberg, 1971). HCN production by *Pseudomonas aeruginosa* occurs after an inception period during late log phase which involves the synthesis of the cyanogenic enzyme system (Castric *et al.*, 1979). A period of active cyanide production follows inception which is, in turn, followed by an abrupt termination which corresponds to the entry of the culture into stationary phase. This sequential process is brought into play and later terminated during the culture cycle by cellular metabolic and environmental stimuli. These stimuli and their mode of action in the regulation of cyanogenesis, and so secondary metabolism, are poorly understood. The present work examines the factors involved in the termination of cyanogenesis in *P. aeruginosa*. The results indicate that 1) termination is probably caused by the inactivation of the cyanogenic enzyme system; 2) this inactivation is probably due to oxygen toxicity; 3) this enzyme system is probably protected during cyanogenesis by cell respiration and by the presence of the metabolic precursor of cyanide, glycine.

III. MATERIALS AND METHODS

A. ORGANISM AND GROWTH MEDIUM

The isolation and storage of *Pseudomonas aeruginosa* 9-D2 have been described previously (Meganathan and Castric, 1977). The complete synthetic medium consisted of L-glutamate (20 mM), glycine (12.5 mM), D, L-methionine (5mM), K_2HPO_4 (5 mM), NaH_2PO_4 (5 mM), $MgSO_4 \cdot 7H_2O$ (2mM), ferric citrate (0.02 mM), and tris (hydroxylmethyl) aminomethane (50 mM). This medium minus glutamate, glycine, and methionine is referred to as the salts solution. The medium was adjusted to a pH of 7.5 at room temperature with concentrated HCl and sterilized by autoclaving.

B. CELL GROWTH

Unless indicated otherwise the synthetic medium was inoculated with an early stationary phase culture giving an initial concentration of 3×10^8 cells per ml. Incubations were performed in rubber-stoppered Fernback flasks containing 1 liter of medium which was rotated at 250 rpm at a temperature of 35°C. Sterile air was passed via a glass delivery tube in the stopper over the surface of the culture at a rate of 3 liters per minute. A second tube vented the air from the flask. A third tube allowed culture sampling.

C. CULTURAL CYANOGENIC CAPACITY

The ability of whole cells to produce hydrogen cyanide is termed the cultural cyanogenic capcity (Castric *et al.*, 1979). To measure this capcity, aliquots of culture were removed, centrifuged at 10,000 × g for 10 minutes at 4°C, and resuspended in a volume of the salts solution giving approximately 2 × 10^{10} cells per ml. Portions of this cell suspension were incubated in the culture apparatus described previously (Castric *et al.*, 1979) containing salts solution, glycine (12.5 mM), and L-glutamic acid (20 mM) in a final volume of 2.0 ml. Culture aeration and HCN collection were carried out by passing air at a rate of 300 ml/min over the concave surface of the stirring culture and to a base trap via an exit delivery tube. After a warm-up period of 3 minutes, cyanide was collected for a period of 15 minutes and was quantitated using the colorimetric method of Asmus and Garschagen (1953). Cyanogenic capacity is expressed as nmoles HCN per 15 minutes incubation per 1 × 10^9 cells.

D. HCN PRODUCTION BY CELL EXTRACTS

Portions of the culture were centrifuged at 10,000 × g for 10 minutes at 4°C. These cells were resuspended in 0.1 M Tris HCl, pH 8.3, and disrupted at 4°C, using four 1 minute bursts, with an Artek Sonic Dismembrator. The suspension produced was clarified by centrifugation at 20,000 × g for 20 minutes at 4°C. The methods involved in the assay of the HCN synthase are similar to those employed by Wissing, 1975; this volume). The apparatus used to assay HCN production by these extracts was that referred to in the previous section. Again the incubation temperature was 35°C but the gas flow rate, either air or nitrogen, was 500 ml per minute. The reaction mixture contained 200 μmol Tris-HCl, 30 μmol glycine, 2.0 μmol phenazine methosulphate, and enzyme preparation, approximately 5 mg of protein in a volume of 2.0 ml and at a pH of 8.3. The reaction was initiated with the addition of phenzine methosulphate after which cyanide was collected for 8 minutes with base trap changes at 2 minute intervals. Cyanide was quantitated as described above.

E. AMINO ACID POOLS.

Culture samples containing 5-25 × 10^{10} cells were centrifuged at room temperature for 5 minutes at 5,000 × g. The supernatant fluid was decanted, and the pellets formed were drained well and resuspended in 50% ethanol. This suspension was stored 12-18 hours at 4°C and centrifuged for 15 minutes at 20,000 × g. The supernatant fluid was decanted, brought to dryness at 50°C in a stream of air, and resuspended in a minimal volume. Amino acid content was measured by applying portions of these samples to a Durrum D-500 amino acid analyzer.

F. CULTURAL OXYGEN LEVELS.

Cultures were grown in 1 liter amounts in the apparatus and under the conditions indicated in a previous section. A Clark type oxygen electrode was periodically inserted through an opening in the side of the flask allowing measurements of oxygen level.

IV. RESULTS

A. CYANOGENIC ACTIVITY OF CELL EXTRACTS

Extracts of *P. aeruginosa* 9-D2, assayed aerobically, were capable of significant production of HCN (Fig. 1). Incuba-

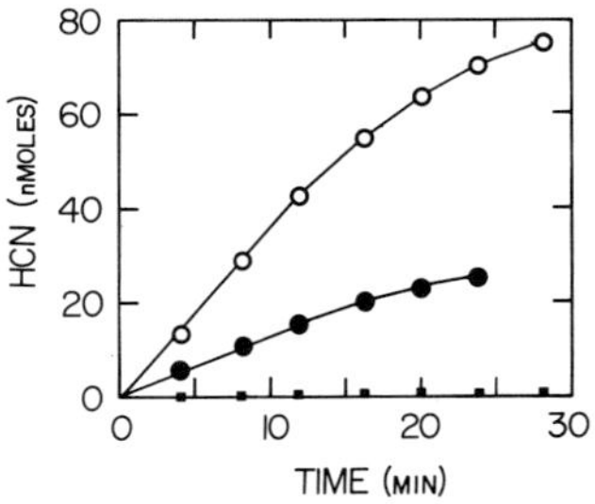

Fig. 1 HCN synthase activity by extracts of *Pseudomonas aeruginosa.* ■ anaerobic conditions; ● aerobic conditions; ○ anaerobic conditions in the presence of 1 mM phenazine methosulphate

tion of these extracts under anaerobic conditions resulted in barely detectable amounts of cyanide. This implicates oxygen as an electron acceptor in the oxidation of glycine to cyanide and carbon dioxide by this organism, as has been previously indicated with whole cells of an unidentified cyanogenic pseudomonad (Wissing, 1974). The inclusion of phenazine methosulphate in the reaction mixture under anaerobic conditions allowed the production of cyanide but here at about three times the rate as that seen under aerobic conditions. The linearity of HCN production by the extract continued for 8 to 12 minutes after which time there was a visible decline in rate. Dichlorophenolindolphenol and potassium ferricyanide in comparable concentrations also supported cyanogenesis under anaerobic conditions by extracts of this organism, but the amounts of HCN produced were significantly lower (results not shown).

The production of HCN by these extracts was dependent on glycine concentration as is indicated by Fig. 2. Here an apparent K_m of 1.7 mM for glycine was observed using the conditions of assay described in Section III. As indicated previously, this activity is proportional to extract concentration and has an optimal pH of 8.3 in 0.1 M Tris HCl buffer (Castric *et al.*, 1979). The agent catalyzing the activity described here is provisionally referred to as HCN synthase.

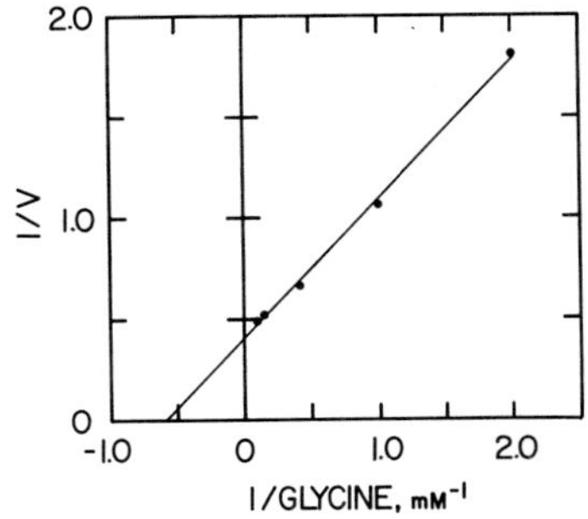

Fig. 2 Determination of the apparent Km for glycine. Velocity is nmoles HCN per min. A crude extract containing 5.0 mg protein per ml was employed. Assay conditions are those described in Section III.

B. LOSS OF CULTURAL CYANOGENIC CAPACITY

The entry of *Pseudomonas aeruginosa* 9-D2 batch cultures into stationary phase was accompanied by an abrupt decline in the capacity of these cells to form cyanide (Fig. 3).

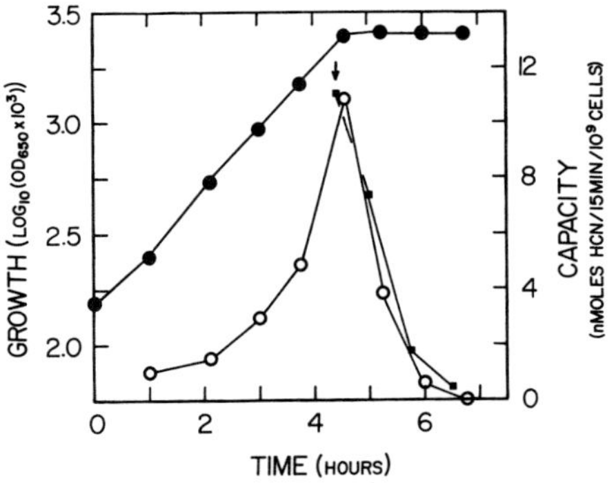

Fig. 3 The influences of chloramphenicol on the decline in cyanogenic capacity of *Pseudomonas aeruginosa*. Chloramphenicol was added, at the time indicated by the arrow, to a final concentration of 0.5 mM. ■ cyanogenic capacity in the presence of chloramphenicol; ○ cyanogenic capacity in the absence of chloramphenicol; ● cell growth.

This loss is paralleled by a decline in enzymatic conversion of glycine to cyanide (Castric *et al.*, 1979) which indicates that some type of metabolic regulation is at work. To establish whether this regulation involved synthesis of an inactivating protein, synthesis of low molecular weight effectors, or an inherent instability of this catalytic system the following experiments were performed.

If the termination of cyanogenesis involves the synthesis of a protein inhibitor, it would be anticipated that this synthesis would take place during the latter part of the period of cyanide production. The addition of chloramphenicol, in amounts sufficient to stop cell growth, did not eliminate the loss of cyanogenic activity as shown in Fig. 3. Further, neither the addition of this inhibitor at various times during this transition period nor the substitution of rifampicin, again in amounts sufficient to inhibit cell growth, prevented the decline in cyanogenic capacity (results not shown). These results indicate synthesis of a protein, such as a modifying enzyme or a protease, is not involved in inhibition.

C. LACK OF INACTIVATING FACTOR IN CELL EXTRACTS

In order to determine whether an inactivating agent is at work in the regulation of HCN biosynthesis, extracts were made of post-cyanogenic cells as well as of cells having the maximum capacity to produce cyanide. As shown in Table I, the ability of these extracts to produce HCN differed greatly but correspond to the cyanogenic capacity of the cells from which the extracts were made. In the presence

Table I The effect of extracts from post-cyanogenic cells on cyanide production by extracts of cyanogenic cells

Extract treatment[(a)]	Activity (nmoles HCN/min)
No treatment	
Extract 1	6.87
Extract 2	0.07
1 hour at 35°C	
Extract 1	6.53
Extract 2	0.07
Extract 1 plus Extract 2	6.20

(a) All steps were performed in the presence of 0.25 M glycine. Extracts were used in 1 ml volumes each. Extract 1 was taken from a culture after 4½ hours of incubation when the $\log_{10}$ $(OD_{650} \times 10^3)$ was 3.25, and when the cyanogenic capacity was 12.2 nmoles HCN/15 min/10^9 cells. Extract 2 was taken from the same culture, but after 6½ hours of incubation when the $\log_{10}$ $(OD_{650} \times 10^3)$ was 3.39, and when the cyanogenic capacity had fallen to 0.4 nmoles HCN/15 min/10^9 cells.

of excess glycine, a point to be discussed subsequently, activity was not lost by incubation of the cyanogenic extracts for 1 h at 35°C. Most significantly, incubation of these cyanogenic extracts with the inactive post-cyanogenic extracts resulted in no loss of the ability of the former to produce HCN.

D. STABILITY OF HCN SYNTHASE ACTIVITY

The HCN synthase, rather than being inactivated after HCN production is complete, may be inherently unstable and only stabilized when its presence is required. This was indicated when actively cyanogenic homogenates were subjected to gel filtration on Sephadex G-25 in the presence and absence of glycine. While gel filtration with glycine included in the elution buffer resulted in no loss of activity, the omission of this amino acid from the buffer resulted in an 80-90% loss of activity (results not shown).

Further, extracts incubated aerobically for 20 minutes at 35°C in the absence of added glycine showed a significant drop in activity (Table II), while extracts incubat-

Table II Influence of incubation conditions on the stability of the HCN synthase of *Pseudomonas aeruginosa*

Treatment[a]	Activity (nmoles/min)
Experiment 1	
Control	7.73
Anaerobic incubation	8.54
Aerobic incubation	1.13
Aerobic incubation in the presence of 15 mM glycine	5.33
Experiment 2	
Control	6.05
Aerobic incubation	0.65
Aerobic incubation in the presence of 1 mM dithiothreitol	3.70

(a) Control samples were assayed at zero time using the procedure indicated in Section III. All other samples were incubated for 20 minutes at 35°C in 9 cm × 2 cm glass tubes. Anaerobic conditions were achieved with a stream of nitrogen gas flowing over the sample at 100 ml per minute. Aerobic conditions involved incubating the samples in unstoppered tubes. The aerobic and anaerobic samples were then assayed using the procedure referred to above.

ed in the same way except under anaerobic conditions showed no loss in activity. Some protection under aerobic conditions was afforded by including the substrate, glycine, in the incubation mixture in a concentration of 15 mM. Incubation of the extracts aerobically in the presence of 1 mM dithiothreitol, but in the absence of glycine, also resulted in a partial protection of the enzyme system. Increasing the levels of dithiothreitol decreased the rate of cyanogenesis possibly by interference with the transfer of electrons to phenazine methosulphate (results not shown).

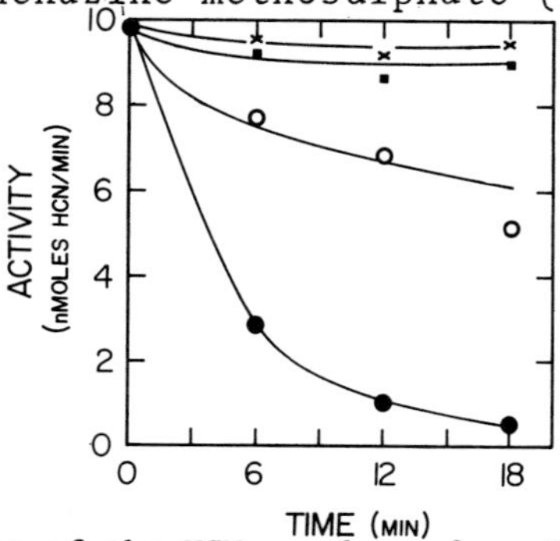

Fig. 4 Inactivation of the HCN synthase from *Pseudomonas aeruginosa*. Samples were incubated as described in Table I. At the times indicated aliquots were removed and were assayed anaerobically using the procedure described in Section III. ■ anaerobic conditions; ● aerobic conditions; O aerobic conditions in the presence of 7.5 mM glycine; x aerobic conditions in the presence of 100 mM glycine.

The rate of inactivation of the HCN synthase in the absence of protective conditions was extremely rapid (Fig. 4). Here it can be seen that under aerobic conditions, activity was lost with a half-life of about 4 minutes. This inactivation was again avoided under anaerobic conditions and by the presence of glycine, this time at levels of 100 mM. Glycine at a concentration of 7.5 mM afforded significant protection of the HCN synthase. This is a concentration which might be anticipated to occur in the intracellular glycine pool of this organism during the period of cyanogenesis.

E. INFLUENCE OF GLYCINE AND OXYGEN ON CYANOGENIC CAPACITY

Since glycine, the metabolic precursor of HCN in *P. aeruginosa* (Castric, 1977), stabilized HCN synthase activity in cell extracts, the levels of intracellular glycine were examined next. Figure 5 shows amino acid pools taken at various points of the culture cycle. Here one can see that glycine levels climbed during the culture cycle and peaked at the same time the cyanogenic enzyme system was most active. Further, the glycine pool declined at the time in which the decline in cyanogenic activity was taking place. While

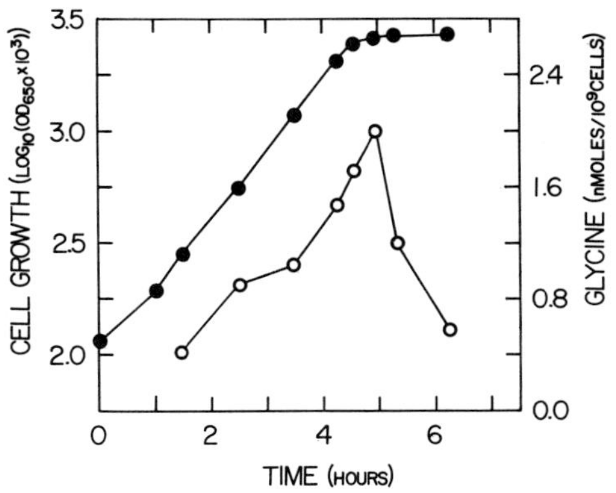

Fig. 5 Variation of intracellular glycine levels in response to growth of *Pseudomonas aeruginosa*. ○ glycine level; ● cell growth.

the internal volume available to glycine cannot be precisely determined, volumes which result in glycine concentrations of 5 to 10 mM at maximum are not unreasonable. These are values which significantly protected the cyanogenic enzyme system from inactivation (Fig. 4).

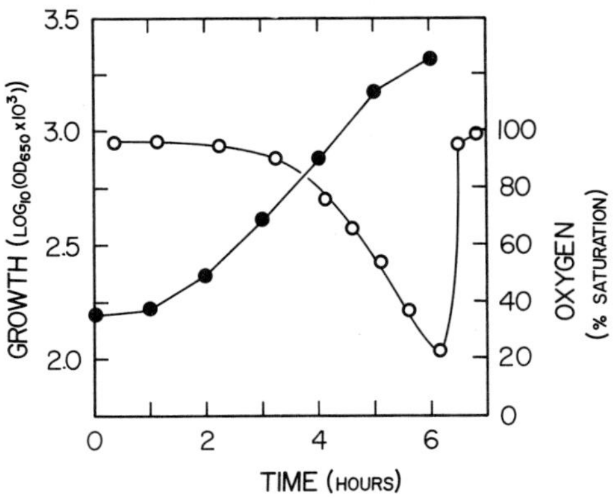

Fig. 6 Variation in cultural oxygen levels in response to growth of *Pseudomonas aeruginosa*. ○ oxygen level; ● cell growth.

If oxygen is detrimental to the cyanogenic apparatus it would be likely that this system would appear at lower oxygen tensions. Figure 6 shows the levels of dissolved oxygen as the culture cycle progresses. Under the conditions of cultivation oxygen concentration decreased continuously until the point at which the culture entered stationary phase. This point corresponds to the time in the culture cycle when the carbon and energy source is depleted and to the point of maximum cyanogenic capacity (Castric *et al.*, 1979). The period of time in which oxygen level of the culture climbs corresponded to the period of inactivation of the HCN synthase which implicates oxygen in the *in vivo* loss of cyanogenic capacity. The experiment presented in Fig. 7 supports this implication. Here the usual decline in culture capacity was avoided by replacing the cultural air flow with nitrogen.

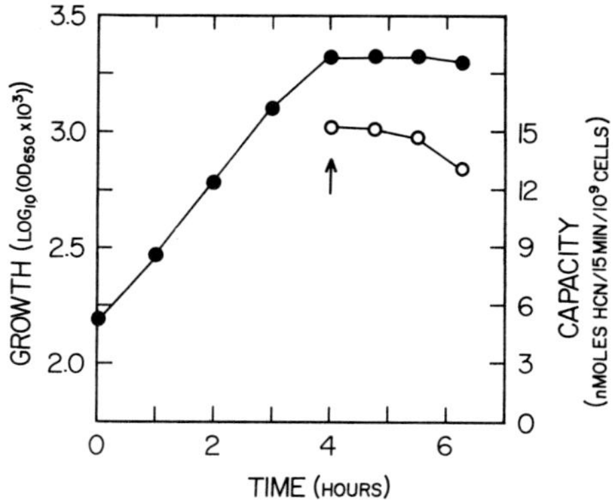

Fig. 7 The influence of imposing anaerobic conditions on the decline in cyanogenic capacity of *Pseudomonas aeruginosa*. Anaerobic conditions were established, at the time indicated by the arrow, by substituting nitrogen for air as the gas flowing through the culture vessel. ○ cyanogenic capacity; ● cell growth.

V. DISCUSSION

Cyanogenesis in *P. aeruginosa*, under the conditions described in this paper, sequentially involved synthesis of the cyanogenic enzyme system, followed by a short period of HCN production, which, in turn, was followed by a loss of the ability of these cells to produce HCN. This loss of cyanogenic ability appeared to be due to an inactivation of the cyanogenic enzyme system rather than to the production of cyanide utilizing enzymes because 1) protein synthesis inhibitors did not prevent the decline in cyanogenic activity 2) mixing of extracts from post cyanogenic cells with extracts from cyanogenic cells did not result in loss of activity. The latter point also indicates that low molecular weight effectors are not produced while the former point indicates that a protein inhibitor is not involved. The HCN synthase seemed to be inherently unstable and required anaerobic conditions or the presence of glycine for stability. Thus, inactivation *in vivo* may result when 1) intracellular glycine levels decline, and 2) oxygen levels increase as would occur when respiration declines due to carbon and energy source depletion. Such conditions occurred as the culture completed the transition between log and stationary phases.

The protective effect of dithiothreitol and glycine to aerobic conditions may indicate that a sulphydryl group at the active site is the labile component of the HCN synthase. The nature of this inactivation cannot be stated with certainty until more is known of this enzyme system. For example, does the HCN synthase transfer electrons from the oxidation of glycine to the terminal electron acceptor or is an intermediate, such as a component of an electron transport system, involved? Inactivation might then be due to the loss of such an obligatory electron carrier and not to damage of the catalytic entity involved in HCN synthesis. This last point does not seem likely since the cyanogenic activity of extracts of an unidentified *Pseudomonad* chromatograph as a discrete peak on gel filtration (Wissing, this volume).

Oxygen sensitivity of enzymes from aerobic bacteria has been previously demonstrated. Although the nitrogenase from aerobic bacteria (Dalton and Postgate, 1969) is the best known example others have been described including the glutamine phosphoribosylpyrophosphate amidotransferase of *Bacillus subtilis* (Turnbough and Switzer, 1975) and the gramicidin S synthetase of *Bacillus brevis* (Friebel and Demain, 1977). The physiological function of this inactivation is obscure but may involve regulation of these enzymes (Switzer, 1977). With *P. aeruginosa* such an inactivation would indicate a relatedness between oxygen levels and particular functions in this organism. Here high cultural or intracellular oxygen levels might signify a state of well-being for this obligate aerobe while lowered levels of oxygen might signal the need for auxillary metabolic functions including secondary metabolism. The reintroduction of oxygen would signal a return to the cell's original state, and so cause the dismantling of the enzymes of secondary metabolism.

VI. ACKNOWLEDGEMENTS

The efforts of Philip Hoschar are gratefully acknowledged. This work was supported by grants BMS 74-16398 and PCM 77-24117 from the National Science Foundation.

REFERENCES

Asmus, E. and Garschagen, H. (1953). *Zeit. Analyt. Chemie* 138, 414-422.

Castric, P.A. (1975). *Can. Microbiol.* 21, 613-618.

Castric, P.A. (1977). *J. Bacteriol.* 130, 826-831.

Castric, P.A., Ebert, R.F. and Castric, K.F. (1979). *Current Microbiol.* 2, 287-292.

Collins, P.A., Rodgers, P.B. and Knowles, C.J. (1980). *J. Gen. Microbiol.* 117, 73-80.

Dalton, H. and Postgate, J.R. (1969). *J. Gen. Microbiol.* 54, 463-473.

Demain, A.L., Kennel, Y.M. and Aharonowitz, Y. (1979). *In:* "Microbial

technology: Current State, Future Prospects" (A. T. Bull, D. C. Ellwood, C. Ratledge, eds.) Twenty-Ninth Symposium of the Society for General Microbiology, pp. 163-185. Cambridge University Press, Cambridge.
Friebel, T.E. and Demain, A.L. (1977). *J. Bacteriol.* 130, 1010-1016.
Knowles, C.J. (1976). *Bact. Rev.* 40, 652-680.
Meganathan, R. and Castric, P.A. (1977). *Arch. Microbiol.* 114, 51-54.
Rodgers, P.B. and Knowles, C.J. (1978). *J. Gen. Microbiol.* 108, 261-267.
Switzer, R.L. (1977). *Ann. Rev. Microbiol.* 31, 135-157.
Turnbough, D.L. and Switzer, R.L. (1975). *J. Bacteriol.* 121, 108-114.
Weinberg, E.D. (1971). *Persp. Biol. Med.* 14, 565-577.
Weinberg, E.D. (1978). *Folia Microbiol.* 23, 496-504.
Wissing, F. (1968). *Physiol. Plant.* 21, 589-593.
Wissing, F. (1974). *J. Bacteriol.* 117, 1289-1294.
Wissing, F. (1975). *J. Bacteriol.* 121, 695-699.

THE ENZYMOLOGY OF CYANIDE PRODUCTION FROM GLYCINE BY A *PSEUDOMONAS* SPECIES. SOLUBILIZATION OF THE ENZYME

FRODE WISSING and KIRSTEN S. ANDERSEN

Department of Chemistry, The Royal Dental College, DK-8000 Aarhus C, Denmark

I. SUMMARY

Solubilization of the cyanide producing enzyme system from a *Pseudomonas* species was investigated. Relative to the activity in whole bacteria 78% of the activity could be obtained by sonication-detergent treatment, 76% of the activity by a freezing-thawing-detergent method and 188% of the activity by lysozyme-detergent treatment. A preparation made by sonication-detergent treatment was purified 9 fold on a Sepharose 6B column. The presence of rhodanese and β-cyanoalanine synthase was established. The K_m value of the solubilized enzyme with respect to glycine was 3×10^{-4} M in the presence of phenazine methosulfate and air. Some evidence that the enzyme may be located on the outer side of the cytoplasmic membrane is given. The HCN producing activity was found to be unstable in the presence of air in both harvested bacteria and enzyme preparations. The putative intermediates in cyanide production, formaldoxime and oxamic acid, did not produce HCN with whole bacteria or enzyme preparations.

II. INTRODUCTION

Some fungi (Ward and Thorn, 1966) and bacteria (Lorck, 1948; Michaels *et al.*, 1965; Wissing, 1974; Castric, 1977; Rodgers and Knowles, 1978) can produce cyanide and carbon dioxide by the oxidation of glycine, the simplest of the amino acids. The conditions under which microorganisms produce cyanide from glycine have been subject to thorough investigations (Michaels and Corpe, 1965; Wissing, 1968, 1975; Brysk *et al.*, 1969; Ward *et al.*, 1971; Niven *et al.*, 1975). The results have been reviewed by Knowles (1976), and Castric (this volume).

Early speculations on how cyanide was produced, based on the following observations with intact cyanogenic bacteria, led to hypothetical reaction schemes for the enzymatic process:

1) glycine is the substrate (Lorck, 1948; Michaels *et al.*, 1965; Wissing, 1968; Castric, 1977; Rodgers and Knowles, 1978)
2) Gly → HCN, molar ratio 1.0:1.1 (Wissing, 1974)
3) HCN and CO_2, product ratio 11%:10% (Michaels *et al.*, 1965)
4) HCN originates from the methylene group and CO_2 from the carboxyl group of glycine (Michaels *et al.*, 1965)
5) the C-N bond in glycine is retained in HCN (Brysk *et al.*, 1969)
6) oxidative conditions are needed (Wissing, 1974; Castric, 1975; Nazly *et al.*, this volume)
7) some flavine inhibitors inhibit HCN production (Wissing, 1974)
8) iron stimulates cyanogenesis (Castric, 1975; Rodgers and Knowles, 1978).

In these hypotheses oxamic acid (Michaels *et al.*, 1965), formaldoxime (Conn, 1973) or iminoacetic acid (Wissing, 1974) could be intermediates:

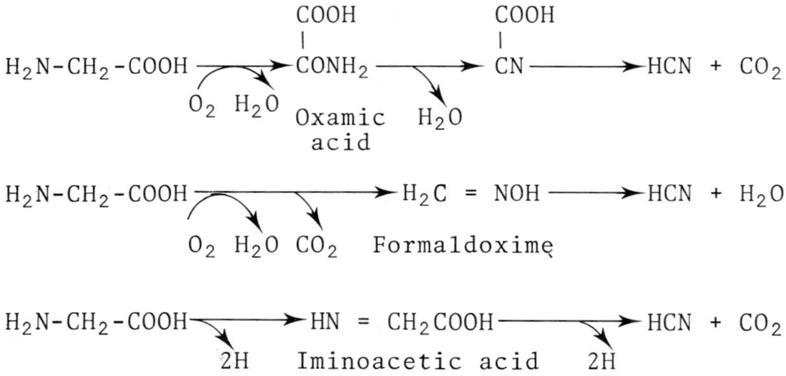

Unfortunately, iminoacetic acid is too unstable to handle, but oxamic acid and formaldoxime have been tested and found to give no cyanide production with the *Pseudomonas* species under investigation here.

Experiments with whole cyanogenic bacteria are limited by the difficulty of interpreting the results obtained, caused, for example by: (i) possible transport problems for glycine through the membrane, depending on the localization of the enzyme, and (ii) the interference of cyanide utilizing enzymes, such as rhodanese, β-cyanoalanine synthase and γ-cyano-α-aminobutyric acid synthase, which have been shown to be present in the cyanogenic *Chromobacterium violaceum* (Rodgers and Knowles, 1978). Therefore, attempts have been made to prepare cell-free extracts which finally resulted in active preparations from a *Pseudomonas* species (Wissing, 1975) and from *Pseudomonas aeruginosa* Castric *et al.*, 1979).

As shown by the investigations reported here, whereas

high aeration was needed during growth of the *Pseudomonas* species, very little oxygen could be allowed to be present during preparation of the enzyme. Oxygenation was again needed during assay of the HCN producing activity. Solubilization of the cyanide producing enzyme will be described, as will the first step in a purification of the enzyme by molecular sieving.

III. METHODS AND MATERIALS

A. GROWTH AND STORAGE OF BACTERIA

The bacterium, a cyanide producing strain C of a *Pseudomonas* species, was maintained by culturing alternatively on nutrient agar or on a succinate-minimal salts agar medium enriched with glycine and ferrichloride (Wissing, 1974). For the experiments, bacteria in the stationary phase of growth, were obtained from cultures grown for 18 h on a liquid medium consisting of 8 g Bacto Nutrient (Difco) and 5 g NaCl/1 distilled water. The pH of the medium was adjusted to 7.5 with NaOH, and a separately autoclaved solution of 10 ml of 20 mmoles glycine, 0.2 mmole $FeCl_3$ and 1 mmole $Na_4P_2O_7$ was also added. During growth the medium was maintained at 20°C, aerated and stirred vigorously. Harvested bacteria were washed and stored in 0.05 M KH_2PO_4/Na_2HPO_4 buffer (pH 7.5) as a 10% wet weight suspension at 0°C in hermetically closed plastic vials. By storage in this manner the bacteria remained in an essentially anaerobic state, due to endogenous respiration, and kept all their HCN producing activity for 3 to 4 weeks if they were washed with water immediately before being resuspended in the appropriate experimental buffers. The cyanide producing activity, with glycine as the substrate, was measured on 2% wet weight suspensions of intact bacteria in 0.1 M Tris-HCl (pH 8.2) without any further additions. Dithiothreitol (DTT) and ethylenediaminetetraacetate (EDTA), which are necessary for solubilized enzyme preparations, caused decreases and variations in the activity of whole bacteria. Phenazine methosulfate (PMS) had no effect on whole bacteria when tested in the presence of air.

B. ANALYSES

The cyanogenic capacity of cell-free extracts was measured in the reaction chamber (Wissing, this volume). It was first filled with 1 ml of 0.1 M Tris-HCl (pH 8.2) buffer which was 1 mM with respect to EDTA and DTT and supplemented with ethanol (1% v/v) and Triton X-100 (0.03% w/v) (which is referred to below as the assay buffer). Either 100 µl of the same buffer or 100 µl of a solution of a test substrate and 1 ml of suitably diluted enzyme was then added. Glycine (44 µmole) and PMS (1.32 µmole) in 100 µl of H_2O were added to give a final reaction volume of 2.2 ml. Cyanide liberated was transferred by aeration to 1 ml 0.1 M NaOH for periods of 4 min (Wissing, this volume) and determined by the method of Epstein (1947). The assays were performed in the dark. For the measurements of activities glycine was not added before a suitably steady state of endogenous HCN production was established in the enzyme preparation. A unit of enzyme is defined as the amount that will produce 1 μmole of HCN per minute at pH 8.2 and 20°C. The specific activity of a preparation is derived from the amount of HCN produced within the first 4 minutes after glycine addition.

β-Cyanoalanine synthase was assayed by the method described by Blumenthal *et al.* (1968). Rhodanese was assayed by the method of Sörbo (1955).

The protein content in enzyme preparations or exhaustively sonicated bacteria was determined according to the method of Bradford (1976) by the Bio-Rad Protein Assay (Bio-Rad Laboratories, Kent, England). This procedure showed only negligible interferences by the DTT and Triton X-100 concentrations applied here.

C. ENZYME SOLUBILIZATIONS

1. *Sonication*

Bacteria were washed with water (0 to 5°C) and resuspended in 0.1 M Tris-HCl (pH 8.2) to give a 10% wet weight suspension. Oleic acid in 100 μl of ethanol was added to 10 ml of the bacterial suspension to give a final concentration of 0.5 mM. The bacteria were placed in an icebath and sonicated for 4 × 1 min, with 30-s intermittent periods for cooling, with an MSE 150-W Ultrasonic Disintegrator Mk2. Metal from the tip of the sonifier and coarse cell-debris were removed by centrifugation at 3000 × g for 10 min. Then 9.5 ml of the supernatant was mixed with 500 μl of the above Tris buffer containing Triton X-100 to give a final concentration of 0.3% (w/v). After standing for 5 min in ice, insoluble material was precipitated by centrifugation at 100,000 × g for 45 min. The resulting supernatant was stored in ice.

2. *Freezing-Thawing*

Bacteria washed with water (0 to 5°C) were resuspended in 0.1 M Tris-HCl (pH 8.2) buffer with EDTA (1 mM), DTT (1 mM), Triton X-100 (0.06% w/v), ethanol (1% v/v) and oleic acid (0.5 mM) to give a 5% (wet weight) suspension. The bacteria were frozen at -20°C. After freezing for 24 h or 48 h the bacteria were placed in a beaker with water at 5°C until thawed and then centrifuged at 100,000 × g for 45 min. The resulting supernatant was stored in ice.

3. *Lysozyme Treatment*

Bacteria were washed with water (0 to 5°C) and resuspended in 0.1 M Tris-HCl (pH 8.2) to give a 2% (wet weight) suspension. A 50 ml portion in a 50 ml conical flask was placed in a water bath at 25°C and stirred magnetically. In sequence, different compounds were added, as solutions in 500 µl Tris buffer or ethanol, in amounts giving the final concentrations indicated in brackets: EDTA (1 mM), DTT (1 mM), lysozyme (0.5 mg/ml), oleic acid in ethanol (0.5 mM) and Triton X-100 (0.06% w/v). After stirring for 15 min the suspension was cooled in ice for 5 min and then centrifuged at 27,000 × g for 20 min. The resulting supernatant was stored in ice.

4. *Sepharose CL-6B Column Chromatography*

The 100,000 × g supernatant containing solubilized enzyme, obtained by the sonication procedure, was applied to a 40 × 2.5 cm Sepharose CL-6B column, which previously had been equilibrated with 1 litre of assay buffer. The column was eluted with the same buffer at a rate of 1.3 ml per min. Fractions of 5 ml were collected. All steps were made at 4°C.

5. *Chemicals*

Triton X-100 was obtained from Carl Roth, Karlsruhe, Germany. Phenazine methosulfate was from British Drug House, oxamic acid from Sigma, formaldoxime-HCl from Fluka, and Sepharose CL-6B from Pharmacia. Whenever possible, all other reagents were of analytical grade; glass distilled water was used throughout.

IV. RESULTS AND DISCUSSIONS

A. OPTIMAL DETERGENT CONCENTRATION

The cyanide producing enzyme is known to be associated with the membrane in *Pseudomonas* species strain C (Wissing, 1975), so various detergents and their combinations with solvents have been tried on preparations of disrupted bacteria. The non-ionic detergent Triton X-100 was used for solubilization of the enzyme from sonicated bacteria. Under the conditions described in "Methods and Materials" a Triton X-100 concentration higher than 0.15% (w/v), which is ten times the critical micelle concentration (Helenius *et al.*, 1979), did not improve the solubilization further. Other non-ionic detergents such as Brij 35, Tween 80 and Tween 20 were found to be less efficient than Triton X-100 in their solubilizing effect on the HCN producing enzyme.

During the different solubilization procedures it was found that oleic acid, when added in ethanol to give a final concentration of 0.5 mM, normally increased the activities in solubilized preparations of the enzyme by about 40%, of which about 20% increase in activity was due to the effect of ethanol alone. Butanol and acetone acted in the same way as ethanol when added to give a 1% (v/v) final concentration, but the stability of the enzyme was impaired. Other lipophilic compounds tested were ubiquinone (Q_{10}), DL-α-tocopherol, linoleic acid and arachidonic acid, all of which showed similar ability to oleic acid in improving activity.

B. OPTIMAL PMS AND DTT CONCENTRATIONS

Whereas the membrane-bound enzyme requires oxygen for cyanide production (Wissing, 1974) the solubilized enzyme is completely dependent on other electron acceptors. Alternatively it can be linked to the respiratory system in the membranes. Phenazine methosulfate was previously found to be the best compound to substitute for oxygen with intact bacteria (Wissing, 1974). Its optimal concentration, for its effect on HCN production by the solubilized enzyme, was found to be 0.3 mM. With whole bacteria 1 mM DTT inhibited the activity of cyanide formation by about 10%, whereas the activity of the solubilized enzyme was doubled in the presence of 1 mM DTT. Experiments to determine its optimal concentration showed that more than 0.5 mM DTT did not increase the activity further.

C. SOLUBILIZATION OF THE ENZYME

The *Pseudomonas* species investigated here does not excrete cyanide producing activity into its surrounding medium. The cell wall has to be modified before active enzyme, in a solubilized state, can be detected. Table I shows the activities and recoveries of cyanogenesis by various preparations in relation to the activity in whole bacteria. Three different procedures to disrupt the bacteria in combination with detergents were tested.

By sonication 58% of the activity could be recovered in the supernatant from ultracentrifugation, when no detergents were added. Addition of both oleic acid and Triton X-100 increased the recovery to 78%. No significant increase in specific activity was obtained since other proteins were solubilized at the same time.

Miozzari *et al.* (1978) have described a permeabilization procedure of microorganisms to obtain membrane located enzymes by freezing and thawing in the presence of low concentration (0.05% w/v) of Triton X-100. By using this method on the cyanide producing bacterium, with 0.06% (w/v) Triton X-100, 76% of the activity could be recovered. Freezing-thawing two times yielded 89% recovery. As shown in "Methods and Materials" oleic acid in ethanol, EDTA and DTT were added to the bacteria before freezing. The specific activity was increased about two times, as much cell material could be removed from this preparation by centrifugation. The nucleic acid content was very low as judged by the orcinol test or by comparing the elution profiles from Sephadex G-200 chromatography of this prep-

Table I Differences in specific activities and recoveries of cyanide formation by different bacterial homogenates prepared by sonication, freezing-thawing or lysozyme treatment.[a]

Method	Preparation	Specific Activity (mU/mg)	Recovery (%)
None	Whole bact.	1.28	100
Sonication	100,000 × g sup.	1.34	58
Sonication + oleic acid	100,000 × g sup.	1.34	64
Sonication + oleic acid + Triton X-100	100,000 × g sup.	1.36	78
None	Whole bact.	1.32	100
Freezing-thawing × 1[b]	100,000 × g sup.	1.45	76
Freezing-thawing × 2[b]	100,000 × g sup.	2.06	89
None	Whole bact.	1.24	100
Lysozyme	27,000 × g sup.	0.73	15
Lysozyme + oleic acid	27,000 × g sup.	2.54	144
Lysozyme + oleic acid + Triton X-100	27,000 × g sup.	2.20	182

[a] Results are based on duplicate experiments

[b] Oleic acid and Triton X-100 were present during freezing-thawing.

aration and of a preparation made by the method of sonication (results not shown).

When lysozyme alone was used to solubilize the enzyme from 2% (wet weight) suspensions of the bacteria 15% of the activity could be recovered. If oleic acid was added 144% recovery was obtained, while further addition of Triton X-100 increased the recovery to 188%. By this method of preparation oleic acid in ethanol, EDTA and DTT were all present from the beginning of the experiment. A non-homogenous suspension occurred during the lysozyme treatment, which made this preparation easier to centrifuge than the other preparations.

It is thus clear that the sonication procedure is advantageous in obtaining a small volume of the enzyme preparation, whereas the lysozyme preparation gives 5 times the volume of extract to the starting volume of the bacteria. However, the lysozyme preparation method is advantageous in that it has nearly double the specific activity of that obtained by the sonication technique.

D. STABILITY OF THE ENZYME

The cyanide producing enzyme system is very unstable. A preparation made by sonication normally loses about half of its activity when stored overnight in ice. It was observed that a preparation, closed with a plastic cap, on standing gradually developed a faint change in its reddish colour to a more yellow colour, beginning with the top of the solution. If samples were withdrawn from these two layers, no activity was left in the yellow fraction but the reddish layer had retained full activity. This is in agreement with the suggestion made by Dr P. A. Castric (personal communication) that oxygen may be deleterious to the enzyme. A possible confirmation of this is given by the experiments shown in Fig. 1, where cyanide production was followed in a lysozyme preparation to which glycine was added after 20 and 40 min respectively. In the experiment in which glycine was added 20 min later than in the first experiment, after a steady endogenous HCN production was established, only 62% of the activity remained. From the insert in Fig. 1 it can be seen that the cyanide production is almost linear for at least 20 min during the assay.

E. HCN UTILIZING ENZYMES

Rhodanese and β-cyanoalanine synthase were found to be present in the bacterium and could be separated from the cyanide producing enzyme by chromatography on a Sepharose CL-6B column as shown in Fig. 2. Purification of up to 9 fold of the HCN producing enzyme was achieved. The specific activities of the rhodanese and the β-cyanoalanine synthase were about 30 and 10 times higher than the specific activity of the cyanide producing enzyme. The nearly

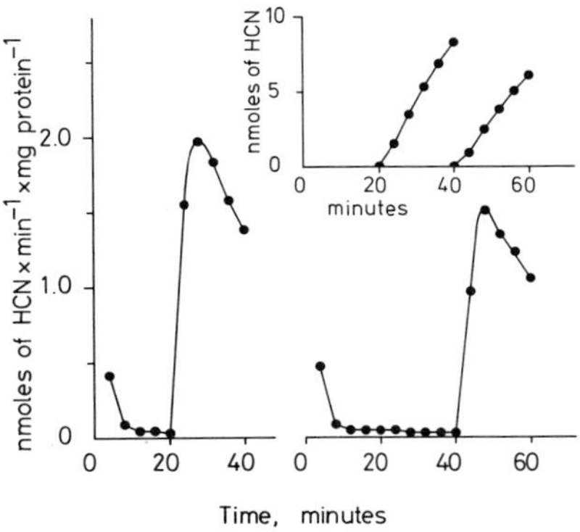

Fig. 1 The effect of different pre-aeration times on the rate of HCN production by the lysozyme-detergent solubilized enzyme. Glycine addition after 40 min of pre-aeration (right hand curve) resulted in a specific activity of about 60% of the activity obtained by 20 min pre-aeration (left hand curve).
The insert shows the time dependence of the accumulation of HCN by the respective experiments.

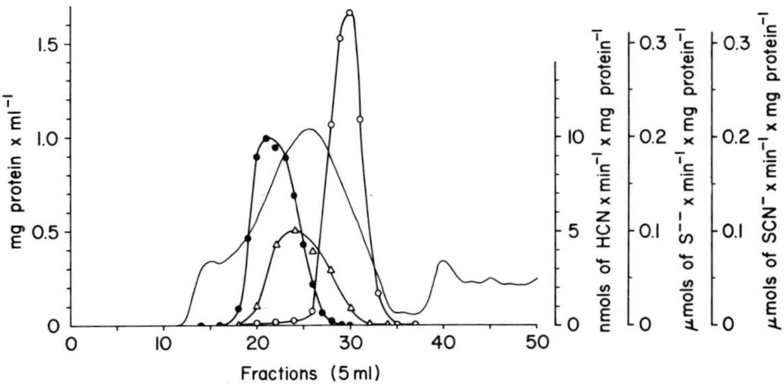

Fig. 2 Sepharose CL-6B column chromatography of an enzyme preparation made by the sonication-detergent treatment of the HCN producing bacterium. Protein elution profile (——), HCN producing activity (●), β-cyanoalanine synthase activity (△), and rhodanese activity (○).

complete separation of rhodanese from the HCN producing activity was associated with the observation that DTT no longer had the effect of increasing the activity of the HCN producing enzyme. Pecci *et al.* (1976) and Costa *et al.* (1977) have observed that rhodanese is inhibited by low concentrations of DTT in a time dependent manner. Table II lists enzymes from different origins which, by their presence, might influence cyanide determinations in crude preparations from cyanogenic organisms. From their optim-

Table II Optimal pH-values for HCN utilization by some enzymes of different origin.[a]

HCN utilizing enzyme	pH-optimum	Reference
Thiosulphate: cyanide sulfurtransferase (2.8.1.1.)	8.6	Sörbo, 1953
3-mercaptopyruvate: cyanide sulfurtransferase (2.8.1.2.)	9.1	Hylin and Wood, 1959
β-cyanoalanine synthase (4.4.1.9.)	9.5	Hendrickson and Conn, 1969
γ-cyano-α-aminobutyric acid synthase	8.3-9.6	Ressler *et al.*, 1973
Formamide hydro-lyase (4.2.1.66)	7-9	Fry and Millar, 1972
HCN metabolized to NH_3 + CO_2	8.5-9	Skowronski and Strobel, 1969
HCN metabolized to α-aminopropionitrile	7.8	Strobel, 1966
HCN metabolized to γ-amino-γ-cyanobutyric acid	8	Strobel, 1967

[a] Compiled from the literature.

al pH ranges it can be seen that they all metabolize cyanide maximally at rather high pH values, close to pH 8-8.5, which is the optimum for HCN production by the *Pseudomonas* species used in this study.

F. LOCALIZATION OF THE ENZYME

The reaction of the enzyme with glycine showed typical Michaelis-Menten kinetics by both whole bacteria (Wissing, 1974) and the solubilized enzyme (Fig. 3). The respective

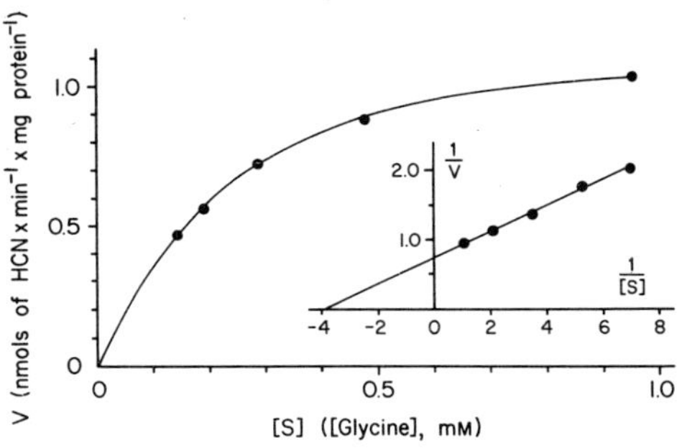

Fig. 3 Kinetics of cyanide production as a function of glycine concentration in the presence of oxygen (air). The enzyme was solubilized by the sonication-detergent treatment of the HCN producing bacterium.

K_m values of 5×10^{-4} M and 2.7×10^{-4} M are very similar. From this one may speculate whether the enzyme is located on the outside of the membrane as greater differences in the values might have been observed if glycine had to penetrate the cytoplasmic membrane before interacting with the enzyme.

Also, the molar ratio of 1:1 for glycine utilization and cyanide production found with whole bacteria (Wissing, 1974) could make a localization of the enzyme on the outer side of the membrane likely, because one might otherwise expect a change in this molar ratio due to interference by rhodanese and β-cyanoalanine synthase. These enzymes are present at 30 and 10 times higher activities respectively than the activity of the HCN producing enzyme.

G. INTERMEDIATES

The putative intermediates in the enzymatic conversion of glycine to HCN and CO_2, oxamic acid and formaldoxime, did not give rise to any HCN production. They were added, with or without PMS, to give 10 mM final concentrations to suspensions of either whole bacteria or solutions of the enzyme prepared by the lysozyme method. The formaldoxime experiment was corrected for the background readings in the Epstein assay, caused by formaldoxime itself.

ACKNOWLEDGEMENTS

This work was supported by the Danish Natural Science Research Council via grant No. 511-7130.

REFERENCES

Blumenthal, S.G., Hendrickson, H.R., Abrol, Y.P. and Conn, E.E. (1968). *J. Biol. Chem.* 243, 5302-5307.
Bradford, M.M. (1976). *Anal. Biochem.* 72, 248-254.
Brysk, M.M., Corpe, W.A. and Hankes, L.V. (1969). *J. Bacteriol.* 97, 322-327.
Bunch, A.W. and Knowles, C.J. (1980). *J. Gen. Microbiol.* 116, 9-16.
Castric, P.A. (1975). *Can. J. Microbiol.* 21, 613-618.
Castric, P.A. (1977). *J. Bacteriol.* 130, 826-831.
Castric, P.A., Ebert, R.F. and Castric, K.F. (1979). *Current Microbiol.* 2, 287-292.
Conn, E.E. (1973). *In* "Nitrogen Metabolism in Plants", Biochemical Society Symposium (T.W. Goodwin and R.M.S. Smellie, eds) Vol. 38, pp. 227-302. Biochemical Society, London.
Costa, M., Pecci, L., Pensa, B. and Cannella, C. (1977). *Biochem. Biophys. Res. Commun.* 78, 596-602.
Epstein, E. (1947). *Anal. Chem.* 19, 272-274.
Fry, W.E. and Millar, R.L.(1972). *Arch. Biochem. Biophys.* 151, 468-474.
Helenius, A., McCastin, D.R., Fries, E. and Tanford, C. (1979). *In* "Methods in Enzymology" (S. P. Colowick and N. O. Kaplan, eds) Vol. LVI, pp. 734-749. Academic Press, New York, San Francisco, and London.
Hendrickson, H.R. and Conn, E.E. (1969). *J. Biol. Chem.* 244, 2632-2640.
Hylin, J.W. and Wood, J.L. (1959). *J. Biol. Chem.* 234, 2141-2144.
Knowles, C.J. (1976). *Bacteriol. Reviews* 40, 652-680.
Lorck, H. (1948). *Physiologia Plantarum* 1, 143-146.
Michaels, R. and Corpe, W.A. (1965). *J. Bacteriol.* 89, 106-112.
Michaels, R., Hankes, L.V. and Corpe, W.A. (1965). *Arch. Biochem. Biophys.* 111, 121-125.
Miozzari, G.F., Niederberger, P. and Hütter, R. (1978). *Anal. Biochem.* 90, 220-233.
Niven, D.F., Collins, P.A. and Knowles, C.J. (1975). *J. Gen. Microbiol.* 90, 271-285.
Pecci, L., Pensa, B., Costa, Mara., Cignini, P.L. and Cannella, C. (1976). *Biochem. Biophys. Acta* 445, 104-111.
Ressler, C., Abe, O., Kondo, Y., Cottrell, B. and Abe, K. (1973). *Biochemistry* 12, 5369-5377.
Rodgers, P.B. and Knowles, C.J. (1978). *J. Gen. Microbiol.* 108, 261-267.
Skowronski, B. and Strobel, G.A. (1969). *Can. J. Microbiol.* 15, 93-98.
Strobel, G.A. (1966). *J. Biol. Chem.* 241, 2618-2621.
Strobel, G.A. (1967). *J. Biol. Chem.* 242, 3265-3269.
Sörbo, B.H. (1953). *Acta. Chem. Scand.* 7, 1137-1145.
Sörbo, B.H. (1955). *In* "Methods of Enzymology" (S. P. Colowick and N.O. Kaplan, eds) Vol.II, pp.334-336. Academic Press, New York.

Ward, E.W.B. and Thorn, G.D. (1966). *Can. J. Botany* 44, 95-104.
Ward, E.W.B., Thorn, G.D. and Starrat, A.N. (1971). *Can. J. Microbiol.* 17, 1061-1066.
Wissing, F. (1968). *Physiologia Plantarum* 21, 589-593.
Wissing, F. (1974). *J. Bacteriol.* 117, 1289-1294.
Wissing, F. (1975). *J. Bacteriol.* 121, 695-699.

CYANIDE PRODUCTION BY HARVESTED *CHROMOBACTERIUM VIOLACEUM*

NAHEED NAZLY, PAULINE A. COLLINS
and CHRISTOPHER J. KNOWLES

*Biological Laboratory, University of Kent,
Canterbury, CT2 7NJ, England*

I. SUMMARY

Cyanide formation by harvested cultures of *Chromobacterium violaceum* was investigated. Cyanogenesis was massively stimulated by addition of glycine to the bacteria. When methionine was also present a higher level of cyanide formation was sometimes observed. Glycine could be replaced by threonine, and, to a lesser extent, serine. The concentration of glycine required for half maximal cyanogenesis was 4.4 x 10^{-5} M. Under anaerobic conditions no cyanide was formed from glycine by suspensions of *C. violaceum* that had been grown aerobically; aeration of the suspensions resulted in immediate cyanogenesis. Addition of electron acceptors such as phenazine methosulfate under anaerobic conditions caused formation of small amounts of cyanide. Cultivation of *C. violaceum* on glucose under anaerobic conditions in the presence of fumarate (as an electron acceptor), glycine and methionine resulted in formation of cyanide.

II. INTRODUCTION

Chromobacterium violaceum and a few pseudomonads are the only non-photosynthetic bacteria known to produce cyanide, whereas many fungi are cyanogenic (Knowles, 1976; Castric, this volume). The alga *Chlorella vulgaris* can form cyanide from D-histidine (Pistorius *et al.*, 1977) and from the oxime of glyoxylic acid (Solomonson and Spehar, 1977, 1979). The cyanobacterium *Anacystis nidulans* forms cyanide from L-histidine (Pistorius *et al.*, 1979).

Cyanide formation by two *Pseudomonas* species, *C. violaceum* and the snow mould fungus (Wissing, 1968; Castric, 1975; Rodgers and Knowles, 1978; Collins *et al.*, 1980; Bunch and Knowles, 1980) exhibits the classical properties of secondary metabolite synthesis (Weinberg, 1971). Cyanide is formed by decarboxylation of glycine by both the bacteria and the snow mould basidiomycete (Michaels and Corpe, 1965; Ward and Thorn, 1966; Ward *et al.*,1971, 1977; Wissing, 1974; Rodgers and Knowles, 1978; Collins *et al.*, 1980; Bunch and Knowles, 1980). Threonine or serine can replace glycine as a precursor of cyanide, although lower yields of cyanide are noted with the latter compound (Castric, 1977; Rodgers and Knowles, 1980; P.A. Collins and C.J. Knowles, unpub. obsv.); presumably they are metabolised to glycine prior to conversion to cyanide. In the bacteria, but not the snow mould fungus, methionine or its various metabolites massively stimulate cyanogenesis from glycine, but methionine is not a precursor of cyanide (Michaels and Corpe, 1965; Castric 1975, 1977; Rodgers and Knowles, 1978; Collins *et al.*, 1980).

In this paper we report the effect of growth conditions on the ability of intact, harvested cells of *C. violaceum* to produce cyanide.

III. MATERIALS AND METHODS

A. ORGANISM AND GROWTH CONDITIONS

Chromobacterium violaceum strain NC1B 9131 was grown routinely at 30°C under aerobic conditions on M9 mineral salts medium as described previously (Rodgers and Knowles, 1978). Glutamate (10 mM) was the carbon and nitrogen source and, as indicated, the medium was supplemented with 2 mM glycine and/or 0.5 mM methionine. In experiments where growth was limited due to carbon depletion from the medium 6 mM glucose was used as the sole source of carbon, and 18.6 mM NH_4Cl and/or 6 mM glycine were provided as the nitrogen sources. Where stated, 0.5 mM methionine was also added to the medium, but it does not act as a source of nitrogen or carbon for growth (Collins *et al.*, 1980). *C. violaceum* was also grown anaerobically at 30°C in 50 ml bottles filled to the neck with M9 salts medium containing 0.1 mg/ml resazurin as an indicator of anaerobiosis. The carbon and nitrogen sources were 20 mM glucose, and 18.6 mM NH_4Cl and/or 6 mM glycine, respectively. Where stated, 10 mM sodium fumarate was used as an electron acceptor.

B. CELL SUSPENSIONS

Bacteria were routinely harvested in the late exponential phase (9 or 14 h after inoculation for glutamate or glucose-containing cultures, respectively). Cultures were centrifuged at 33,000 g for 5 min at 4°C and washed twice in carbon and nitrogen-free M9 salts medium. The cells were finally resuspended in M9 salts (C- and N-free) at approximately 5-fold the growth concentration.

C. CYANIDE PRODUCTION

Production of cyanide by harvested bacteria was determined in two ways. Experiments on the effect of time of harvesting on the ability of the bacterium to produce cyanide were carried out in shake flasks. Cells were suspended at 0.3 to 0.5 mg dry wt/ml in 100 ml M9 salts containing 10 mM glutamate, 2 mM glycine, 0.5 mM methionine and 25 μg/ml chloramphenicol in 250 ml conical flasks. They were incubated in a gyrotary shaker (250 rpm) at 30°C. Samples were removed every hour for 6 h and assayed for cyanide formation. Maximal production occurred after 3-5 h incubation.

All other experiments to determine cyanide production involved the use of a slight modification of the apparatus designed by Wissing (1974, this volume). The rubber stopper was replaced by a glass stopper fitted with a Suba-seal, an air inlet with the tube extended to immediately above the surface of the reaction suspension, and an air/cyanide outlet which was connected to a trap containing 1.05 ml 1M NaOH. A 1 ml suspension of *C. violaceum* (about 2 mg dry wt) was added to the reaction chamber and equilibrated for 30 min. at 30°C to obtain the endogenous rate of cyanide production. A constant stream of air (0.8 litre/min) was used, giving a recovery of 95% of the cyanide produced in 5 min. by the stirred suspension. After the preincubation, 25 μg/ml chloramphenicol and substrate amino acids were added via the Suba-seal. Cyanide produced was trapped at 2-5 min. intervals for a duration of 25 min. The trapped cyanide was neutralised and assayed by the Epstein (1947) method.

D. GROWTH AND DRY WEIGHT

Bacterial growth was measured by the absorbance at 750 nm using 10 mm cuvettes in a Pye-Unicam SP500 spectrophotometer. The dry weights of bacteria were obtained by comparison with a standard curve of absorbance against dry weight. Duplicate 5 ml samples (at various absorbance values) of a 9 h glutamate-grown culture were harvested by centrifugation at 6000 g for 20 min in preweighed test tubes. The pellets were washed in 0.15 M NaCl and then in distilled water. The bacteria were dried to constant weight at 105°C.

IV. RESULTS AND DISCUSSION

Previous studies on cultures of *C. violaceum* grown aerobically on a mineral salts medium containing glutamate as the carbon and nitrogen source, in the presence of glycine and methionine, have shown that maximum growth and cyanide production were obtained about 10 h and 12 h after inoculation, respectively (Rodgers and Knowles, 1978). Addition of an inhibitor of protein synthesis (chloramphenicol) to the growing cultures indicated that the enzyme system involved in cyanide synthesis from glycine was induced during the late-exponential phase of growth. The data given in Table I supports this supposition. Cells were grown on 10 mM glutamate and harvested at various times after inoculation. The ability to produce cyanide, when incubated with glutamate, glycine and methionine in the presence of chloramphenicol, was greatest for bacteria harvested 7 to 9 h after inoculation. The apparently lower level of cyanogenesis by cells grown for longer than 9 h may have been due to induction of enzymes for cyanide degradation at about this time (Rodgers and Knowles, 1978). β-cyanoalanine synthase is probably the most important of these enzymes (Rodgers, this volume).

Table I The effect of time of harvesting of *C. violaceum* on the ability of harvested cells to produce cyanide

Time of harvesting (h)	Maximum cyanide produced by harvested cells (μmoles / g dry wt)
5.5	263
7.0	798
9.0	1045
11.0	92

C. violaceum was grown on M9 mineral salts containing 10 mM glutamate. Cyanide production by harvested bacteria was determined in the presence of 10 mM glutamate, 2 mM glycine, 0.5 mM methionine and 25 μg/ml chloramphenicol as described in the Methods.

Castric *et al.* (1979), from measurements of the activities of cell-free extracts and intact cells, have shown an analogous increase in specific activity of the cyanide synthesising system of *P. aeruginosa* in the late-exponential phase of growth, prior to the onset of active cyanogenesis at the start of the stationary phase.

Further experiments on *C. violaceum* grown aerobically on glutamate were performed on cultures that had been harvested 9 h after inoculation. For cultures grown on glucose the time of harvesting was also selected to give optimal cyanogenesis (14 h after inoculation).

Figure 1 shows the initial rate of cyanide formation by harvested bacteria that had been grown on glutamate. After an initial low level of cyanogenesis, little

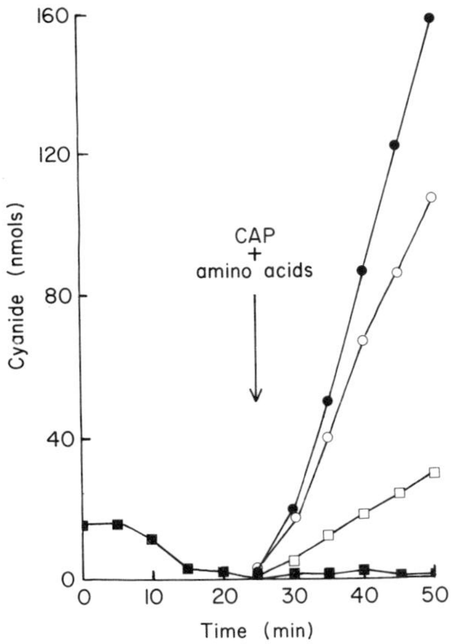

Fig. 1 The production of cyanide by suspensions of *C. violaceum* that had been grown on glutamate. At the time shown by the arrow 25 μg/ml chloramphenical plus 0.5 methionine (□), 2 mM glycine (○), or 2 mM glycine and 0.5 mM methionine (●) were added. No additions (■).

further cyanide was formed. Addition of methionine to the suspension gave a low rate of cyanide production, but addition of glycine caused a much greater rate of cyanogenesis. A somewhat higher rate of cyanogenesis occurred when both glycine and methionine were present. This increment over the rate found with glycine alone was variable and often there was little or no increase in the rate of cyanide formation when methionine was also present (e.g. Fig. 3). When cyanide production was measured over a 3-5 h period it was found that the total amount formed was also in the order: + glycine + methionine ⩾ + glycine ⩾ + methionine (not shown). These observations were somewhat unexpected as it had been shown with growing cultures that both glycine and methionine were needed for massive cyanogenesis (Michaels and Corpe, 1965; Rodgers and Knowles, 1978). Since methionine seems to regulate the activity of the cyanide synthesising enzyme(s) and β-cyanoalanine synthase (Rodgers and Knowles, 1978; Rodgers, this volume) it could be that the intracellular level of methionine in the harvested bacteria was at (or almost at) the optimal level for maximal cyanogenesis to occur.

Table II shows the effect of inclusion of glycine and/or methionine in the glutamate-containing growth medium on the ability of harvested bacteria to produce cyanide

Table II The rate of cyanide production by whole cells of *C. violaceum* grown on glucose or glutamate.

Growth conditions	Cyanogenesis by harvested bacteria (nmoles/min/(mg dry wt))
Glutamate	2.8
Glutamate, glycine	1.8
Glutamate, methionine	2.9
Glutamate, glycine, methionine	2.1
Glucose, glycine, methionine	0.3
Glucose, glycine, methionine, NH_4Cl	1.3

The concentrations of the compounds used in the growth medium were 10 mM glutamate, 6 mM glucose, 2 mM glycine, 0.5 mM methionine, 18.6 mM NH_4Cl. Bacteria were harvested after 9 or 14 h when grown on glutamate or glucose, respectively. Cyanide production by harvested bacteria was measured as described in the Methods, in the presence of 2 mM glycine, 0.5 mM methionine and 25 μg/ml chloramphenicol.

in the presence of glycine and methionine. Addition of methionine to the growth medium had no effect on the ability of the harvested bacteria to form cyanide. In contrast, addition of glycine to the growth medium apparently partially reduced the ability of harvested bacteria to form cyanide, despite the fact that it was the substrate for cyanogenesis. These observations support our previous tentative conclusions that (a) methionine has a stimulatory rather than an inductive effect on cyanogenesis, and (b) glycine may partially repress formation of the cyanide-producing enzyme system (Collins *et al.*, 1980). Clearly a technique for obtaining cell-free extracts able to form cyanide is required to confirm or disprove these suppositions.

We have shown (Collins *et al.*, 1980) that glucose-grown cultures of *C. violaceum* formed less cyanide from glycine when it was the sole source of nitrogen than when NH_4Cl was also present in the growth medium. A similar effect has been noted with harvested cells (Table II). Harvested bacteria from cultures grown on glucose in the presence of glycine and methionine had about half the capacity to produce cyanide than did bacteria that had been grown on glutamate, glycine and methionine. Although this suggests some catabolite repression of cyanogenesis in the glucose-grown cultures, the level of cyanide formed during growth was similar (Collins *et al.*, 1980).

The effect of variation of glycine concentration on the rate of formation of cyanide by bacteria that had been grown on glutamate is shown in Fig. 2. The maximal rate

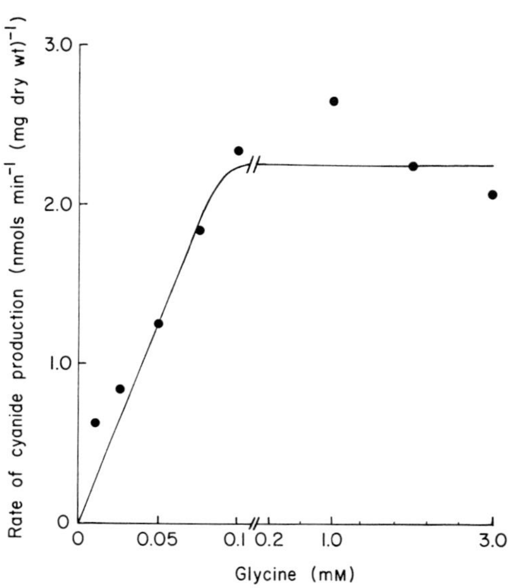

Fig. 2 The effect of variation of glycine concentration on the rate of production of cyanide by suspensions of *C. violaceum* that had been grown on glutamate.

of synthesis of cyanide was 2.2 nmoles/min/(mg dry wt) at a saturating concentration of glycine of about 2 x 10^{-4} M and half maximal activity at 4.4 x 10^{-5} M glycine. This compares with the "apparent K_M" of 5 x 10^{-4} M for glycine reported by Wissing (1974) for a *Pseudomonas* species. It should be remembered that the limiting factor could be something other than the cyanide-forming system, e.g. the affinity of a transport system for glycine entry into the bacteria. At low concentrations of added glycine about 70% of it was converted to cyanide (not shown), indicating that under these conditions cyanide is the principal metabolite. Wissing (1974) found a 1:1 ratio of glycine added to cyanide formed for his *Pseudomonas* species.

Cyanogenesis in growing cultures of *C. violaceum* occurred when threonine was used instead of glycine, presumably due to its conversion to glycine (Collins *et al.*, 1980). However, serine, which is metabolised to glycine and a carbon-one unit by serine hydroxymethyl-transferase (P.A. Collins and C.J. Knowles, unpub. obsv.), is a poor substitute for glycine. This trait was also seen with harvested bacteria (Fig. 3). Cyanide was produced at a similar rate from both glycine and threonine in the presence or absence of methionine. A similar rate of cyanogenesis was noted for the first few minutes after addition of serine plus methionine to the bacteria, but

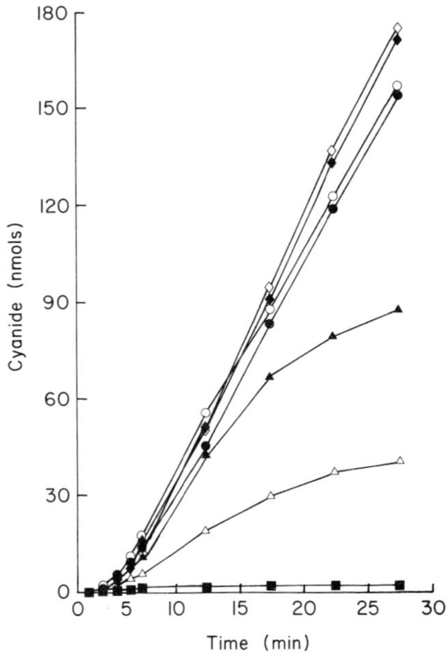

Fig. 3 The production of cyanide by suspensions of *C. violaceum* that had been grown on glutamate. At the start of the experiment 25 μg/ml chloramphenicol plus 2 mM threonine (◇), 2 mM threonine and 0.5 mM methionine (◆), 2 mM glycine (●), 2 mM glycine and 0.5 mM methionine (○), 2 mM serine (△), 2 mM serine and 0.5 mM methionine (▲). No additions (■).

the observed rate of cyanide formation soon decreased. A possible reason for this could have been its removal via β-cyanoalanine synthase (Rodgers and Knowles, 1978):

$$\text{serine} + HCN \rightarrow \beta\text{-cyanoalanine} + H_2O$$

Wissing (1974, 1975) showed that oxygen was required for cyanogenesis by a *Pseudomonas* species. Other electron acceptors, such as phenazine methosulfate (PMS), 2-6-dichlorophenolindophenol (DCIP) and methylene blue (MB), could replace oxygen to give a partial stimulation of cyanide formation. Figure 4 shows that little cyanide was produced from glycine by harvested suspensions of *C. violaceum* when they were incubated under anaerobic conditions. Initiation of continuous aeration of the bacteria resulted in an immediate, large stimulation of cyanogenesis. A small amount of cyanide was formed when a little PMS, DCIP or fumarate was added to the anaerobic bacteria, but nitrate was ineffective. Presumably more cyanide was not formed on addition of PMS, DCIP or fumarate as they were also reduced by other reactions.

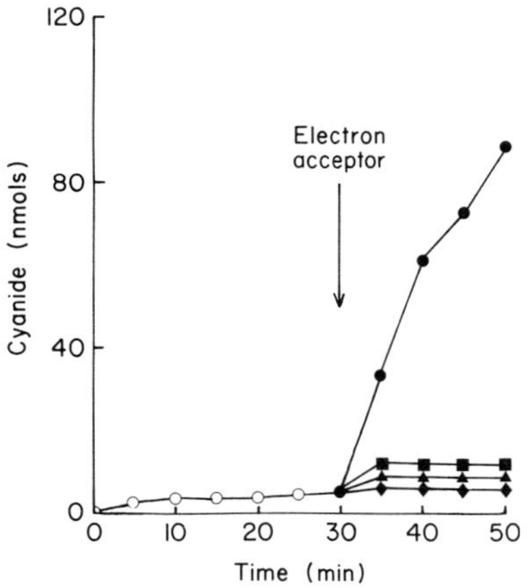

Fig. 4 The production of cyanide by suspensions of *C. violaceum* that had been grown on glutamate. At the start of the experiment 25 μg/ml chloramphenicol, 2 mM glycine and 0.5 mM methionine were added and the suspension incubated under a stream of nitrogen (0.8 litre/min). After 30 min the nitrogen was replaced by air (0.8 litre/min) (-●-) or 0.4 or 4 mM phenazine methosulfate (■), 0.4 mM 2,6-dichlorophenol indophenol (▲) or 10 mM fumarate (◆) was added with a continued flow of nitrogen.

This possibility is supported by the observation that addition of more PMS a few minutes later (not shown) caused an extra small amount of cyanide formation. This suggests that PMS, DCIP and fumarate can act as electron acceptors for cyanogenesis but very much less efficiently than oxygen.

There could be an indirect link between cyanogenesis and oxygen, i.e. the oxygen could be needed to promote respiration and hence stimulate metabolic activity in general. Since cyanide is more oxidised than glycine, an electron acceptor will be needed for cyanogenesis to occur, either with oxygen as the direct acceptor (via an oxygenase, peroxidase, etc.) or, as indicated by the above experiments, via linkage to the respiratory system.

The production of cyanide by anaerobic cultures of *C. violaceum* (Fig. 5) confirms that oxygen is not essential for cyanogenesis. The bacterium is unable to grow on glutamate under anaerobic conditions. With glucose as the carbon source, and either glycine plus NH_4Cl (Fig. 5a) or glycine (Fig. 5b) as the nitrogen sources, only low growth was observed unless fumarate was present as an electron acceptor. Nitrate was unable to act as an electron acceptor. In the culture containing NH_4Cl more cyanide was produced when glycine and methionine were present (Fig. 5c). Unlike aerobic cultures

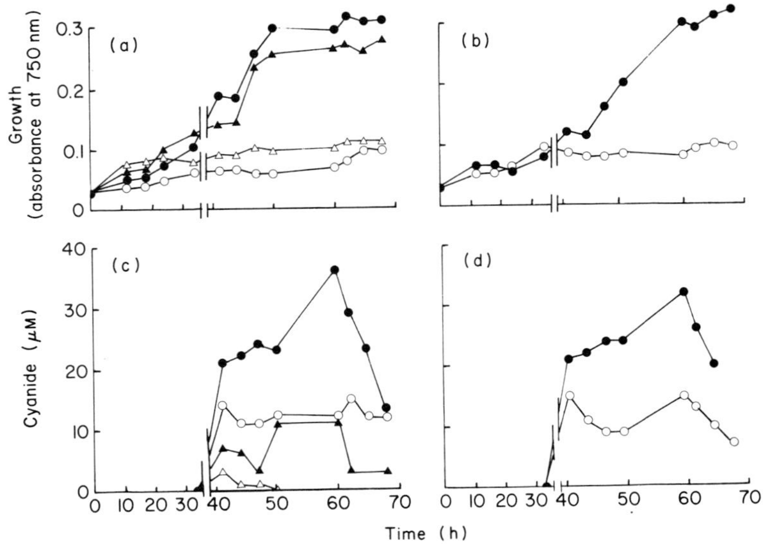

Fig. 5 Growth (a,b) and cyanide production (c,d) by cultures of *C. violaceum* incubated under anaerobic conditions on 20 mM glucose. In (a,c) the cultures contained 20 mM NH_4Cl, whereas in (b,d) no ammonium salt was present. The following were also added: 2 mM glycine, 0.5 mM methionine and 10 mM sodium fumarate (●); fumarate (▲); 2 mM glycine and 0.5 mM methionine (○); no further addition (△).

(Collins *et al.*, 1980), the use of glycine as the sole source of nitrogen did not substantially reduce the level of cyanide formation.

ACKNOWLEDGEMENTS

This work was supported by the Science Research Council via grant no. GR/A/11543 to C.J.K. We thank Dr A.W. Bunch and Dr P.B. Rodgers for helpful discussions.

REFERENCES

Bunch, A.W. and Knowles, C.J. (1980). *J. Gen. Microbiol.* 116, 9-16.
Castric, P.A. (1975). *Can. J. Microbiol.* 21, 613-618.
Castric, P.A. (1977). *J. Bacteriol.* 130, 826-831.
Castric, P.A., Ebert, R.F. and Castric, K.F. (1979). *Current Microbiol.* 2, 287-292.
Collins, P.A., Rodgers, P.B. and Knowles, C.J. (1980). *J. Gen. Microbiol.* 117, 73-80.

Epstein, J. (1947). *Anal. Chem.* 19, 272-274.
Knowles, C.J. (1976). *Bacteriol. Rev.* 40, 652-680.
Michaels, R. and Corpe, W.A. (1965). *J. Bacteriol.* 89, 106-112.
Pistorius, E.K., Gewitz, H.-S., Voss, H. and Vennesland, B. (1977). *Biochim. Biophys. Acta* 481, 384-394.
Pistorius, E.K., Jetschmann, K., Voss, H. and Vennesland, B. (1979). *Biochim. Biophys. Acta* 585, 630-642.
Rodgers, P.B. and Knowles, C.J. (1978). *J. Gen. Microbiol.* 108, 261-267.
Solomonson, L.P. and Spehar, A.M. (1977). *Nature* 265, 374-375.
Solomonson, L.P. and Spehar, A.M. (1979). *J. Biol. Chem.* 254, 2176-2179.
Ward, E.W.B. and Thorn, G.D. (1966). *Can. J. Bot.* 44, 95-104.
Ward, E.W.B., Thorn, G.D. and Starratt, A.N. (1971). *Can. J. Microbiol.* 17, 1061-1066.
Ward, E.W.B., Starratt, A.N. and Robinson, J.R. (1977). *Can. J. Bot.* 55, 2065-2069.
Wissing, F. (1968). *Physiol. Plant.* 21, 589-593.
Wissing, F. (1974). *J. Bacteriol.* 117, 1289-1294.
Wissing, F. (1975). *J. Bacteriol.* 121, 695-699.

CYANIDE DEGRADATION BY *CHROMOBACTERIUM VIOLACEUM*

PAUL B. RODGERS

*Group Research and Development,
Philip Lyle Memorial Research Laboratory,
The University, Whiteknights, Reading, Berks., England*

I. SUMMARY

Cyanide degradation was studied in cultures of *Chromobacterium violaceum* grown on L-glutamate, as sole carbon and nitrogen source, either alone or supplemented with glycine and/or L-methionine. *C. violaceum* had previously been shown to possess the cyanide-degrading enzymes β-cyanoalanine synthase, γ-cyano-α-aminobutyric acid synthase and rhodanese. The fate of degraded cyanide was followed through the use of radiolabelled cyanide. Radioactivity could be detected in β-cyanoalanine, which accumulated in the growth medium, but not in γ-cyano-α-aminobutyric acid or thiocyanate, suggesting that β-cyanoalanine synthase is the major route for cyanide degradation in this organism. Radioactivity could not be detected in possible metabolites of β-cyanoalanine, such as asparagine or aspartate, indicating that β-cyanoalanine formation is a pathway of cyanide degradation rather than cyanide utilisation. Formation of β-cyanoalanine by cultures grown on combinations of glutamate, glycine and methionine was quantified. Cultures grown under high cyanide-producing conditions, i.e. on glutamate plus glycine and methionine, produced the largest amount of β-cyanoalanine and the increase in β-cyanoalanine concentration of the growth medium correlated with a decrease in the cyanide concentration of the growth medium.

II. INTRODUCTION

Chromobacterium violaceum is one of a small number of bacteria that have been found to produce inorganic cyanide (see Castric, this volume). The substrate for cyanide production is glycine, and methionine stimulates the process through an unknown mechanism (Michaels and Corpe, 1965). Inclusion of glycine and L-methionine in the medium of *C.*

violaceum growing on L-glutamate as sole carbon and nitrogen source resulted in a six-fold stimulation of cyanide production (Rodgers and Knowles, 1978). Maximal cyanogenesis in growing cultures occurred during the transition from exponential growth to the stationary phase of growth, after which the cyanide content of the growth medium decreased (Rodgers and Knowles, 1978). This decrease in the cyanide concentration appears to be correlated with the induction of three cyanide-utilising enzymes in the early stationary phase of growth (Rodgers and Knowles, 1978). These enzymes are β-cyanoalanine synthase (EC 4.4.1.9), γ-cyano-α-aminobutyric acid synthase (EC 4.4.1) and rhodanese (EC 2.8.1.1, thiosulphate : cyanide sulphur-transferase). Prevention of induction of the cyanide-utilising enzymes had little effect on the level of cyanogenesis by *C. violaceum* but inhibited the decrease in the cyanide content of the medium, suggesting that this decrease is due to further metabolism of cyanide. However, this hypothesis is based on observations of the *in vitro* activities of the cyanide-utilising enzymes. The present study is an attempt to estimate the *in vivo* activities of these enzymes and to identify the products of cyanide degradation by *C. violaceum.*

III. MATERIALS AND METHODS

A. ORGANISM AND GROWTH CONDITIONS

Chromobacterium violaceum NCIB 9131 was grown aerobically at 30°C as described previously (Rodgers and Knowles, 1978).

B. IDENTIFICATION OF AMINO ACIDS PRESENT IN GROWTH MEDIA

Amino acids present in the growth medium were separated by cellulose or silica gel thin layer chromatography (Eastman Chromagram precoated plates). Samples of stationary phase cultures, from which bacteria had been removed by centrifugation, and of amino acid standards (1mM), were chromatographed. The volumes applied were 10μl of the media samples and 5μl of the standards. The solvent used for cellulose plates was methanol : pyridine : water (20 : 1 : 5 v/v) or acetone : pyridine : ammonia : water (30 : 45 : 5 : 20 v/v) whereas that for silica gel plates was n-propanol : 31.5% (w/w) ammonia (70 : 30 v/v). Plates were developed by spraying with 0.25% ninhydrin in acetone and heating at 110°C for 20 min.

C. DISTRIBUTION OF RADIOACTIVITY FROM RADIOLABELLED KCN

The distribution of radioactivity from labelled KCN was determined by addition of 4 μCi [^{14}C]-KCN (specific activity 1 μCi/μmole) to 100 ml bacterial cultures during the stationary phase of growth. At intervals 3ml samples were removed from the culture and the radioactivity present in bacteria and the medium, both as cyanide and its non-volatile products, was determined. A 1 ml aliquot of the culture sample was collected on a 0.45 μm Millipore filter and washed with 15 ml sterile growth medium. The filter was immersed in 0.5 ml water and mixed with 5 ml PCS scintillation fluid (Phase Combining System). Radioactivity was measured using a scintillation counter.

Bacteria were removed from the other 2 ml of the culture sample by centrifugation. The total amount of radioactivity present in the culture fluid was determined after mixing a 0.5 ml aliquot of the supernatant with 5 ml PCS. A further 1.0 ml of the supernatant was split into two fractions, one containing cyanide and the other its non-volatile derivatives. This was achieved by stirring the solution under a stream of air. Cyanide, and presumably any carbon dioxide dissolved in the medium, was trapped in 1.0 ml 1M NaOH. Radioactivity remaining in the medium after cyanide had been removed was measured after mixing 0.5 ml of the treated medium with 5 ml PCS. In order to measure the radioactivity present in the volatile fraction as cyanide, 0.5 ml of the NaOH trap was neutralised with 0.5 ml 1 M HCl, and 0.5 ml of the neutral solution mixed with 5 ml PCS (PCS is immiscible with aqueous solutions at alkaline pH values). If significant quantities of cyanide were being converted to carbon dioxide there would be little change in the amount of radioactivity in the NaOH trap. Because the radioactivity levels dropped at comparable rates to the fall in culture concentration of cyanide it was concluded that no significant conversion of cyanide to carbon dioxide was taking place.

D. INCORPORATION OF RADIOACTIVITY FROM RADIOLABELLED KCN INTO AMINO ACIDS

Incorporation of radioactivity from [^{14}C]-KCN into amino acids was measured by addition of 8μCi [^{14}C]-KCN (specific activity 1μCi/μmole) to cultures in the stationary phase of growth. The total radioactivity in the culture fluid and the distribution of this between the volatile and non-volatile fractions of the medium were determined as described above. The distribution of radioactivity between amino acids was measured by preparing dinitrophenyl (DNP) derivatives of the medium amino acids, separating them by silica gel thin layer chromatography and counting the radioactivity in the derivatives. Aliquots (100 μl) of cyanide-free medium were mixed with 10 μl 1M K_2CO_3 and 15 μl of a 10% (w/v) solution of 1-fluoro-2-dinitrobenzene in absolute ethanol, and incubated in the dark for 1h at 70°C. After cooling, the mixture was acidified with 50μl of concentrated HCl and the DNP-amino acids extracted with diethylether, thus separating the sample into organic and aqueous phases. The radioactivity in the aqueous phase was counted after diluting 25 μl samples to 0.5 ml with water and mixing with 5 ml PCS.

Ether was removed from the organic phase by aeration and the sample freeze-dried, followed by resuspension in 25 μl methanol. Three 5 μl aliquots were taken. One was diluted to 0.5 ml with water and its radioactivity measured after mixing with 5 ml PCS. The other two aliquots were applied to silica gel thin layer plates. One spot was scraped off immediately and its radioactivity counted after mixing with 0.5 ml water and 5 ml PCS; this allowed an estimation to be made of the amount of sample lost during the process of application to thin layer plates. The other spot was subjected to chromatography, using a solvent of chloroform : methanol : glacial acetic acid (85 : 13 : 2 v/v), after which sequential 1 cm squares were removed from the chromatogram and the amount of radioactivity in each square counted as above. Radioactive amino acids were identified by comparing those squares containing radioactivity with the position of DNP-amino acid standards run concurrently with the unknowns. Quenching of scintillation by DNP-amino acids, due to their bright yellow colour, was corrected by use of a quench curve.

E. β-CYANOALANINE ASSAY

The β-cyanoalanine content of culture growth media was assayed as follows. The growth medium amino acids were separated using silica gel thin layer chromatography as described above. The plate was developed by dipping in a mixture of 1% ninhydrin in acetone (100 vol) and a solution of 1 g cadmium acetate in 100 ml glacial acetic acid and 50 ml water (15 vol), and heating at 100°C for 5 min. Blue spots corresponding to β-cyanoalanine were scraped off into 1 ml absolute ethanol, left to stand for 30 min and centrifuged to remove silica gel. The absorbance of the solution was read at 640 nm and β-cyanoalanine content estimated by means of a standard curve constructed from β-cyano-alanine treated as outlined above.

F. OTHER ASSAYS

The method used for assay of β-cyanoalanine synthase in cell extracts was that of Hendrickson and Conn (1969), as modified by Rodgers and Knowles (1978). Cell extracts were prepared as described previously (Rodgers and Knowles, 1978). Cyanide was assayed by the method of Epstein (1947). Thiocynate was assayed by the methods of Epstein (1947) and Sorbo (1953).

G. CHEMICALS

Chloramphenicol and β-cyanoalanine were obtained from Sigma; [^{14}C]-KCN from the Radiochemical Centre, Amersham; PCS from Hopkin and Williams. Chloramphenicol was dissolved in water to a concentration of 25 μg/ml and filter sterilised using a 0.45 μm Millipore filter. Whenever possible, all other reagents were of analytical grade; glass-distilled water was used throughout.

IV. RESULTS AND DISCUSSIONS

The *in vivo* activities of the cyanide-utilising enzymes were studied by examining the distribution of radioactive products derived from [^{14}C]-KCN added to bacterial cultures. Preliminary experiments in which [^{14}C]-KCN was added to stationary phase cultures indicated that 59-85% of added cyanide was converted to non-volatile derivatives which accumulate in the growth medium (Table I). Less than 2% of

Table I Distribution of radioactivity from [^{14}C]-KCN added to stationary phase cultures (12h)of *C. violaceum*. The effect of adding 50 μg ml^{-1} chloramphenicol in late exponential phase (10 h).

Per cent total radioactivity in culture present as:

Growth medium	Chloramphenicol	Residual cyanide in medium	Non-volatile derivatives of cyanide in medium	Cell components
Glu, gly + met	-	9	85	1
Glu, gly + met	+	31	75	1
Glu	-	38	59	2
Glu	+	26	76	1

4μCi [^{14}C]-KCN were added and cultures incubated for 8 h before samples were taken for analysis of distribution of radioactivity. *C. violaceum* was grown on 10 mM L-glutamate, either alone or supplemented with 2 mM glycine and 0.5 mM L-methionine.

the total radioactivity was found in cells; indicating that there was little or no incorporation of the products of cyanide metabolism, or cyanide itself, into cellular components. Addition of chloramphenicol to cultures before [^{14}C]-KCN addition had only a small effect on the formation of non-volatile derivatives (Table I), despite the fact that addition of chloramphenicol at this point during growth inhibits induction of the three cyanide-utilising enzymes (Rodgers and Knowles, 1978). This failure of chloramphenicol to inhibit the conversion of cyanide to non-volatile derivatives is surprising, but may be due to non-specific reactions of cyanide with compounds excreted by stationary phase bacteria. For example, cyanide reacts readily with keto groups to form cyanohydrins. Such reacttions would be unaffected by a protein synthesis inhibitor.

Previous workers found that stationary phase *C. violaceum* cells resuspended in succinate, serine and [^{14}C]-KCN incorporated radioactivity into β-cyanoalanine and asparagine, both of which accumulated in the incubation medium (Brysk *et al.*, 1969). Radiolabelled aspartate was found in the cells, suggesting that cyanide is metabolised to aspartate via β-cyanoalanine and asparagine. Other experiments, in which washed, resuspended, early exponential phase *C. violaceum* cells were incubated with cyanide plus glycine, demonstrated an accumulation of γ-cyano-α-aminobutyric acid and β-cyanoalanine in the supernatant fluid (Brysk and Ressler, 1970).

In the present study β-cyanoalanine could be detected in the medium of cultures grown on glutamate supplemented with glycine and/or methionine, but not in cultures grown on glutamate alone. Asparagine, aspartate and γ-cyano-α-aminobutyric acid could not be detected in any growth media. Addition of [^{14}C]-KCN to stationary phase cultures grown on glutamate, either alone or supplemented with glycine and methionine (i.e. low and high cyanide producing conditions respectively), resulted in the accumulation of radioactivity in β-cyanoalanine present in the growth medium but not in any other amino acid (Fig. 1a and 1c). The addition of chloramphenicol before [^{14}C]-KCN addition, although it did not inhibit the conversion of cyanide to all non-volatile derivatives, inhibited the formation of β-cyanoalanine; particularly by bacteria grown under high cyanide producing conditions (Fig. 1b and 1d). This confirms the hypothesis made from earlier *in vitro* observations that the effect of chloramphenicol upon the cyanide content of the growth medium is mediated through an inhibition of cyanide utilisation (Rodgers and Knowles, 1978).

Failure to detect γ-cyano-α-aminobutyric acid and asparagine in growth media, taken with the lack of incorporation of radiolabel from [^{14}C]-KCN into cell components, suggests that β-cyanoalanine is the major product of cyanide degradation in the growth conditions used in the present study. This conclusion is strengthened by an inability to detect thiocyanate, a product of both the γ-cyano-α-aminobutyric acid synthase (Rassler *et al.*, 1973) and rhodanese reactions (Sorbo, 1953) in any growth media. It is suggested that cyanide is metabolised predominantly to β-cyanoalanine which accumulates in the growth medium and is not metabolised further to asparagine or aspartate. Consequently it is a path of cyanide degradation rather than one of cyanide assimilation into proteinaceous amino acids.

The production of β-cyanoalanine by cultures of *C. violaceum* was quantified (Fig. 2). In all growth media where β-cyanoalanine could be detected, the amino acid began to accumulate as the medium cyanide concentration reached a maximum, and peaked at a point in the stationary phase of

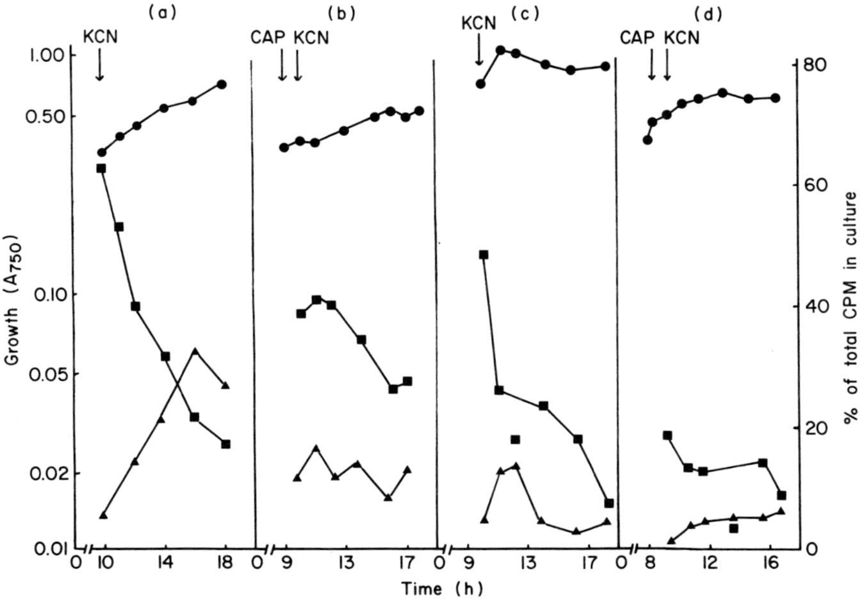

Fig. 1 Conversion of cyanide to β-cyanoalanine by cultures of *C. violaceum* growing on 10 mM L-glutamate, either alone (c,d) or supplemented with 2 mM glycine and 0.5 mM L-methionine (a,b), in the absence (a,c) or presence (b,d) of chloramphenicol (CAP). Growth (- ● -) and the percentage of total radioactivity present as cyanide (- ■ -) and β-cyanoalanine (- ▲ -) were followed. Fifty μg/ml CAP and 8 μCi [^{14}C]-KCN were added at the times indicated by the arrows.

growth when the cyanide concentration was essentially zero. Cultures grown on glutamate plus glycine and methionine accumulated the highest concentration of β-cyanoalanine (320 μM) which is considerably higher than the maximum concentration of cyanide (200 μM) attained by these cultures (Fig. 2c). This may indicate that cyanide is being converted to β-cyanoalanine at a faster rate than cyanide formation from glycine, consequently not all cyanide produced is detected.

Although no β-cyanoalanine could be detected in cultures grown on glutamate alone, [^{14}C]-KCN incorporation experiments indicated that some cyanide is converted to β-cyanoalanine by these cultures (Fig. 1c). Presumably the amount of β-cyanoalanine formed is below the detection limits of the assay (1 μM). In earlier experiments with cell extracts it was found that cells grown on glutamate alone had higher β-cyanoalanine synthase activity than cells grown on glutamate plus glycine and methionine (Rodgers and Knowles, 1978). The small amount of β-cyano-

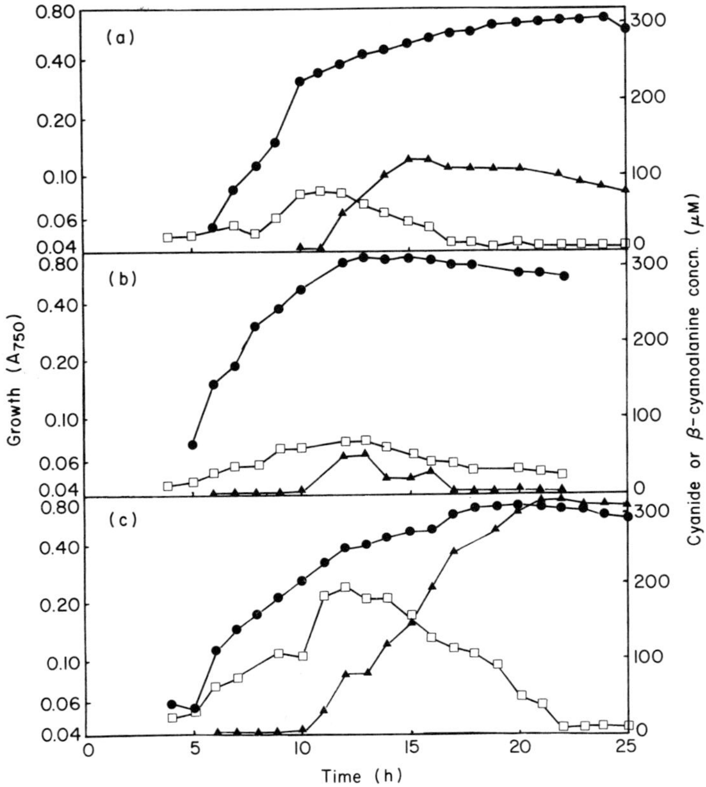

Fig. 2 Accumulation of cyanide and β-cyanoalanine in the medium of *C. violaceum* cultures growing on 10 mM L-glutamate supplemented with (a) 2 mM glycine, (b) 0.5 mM L-methionine, (c) 2 mM glycine and 0.5 mM L-methionine. Growth (- ● -), cyanide (- □ -) and β-cyanoalanine (- ▲ -) concentrations were followed.

alanine formed by cultures grown on glutamate alone, compared to those grown on glutamate plus glycine and methionine, is presumably due to the very low concentrations of cyanide produced by the former cultures.

The concentration of cyanide produced by cultures grown on glutamate and glycine or glutamate and methionine is similar (around 70 μM) but the concentration of β-cyanoalanine accumulated by the former cultures is 120 μM compared to 50 μM by the latter cultures (Fig. 2a and b). Experiments with cell extracts show that methionine inhibits β-cyanoalanine synthase by up to 80% (Fig. 3) whereas identical concentrations of glycine do not inhibit the enzyme. This phenomenon may provide an explanation for the difference in β-cyanoalanine production between cultures grown

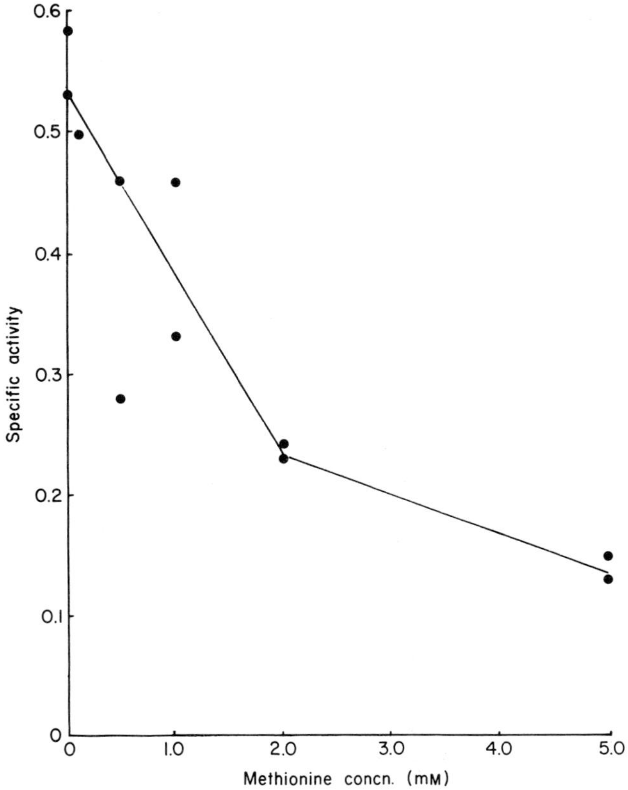

Fig. 3 Effect of methionine on β-cyanoalanine synthase activity of *C. violaceum* extracts. Extracts were prepared from stationary phase cells grown on 10 mM L-glutamate alone. Specific activity units - nmoles H_2S produced/min/(mg protein).

on glutamate and glycine or glutamate and methionine. Cultures grown under high cyanide producing conditions produce elevated amounts of β-cyanoalanine despite the presence of methionine (Fig. 2c). In these cultures, despite the partial inhibitory effect of methionine on β-cyanoalanine synthase, the higher level of β-cyanoalanine may be due to the much higher concentration of cyanide present.

This study suggests that β-cyanoalanine is the major product of cyanide degradation by *C. violaceum* grown on glutamate supplemented with glycine and/or methionine. The concentration of cyanide accumulating in cultures of cyanogenic bacteria is a function of the relative rates of cyanide synthesis and degradation (plus of course volatilisation), a fact not always taken into account during studies on cyanide biosynthesis. Factors which decrease the rate of cyanide degradation, such as chloramphenicol or methionine, may appear to stimulate cyanide production by bacterial cultures. Indeed, the addition of 0.5 mM L-methionine to late exponential phase cultures of *C. violaceum* growing on glutamate, either alone or supplemented with glycine, causes a two-fold increase in the maximum concentration of cyanide accumulated by these cultures (Rodgers, 1978). This is not to say that the stimulatory effect of methionine on cyanide production is wholly explained by its inhibitory effect on β-cyanoalanine synthase.

Little is known about the enzymology of the β-cyanoalanine synthase from *C. violaceum*. The enzyme has been purified from higher plants where the substrate for the reaction has been shown to be L-cysteine (Hendrickson and Conn, 1969; Akopyan and Goryachenkova, 1976). The substrate for the bacterial enzyme is not known. In two acyanogenic bacteria, *Escherichia coli* and *Bacillus megaterium*, which contain β-cyanoalanine synthase activities, these reactions have been shown to be secondary activities of enzymes of the cysteine biosynthetic pathway (Dunnill and Fowden, 1965; Castric and Conn, 1971). Recent work suggests that the substrate for *C. violaceum* β-cyanoalanine synthase is either L-serine or *O*-acetyl-L-serine rather than L-cysteine (P. B. Rodgers, unpubl. obs.).

ACKNOWLEDGEMENTS

I wish to thank Drs Chris Knowles and Alan Bunch for many useful discussions.

REFERENCES

Akopyan, T.N. and Goryachenkova, E.V. (1976). *Biochem. (Biokhimiya)* 41, 746-753.

Brysk, M.M., Corpe, W.A. and Hankes, L.V. (1969). *L. Bact.* 97, 322-327.

Brysk, M.M. and Ressler, C. (1970). *J. Biol. Chem.* 245, 1156-1160.

Castric, P.A. and Conn, E.E. (1971). *J. Bact.* 108, 132-136.

Dunnill, P.M. and Fowden, L. (1965). *Nature* 208, 1206-1207.

Epstein, J. (1947). *Analyt. Chem.* 19, 272-274.

Hendrickson, H.R. and Conn, E.E. (1969). *J. Biol. Chem.* 244, 2632-2640.

Michaels, R. and Corpe, W.A. (1965). *J. Bact.* 89, 106-112.

Ressler, C., Abe, O., Kondo, Y., Cottrell, B. and Abe, K. (1973). *Biochem.* 12, 5369-5377.

Rodgers, P.B. (1978). *Ph.D. Thesis*, University of Kent, Canterbury, U.K.

Rodgers, P.B. and Knowles, C.J. (1978). *J. Gen. Microbiol.* 108, 261-267.

Sörbo, B.H. (1953). *Acta Chem. Scand.* 7, 1129-1136.

THE EFFECT OF GROWTH CONDITIONS ON CYANOGENESIS BY THE SNOW MOULD FUNGUS

ALAN W. BUNCH and CHRISTOPHER J. KNOWLES

Biological Laboratory, University of Kent, Canterbury CT2 7NJ, England

I. SUMMARY

Cyanide is produced from glycine when the snow mould basidiomycete is grown in a medium containing glycine and either acetate or glucose as the carbon and energy source. In the glucose containing medium cyanide is produced from the methylene carbon of glycine and appears at the end of the growth phase. Carbon dioxide is formed from the carboxyl group of glycine both during growth and the period of cyanogenesis (Bunch and Knowles, 1980). In contrast, in the acetate-containing medium cyanide is derived from both the methylene and carboxyl groups of glycine, and cyanide is formed throughout the growth of the culture. Little CO_2 is formed from glycine. In a medium containing both glucose and acetate, the glucose is utilised before the acetate and cyanogenesis commences coincident with the utilisation of acetate. Addition of the potential methyl-group donors, betaine and N,N-dimethylglycine to the glucose plus glycine-containing medium partially represses growth and shifts cyanogenesis to the growth phase. Their addition to a medium containing only glucose has no effect on growth or cyanogenesis.

II. INTRODUCTION

Microbial metabolism can be separated into primary and secondary metabolism. Secondary metabolite production by batch cultures has several typical characteristics (Drew and Demain, 1977; Weinberg, 1977, 1978). Most of these characteristics are exhibited during cyanide production by the snow mould fungus (Ward and Thorn, 1966; Bunch and Knowles, 1980) and other cyanogenic microorganisms (Wissing, 1968; Castric, 1975; Rodgers and Knowles, 1978; see also Knowles, 1976; Castric, this volume).

The most noticeable feature of secondary metabolite synthesis is that they are usually produced towards the end of the growth phase of batch cultures, i.e. during the idiophase. It has been proposed that this reflects repression or inhibition of the enzymes involved in secondary metabolism by the catabolism of rapidly utilised carbon sources such as glucose (Demain *et al.*, 1979).

Cyanide production during batch culture of the snow mould fungus with glucose as the carbon source occurs only during the idiophase even when stimulated by the inclusion of glycine, the precursor of cyanide, in the growth medium (Bunch and Knowles, 1980). The C-1 atom of glycine is converted to CO_2 both during growth (the trophophase) and in the idiophase, whereas the C-2 atom is catabolised to cyanide only during the idiophase. Little cyanide is produced from the C-1 atom of glycine, or CO_2 from the C-2 atom (Bunch and Knowles, 1980).

When the snow mould is grown on the less rapidly utilised carbon source, acetate, cyanide production occurs both during the trophophase and the idiophase. The inclusion of glycine in the medium stimulates cyanide production throughout the incubation(Bunch and Knowles, 1980).

In this paper we report that there are other factors that affect the onset of cyanogenesis by glucose and acetate-containing cultures of the snow mould. The significance of cyanide catabolism to CO_2 during growth of acetate-containing cultures is also assessed.

III. METHODS

A. GROWTH OF SNOW MOULD FUNGUS

The W_2 isolate of the snow mould fungus was obtained from Dr E. W. B. Ward. It was grown in shake cultures in the defined medium described by Ward and Thorn (1966), except that the carbon source was either 10 mM glucose or 30 mM acetate. Vitamins and amino acids were filter sterilised. Growth conditions and inoculum preparation were as described previously (Bunch and Knowles, 1980). Glucose was measured by the glucose oxidase method (Niven *et al.*, 1977) and acetate by the procedure of Holt and Bergmeyer (1974). Cyanide present in the growth medium was assayed by the method of Epstein (1947).

B. METABOLISM OF [^{14}C] GLYCINE.

Cultures (50 ml) were grown with 30 mM acetate plus 10 mM glycine, to which was added 10 μCi of either [1-^{14}C] glycine (56 mCi mmol^{-1}) or [2-^{14}C] glycine (54 mCi/mmol) in a flask fitted with a centre well. After a fixed period the rate of $H^{14}CN$ and $^{14}CO_2$ production was measured, together with residual [1 or 2-^{14}C] glycine concentration, as described earlier (Bunch and Knowles, 1980).

C. METABOLISM OF $K^{14}CN$.

The ability of the snow mould fungus to metabolise cyanide to CO_2 was determined after transferring cultures (50 ml) to small conical flasks fitted with a centre well. To the main compartment of each flask was added 2μCi $K^{14}CN$ (59.3 mCi/mmd) and to the centre well 1 ml 4M KOH. The flasks were stoppered and incubated for 24 h at 15°C on an orbital shaker at 275 rev./min. Radioactive CO_2 and cyanide in the centre well and the growth medium were then assayed (Bunch and Knowles, 1980).

D. MATERIALS

Radioactive chemicals were obtained from the Radiochemical Centre, Amersham. Radioactive glycine was checked for purity by thin layer chromatography (t.l.c.) in butanol/water/acetic acid (120 : 50 : 30 by vol.). Radiolabelled cyanide was checked for purity by t.l.c. in butanol saturated with water (Oró and Kiball, 1962). Phase combining system (PCS) was obtained from Amersham Corp., Arlington Heights, Ill., U.S.A. Wherever possible all other reagents were of analytical grade; glass-distilled water was used throughout.

IV. RESULTS

In previous studies it was shown that cyanide was produced only during the idiophase by cultures of the snow mould fungus grown in a medium containing 10 mM glucose as the carbon source, in the presence (Fig. 1a) or absence (Fig. 1b) of 10 mM glycine (Bunch and Knowles, 1980). The maximum growth yield of the 50 ml cultures was 60-70 mg. dry wt of fungus. Growth ceased due to depletion of glucose from the medium. Glycine could not be used as a carbon source. When 30 mM acetate replaced glucose as the carbon source in the presence (Fig. 1c) or absence (Fig. 1d) of 10 mM glycine, cyanide production occurred both during the trophophase and the idiophase. The maximum yield (40-45 mg. dry wt) of the 50 ml cultures was lower than the glucose-grown cultures and neither acetate nor the nitrogen source, asparagine, was completely depleted from the medium at the time when growth stopped.

The presence of either 10 mM betaine (Fig. 2a) or 10 mM N,N-dimethylglycine (Fig. 2b) in media containing 10 mM glucose and 10 mM glycine resulted in a reduction in the maximum fungal yield of the 50 ml cultures, as well as causing cyanide production throughout the trophophase and the idiophase. Neither betaine nor N,N-dimethylglycine had any effect on growth or cyanogenesis when glycine was absent from the glucose-containing medium. For clarity the amount of cyanide lost by volatilisation is not shown, but is proportional to the concentration of cyanide in the growth medium (see Bunch and Knowles, 1980).

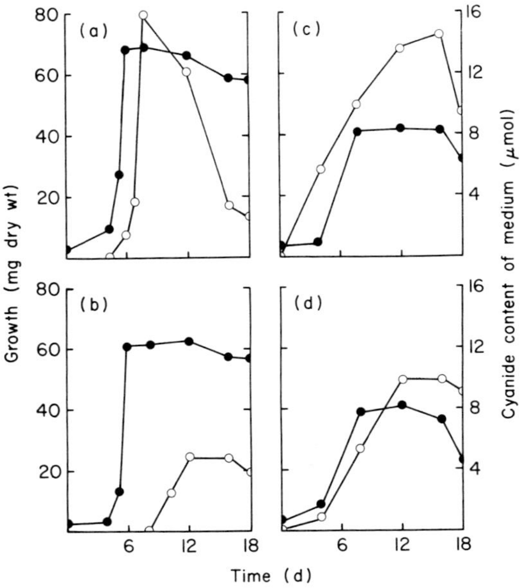

Fig. 1 The formation of cyanide during growth on 10 mM glucose (a,b) or 30 mM acetate (c,d) in the presence (a,c) or absence (b,d) of 10 mM glycine. The changes in culture dry wt (-●-) and cyanide concent of the growth medium (-○-) are given for 50 ml cultures. From Bunch and Knowles, (1980); diagrams reproduced by courtesy of the *Journal of General Microbiology*.

Cultures (50 ml) of the snow mould fungus grown in a medium containing both 10 mM glucose and 30 mM acetate started to produce cyanide 8d after inoculation, when all the glucose had been depleted from the medium (Fig. 3). Acetate began to be used only after the glucose had been consumed. It continued to be used until 12d., despite growth terminating 10d after inoculation. No correlation was evident between the pH of the medium and cyanide formation.

It has been shown that the C-2 atom of glycine rather than the C-1 atom is incorporated into cyanide without breakage of the carbon-nitrogen bond, for cultures of the snow mould fungus grown in the glucose-containing medium (Ward *et al.*, 1977; Bunch and Knowles, 1980). However, metabolism of glycine during growth of acetate-containing cultures resulted in equal amounts of $H^{14}CN$ being produced from either [1-^{14}C] or [2-^{14}C] glycine (Fig. 4). Unlike the glucose-containing cultures (Bunch and Knowles, 1980), the acetate-containing cultures caused little formation of $^{14}CO_2$ from [1-^{14}C] or [2-^{14}C] glycine (Fig. 4).

We have previously shown that cyanide is degraded to CO_2 by glucose-containing cultures, with maximal activity

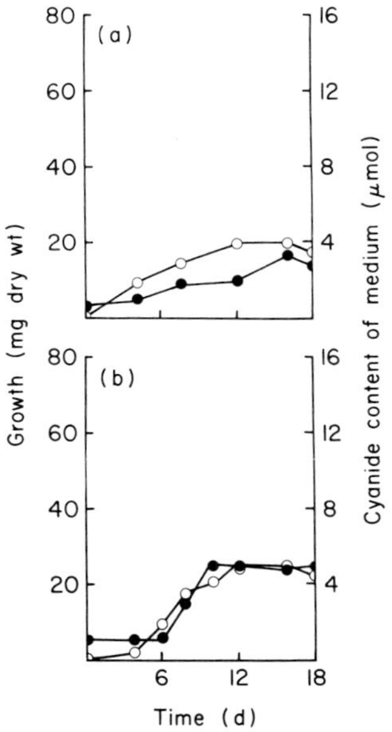

Fig. 2 The formation of cyanide (-○-) during growth (-●-) of 50 ml cultures on 10 mM glucose in the presence of 10 mM glycine and either 10 mM betaine (a) or 10 mM N,N-dimethylglycine (b).

in the idiophase, coincident with the optimal cyanide-producing activity (Bunch and Knowles, 1980). In contrast, the production of CO_2 from cyanide was maximal during the early stages of growth by cultures grown with acetate as the carbon source, not during the period of maximum cyanide production (Fig. 5). Only very small amounts of $H^{14}CN$ were incorporated into alanine, glutamate, β-cyanoalanine and formamide (< 1%). Of the total amount of radioactivity taken up by the fungal cells (< 1% of the total radioactivity) most (80%) was recovered as cyanide.

V. DISCUSSION

The work presented in this and the previous paper (Bunch and Knowles, 1980) reveals wide differences in the metabolism of cyanide by the snow mould fungus, depending on the growth conditions. Thus cyanide is produced only at the end of the growth phase when glucose is the carbon source, but both during and after growth on acetate. Inclusion of other compounds in the growth medium can also be important. Addition of betaine or N,N-dimethylglycine to cultures containing glucose and glycine causes a shift in cyanogenesis to the growth phase, as well as partially inhibiting growth. It is noteworthy that betaine and N,N-dimethylglycine, like methionine (which is a stimula-

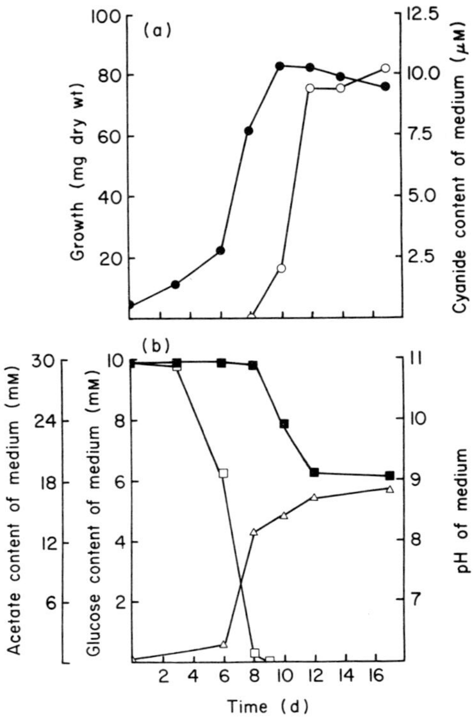

Fig. 3 Growth (-●-), cyanide (-○-) and pH (-△-), acetate (-■-) or glucose (-□-) content of the medium for a 50 ml culture growing on 10 mM glucose plus 30 mM acetate.

tor of bacterial cyanogenesis, Rodgers and Knowles, 1978; Collins, Rodgers and Knowles, 1980), require carbon-one units for their synthesis. Moreover, they can also act as methyl-group donors. It seems likely therefore that microbial cyanogenesis is closely associated with carbon-one as well as glycine metabolism.

Cyanide production by cultures containing both glucose and acetate begins only after glucose has been utilised (Fig. 3). This would seem to indicate catabolite repression of cyanogenesis by glucose (*cf.* Demain *et al.*, 1979). However, there is an alternative possibility which could also account for the effects of betaine and N,N-dimethylglycine. The different patterns of cyanide formation observed (Figs. 1, 2, 3) could reflect varying pathways and rates of demand for glycine depending on the growth conditions. In addition, the pathway of glycine (and serine) production could also affect the provision of carbon-one units via the tetrahydrofolate pool. Cyanogenesis would then be a method for removal of excess glycine, or serve either to prevent over or under provision of carbon-one units.

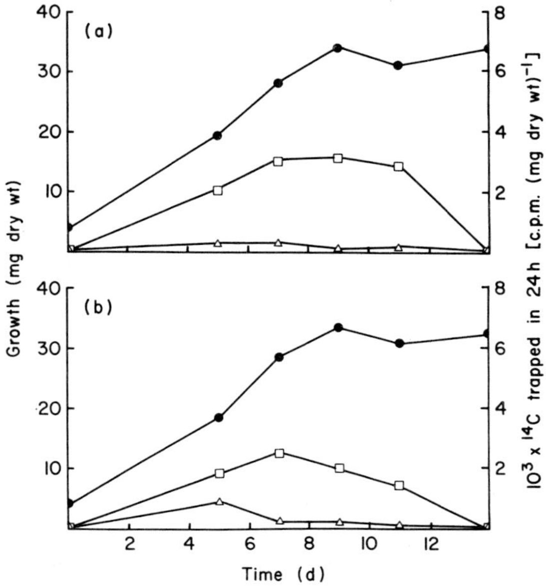

Fig. 4 Metabolism of [2-^{14}C] glycine (a) or [1-^{14}C] glycine (b) during growth of a 50 ml culture on 30 mM acetate plus 10 mM glycine Growth (-●-) $^{14}CO_2$ production (-Δ-) and $H^{14}CN$ production (-□-). Each point represents the total ^{14}C trapped during the previous 24h.

The metabolism of glycine appears to be different in media containing glucose or acetate plus glycine. In the former case CO_2 is produced from the carboxyl carbon of glycine (Bunch and Knowles, 1980) whereas on acetate plus glycine little CO_2 is released into the medium (Fig. 4). This could reflect a greater reequirement for CO_2 for growth of the fungi on acetate. This possibility is perhaps supported by the capacity of acetate plus glycine grown fungi to produce CO_2 from cyanide during the growth phase (Fig. 5). A further difference in the metabolism of glycine under the different growth conditions is that cyanide is produced only from the methylene carbon of glycine during growth on glucose plus glycine but from both the methylene and carboxyl carbons of glycine during growth on acetate plus glycine. The latter observation suggests that a symmetrical intermediate is formed. One possibility could be the reversible conversion of glycine to oxalate via glyoxylate.

When many microorganisms are grown on acetate as their source of carbon and energy they induce the enzymes of the glyoxylate cycle as the major catabolic pathway (Kornberg, 1966). If this occurs in the snow mould fungus, glycine could be produced by amination of glyoxylate.

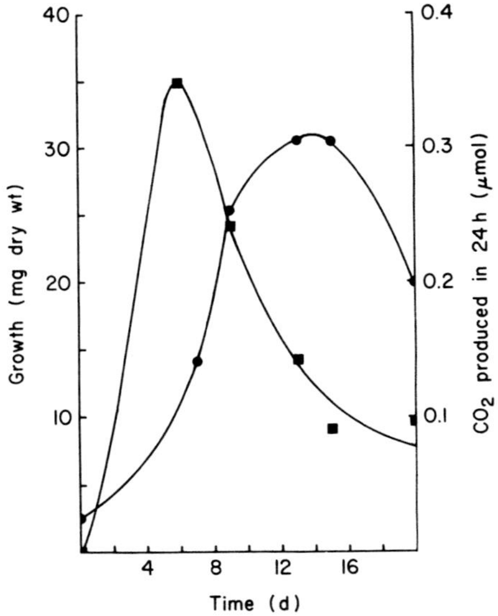

Fig. 5 The production of $^{14}CO_2$ from [^{14}C] cyanide by 50 ml cultures grown in media containing 30 mM acetate. Growth (-●-) and the rate of $^{14}CO_2$ production from $K^{14}CN$ (- ■ -) added 24h prior to the time shown.

Carbon-one units would then have to be derived in some manner other than the usual route of conversion of serine to glycine and methylene tetrahydrofolate (which could be operating during growth on glucose). A likely route would be conversion of glyoxylate to oxalate and formate, thereby explaining the randomisation of the radioactivity during conversion of glycine to cyanide during growth on acetate.

ACKNOWLEDGEMENTS

This work was supported by the Science Research Council via a Ph.D. studentship to A. W. Bunch and grants No. GR/A/11543 and GR/A/79598 to C. J. Knowles.

REFERENCES

Bunch, A.W. and Knowles, C.J. (1980). *J. Gen. Microbiol.* 116, 9-16.

Castric, P.A. (1975). *Can. J. Microbiol.* 21, 613-618.

Collins, P.A., Rodgers, P.B. and Knowles, C.J. (1980). *J. Gen. Microbiol.* 117, 73-80.

Demain, A.L., Kennel, Y.M. and Aharonowitz, Y. (1979). *Symp. Soc. Gen. Microbiol.* 29, 163-185.

Drew, S.W. and Demain, A.L. (1977). *Ann. Rev. Microbiol.* 31, 343-356.

Epstein, J. (1947). *Anal. Chem.* 19, 272-274.

Holt, G. and Bergmeyer, H.U. (1974). *In* "Methods of Enzymatic Analysis", (H. U. Bergmeyer, Ed.), 2nd edn., p.1528-1532. Academic Press, New York and London.

Knowles, C.J. (1976). *Bacteriol. Rev.* 40, 652-680.

Kornberg, H.L. (1966). *Essays in Biochemistry.* 2, 1-31.

Niven, D.F., Collins, P.A. and Knowles, C.J. (1977). *J. Gen. Microbiol.* 98, 95-108.

Oró, J. and Kiball, A.P. (1962). *Arch. Biochem. Biophys.* 96, 293-313.

Rodgers, P.B. and Knowles, C.J. (1978). *J. Gen. Microbiol.* 108, 261-267.

Ward, E.W.B. and Thorn, G.D. (1966). *Can. J. Bot.* 44, 95-104.

Weinberg, E.D. (1977). *In* "Microorganisms and Minerals", (Weinberg, E.D., ed.), p.289-316. Marcel Dekker, New York.

Weinberg, E.D. (1978). *Folia Microbiol.* 23, 496-504.

Wissing, F. (1968). *Physiol. Plant.* 21, 589-593.

HYDROGEN CYANIDE METABOLISM BY FUNGAL PATHOGENS OF CYANOGENIC PLANTS

WILLIAM E. FRY and DONALD F. MYERS*

Department of Plant Pathology, Cornell University, Ithaca, New York 14853, U.S.A.

I. HYDROGEN CYANIDE AND PLANT DISEASE

The survival value to microorganisms of HCN metabolizing pathways is not yet well defined (Knowles, 1976). These pathways are presumably important in environments where HCN is found in significant concentrations. Diseased cyanogenic plants provide such an environment, and are potentially useful for studying the significance of these pathways. When a cyanogenic plant is stressed, such as during the development of disease, HCN is released due to the degradation of cyanogenic glycosides (Conn, 1973; Millar and Higgins, 1970). The released HCN might interact with the pathogen and/or it might interact with host plant cells and thereby cause or contribute to the symptoms of toxicity observed. HCN produced as a result of snow mould of alfalfa apparently contributes to symptoms on alfalfa (see Bunch and Knowles, this volume; Colotelo and Ward, 1961 and Lebeau and Dickson, 1955). It is the nature of the interaction between HCN and various fungi during pathogenesis of cyanogenic plant tissues that is the subject of this review.

To a plant pathologist, knowledge of the mechanism by which a pathogen copes with HCN is an intriguing objective because it may help us to understand why some fungi are able to cause disease in cyanogenic plants while others are not. There have been two general approaches to studying the role of HCN in disease. The first approach has been to study an incompatible interaction (the resistant interaction) and to test the hypothesis that incompatibility is due in part to an inhibitor (e.g. HCN). The second approach has been to study a compatible interaction (the susceptible interaction) and test the hypothesis

*Present address: Department of Plant Pathology, University of California, Davis, CA 95616, U.S.A.

that a mechanism which enables a pathogen to cope with HCN functions *in vivo* and is necessary for pathogenicity or virulence.

For at least 50 years plant pathologists have considered the first approach and speculated that the resistance of cyanogenic plants to certain microbial pathogens may be related to the plant's HCN content (Robinson, 1930; Timonin, 1941; Reynolds, 1924). They hypothesized that plants containing higher levels of cyanogenic glycosides should be more disease-resistant than plants containing lower levels of glycosides. Indeed, some researchers have found positive correlations between high levels of cyanogenic glycosides and disease resistance in some host-parasite interactions (Snyder, 1950; Wilkinson and Millar, 1978). However, others have not found positive correlations. For example, Trione (1960) was unable to associate resistance to *Fusarium oxysporum* f. sp. *lini* in flax to high levels of cyanogenic glycosides. We suggest that this approach may not be particularly useful because the microorganisms in these compatible interactions have probably developed mechanisms to cope with the HCN in their environments.

In the late 1960s Millar and coworkers (Millar and Higgins, 1970; Fry and Millar, 1971a; Fry and Millar, 1971b) began an investigation of the second approach by testing the relative HCN tolerance of pathogens of cyanogenic and noncyanogenic plants. By determining the ability of four *Stemphylium* species to grow in HCN-containing media, they showed that *Stemphylium loti*, a pathogen of the cyanogenic plant *Lotus corniculatus*, was more tolerant to HCN than other *Stemphylium* species pathogenic on noncyanogenic or weakly cyanogenic plants. However, when the immediate response to HCN was determined, *S. loti* appeared as sensitive to HCN as the nontolerant fungi. Tolerance was induced by exposing the fungus to minute concentrations of HCN (0.1-1.0 mM). Once adapted, *S. loti* was insensitive to HCN concentrations of 25 mM, while other species remained sensitive. Subsequently, it was learned that tolerance to HCN could be induced in many fungi (Fry and Evans, 1977).

II. MECHANISMS OF HCN TOLERANCE IN FUNGI

The enhanced tolerance to HCN in fungal pathogens of cyanogenic plants was associated with their ability to metabolize HCN (Fry and Millar, 1971b). Although the mechanism of tolerance in these fungi was unknown initially, a variety of mechanisms had been identified previously in other microorganisms. Some fungi incorporated HCN into amino acids such as alanine, glutamate and asparagine (Strobel, 1964; Allen and Strobel, 1966). *Fusarium solani* converted HCN to ammonia enzymatically and presumably also to carbon dioxide (Shimizu and Taguchi, 1969). *Rhizoctonia solani* incorporated HCN into propionaldehyde to yield α-amino-butyronitrile and α-aminobutyric acid (Mundy *et al.*, 1973). Another candidate for HCN metabolism was β-cyanoalanine synthase, which occurs commonly in higher plants and some bacteria and catalyzes the formation of β-cyanoalanine and hydrogen sulfide from HCN and cysteine (Akopyan *et al.*, 1975; Dunnill and Fowden, 1965). Finally rhodanese, which catalyses the metabolism of HCN to thiocyanate in the presence of a sulfur donor, is widely distributed among organisms (Westley, 1973) and might enable fungi to detoxify HCN.

To identify the mechanism of HCN metabolism in *S. loti*, ^{14}C-labelled HCN was fed to conidia (Fry and Millar, 1972). After adaptation for 2 h in 0.1 mM KCN, *S. loti* spores could metabolize all HCN within a 2 mM solution. Most of the ^{14}C remained in the supernatant and negligible counts were found in the conidia themselves or in the CO_2 formed by the conidia. The labelled product was uncharged, insoluble in organic solvents, slightly volatile, and difficult to separate from water. Base hydrolysis of the product yielded ammonia. The hydrolosis product was distilled at acid pH, trapped in a mild base, dried, and the infra-red spectrum of the hydrolysis product was obtained. This spectrum and that of standard sodium formate were identical (Fry and Millar, 1972), suggesting that formamide was the product of HCN metabolism. Cell-free extracts of adapted conidia of *S. loti* could accomplish the same reaction. The new enzyme activity was named formamide hydrolyase (FHL).

III. CHARACTERISTICS AND PURIFICATION OF FORMAMIDE HYDROLYASE

Conversion of HCN to formamide has a 1 : 1 stoichiometry and is observed whether the reaction is catalyzed by extracted enzyme or by whole conidia (Fry and Millar, 1972; Fry and Munch, 1975). The equilibrium for the reaction appears to be directed towards formamide, because HCN production has not been detected after incubating the enzyme with formamide under various conditions (Fry, unpublished). The pH optimum for enzyme activity is between pH 7 and pH 9 and the enzyme has an estimated K_m of 27 mM (Fry and Munch, 1975). Further fungal metabolism of formamide has not been observed (Fry and Myers, unpublished).

Initial attempts to purify FHL were not particularly successful (Fry and Millar, 1972; Fry and Munch, 1975). The enzyme was inactivated during ammonium sulfate fractionation, but could be concentrated by ultrafiltration. Although the enzyme passed through a column of Sephadex G-100 in the void volume and was absorbed onto DEAE Sephadex, relatively little purification was accomplished. Because the enzyme was at least partially excluded in Biogel A1 5M, which purportedly has an exclusion limit of 15 million daltons, its activity may be associated with a membrane or particle (Fig. 1). This possibility was ex-

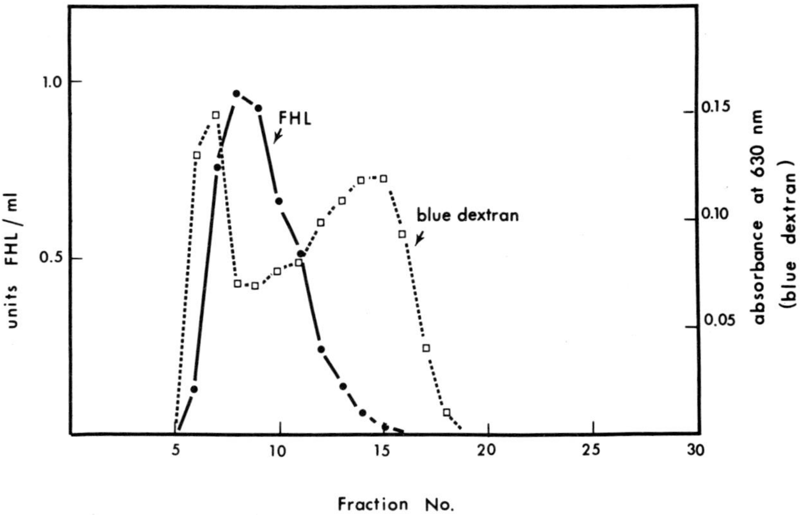

Fig. 1 Elution pattern of formamide hydro-lyase through a column of Bio-Gel A-15 M. Column size was 1.5 × 43.5 cm, and the eluant was collected in 3.3 ml fractions. The first appearance of Blue Dextran 2000 (average molecular weight of 2,000,000) indicates the void volume of the column. The amount of protein detectable in the fractions was below the limits of protein estimation. Data are from Fry and Munch (1975).

plored further by centrifugation and detergent separation techniques. Although the enzyme remained soluble after centrifugation at 100,000 g for 90 min, it was pelleted in an isotonic medium after centrifugation at 200,000 g for 200 min (Table I). Efforts to separate enzyme activi-

Table I Location of FHL activity in fractions of homogenates of HCN-induced *Gloeocercospora sorghi* after differential centrifugation.

Source			FHL Activity
1,000 × g	20 min.	Pellet	0.47
10,000 × g	20 min.	Pellet	0.35
30,000 × g	30 min.	Pellet	0.84
200,000 × g	200 min.	Pellet	18.40
200,000 × g	200 min.	Supernatant	0.89

ty from the large molecular weight moiety with mild detergents such as Triton have been unsuccessful. Thus its molecular weight and possible association with a particle or membrane remain to be determined.

The enzyme is quite stable, retaining activity for days at room temperature, for weeks at 4 C and for months when frozen. Activity of FHL was unaffected by EDTA, mercaptoethanol and thiocyanate, but was inhibited at concentrations of 10 mM fluoride and azide.

IV. INDUCTION AND REGULATION OF FORMAMIDE HYDROLYASE

The effect of formamide on induction of FHL was also determined (Fry *et al.*, unpublished). Mycelium of *Gloeocercospora sorghi* (a fungus which produces large quantities of FHL when adapted to HCN) was incubated with different concentrations of formamide with or without 1.0 mM HCN (Fig. 2). Instead of repressing enzyme induction as might be ex-

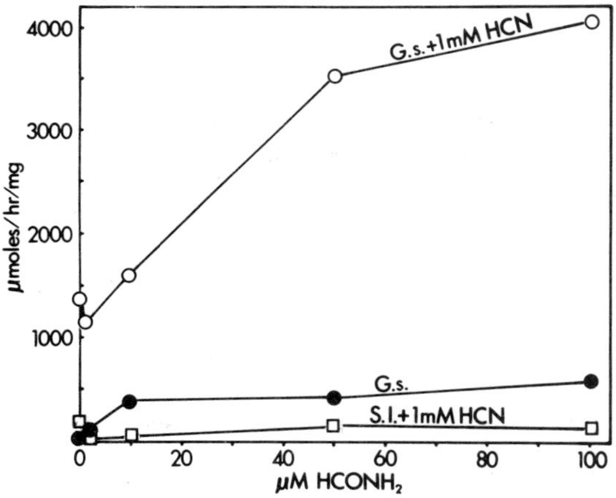

Fig. 2 Activities of formamide hydro-lyase produced by *Gloeocercospora sorghi* and *Stemphylium loti* with and without HCN in increasing concentrations of formamide. No FHL was detected in *S. loti* in the absence of HCN.

pected, formamide enhanced the amount of FHL produced by *G. sorghi* either in the presence or absence of HCN. Similar results were obtained with *S. loti*.

Although HCN was always an efficient inducer of FHL (Table II), the enzyme was apparently not regulated in an identical way in all fungi tested. *Fusarium solani* f. sp. *pisi* and *S. loti* produced little or no constitutive FHL activity, whereas *G. sorghi* and *Helminthosporium maydis* produced significant constitutive activity. Because of these differences we determined the effects of various nitriles and poisons on induction. Acetonitrile, propion-

Table II Formamide hydrolyase activity in cells of four fungi treated with various chemicals

	FHL Activity (μmoles $HCONH_2$/mg/hr)			
Chemical[1]	F.s.p.[2]	G.s.[2]	H.m.[2]	S.l.[2]
H_2O	0	44	38	2
HCN (1.0 mM)	158	1240	841	129
H_3CCN (1.0 mM)	0	52	66	0
H_5C_2CN (1.0 mM)	0	64	22	2
NaN_3 (1.0 mM)	0	780	16	1
NaSCN (1.0 mM)	0	83	22	2
$HCONH_2$ (100 mM)	26	895	23	4
Antimycin A (0.01 mM)	0	1357	133	1

[1]Fungi were exposed to each chemical at the indicated concentration for 18 hours prior to assay.

[2]The fungi tested were: *Fusarium solani* f. sp. *pisi*, *Gloeocercospora sorghi*, *Helminthosporium maydis*, and *Stemphylium loti*.

itrile, and thiocyanate did not enhance FHL activity in any of the fungi. However, sodium azide enhanced FHL activity in *G. sorghi* but not in the other three fungi. Formamide enhanced FHL activity in *F. solani* f. sp. *pisi* and in *G. sorghi*, but not in *H. maydis* or *S. loti*. Antimycin A enhanced FHL activity in *G. sorghi* and *H. maydis* but not in *S. loti* or *F. solani* f. sp. *pisi*. Apparently, compounds which poison or stress *G. sorghi* will enhance its FHL activity. For example, in some experiments fragmenting the mycelium of *G. sorghi* in buffered medium enhanced FHL activity slightly. The significance of these regulatory differences to the survival of these fungi in their natural environments or in environments containing HCN is unknown.

V. ASSOCIATION OF HCN METABOLISM WITH PATHOGENICITY

To estimate the extent to which the ability to produce FHL was associated with fungal pathogens, we assayed 30 different fungi: members of the Phycomycetes, Ascomycetes, Basidiomycetes, and Deuteromycetes (Fry and Evans, 1977). The fungi in this group consisted of known pathogens of cyanogenic plants, fungi not known to be pathogens of cyanogenic plants but pathogenic to non-cyanogenic plants, and fungi not known to be plant pathogens. All of the fungi which were pathogens of cyanogenic plants produced HCN-induced FHL, although the amount of FHL produced varied considerably. Among the pathogens of non-cyanogenic plants, some contained FHL but others did not. In addition, these FHL activities were induced by HCN. Finally, with a single exception fungi which were not known plant pathogens were generally incapable of producing FHL. These results are consistent with the hypothesis that pathogens of plants that are strongly cyanogenic must have a means to cope with the HCN they encounter, and that FHL is the enzyme responsible for this ability.

VI. FUNGAL METABOLISM OF HCN IN VIVO

Though the ability of fungi to detoxify HCN via FHL is closely associated with fungal pathogenicity to cyanogenic plants, this association is not sufficient to prove that the cyanogenic glycosides are actually metabolized to produce HCN *in vivo* and that FHL is functioning *in vivo*. Infected plant tissues contained less cyanogenic glycoside than healthy tissues (Balasubramanian and Rangaswami, 1963; Fry and Munch, 1974), but the metabolizing-enzymes involved and the quantification and kinetics of this loss were unknown. These aspects were determined by investigating target leaf spot of sorghum caused by *G. sorghi* (Myers and Fry, 1978a; 1978b). The primary leaves of 8 to 10-day-old sorghum plants were inoculated, and the macroscopic appearance of the leaves, the progress of the fungal pathogen, the content of cyanogenic glycoside, and the activities of various enzymes were monitored periodically for 3.5 days. Within 48 hours after inoculation the tissue was at least 50% necrotic and fungal hyphae had begun to ramify throughout the tissue. By 84 hours after inoculation the pathogen had colonized the tissue extensively and the tissue was nearly completely necrotic. A steady decline in the cyanogenic glycoside content of leaves occurred, beginning between 12 and 24 hours after inoculation (Fig. 3). At 84 hours after inoculation only about 15% of the initial total cyanogenic glycoside in these leaves could be detected. About 15% of the initial cyanogenic glycoside was metabolized and the HCN was volatilized (Fig. 3). There are at least four possibilities for the cyanogenic glycoside which disappeared: (i) glycoside was metabolized to HCN which was bound to host or pathogen cell constituents; (ii) glycoside was metabolized to HCN which was metabolized destructively by host or pathogen enzymes; (iii) glycoside was metabolized to HCN which was incorporated by host or pathogen enzymes into metabolically active products; (iv) glycoside was metabolized by a pathway that did not produce HCN. We investigated the second and third possibilities. We first assessed the activities of the cyanogenic glycoside-metabolizing enzymes in homogenates of

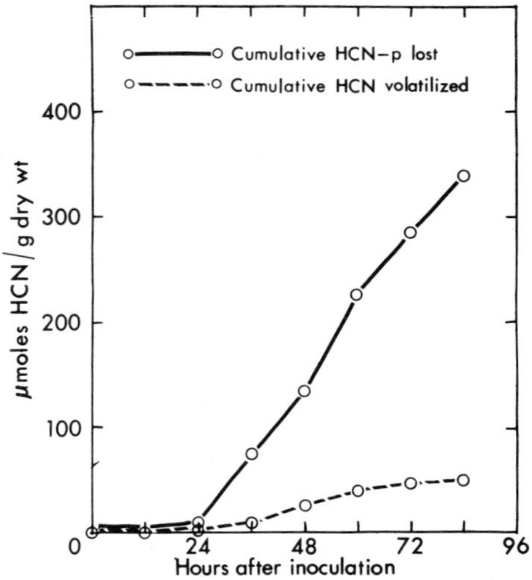

Fig. 3 Cumulative hydrogen cyanide potential (HCN-p) lost and cumulative HCN volatilized from primary leaves of the sorghum cultivar, Grazer, infected by *Gloeocercospora sorghi*. Values are accumulative and expressed as µmoles HCN/g leaf dry wt. Data are from Myers and Fry, 1978a.

infected leaves (Fig. 4) (Myers and Fry, 1978c). Activities of oxynitrilase were nearly constant during the first 84 hours after inoculation. Activity of the β-glucosidase measured against dhurrin (the cyanogenic glycoside in sorghum) increased dramatically during the first 36 hours after inoculation and stabilized thereafter, although the maximal activity was less than that of the oxynitrilase. We suggest that this increase in β-glucosidase activity could be explained by contributions of β-glucosidase from the pathogen. Pathogen production of β-glucosidase has been demonstrated in diseases of other cyanogenic plants (Millar and Hemphill, 1978; Wilkinson and Millar, 1979). Also, during its early stages of development the pathogen apparently caused a change in the permeability of both underlying and more distant host cells as evidenced by the water-soaking in these tissues (Myers and Fry, 1978b). These changes may facilitate the release of dhurrin from its storage site in the vacuole (Saunders *et al.*, 1977; Saunders and Conn, 1978), and make its metabolism by β-glucosidase and oxynitrilase more likely.

Activities of HCN-metabolizing enzymes also were assessed in infected plant tissues (Myers and Fry, 1978c). Rhodanese and β-cyanoalanine synthase activities were detected both in healthy tissues and in inoculated tissues, but their activities decreased slightly during disease development (Fig. 5). Neither enzyme activity could be demonstrated in *G. sorghi*.

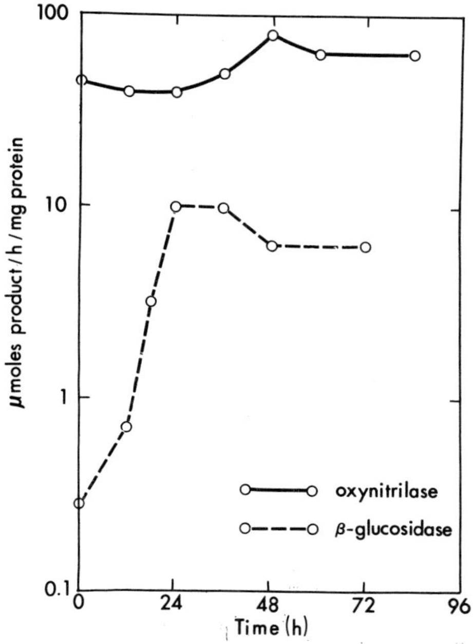

Fig. 4 Oxynitrilase and β-glucosidase specific activities in extracts of diseased sorghum during development of *Gloeocercospora sorghi* in sorghum primary leaves inoculated 6 days after leaf emergence. Data are from Myers and Fry (1978c).

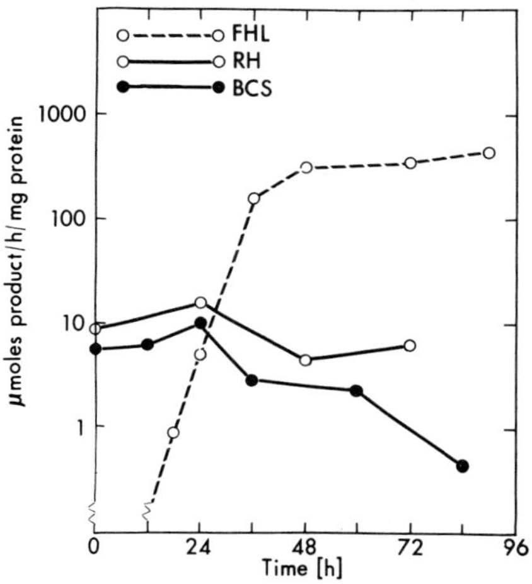

Fig. 5 Formamide hydrolyase (FHL), rhodanese (RH), and β-cyanoalanine synthase (BCS) specific activities in extracts of diseased sorghum during the development of *Gloeocercospora sorghi* in sorghum primary leaves inoculated 6 days after leaf emergence (Myers and Fry, 1978c).

On the basis of these activities and substrate availability, we hypothesized that FHL was the enzyme most likely to be responsible for HCN metabolism in diseased sorghum. Formamide hydrolyase activity could not be detected in healthy sorghum tissue or before 18 hours after inoculation. However, within 18 to 24 hours, FHL activity was detected and increased approximately 200-fold between 24 and 48 hours after inoculation (Fig. 5). The activity of FHL was at least 10-fold greater in infected tissue than either rhodanese or β-cyanoalanine synthase, and the rapid increase in FHL activity was associated closely in time with the decline in HCN potential (Fig. 6).

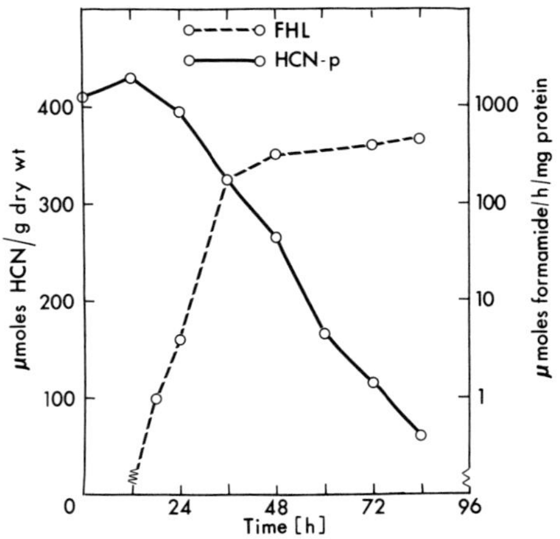

Fig. 6 Hydrogen cyanide potential (HCN-p) of diseased sorghum and formamide hydrolyase (FHL) specific activity in extracts of diseased sorghum during the development of *Gloeocercospora sorghi* in sorghum primary leaves inoculated 6 days after leaf emergence.

The correlation between FHL activity and cyanogenic glycoside content is striking if FHL activity in inoculated leaves of differing initial concentrations of dhurrin is examined (Table III). Two or three days after inoculation, all leaves were infected to the same extent and at about similar rates. Formamide hydrolyase activity was highest in infected tissues which initially had high levels of cyanogenic glycoside, was intermediate in tissues which initially had intermediate levels of cyanogenic glycoside, and was not detectable in tissues with very low or undetectable glycoside levels. While these correlations do not absolutely prove that FHL is responsible for HCN metabolism in diseased sorghum, they support our hypothesis that it is. Also, changes in the activities of rhodanese and β-cyanoalanine synthase did not correlate with the decrease in cyanogenic glycoside. Furthermore, the need for additional substrates at concentrations com-

Table III Maximum specific activity of formamide hydrolyase (FHL) (48 to 96 hours after inoculation with *Gloeocercospora sorghi*) in extracts of sorghum leaves differing in initial hydrogen cyanide potential (HCN-p) prior to inoculation

Leaf position[1]	Plant age (wk)	HCN-p[2] µmoles HCN/g dry wt	Specific activity[3] moles formamide/ hour/mg protein
1	1.5	464.8	340.0
2	1.5	144.0	156.7
3	1.5	49.3	46.2
7	5	9.9	2.2
8	7	3.2	0
9	9	0	0

[1]Leaf 1 was the first true leaf produced; leaf 2 was the second leaf, etc.

[2]The HCN-p was determined by the chloroform-base method using microdiffusion dishes as described in Myers and Fry, 1978a.

[3]HCN-p and FHL specific activities were ranked from highest to lowest and a correlation coefficient computed (r = .9867). The correlation was significant (P = 0.05).

parable to HCN probably would limit the activities of all enzymes except FHL in diseased sorghum.

Although we have hypothesized that FHL is primarily responsible for HCN metabolism in infected sorghum, we could not detect the product of its activity, formamide, in extracts of diseased sorghum (Myers and Fry, 1978c). However, diseased leaves could metabolize formamide from solution 16-fold faster than necessary to remove all the formamide available from HCN produced by the leaves (Table IV). Since surface sterilization significantly reduced the formamide metabolized by diseased leaves and since *G. sorghi* apparently does not metabolize formamide (W. E. Fry, unpublished), another microorganism associated with the lesion may be involved. Indeed, a *Pseudomonas* sp. isolated from lesions on sorghum caused by *G. sorghi* converted formamide to carbon dioxide and ammonia and could use formamide as a sole carbon and nitrogen source (Thatcher and Weaver, 1976).

Table IV Metabolism of formamide by healthy or diseased sorghum leaves

Leaf treatment[1]	Formamide metabolized	
	Healthy µmoles/flask (%)	Diseased µmoles/flask (%)
no treatment	17 (7) B[2]	80 (32) C
surface-sterilized[3]	15 (6) B	25 (10) B
autoclaved[4]	0 (0) A	0 (0) A

[1]Ten primary leaves (.0125 g dry wt) were incubated in 10-ml aliquots of a solution containing 250 µmoles formamide and salts. Flasks were incubated 8 days under fluorescent light at 25°C on a rotary shaker at 100 rev/min. Formamide in these solutions was measured colorimetrically on the eighth day of incubation after forming the hydroxamic acid derivative. Data are from Myers and Fry (1978c).

[2]Numbers followed by the same letter in a column are not significantly different (Duncan's Multiple Range Test, P = 0.05).

[3]Leaves were surface sterilized for 2 min in 10% bleach in 0.15% Tween 20 prior to incubation.

[4]Leaves were autoclaved for 20 min at 1 atmosphere gauge pressure (16 psi) prior to incubation.

VII. CONCLUSIONS AND FUTURE GOALS

We suggest that interactions between fungal pathogens and cyanogenic plants offer useful systems both to assess the role of HCN metabolism in fungi and the importance of cyanogenesis to the survival of these plants. We do not suggest that the ability to metabolize HCN via FHL will enable a fungus to be a pathogen of cyanogenic plants. However, the ability to produce FHL may be one of many necessary characteristics for successful pathogenicity. Other factors may also be necessary. For example, Rissler and Millar (1977) have shown that the initial production of FHL by *S. loti* may depend on activity of an alternate terminal oxidase (ATO) when the cytochromes of the electron transport system are blocked. Both FHL and ATO may be necessary for successful fungal pathogenesis of cyanogenic plants.

The necessity (for pathogenicity) of an HCN-insensitive oxidase or an HCN detoxification mechanism could be tested through the use of mutants. By exposure of fungal cells to chemical mutagens, mutants incapable of producing FHL should arise. The mutant should be backcrossed to the wild-type parent to produce isolates near-isogenic with the wild type, but which specifically lack the ability to produce FHL. The cyanide sensitivity and pathogenicity of these isolates then could be compared to the wild-type. If the near-isogenic mutant were less tolerant of HCN and less pathogenic than the wild-type, the hypotheses that the cyanogenic glycosides have a defence function in plants, and that FHL is a mechanism which enables fungi to overcome this defence mechanism would be well supported. Unfortunately, initial efforts to select these mutants from a mutagenized population have not been successful (Fry, unpublished).

REFERENCES

Akopyan, T.N., Braunstein, A.E. and Goryachenkova, E.V. (1975). *Proc. Natl. Acad. Sci. U.S.A.* 72, 1671-16

Allen, J. and Strobel, G.A. (1966). *Can. J. Microbiol.* 12, 414-416.

Balasubramanian, A. and Rangaswami, G. (1963). *Curr. Sci. (Bangalore)* 32, 223.

Colotelo, N. and Ward, E.W.B. (1961). *Nature* 189, 242-243.

Conn, E.E. (1973). *In* "Chronic Cassava Toxicity" (B. Nestel and R. MacIntyre, eds), pp.55-63 International Development Research Centre, Ottawa, Canada.

Dunnill, P.M. and Fowden, L. (1965). *Nature (London)* 208, 1206-1207.

Fry, W.E. and Evans, P.H. (1977). *Phytopathology* 67, 1001-1006.

Fry, W.E. and Millar, R.L. (1971a). *Phytopathology* 61, 501-506.

Fry, W.E. and Millar, R.L. (1971b). *Phytopathology* 61, 494-500.

Fry, W.E. and Millar, R.L. (1972). *Arch. Biochem. Biophys.* 151, 468-474.

Fry, W.E. and Munch, D.C. (1974). *Proc. Am. Phytopathol. Soc.* 1, 34.

Fry, W.E. and Munch, D.C. (1975). *Physiol. Plant Pathol.* 7, 23-33.

Knowles, C.J. (1976). *Bacteriol. Reviews* 40, 652-680.

Lebeau, J.B. and Dickson, J.G. (1955). *Phytopathology* 45, 667-673.

Millar, R.L. and Hemphill, R. (1978). *Physiol. Plant Pathol.* 13, 259-270.

Millar, R.L. and Higgins, V.J. (1970). *Phytopathology* 60, 104-110.

Mundy, B.P., Liu, F.H.S. and Strobel, G.A. (1973). *Can. J. Biochem.* 51, 1440-1442.

Myers, D.F. and Fry, W.E. (1978a). *Phytopathology* 68, 1037-1041.

Myers, D.F. and Fry, W.E. (1978b). *Phytopathology* 68, 1147-1157.

Myers, D.F., and Fry, W.E. (1978c). *Phytopathology* 68, 1717-1722.

Reynolds, E.S. (1924). *Am. J. Bot.* 11, 215-217.

Rissler, J.F. and Millar, R.L. (1977). *Plant Physiol.* 60, 857-861.

Robinson, M.E. (1930). *Biol. Rev. (Cambridge Phil. Soc.)* 5, 120-141.

Saunders, J.A. and Conn, E.E. (1978). *Plant Physiol.* 61, 154-157.

Saunders, J.A., Conn, E.E. and Stocking, C.R. (1977). *Plant Physiol.* 59, 647-652.

Shimizu, T. and Taguchi, H. (1969). *J. Ferment. Technol.* 47, 638-643.

Snyder, E.B. (1950). PH.D. Thesis, University of Wisconsin, Madison, 86 pp.

Strobel, G.A. (1964). *Can. J. Biochem.* 42, 414-416.

Thatcher, R.C. and Weaver, T.L. (1976). *Science* 192, 1234-1235.

Timonin, M.I. (1941). *Soil Sci.* 52, 395-414.
Trione, E.J. (1960). *Phytopathology* 50, 482-486.
Westley, J. (1973). *In* "Advances in Enzymology" (A. Meister, ed.), Vol. 39, pp.327-368. Interscience, John Wiley and Sons, New York.
Wilkinson, H.T. and Millar, R.L. (1978). *Can. J. Bot.* 56, 2491-2496.
Wilkinson, H.T. and Millar, R.L. (1979). *Can. J. Bot.* 57, 69-73.

ENZYMIC HYDROLYSIS OF NITRILES

PETER CHAMBERLAIN* and R. MURRAY MACKENZIE

Department of Molecular and Life Sciences,
Dundee College of Technology,
Bell Street, Dundee, DD1 1HG, Scotland

I. CHEMICAL HYDROLYSIS OF NITRILES

The hydrolysis of organic nitriles to amides and acids is a well known, synthetically useful, chemical reaction.

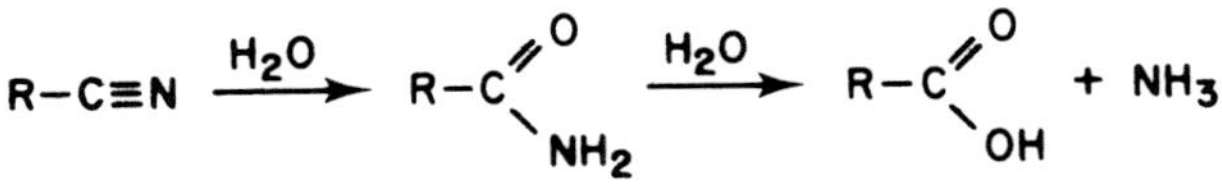

It has been comprehensively reviewed (Schaefer, 1970). The reaction is usually brought about by acid or alkaline catalysis, when the hydrolysis of the intermediate amide is faster than that of the nitrile. However various techniques are available for the isolation of the intermediate amide in good yield (Schaefer, 1970; Hall and Gisler, 1976).

Amides may also be prepared in good yield by reaction of the nitrile with hydrogen peroxide under mildly alkaline conditions

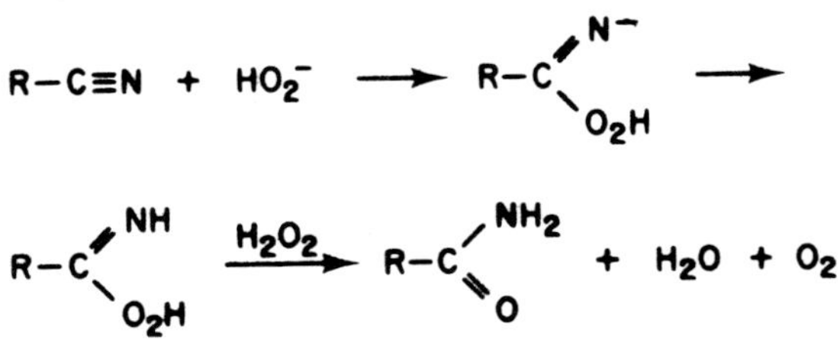

(A)

The intermediate peroxyimidic acid (A) is a useful oxidizing agent which may be reduced under a variety of cond-

---

*Present address: Allied Colloids Ltd., P.O. Box 38, Low Moor, Bradford.

itions (Schaefer, 1970).

Acids may be obtained by heating amides with sodium peroxide

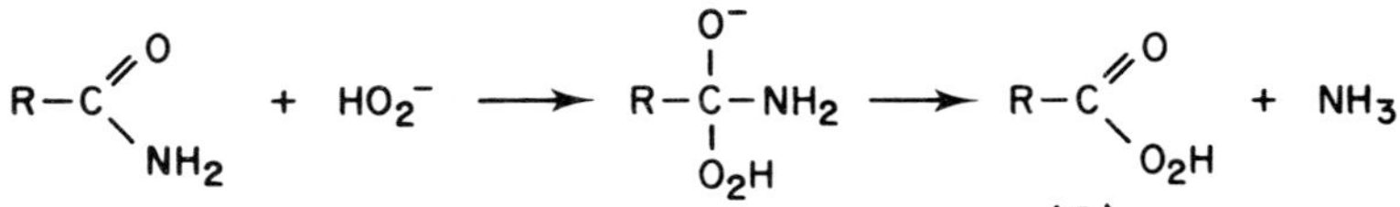

(B)

Under the reaction conditions employed, the peroxycarboxylates (B) decompose (Vaughan and Robbins, 1975). The conversion of nitriles to hydroxamic acids (C) by hydrogen peroxide

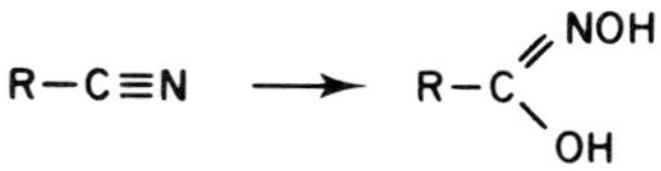

(C)

and thence to carboxylic acids has been claimed (Oliveri-Mandala, 1922).

There are several reports of the hydrolysis of nitriles catalysed by metal ions. For example, the second-order rate constant for the alkaline hydrolysis of the nickel (II) complex of (D) is 10^7 times greater than for the free ligand (Breslow *et al.*, 1967). It is proposed that nickel can bond to the developing imino anion in the transition-state leading to (E).

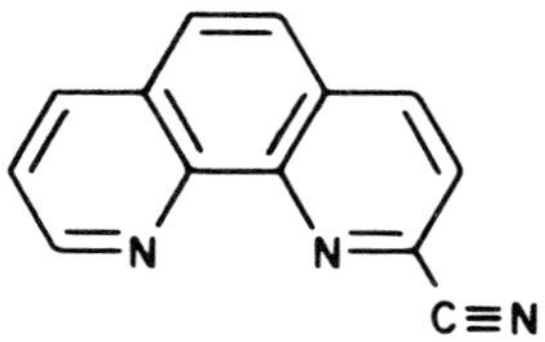

(D)

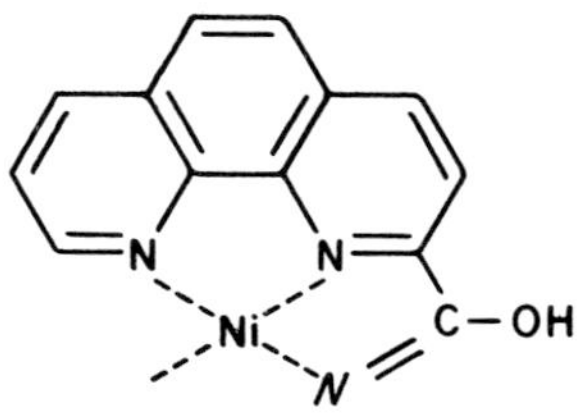

(E)

Benzonitrile and 3- and 4-cyanophenols complexed to pentamminecobalt (III) are readily hydrolysed to the amide in alkali (Pinnell *et al.*, 1972). Base-catalysed hydrolysis of acetonitrile to the amide is increased by about 10^8 on complexation with pentammineruthenium (Zanella and Ford, 1974).

Hydrolysis of nitriles to amides has been achieved using chloropentammineruthenium (III) chloride. Copper (II) and nickel (II) ions catalyse the hydration of the cyano group in 2-cyanopyridine to the corresponding amide (Barnard, 1969; Kamaya *et al.*, 1971). Furthermore, Bennett and Yoshida (1973) have reported the conversion of nitriles to amides by catalysis involving various platinum, rhodium and iridium complexes. Other techniques for the conversion of nitriles to amides include catalysis by nickel metal (Watanabe and Sakai, 1966), and by wet manganese dioxide in dichloromethane (Cook *et al.*, 1966).

II. BIOLOGICAL REACTIONS OF NITRILES

Until recently, the above transformations were thought to be largely within the chemical domain. Indeed, the number of naturally occurring nitriles is relatively restricted. However there is now rapidly increasing evidence for the existence of enzymes capable of converting nitriles to amides and/or acids. One can further speculate that such nitrilase enzymes could have played an important part in the early evolution of life. The role of HCN in prebiotic evolution is reviewed by Oró and Lazcano-Araujo in this volume. Hydrogen cyanide and cyanide ion can be incorporated into organic molecules, and hydrolysis of the resulting nitrile group can produce acids, including those of biological importance. Early primitive earth simulations showed that amino acids could have been formed without life. For example, Miller (1953) suggested a Strecker synthesis for glycine production.

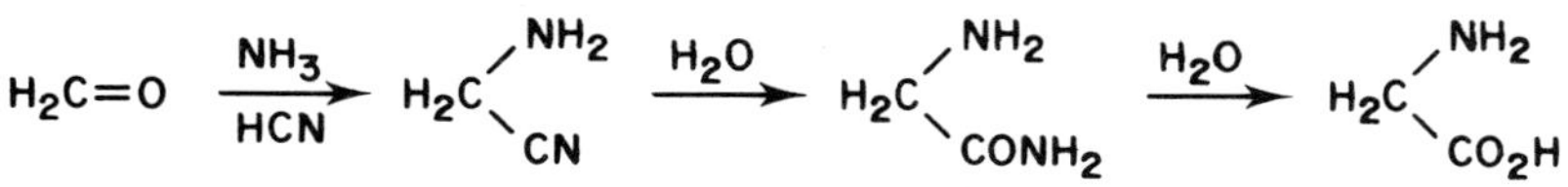

In addition, the triple bond in the C≡N group allows many molecules to undergo addition reactions, giving higher molecular weight compounds. Thus, cyanide polymerization may have been involved in the production of important biological molecules, for example adenine, $H_5C_5N_5$. Indeed, the addition of HCN to the photoisomerized tetramer has provided an industrial process for the synthesis of adenine.

These considerations perhaps make it less surprising that many nitrilase enzymes are now being found, and that they are usually of microbial, or to a lesser extent, of green plant origin. Microorganisms are often more chemically versatile than higher forms of life, and the respiration rate of some single cell organisms is affected little, or not at all by cyanide (Henry, this volume).

It is important, at this stage, to clarify the meaning of the word 'nitrilase'. In this article, we have defined a nitrilase as an enzyme capable of converting a nitrile to the corresponding amide and/or acid. This action is very diferent from that of the 'oxynitrilase' mandelonitrilase, found in bitter almonds (Becker *et al.*, 1963). This enzyme attacks mandelonitrile which is formed from amygdalin by the action of emulsin, yielding benzaldehyde and hydrogen cyanide:

$$C_6H_5-\underset{\displaystyle OH}{\underset{|}{CH}}-CN \longrightarrow C_6H_5-CHO + HCN$$

It is also important to distinguish between those nitrilases which hydrolyse the nitrile directly to the acid, using two molecules of water, and those which produce the amide. They may, or may not, be associated in a reaction chain with an amidase, a separate enzyme. Hence the acid may be produced from the nitrile by one enzyme or by two. *Fusarium solani* for example, can use benzonitrile as sole source of carbon and nitrogen, and the enzyme in this organism converts the nitrile to benzoic acid. Benzamide was not detected, nor could benzamide act as a substrate for the enzyme (Harper, 1977).

In contrast, a *Pseudomonas* group (III) organism (N.C.I.B. 10477) was found to metabolise 2-^{14}C-acetonitrile, leading to the normal intermediates of the Krebs cycle (Firmin and Gray, 1976). The authors suggested that acetonitrile was converted to the amide, then the acid. They showed that 2-^{14}C-acetamide could accumulate after addition of the nitrile, and that labelled acetonitrile and acetate both led to exactly the same labelled Krebs cycle intermediates. They suggested, but did not show, that the cells contained an amidase. Earlier work had shown the presence of amidase in *Pseudomonas aeruginosa*, which can grow on acetamide as sole carbon source. Mutants of this organism were produced (Skinner and Clarke, 1968) which demonstrated that acetamide was converted to acetate by acetamidase, then to acetyl coenzyme A by acetic thiokinase. This, and other work, (Brammer and Clarke, 1964) showed that the acetamidase was inducible, and group specific for aliphatic amides (aliphatic acylamide amidohydrolase EC.3.5.1.4.).

A third situation was found (Hook and Robinson, 1964; Robinson and Hook, 1964) with an enzyme isolated from a *Pseudomonas* species capable of growing on the naturally occurring cyanopyridine, ricinine (F). This enzyme catalysed production of the acid, together with a small amount of amide, although the amide was not a substrate for the enzyme.

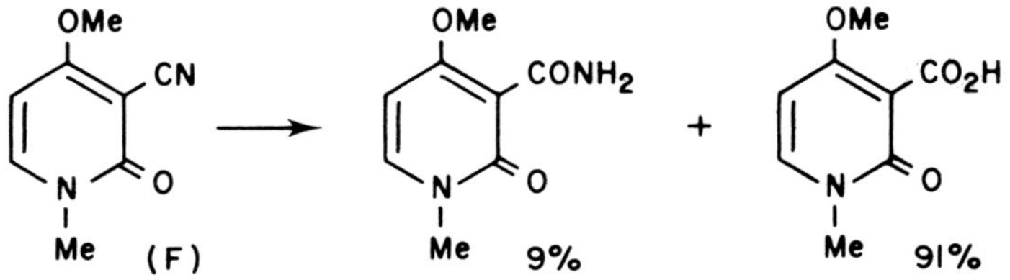

A nitrile, its associated amide, and acid, are all at the same oxidation level, and thus the overall reaction in each case is a hydrolysis. Thus it would appear that these reactions proceed via a simple hydrolytic mechanism. However, the possibility cannot be excluded that a biological oxidation/reduction mechanism may be found. A well known chemical analogy here is the conversion of nitriles to amides by hydroperoxide anion discussed earlier. No enzymic example has been reported, nor is there any confirmation, as yet, of the involvement of metal ions as co-factors in the reactions, though once again there is a good chemical analogy.

Although this article is concerned with the enzymic hydrolysis of nitriles, it should be noted that nitriles can be involved in other biological reactions. The action of mandelonitrilase has already been mentioned, and this type of degradation of a cyanhydrin to a carbonyl compound and hydrogen cyanide is found in fungi, plants and the arthropods. The hydroxynitrilase of sorghum is of particular interest (Conn *et al.*, 1966).

There is also evidence, partly indirect, for α-hydroxylation of nitriles. In green plants, nitriles can give rise to acids containing one less carbon atom (Chamberlain and Wain, 1973), and the metabolism of 3-indolylacetonitrile involves production of 3-indolealdehyde (Fawcett *et al.*, 1958).

Another reaction type involving nitriles is found in the young shoots and cotyledons of the blue lupin (Hendrickson and Conn, 1971). The enzyme β-cyanoalanine synthase catalyses the reaction.

$$\text{L-cysteine} + \text{HCN} \longrightarrow \beta\text{-cyanoalanine} + H_2S$$

Subsequent hydrolysis would yield asparagine and aspartic acid. It is interesting to note that the *Pseudomonas* species containing ricinine nitrilase (Hook and Robinson, 1964) contains another enzyme which converts β-cyanoalanine to aspartic acid, without the intermediacy of asparagine.

III. NITRILE HYDROLYSIS IN FUNGI

Nitrilase activity in fungi, though less widely reported than in bacteria, may eventually prove to be widespread. Yamaguchi (1934) suggested that many bacteria and moulds were not sensitive to cyanide and that mould growth and respiration were increased by cyanide addition. Pett (1937) found that yeast could grow, and be repeatedly subcultured, in the presence of cyanide. This led to a high respiration rate, increased flavin content, and production of a blue fluorescing pigment.

Many of the earlier reports did not attempt to show that enzymic nitrile hydrolysis occurred. However, Thimann and Mahadevan (1964) showed that 3-indolylacetonitrile could be converted to 3-indolylacetic acid by several *Fusarium* species, *Aspergillus niger*, and *Penicillium chrysogenum*.

Shimizu and Taguchi (1969) showed that cyanide led to the development of a cyanide degrading mechanism in *Fusarium solani*. This organism has also been implicated in the biodegradation of the herbicides bromoxynil (G) and ioxynil (H).

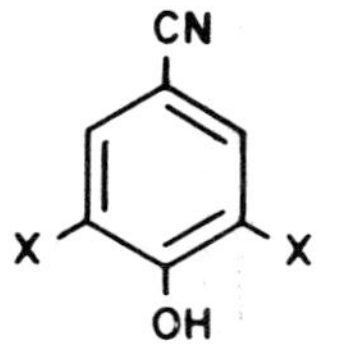

(G) X = Br
(H) X = I

Harper (1977) isolated a strain of *Fusarium solani* from bromoxynil-treated soil. The purified nitrilase enzyme was found to hydrolyse benzonitrile to benzoic acid and ammonia. It showed a broad specificity, and Harper suggested that it played an important part in the breakdown of nitrile herbicides. He found a molecular weight of 620,000 with the enzyme composed of eight subunits (MW 76,000). The enzyme was susceptible to inhibition by thiol-specific reagents, and showed a broad pH optimum from 7.8 to 9.1.

An example of the potential role of nitrile hydrolysis in microbial metabolism was obtained by Strobel (1966) who fed $H^{14}CN$ to a psychrophilic *Basidiomycete*, and found that it produced 1-^{14}C-α-aminopropionitrile. He obtained evidence that the nitrile was produced from formaldehyde and ammonia, and that hydrolysis of the nitrile produced alanine. In a later paper (Strobel, 1967) it was shown that the organism produced 4-amino-4-cyanobutanoic acid and that nitrilase hydrolysis then produced glutamic acid. Thus nitrile hydrolysis in this organism led into the central metabolic pathway. Subsequently, Bunch and Knowles (1980) found that in the snow mould, carbon dioxide was the major product of cyanide metabolism, with little formation of the amino acids found by Strobel. However, the possibility remains that a route from cyanide to a nitrile, and nitrile hydrolysis is an important potential pathway in microbial metabolism, to yield energy, carbon as required, and ammonia.

Fukuda *et al.* (1973) found evidence for the formation of L-α-hydroxyacids from DL-hydroxynitriles by *Torulopsis Candida*. The yields of acid were less than 50%. Hence it is not possible to distinguish between two possibilities, a specific nitrilase which selectively hydrolyses the L-hydroxynitrile, or hydrolysis of both enantiomers, followed by further metabolism of the D-hydroxyacid.

IV. NITRILE HYDROLYSIS IN PLANTS

Interest in nitrile hydrolysis in green plants increased after the study of growth stimulation caused by nitrile derivatives of natural plant growth substances. Jones *et al.* (1952) and Henbest *et al.* (1953) isolated indoleacetonitrile from cabbage, and showed it to be an auxin active in oat and wheat coleoptiles.

Fawcett *et al.* (1955) found that several nitriles were active in promoting growth in wheat, and that 3-indoleacetonitrile showed little activity in pea, but was highly active in wheat. They found 3-indolylcarboxylic acid in both pea and wheat, and suggested that this was due to α-oxidation of the nitrile.

The first evidence for hydrolysis of nitriles was produced by Thimann and Mahadevan (1963) who demonstrated the presence of a nitrilase in grasses, cabbage, radish, and the banana family. The enzyme was not widespread, being found only in the above mentioned groups from twenty-one families tested. The enzyme, partially purified from barley leaves, was found to be soluble, pH optimum near 7, with an activation energy of 58.8 kJ/mole and a Michaelis constant for indoleacetonitrile of 5.1×10^{-5} M at 25°C. It was susceptible to thiol-specific reagents, and slowly inactivated at 35°C in air. Conversion of indoleacetonitrile to the corresponding acid was quantitative, did not require air, and did not proceed via the amide. The authors suggested that the enzyme catalysed a two-stage hydrolytic reaction, in which the intermediate amide stage remained bound to the enzyme, with further hydrolysis liberating the enzyme, the acid and ammonia.

V. NITRILE HYDROLYSIS IN BACTERIA

Reports of nitrile hydrolysis in bacteria are increasing rapidly, and nitrilase activity is now well established. Early reports (Ponsetti *et al.*, 1956; Giza *et al.*, 1963) suggested that aminoacetonitrile and β-cyanoalanine could be hydrolysed and the discovery of a nitrilase enzyme in plants by Thimann and Mahadevan strengthened this possibility. Then Hook and Robinson, (1964) found and purified a bacterial enzyme which hydrolysed the nitrile group of the naturally-occurring compound ricinine. The enzyme, ricinine nitrilase, was prepared from a species of *Pseudomonas* isolated from soil by enrichment culture, using ricinine as sole carbon source. As previously described, the nitrile was hydrolysed to the acid, along with a small amount of amide, though the amide was not a substrate for the enzyme. They therefore proposed a common intermediate (Equation 1), produced by nucleophilic attack by the enzyme (X might be sulphur or oxygen) on the nitrile, followed by hydration.

Ammonia could then be liberated, yielding the acyl enzyme. The acid is then formed by hydrolysis (Equation 2). Alternatively, the enzyme could act as the leaving group, yielding the amide (Equation 3).

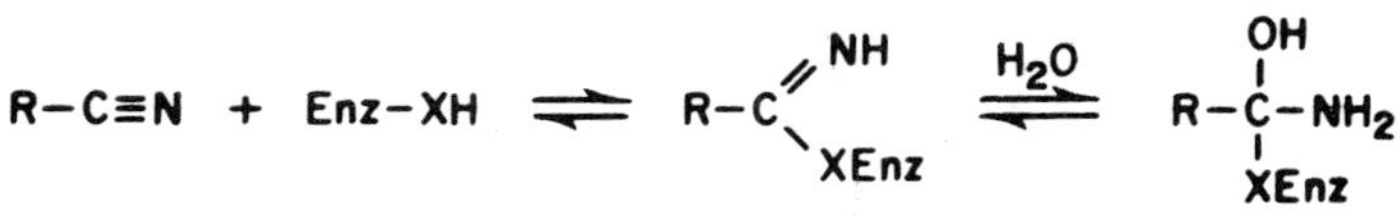

(Equation 1)

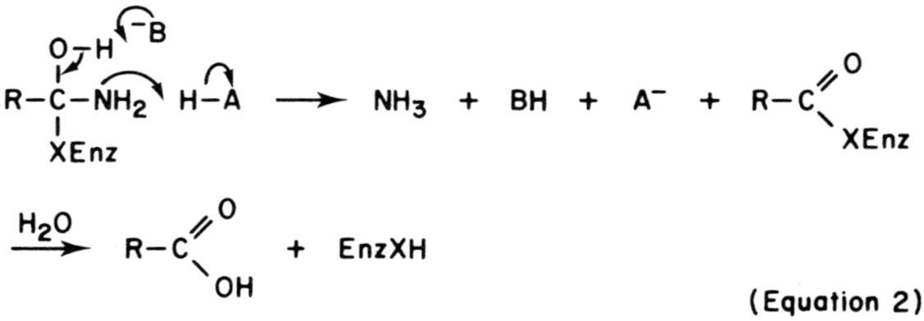

(Equation 2)

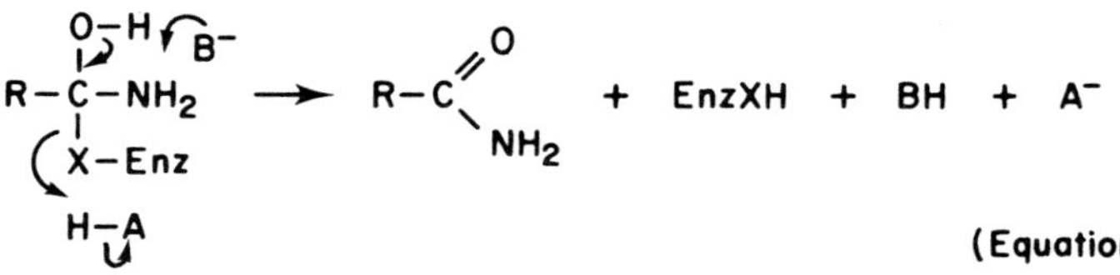

(Equation 3)

(The result, however, could be due to the presence of a reversible amidase.)

The chemical feasibility of this proposal was tested by Cordes and Zervos (1971), by studying the hydrolysis of N-benzyl-3-cyanopyridinium bromide catalysed by mercaptoethanol. Under neutral or slightly acidic conditions, the amide was produced, but at the lower pH, substantial quantities of acid were produced as well.

Hook and Robinson confirmed that ricinine nitrilase was a distinct enzyme from that found by Thimann and Mahadevan. With a purity of 80-90%, the enzyme was stable at 0° at pH 9.5 to 10.5 but was unstable at lower pH. Its optimum was at pH 7.4 to 8.8 with a K_m for ricinine of 1.9×10^{-5}M. The enzyme had a narrow specificity; it hydrolysed a number of analogues of ricinine, but was inactive with nicotinonitrile, phenylacetonitrile, mandelonitrile, indoleacetonitrile, acetonitrile and cyanoacetamide.

By 1969, the potential industrial use of nitrile hydrolysis was recognized. Mimura *et al.* (1969), isolated, from activated sludge, two examples of *Corynebacterium nitrophilus* capable of growth on acetonitrile. One of these organisms was found to tolerate up to 3% acetonitrile in the medium, though growth was limited by the large amount of ammonia produced. In addition to several nitriles, growth was obtained on tridecane, pentadecane and hexadecane, but not on aromatic nitriles.

Fukuda *et al.* (1971) isolated an organism from soil capable of growing on 4% acetonitrile as sole carbon source, a very high tolerance to a compound generally considered to be toxic. This organism was able to utilize many aliphatic nitriles, either as carbon source, or, in presence of glucose, as nitrogen source. DL-α-aminopropionitrile was converted to alanine.

Interest in *Corynebacteria* continued when Grant (1973) studied a culture of *Corynebacterium pseudodiphtheriticum*

N.C.1.B. 10803, which grew aerobically on a large number of carbon sources. It is interesting that this organism was originally isolated because of its ability to grown on the amides, phenacetin (*p*-acetamidophenetole) and paracetamol (*p*-acetamidophenol). The organism grew on some amino acids, some sugars, Krebs cycle compounds, higher straight-chain alkanes, alcohols, carboxylic acids and aliphatic nitriles and amides. The author suggested that nitriles were hydrolysed to amides, then to acids and ammonia. He found that the organism did not grown on phenylacetonitrile, although phenylacetic acid was utilized, suggesting the presence of a nitrilase specific for aliphatic nitriles.

A further step forward occurred with the demonstration by Firmin and Gray (1976) that the pathway of acetonitrile degradation was almost certainly hydrolytic, through acetamide to acetic acid and the Krebs cycle. Their test organism, a *Pseudomonas* species, was isolated from air by its ability to grow on acetonitrile. As already mentioned, the presence of an amidase in *Pseudomonas aeroginosa* had been demonstrated previously (Brammer and Clarke, 1964; Skinner and Clarke, 1968).

Nocardia rhodochrous has also yielded interesting results. DiGeronimo and Antoine (1976) isolated a culture of this organism (LL100 - 21) from barnyard soil, by its ability to grown on 4% acetonitrile as both carbon and nitrogen source, although they found that the enriched culture would not tolerate more than 3% acetonitrile. They found that the nitrilase was an inducible enzyme. The cells originally obtained by acetonitrile enrichment were grown on a glucose medium. Subsequent exposure of these cells to acetonitrile produced no growth, and little or no nitrile hydrolysis, although the parent and control cells showed strong nitrilase activity.

This demonstration of the inducible nature of nitrilase was in contrast to the claim of Fukuda *et al.* (1971) that their nitrilase was constitutive. The Japanese workers had isolated their culture by growth on acetonitrile, and did not use an intermediate glucose growth stage.

Harper (1977) published a very comprehensive paper dealing with C-N cleavage by *Nocardia rhodochrous* N.C.1.B. 11216. The organism was isolated from river mud by enrichment, based on its ability to use benzonitrile as sole source of carbon, nitrogen and energy. The labile enzyme was highly purified and shown to catalyse the conversion of benzonitrile to benzoic acid without formation of benzamide, nor was benzamide a substrate for the enzyme. A range of meta- and para- substituted aromatic nitriles were also hydrolysed, though not aliphatic nitriles. The enzyme is unusual in that it has a time-dependent substrate-activated process in which the substrate catalyses the association of inactive subunits of M.W. 45,000 to form a 12-unit active enzyme of M.W. 560,000. The time of association is at a minimum at pH 7.3. The associated enzyme has an optimum pH of 8, a K_m for benzaldehyde of 4×10^{-3} M, and an activation energy of 51.8 kJ/mole. Harper discussed the possible role of the substrate activated association process, suggesting a metabolic regulation function.

The enzyme, like that of Thimann and Mahadevan (1964), is inhibited by thiol specific reagents. Both enzymes hydrolyse the nitrile to the acid, requiring two water molecules, without forming any free amide. Both Harper (1977) and Thimann and Mahadevan (1964) suggested as a possible mechanism, mucleophilic attack on the nitrile carbon atom by a thiol group at the active site of the enzyme. The resulting enzyme-imino-thioether is hydrolysed via a hydroxyamino thioether to the thioester. Further hydrolysis yields the acid. This is similar to the mechanism proposed by Hook and Robinson (Equations 1 and 2, where X = S).

Harper's enzyme, specific for nitrile groups attached to an aromatic ring, is not related to the enzyme found in *Nicardia* by DiGeronimo and Antoine (1976). It is tempting to consider the possibility that both enzymes were potentially present in the test organisms of Harper and of DiGeronimo and Antoine, and that the enzyme actually found arose through substrate induction. Since most workers use substrate enrichment techniques to isolate organisms, it is not easy to decide whether a nitrilase is constitutive or induced.

Beginning in 1976, French workers have published a series of papers (Arnaud *et al.*, 1976, 1977). They isolated eighteen strains of widely differing taxonomy using the ability to grow on acetonitrile. These strains, belonging to *Bacillus*, *Bacteridium*, *Micrococcus* and *Brevibacterium*, were found to hydrolyse many nitriles and amides, both aliphatic and aromatic. Of these strains, *Brevibacterium R312* was most closely studied. Arnaud *et al.* (1977) isolated this strain, grew it on a yeast extract medium containing acetonitrile, acetamide or ammonium acetate, and maintained the culture on a medium based on yeast and malt extract, bacto-peptone and glucose. The cells were disrupted ultrasonically, and the enzyme found to be in the soluble 180,000 g ultracentrifuge supernatant. The enzyme was active between pH 5 and 10, optimum pH 7; optimum temperature 30° to 35°, with denaturation beginning at 35°; K_m for acetonitrile was 2.5×10^{-2} M. The enzyme was also found to be precipitated between 40 and 50% ammonium sulphate saturation. Dialysis of the 180,000 g supernatant fraction against water or phosphate (pH 7.3) led to a loss in activity, suggesting either that the enzyme requires a dialysable co-factor, or that it is formed by association of inactive components.

The authors were strongly of the view that the enzyme was constitutive, disagreeing with the conclusion of DiGeronimo and Antoine (1976) that their nitrilase from *Nocardia rhodochrous* was induced. The French workers based their criticism on the argument that DiGeronimo and

Antoine were dealing with two enzymes, a constitutive nitrilase and an induced amidase. Their argument that the nitrilase of *Brevibacterium* was constitutive was based on the fact that, during exponential growth, nitrilase activity was found whether or not acetonitrile was present. It should be noted however that the French workers first isolated their organism because of its ability to grown on acetonitrile. They also found that nitrilase activity decreased at the end of the exponential phase and was practically zero in the stationary phase. The case, in Scottish parlance, might be considered 'not proven', and it may be true that, once nitrilase biosynthesis is switched on, it persists for some time, with or without the substrate.

The potential use of *Brevibacterium R312* in the industrial field was recognised by the French workers in patent applications (Commeyras *et al.*, 1973; Commeyras *et al.*, 1977), describing production of amides and carboxylic acids, including racemic amino acids. The same group (Arnaud *et al.*, 1980) published a review of bioconversions of nitriles and their applications. The review listed the naturally occurring nitriles, and current industrial processes leading from nitriles to amides or acids. It was suggested that there is a large potential field for the biological hydrolysis of nitriles, and that certain nitriles are much less expensive than the corresponding amides. Biological hydrolysis can be carried out at moderate pH, room temperature, and with low energy consumption, avoiding production of by-products. There is also the possibility of stereoselective synthesis of single enantiomers.

The review described a study of nitrilase activity in whole cells of *Brevibacterium R312*, indicating that the enzyme was group specific only, i.e. it was capable of hydrolysing a very wide variety of nitriles. A study of amidase activity was also described, again using whole cells; once again it was found that the amidase hydrolysed a wide range of amides. Of the amides tested, only the vinylic acrylamide and methacrylamide and the lactams, caprolactam and α-amino-ε-caprolactam were not hydrolysed. Racemic α-amino and α-hydroxy acids were obtained from the corresponding amides. The amidase, like the nitrilase, was in the 180,000 g supernatant, and precipitated by 35 to 65% ammonium sulphate. It showed activity between pH 3 and 11, with an optimum at pH 7, and an optimum temperature between 60° and 70°. Activity was lost by dialysis and increased by EDTA (unlike the nitrilase).

A very interesting description was given of the isolation of a mutant resistant to fluoracetamide. Wild type strain R312 was unable to grow on this compound because it produced toxic fluoracetic acid, by hydrolysis. The mutant lacked the wide-range non-specific amidase but could hydrolyse certain amides, including nicotinamide, urea, formamide and α-amino amides, yielding the L-α-amino acid. The enzyme had a specific L-α-amino amidase activity, and did not hydrolyse the corresponding D enantiomer.

VI. CONCLUSION

Though nitrilase enzymes have been discovered only comparatively recently, they are known to occur in green plants, fungi and bacteria. Reports of their occurrence, especially in bacteria, are increasing. It is reasonable to assume that a significant number still await discovery.

Nitrilases may be divided into two groups. The first group produce the amide, which may be converted subsequently to an acid by an amidase. This group includes enzymes with the ability to hydrolyse a wide variety of structurally-diverse nitriles. The second group produce the acid directly without liberating the amide. (In one case a small amount of amide is produced as by-product.) The few enzymes in this category are specific for a narrow structural range of nitriles, and these are aromatic or heterocyclic. There has been some speculation on the mechanisms of nitrile hydrolysis, though no comparative study of the two groups.

As might be expected in a new area, there is a scarcity of systematic information. For example, there has been no attempt to isolate and characterise taxonomically a range of nitrile-utilizing bacteria; little is known about the enzymology of the synthesis or degradation of nitriles; one group has suggested that acetonitrilase is inducible, while others have concluded it is constitutive; the cellular location of nitrilases is unknown.

Nitrilase enzymes are recognized as having considerable commercial potential as well as general scientific interest.

REFERENCES

Arnaud, A., Galzy, P. and Jallageas, J.L. (1976). *Rev. Ferment. Ind. Aliment* 31 (2), 39.

Arnaud, A., Galzy, P. and Jallageas, J.L. (1976). *C.R. Hebd. Séances Acad. Sci. Paris Series D* 283 (5), 71.

Arnaud, A., Galzy, P. and Jallageas, J.L. (1977). *Agri. Biol. Chem.* 41 (11), 21 3.

Arnaud, A., Galzy, P. and Jallageas, J.L. (1980). *Adv. in Biochem. Eng.* 14, Microbiol Metabolism (A. Fiechter, ed.)

Barnard, P.F.B. (1969). *J. Chem. Soc. A.* 2140.

Becker, W., Benthen, V., Eschenhof, E. and Pfeil, E. (1963) *Biochem. Z.* 337, 156.

Bennett, M.A. and Yoshida, T. (1973). *J. Amer. Chem. Soc.* 95, 3030.

Brammar, W.J. and Clarke, P.H. (1964). *J. gen. Microbiol.* 37, 307.

Breslow, R., Fairweather, R. and Keana, J. (1967) *J. Amer. Chem. Soc.* 89, 2135.

Bunch, A.W. and Knowles, C.J. (1980). In press.

Chamberlain, K. and Wain, R.L. (1973). *Ann. Applied Biol.* 75, 409.

Commeyras, A., Arnaud, A., Galzy, P. and Jallageas, J.L. (1973). Demande de Brevet D'invention, No. 73, 33613.
Commeyras, A., Arnaud, A., Galzy, P. and Jallageas, J.L. (1977). U.S. Patent 4,000,081.
Cook. M.J., Forbes, E.J. and Khan, G.M. (1966). *Chem. Commun.* 121.
Cordes, E.H. and Zervos, C. (1971). *J. Org. Chem.* 36, 1661.
Diamond, S.E., Grant, B., Tan, G.E. and Taube, H. (1974). *Tetrahedron Lett.* 4025.
DiGeronimo, M.J. and Antoine, A.D. (1976). *Applied and Env. Microbiol. (June)*, 900.
Fawcett, C.H., Seeley, R.C., Taylor, H.F., Waine, R.L. and Wightman, F. (1955). *Nature*, 176, 1026.
Fawcett, C.H., Taylor. H.F., Wain, R.L. and Wightman, F. (1958). *Proc. Roy. Soc. (London)* B148, 543.
Firmin, J.L. and Gray, D.O. (1976). *Biochem. J.* 158, 223.
Fukuda, Y., Fukui, M., Harada, T. and Izumi, Y. (1971) *J. Ferment. Technol.* 49, 1011.
Fukuda, Y., Harada, T. and Izumi, Y. (1973). *J. Ferment. Technol.* 51, 393.
Giza, Y.H., Rutzkin, H. and Ressler, C. (1963). *Fed. Proc.* 22, 651.
Grant, D.J.W. (1973). *Antoinie van Leeuwenhock*, 39, 273.
Hall, J.H. and Gisler, M. (1976). *J. Org. Chem.* 41, 3769.
Harper, D.B. (1977a). *Biochem. J.* 165, 309.
Harper, D.B. (1977b). *Biochem. J.* 167, 685.
Henbest, H.B., Jones, E.R.H. and Smith, C.J. (1953). *J. Chem. Soc.* 3796.
Hendrickson, H.R. and Conn, E.E. (1971). *Methods in Enzymology XVII B*, 233.
Hook. R.H. and Robinson, W.G. (1964). *J. Biol. Chem.* 239, 4263.
Jones, E.R.H., Henbest, H.B., Smith. G.J. and Bentley, J.A. (1952). *Nature*, 159, 485.
Komaya, S., Suzuki, S. and Watanabe, K. (1971). *Bull. Chem. Soc. Japan* 44, 1440.
Miller, S.L. (1953). *Science* 117, 528.
Mimura, A., Kawano, T., Yamaga, K. (1969). *J. Ferment. Technol.* 47, 631.
Oliveri-Mandala, E. (1922). *Gazz. Chim. Ital.* 52(1), 107.
Pett, L.B. (1936). *Biochem. J.* 30, 1438.
Pinnell, D., Wright, G.B. and Jordan, R.B. (1972). *J. Amer. Chem. Soc.* 94, 6104.
Ponsetti, I.V., Wawzanek, S., Franklin, W.E., Winnick, R.E., Winnick, T. (1956). *Proc. Soc. Exptl. Biol. Med.* 93, 515.
Robinson, W.G. and Hook, R.H. (1964). *J. Biol. Chem.* 239, 4257.
Schaefer, F.C. (1970). *In* "The Chemistry of the Cyano Group" (S.Patai and Z. Rappoport, eds.) pp. 240-395. Wiley Interscience, and references cited therein.
Seely, M.K., Criddle, R.S. and Conn, E.E. (1966). *J. Biol. Chem.* 241, 4457.
Skinner, A.J. and Clarke, P.H. (1968). *J. gen. Microbiol.* 50, 183.
Shimizu, T. and Taguchi, H. (1969). *J. Ferment. Technol.* 47, 639.
Strobel, G.A. (1966). *J. Biol. Chem.* 241, 2618.
Strobel, G.A. (1967). *J. Biol. Chem.* 242, 3265.
Thimann, K. and Mahadevan, S. (1964). *Arch. Biochem. Biophys.* 105, 133.

Vaughan, H.L. and Robbins, M.D. (1975). *J. Org. Chem.* 40, 1187.
Watanabe, K. and Sakai, K. (1966). *Bull. Chem. Soc. Japan.* 39, 8.
Yamagutchi, I. (1934). *Benz. yes. Physiol.* 83, 412.
Zanella, A.W. and Ford, P.C. (1974). *J. Chem. Soc. Chem. Commun.* 795.

HCN PRODUCTION BY MICROALGAE

BIRGIT VENNESLAND, ELFRIEDE K. PISTORIUS and HANS-SIEGFRIED GEWITZ

Forschungsstelle Vennesland der Max-Planck-Gesellschaft, Harnackstrasse 23, D-1000 Berlin 33, Germany

I. INTRODUCTION

In the present review, we use the term HCN to refer collectively to hydrogen cyanide and the cyanide ion, when there are no clear grounds for choosing between them.

Our interest in HCN production by algae began with the observation that the molybdoprotein, nitrate reductase, could be converted reversibly into an inactive cyanide complex *in vivo*, in the unicellular green alga *Chlorella vulgaris* (for further details see Solomonson, this volume). The HCN needed for the inactivation process did not have to be added externally, but was provided by the living cells. The present paper summarizes the available information about how *Chlorella* and other algae make HCN.

The cyanogenic glucosides, which are widely distributed in higher plants, have never been reported to occur in microalgae (see Seigler, this volume). We have likewise found no evidence for their presence there. Although, as we shall see, certain amino acids may serve as precursors of HCN in algae, the mechanism of HCN formation appears to be different from the metabolic route established for the conversion of amino acids to cyanogenic glucosides (see Møller, this volume). Compounds other than amino acids may also operate as precursors of HCN in algae.

II. CONDITIONS FAVOURING REVERSIBLE INACTIVATION OF *CHLORELLA* NITRATE REDUCTASE

Our initial approach to the problem of the biogenesis of HCN was to make a study of the effect of various environmental variables on the reversible inactivation of the nitrate reductase enzyme in *Chlorella vulgaris in vivo* (Pistorius *et al.*, 1976). The criterion of reactivation by ferricyanide was employed to identify the HCN complex of the enzyme *in vitro*.

The inactivation was partially prevented by nitrate and CO_2, and was particularly favoured by high O_2 concentrations and high light intensities. It was also favoured by

Mn^{2+} ions, in the sense that Mn^{2+} deficient cells formed little inactive enzyme. The effect of nitrate could be explained by a direct effect on the inactivation reaction. It is the reduced form of the enzyme that forms an HCN complex, and nitrate keeps the enzyme in the oxidized state. The addition of ammonium salts to cells reducing nitrate also caused enzyme inactivation, to the same extent as nitrate removal. We attribute this effect of ammonia to the fact that added ammonium ions inhibit nitrate uptake (Pistorius *et al.*, 1978). In the case of the effects of O_2, light and Mn^{2+}, however, it seemed possible that these agents were affecting HCN production more directly.

This was confirmed in experiments with *Chlorella* extracts and with grana preparations from spinach (*Spinacea oleracea*) and from New Zealand spinach (*Tetragonia expansa*) (Gewitz *et al.*, 1976a, 1976b). In these experiments, the biological material was placed in the main compartment of a Warburg manometer flask, and the HCN was collected by distillation into alkali placed in the central well and then determined by specific chemical methods. In general, no detectable HCN was obtained from unsupplemented preparations incubated in the dark; but when the samples were illuminated in O_2, small amounts of HCN were often observed. Addition of Mn^{2+} and peroxidase stimulated this HCN production. Sonication of the biological material also led to HCN formation. From such evidence we surmised that HCN must be formed from nitrogenous precursors by an oxidative or peroxidative process (Gewitz *et al.*, 1976a, 1976b).

III. D-HISTIDINE, AN HCN PRECURSOR IN *CHLORELLA*

In the next stage of the investigation various possible nitrogenous precursors were added to French Press extracts of *Chlorella vulgaris* or to green grana preparations from leaves, to see if they caused an increase in HCN production and so might be identified as HCN precursors. All of the naturally occurring amino acids were tested. The results suggested that histidine was the most effective, though not necessarily the exclusive precursor of HCN in green cells (Gewitz *et al.*, 1976b).

Further studies of the HCN production from histidine in the presence of *Chlorella* extracts revealed that D-histidine was more effective than L-histidine. The production of HCN from D-histidine was then found to depend on a soluble D-amino acid oxidase present in *Chlorella* (Pistorius *et al.*, 1977; Pistorius and Voss, 1977). The action of this oxidase alone, however, did not elicit HCN formation. Another component was necessary. A particulate preparation from *Chlorella* was effective as the second component, which we have called a cofactor for HCN production by the amino acid oxidase system. Horseradish peroxidase proved to be a convenient substitute for this particulate fraction.

It should be noted that the amino acid oxidase-peroxidase system operates effectively in the dark. Illuminated washed green particles from *Chlorella* and from leaves form HCN from histidine also, but this light-dependent reaction showed no stereospecificity for the substrate. It operates equally well with L-histidine or D-histidine, and histamine is slightly more effective as a substrate (Gewitz *et al.*, 1976b). No further work has yet been done on the light-dependent system, but an extensive study has been made of the dark production of HCN by the amino acid oxidase-peroxidase system.

IV. HCN PRODUCTION BY THE AMINO ACID OXIDASE-PEROXIDASE SYSTEM

The D-amino acid oxidase of *Chlorella vulgaris* has been partially purified and characterized as a flavoprotein (Pistorius and Voss, 1977). It has been resolved into an inactive apoenzyme which can be reactivated by added FAD. It catalyzes the oxidation of a wide variety of D-amino acids (and of glycine), with reduction of O_2 to H_2O_2 and liberation of ammonia from the α-amino group. This enzyme is in every way a typical amino acid oxidase, with very high specificity for the steric configuration of the α-carbon atom, and high tolerance for chemical variability in the R group. Among the best substrates for oxidation are D-leucine and D-methionine, but these substrates yield no HCN.

The capacity to cause HCN formation from histidine on supplementation with a suitable cofactor is apparently shared by all amino acid oxidases. The D-specific kidney enzyme, the L-amino acid oxidase from snake venom, and the *Chlorella* D-amino acid oxidase all catalyze the HCN-forming reaction, in approximate proportion to their ability to oxidize histidine (Pistorius *et al.*, 1977). For convenience, the mechanism of the reaction has been studied mainly with commercially available snake venom L-amino acid oxidase and horse-radish peroxidase (Gewitz *et al.*, 1980).

The reaction is always mixed. Even under conditions optimal for HCN formation, a portion of the histidine is degraded normally as in the absence of peroxidase. At very high buffer concentrations, however, the HCN formed amounts to as much as 70% of the histidine oxidized. The HCN-forming reaction is accompanied by extra O_2 consumption and there are side reactions which interfere with accurate stoichiometric measurements, but a major product of the oxidation appears to be imidazole aldehyde (accompanied by imidazole carboxylic acid). Though the HCN production is inhibited by catalase, the amount of H_2O_2 formed does not appear to be altered by the presence of peroxidase. This is explained by assuming that H_2O_2 is used and then regenerated in the HCN-forming reaction. A plausible reaction sequence is pictured in Fig. 1.

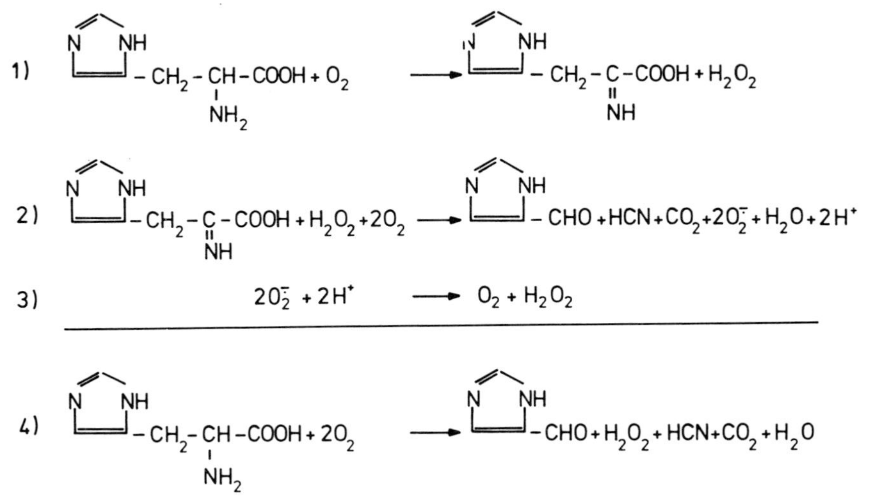

Fig. 1 The production of HCN from histidine in the amino acid oxidase-peroxidase system.

The first step in the reaction is catalyzed by the amino acid oxidase alone, and involves the oxidation of the amino acid to an imino acid, with reduction of O_2 to H_2O_2, as shown in Fig. 1, equation 1 (Bright and Porter, 1975). Normally, in the absence of peroxidase, the imino acid is rapidly hydrolysed non-enzymatically to the keto acid and ammonia. To the extent that this hydrolysis occurs, the reaction product is imidazole pyruvic acid, which in turn reacts non-enzymatically with H_2O_2 to give imidazole acetic acid and CO_2. In the presence of peroxidase, however, some of the imino acid is further oxidized as shown in Fig. 1, equation 2. Two molecules of O_2 are reduced to superoxide anion, and H_2O_2 is reduced to water, thus removing the 4 electrons involved in the conversion of the imino acid to imidazole aldehyde, HCN and CO_2. The superoxide anion then dismutes to H_2O_2 and O_2 (Fig. 1, equation 3). The net reaction is shown in Fig. 1, equation 4.

Added superoxide dismutase stimulates the reaction to a small extent. $O_2^{\cdot-}$ or some form of activated oxygen can be detected by the capacity of the system to cause a stoichiometric concomitant conversion of added hydroxylamine to nitrite.

Histidine is not the only amino acid that yields HCN in the amino acid oxidase-peroxidase system. The other aromatic amino acids, tryptophan, phenylalanine and tyrosine, share this property with histidine, though the latter gives decidedly higher yields. Added peroxidase causes a marked increase in the amount of O_2 taken up when one of the aromatic amino acids is the substrate of amino acid oxidase, but not when the substrate is a non-aromatic ami-

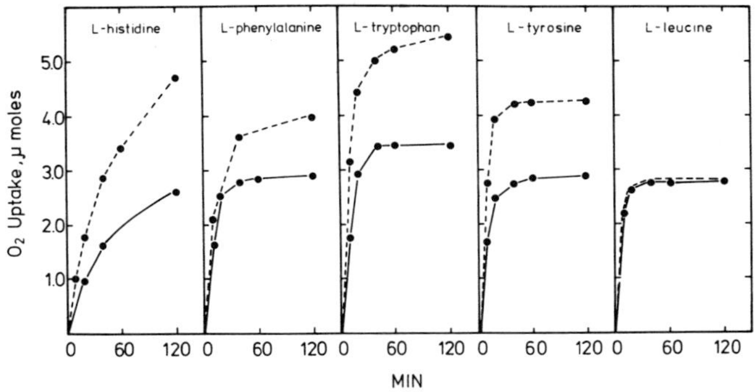

Fig. 2 Effect of peroxidase on O_2 uptake with amino acid oxidase and various substrates.

The reaction mixtures all contained 0.2 U L-amino acid oxidase from snake venom and 3 μmoles of the indicated amino acid, in 1.2 ml of 350 nM HEPPS buffer, pH 7.5. Measurements were made manometrically. The solid line shows the reaction in the absence of peroxidase. The dashed line shows the reaction with 40 μg horse-radish peroxidase added. For further details, see Gewitz *et al.*, 1980.

no acid, as shown in Fig. 2. The extra O_2 consumption observed with the aromatic amino acids was in every case more than enough to account for the HCN formation by a mechanism such as that shown in Fig. 1.

In addition to peroxidase and a cell particulate fraction, substances capable of acting as cofactors for HCN production by the amino acid oxidase system include cytochrome c and a wide variety of redox ions (Pistorius *et al.*, 1977; Gewitz *et al.*, 1980). Vanadium salts added to *Chlorella vulgaris* cells stimulate HCN production, perhaps by exerting such a cofactor effect (Ramadoss, 1979).

V. HCN PRODUCTION BY CYANOBACTERIA (BLUE-GREEN ALGAE)

In a small survey of the cyanobacteria (the procaryotic blue-green algae) *Anacystis nidulans* was found to be a particularly effective HCN former when incubated with histidine. The preferred substrate was L- rather than D-histidine, though both were effective, especially on illumination.

We have never obtained HCN from intact *Chlorella* cells in the dark, though traces were observed in light (Gewitz *et al.*, 1976b). In comparison, the dark production of HCN from L-histidine by *Anacystis nidulans* was striking. Oxygen was necessary for the reaction. Cofactor effects of peroxidase or metal ions could be demonstrated with intact cells, as shown in Table I. As expected, an active L-amino acid oxidase could be demonstrated in the cells (Pistorius and Voss, 1980). A stimulation of O_2 consumption by added amino acids was also observed (Pistorius *et al.*, 1979). The cofactor effect of added peroxidase on in-

Table I HCN formation by intact cells of *Anacystis nidulans*. The experiments were performed in Warburg vessels containing alkali in the center trough to collect the HCN formed. The reaction mixture contained in a total volume of 3 ml : 30 μmoles potassium phosphate buffer, pH 7.0, 45 μl *Anacystis* cells and the additions as indicated: 20 μmoles L-histidine, 100 μg peroxidase, 90 nmoles $VOSO_4$, 45 nmoles $(NH_4)_6Mo_7O_{24}$ or 45 nmoles Na_2WO_4. The samples were shaken in O_2 at 20°C for 3 hrs.

Additions	HCN found, nmoles
None	0
L-His	6.1
Peroxidase	0.2
L-His, Peroxidase	50.1
L-His, $VOSO_4$	33.5
L-His, $(NH_4)_6Mo_7O_{24}$	26.7
L-His, Na_2WO_4	20.7

tact cells suggests that an imino acid product of histidine oxidation is excreted or that the amino acid oxidase is rather externally located.

For comparison with Table I, some results obtained with cell suspensions of two other blue-green algae, incubated with histidine in the dark, are shown in Table II. These data suggest that amino acid oxidases can probably be found in *Nostoc muscorum*, and possibly in *Plectonema boryanum*. *Anabaena variabilis* and *Anabaena cylindrica* (not shown) gave less than 0.1 nmole HCN under similar conditions, but we do not believe this means that HCN formation is absent.

Nitrogenase, the enzyme of nitrogen fixation, can reduce HCN. Thus, cells containing nitrogenase, as many *Anabaena* species do, may give off little HCN even if they form it. It has, in fact, been suggested that nitrogenase evolved originally from an enzyme which reduced and thereby detoxified HCN (Silver and Postgate, 1973).

The L-amino acid oxidase of *Anacystis nidulans* has been purified to homogeneity (Pistorius and Voss, 1980). It has a molecular weight of 98,000 and contains one molecule of FAD per molecule of intact enzyme, and two subunits of equal size. The substrate specificity of this enzyme is unusual. It acts only on basic amino acids. L-argenine, L-lysine and L-ornithine are the preferred substrates, with L-histidine being oxidized at a rate that is about 1% of the rate of oxidation of arginine. The turnover number is

Table II HCN formation by intact cells of *Plectonema boryanum* and *Nostoc muscorum*. The conditions were as in Table I, except that the following additions were made as indicated: 30 μl *Plectonema boryanum* or *Nostoc muscorum* cells, 60 μmoles L-histidine or D-histidine, and 40 μg peroxidase.

Additions	*Plectonema boryanum* HCN found, nmoles	*Nostoc muscorum* HCN found, nmoles
None	0.10	0.11
L-His	0.22	0.20
L-His, Peroxidase	0.26	1.12
D-His	0.24	0.52
D-His, Peroxidase	0.26	1.34

26,000 for arginine - an unusually high value for an amino acid oxidase. This enzyme also has an unusual set of inhibitors: divalent cations and orthophenanthroline. All divalent cations tested were effective, in the sequence $Cu^{2+} > Zn^{2+} > Cd^{2+} > Mn^{2+} > Co^{2+} > Mg^{2+} > Ca^{2+} > Ba^{2+} > Ni^{2+} > Sr^{2+}$. The inhibitory effect of orthophenanthroline led to a search for a metal ion, which has been identified as Zn, firmly bound to the enzyme (Pistorius, unpublished).

VI. HCN PRODUCTION FROM GLYOXYLATE-HYDROXYLAMINE IN *CHLORELLA*

As previously mentioned, high light intensity combined with high O_2 pressures and low CO_2 tensions favour HCN production in *Chlorella vulgaris*, as measured by the formation of the HCN complex of nitrate reductase (Pistorius *et al.*, 1976). These same conditions also stimulate glycolate excretion by the same *Chlorella* cells (Warburg and Krippahl, 1960). Since small amounts of HCN added externally had the same stimulatory effect on glycolate excretion as high O_2 tension, it was proposed that the internal production of HCN mediated the stimulatory effect of O_2 (Vennesland and Jetschmann, 1976). Glycolate is presumably excreted, because its metabolism is blocked, and this could be caused by HCN at the glycine level where pyridoxal phosphate enzymes are involved (see Solomonson, this volume).

The first product of glycolate oxidation is glyoxylate. Solomonson and Spehar (1977, 1979) have described an enzyme system which is present in soluble form in *Chlorella* extracts and makes HCN from glyoxylate and hydroxylamine. This reaction requires Mn^{2+} and ADP. The Mn^{2+} requirement could account for the fact that the capacity to form HCN-inactivated nitrate reductase is impaired in Mn^{2+}-deficient cells (Pistorius *et al.*, 1976). Solomonson and Spehar (1977) proposed that the formation of HCN by this route could provide for a coordinate regulation of photosynthetic CO_2 fixation and nitrate reduction by way of the ribulose-diphosphate carboxylase-oxygenase catalyzed reactions. In brief, phosphoglycolate is formed preferentially from ribulose diphosphate when O_2 tension is high and CO_2 tension is low, and the accumulation of pentose diphosphate is assured by high light intensity. The phosphoglycolate gives glycolate, which is oxidized to glyoxylate, one of the substrates of the HCN-forming reaction. Thus, the HCN produced can inactivate nitrate reductase when the carbon skeletons necessary for combining with NH_3 are in short supply.

The glyoxylate-hydroxylamine system has also been studied on spinach leaf extracts (see Solomonson and Spehar, this volume).

VII. THE PRODUCTION OF HCN FROM UNPHYSIOLOGICAL PRECURSORS

A variety of oximes and nitriles were tested as potential precursors of HCN (see Davies, this volume, for similar experiments with animal tissues). All compounds tested yielded at least a little HCN when incubated with illuminated grana, especially if supplemented with Mn^{2+} and peroxidase. Among the best HCN formers we encountered was malonodinitrile, which formed an autoxidizing system with Mn^{2+} and peroxidase alone, and gave much HCN as shown in Table III. The table also shows the results with glyoxylic acid oxime, which gave a stimulated HCN production in the presence of illuminated grana. Though indolacetonitrile occurs in some plants (Ferris, 1970), there is no evidence that the results of Table III have any physiological significance. But the compounds FCCP (carbonylcyanide *p*-trifluoromethoxy-phenylhydrazone) and CCCP (carbonylcyanide *m*-chlorophenyl-hydrazone) widely used as uncoupling agents in bioenergetic studies, may be regarded as derivatives of malonodinitrile, and have been found to be active HCN precursors. This HCN production is stimulated by illuminated grana or by illuminated *Chlorella* cells, and by O_2 (Pistorius *et al.*, 1975). Comparison of FCCP with CCCP showed that the former was twice as effective an HCN precursor as the latter (Table IV). Since FCCP is proportionately more effective as an uncoupling agent than CCCP, the results suggest that the chemical uncoupling action may be associated with release of HCN. It is also clear that these inhibitors must be degraded during the uncoupling action.

Ferricyanide is another reagent frequently employed in biochemical studies. It and its reduction product, ferrocyanide, both dissociate HCN. Though the amounts involved are small (relative to ferricyanide concentration) because the dissociation is slow, the HCN formed is quite

Table III Formation of cyanide from glyoxylic acid oxime and malonodinitrile. All samples contained 150 μmoles of potassium phosphate buffer, pH 6.5, and 10 μmoles glyoxylic acid oxime or 10 μmoles malonodinitrile as indicated, in a total volume of 3 ml, and the following additions, as indicated: grana preparation from New Zealand spinach containing 0.2 mg chlorophyll, 0.5 mg peroxidase, and 1 μmole $MnSO_4$. The samples were shaken for 3 hr in red light or in the dark, in air or in argon as indicated.

Additions	Gas Phase	HCN found, nmoles			
		Dark		Red light	
		-grana	+grana	-grana	+grana
A. From malonodinitrile					
None	Air	0.4	56	0.4	312
Mn^{2+}	Air	1.0	52	1.4	376
Peroxidase	Air	2.6	62	0.2	1056
Mn^{2+}, Peroxidase	Air	1365.0	410	1400.0	1030
Mn^{2+}, Peroxidase	Argon	0.7	22	0.8	13
B. From glyoxylic acid oxime					
None	Air	-	0.10	0.01	2.9
Mn^{2+}	Air	-	0.08	0.01	23.8
Peroxidase	Air	-	0.22	0.00	3.2
Mn^{2+}, Peroxidase	Air	0.08	0.23	0.02	66.0
Mn^{2+}, Peroxidase	Argon	-	0.20	0.00	0.16

sufficient, for example, to cause complete cessation of nitrate uptake and inactivation of cellular nitrate reductase when ferricyanide is added (to a concentration of 3×10^{-4} M) to a growing *Chlorella* culture (Pistorius *et al.*, 1978). This response of nitrate reductase in intact cells to ferricyanide addition is exactly the opposite of that observed when the ferricyanide is added directly to the HCN-inactivated enzyme, which is activated by oxidation. Ferricyanide itself does not penetrate into the intact cells (Warburg and Krippahl, 1955). It has no access to the intracellular inactive enzyme and cannot oxidize it. But the HCN dissociated from the ferricyanide penetrates the cells readily. There appear to be no membrane barriers to HCN in *Chlorella*.

Table IV Formation of cyanide from FCCP and CCCP. The Warburg vessels containing 200 μmoles potassium phosphate, pH 7.0, 50 μmoles KCl, washed broken chloroplasts from New Zealand spinach (0.2 mg chlorophyll) and the indicated amounts of FCCP and CCCP in a total volume of 3 ml. The vessels were shaken for 1 hr in red light and air.

Additions	nmoles	HCN found, nmoles
None	-	0.0
FCCP	30	8.0
FCCP	75	25.2
FCCP	150	40.4
CCCP	30	4.2
CCCP	75	12.0
CCCP	150	25.6

VIII. THE PHYSIOLOGICAL ROLE OF HCN PRODUCTION: GENERAL

It was initially surmised that HCN plays a role in the regulation of nitrate reduction in algal cells, particularly in *Chlorella* (Gewitz *et al.*, 1974). The formation of a relatively stable HCN-inactivated enzyme has been demonstrated in *Chlorella fusca* (Gewitz *et al.*, 1978) as well as in *Chlorella vulgaris* (Lorimer *et al.*, 1974). The data since obtained with other species do not, however, permit the conclusion that the formation of a stable, HCN-inactivated nitrate reductase *in vivo* is a wide-spread phenomenon. Though, to our knowledge, all nitrate reductases are inhibited by HCN, the strength of HCN binding seems to be variable with enzymes from different sources (Leong and Shen, 1979). It should be emphasized also that the nitrate reductase activity levels of plant and algal cells are subject to wide fluctuations, most of which cannot be ascribed to HCN (Hewitt *et al.*, 1979; Vennesland, 1981).

When *Chlorella vulgaris* cells are transferred from nitrate to ammonia, much HCN-inactivated enzyme is formed. The total nitrate reductase (inactive plus active) gradually declines to a very low level, and the active enzyme declines significantly faster than the HCN-inactivated enzyme (Vennesland, 1981). This suggests that the latter is more stable intracellularly than the former, and that the HCN-inactivation thus possibly involves a mechanism for conserving the molybdoprotein.

The production of HCN by *Chlorella vulgaris* may be regarded as a response to certain types of chemical or environmental stress. If the oxygen tension is high and the cells get much light in the absence of CO_2 and nitrate, so that the light can have no purposeful chemical reducing effect, then HCN production seems to be maximized, and could serve as a stop signal for a variety of metabolic processes. Normal cyanide sensitive respiration stops, CO_2 uptake stops and the carboxylation of ribulose-diphosphate yields to the oxidative production of glycolate as already mentioned. HCN also inhibits nitrate uptake. Many of the enzyme catalyzed reactions involving amino acids should likewise be inhibited (see Solomonson, this volume). Eventually, the *Chlorella* cells recover from a bout with HCN production, just as they recover from HCN administered externally in moderate amounts. The conversion of HCN to the β-carboxamide group of asparagine has been observed in *Chlorella* as well as in higher plant species (Fowden and Bell, 1965). This asparagine formation occurs by way of β-cyanoalanine. If the latter compound is treated with amino acid oxidase, then a release of HCN by a β-elimination reaction has been shown to take place (Miura *et al.*, 1980). [This cannot account for the toxic effects of β-cyanoalanine, when it is administered to animals. β-cyanoalanine is a lathyrogen, a neurotoxic substance (see Ferris, 1970 for review)].

It is far too early to claim that all green cells and quite a few that are not green can make HCN, at least in traces. At present we rather expect this to be true, mainly because we have not yet found any green cells from which we could not elicit a little HCN. Conditions that favour photooxidative processes favour HCN production. One can argue that such processes are destructive, that they are a prelude to, or an accompaniment of cell death. That may be.

Two different types of algal enzyme systems have been found, however, which can operate in the dark to produce HCN. The system studied by Solomonson and Spehar depends on glyoxylate, which is known to be present, and on hydroxylamine, which has frequently been reported to occur, though its biological role is not clear at present, since it is no longer regarded as an intermediate in the reduction of nitrate to ammonia (Hewitt, 1975; Vennesland and Guerrero, 1979). The L-amino acid oxidase of *Anacystis nidulans*, on the other hand, has naturally occurring substrates. The role of this oxidase in cell metabolism is still being studied and it is not possible to estimate what proportion of intracellular histidine might normally be oxidized by the HCN-producing path. We would guess very little, perhaps often none. For optimal production of HCN by intact cells from externally offered histidine in the dark, it is necessary to omit the inhibitory divalent cations from the medium (Pistorius, unpublished).

In the case of the D-amino acid oxidase system of *Chlorella*, our ignorance is even more profound, since nothing is known about the occurrence or formation of D-histidine in *Chlorella*. The D-amino acid oxidases are widely distributed and have long been studied, but may still be regarded as enzymes in search of a function. It has recently been suggested that their true substrates may not be the naturally occurring amino acids, but condensation products of amines and glyoxylate (Hamilton *et al.*, 1979). It was proposed that the products of such enzyme reactions behaved as metabolic effectors to modify the reactivity of proteins or nucleic acids. The HCN formed from aromatic amino acids might also play a regulatory role.

There is little clear information available yet about the process of HCN formation in illuminated grana, though *in vivo* experiments have repeatedly shown that light stimulates the release of HCN, the apparently greater complexity of the photochemical reactions examined led us to study dark reactions first.

These dark reactions are probably not limited to green cells. It has been proposed that the formation of HCN may contribute to the toxicity of snake venom, and account for the fact that most snake venoms contain very high levels of L-amino acid oxidase. The enzyme itself is harmless on injection, but the tissue destruction caused by other venom components is probably necessary to provide the required substrates and cofactors for the HCN production (Pistorius *et al.*, 1977).

There is indirect evidence available that HCN may be formed from histidine in the hepatopancreas of mussels (*Mytillus edulis* L.). Thus, Thoai *et al.* (1954) identified imidazole aldehyde, imidazole alcohol and imidazole carboxylic acid as products of histidine degradation by this tissue. We regard the alcohol and carboxylic acid as products of the aldehyde.

Finally, attention is called to the evidence that HCN production occurs during phagocytosis by polymorphonuclear leucocytes (Stelmaszyńska and Zglicziński, this volume). The chlorination reactions catalyzed by myeloperoxidase seem to be responsible - a different type of reaction from those described in the present paper.

REFERENCES

Bright, H.J. and Porter, D.J.T. (1975). *In* "The Enzymes" (3rd ed. Boyer, P.D., ed) pp. 421-505 Academic Press, New York - San Francisco - London.

Ferris, J.P. (1970). *In* "The Chemistry of the Cyano Group" (Z. Rapport, ed) pp. 717-742. Interscience Publishers, London, New York, Sydney, Toronto.

Fowden, L. and Bell, E.A. (1965). *Nature* 206, 110-112.

Gewitz, H.S., Lorimer, G.H., Solomonson, L.P. and Vennesland, B. (1974). *Nature* 249, 79-81.

Gewitz, H.S., Pistorius, E.K., Voss, H. and Vennesland, B. (1976a). *Planta (Berl.)* 131, 145-148.

Gewitz, H.S., Pistorius, E.K., Voss, H. and Vennesland, B. (1976b).

Planta (Berl.) 131, 149-153.
Gewitz, H.S., Piefke, J. and Vennesland, B. (1978). *Planta (Berl.)* 141, 323-328.
Gewitz, H.S., Piefke, J., Langowska, K. and Vennesland, B. (1980). *Biochim. Biophys. Acta* 66, 11-26.
Hamilton, G.A., Buckthal, D.J., Mortensen, R.M. and Zerby, K.W. (1979) *Proc. Natl. Acad. Sci. USA* 76, 2625-2629.
Hewitt, E.J. (1975). *Ann. Rev. Plant Physiol.* 26, 73-100.
Hewitt, E.J., Hucklesby, D.P., Mann, A.F., Notton, B.A., Rucklidge, G.J. (1979). *In* "Nitrogen Assimilation of Plants" (E.J. Hewitt and C.V. Cutting, eds), pp. 255-287. Academic Press, London - New York - San Francisco.
Leong, C.A. and Shen, T.C. (1979). *Experientia* 35, 584-585.
Lorimer, G.H., Gewitz, H.S., Völker, W., Solomonson, L.P. and Vennesland, B. (1974). *J. Biol. Chem.* 249, 6074-6079.
Miura, R., Shiga, K., Miyake, Y., Watari, H. and Yamano, T. (1980). *J. Biochem.* 87, 1469-1481.
Pistorius, E.K., Gewitz, H.S., Voss, H. and Vennesland, B. (1975). *FEBS Lett.* 59, 162-165.
Pistorius, E.K., Gewitz, H.S., Voss, H. and Vennesland, B. (1976). *Planta (Berl.)* 128, 73-80.
Pistorius, E.K. and Voss, H. (1977). *Biochim. Biophys. Acta* 481, 395-406.
Pistorius, E.K., Gewitz, H.S., Voss, H. and Vennesland, B. (1977). *Biochim. Biophys. Acta* 481, 384-394.
Pistorius, E.K., Funkhouser, E.A. and Voss, H. (1978). *Planta (Berl.)* 141, 279-282.
Pistorius, E.K., Jetschmann, K., Voss, H. and Vennesland, B. (1979). *Biochim. Biophys. Acta* 585, 630-642.
Pistorius, E.K., and Voss, H. (1980). *Biochim. Biophys. Acta* 611, 227-240.
Ramadoss, C.S. (1979). *Planta (Berl.)* 146, 539-544.
Silver, W.S. and Postgate, J.R. (1973). *J. Theor. Biol.* 40, 1-10.
Solomonson, L.P. and Spehar, A.M. (1977). *Nature* 265, 373-375.
Solomonson, L.P. and Spehar, A.M. (1979). *J. Biol. Chem.* 254, 2176-2179.
Thoai, Ng.-V., Glahn, P.E., Hedegaard, J., Manchon, P. and Roche, J. (1954). *Biochim. Biophys. Acta* 15, 87-94.
Vennesland, B. and Jetschmann, K. (1976). *Planta (Berl.)* 128, 81-84.
Vennesland, B. and Guerrero, M.G. (1979). Encyclopedia of Plant Physiology (new series), Vol. 6, Gibbs, M. and Latzko, E., eds., pp. 425-444, Springer, Berlin - Heidelberg - New York.
Vennesland, B. (1981). *In* "Biochemistry and Physiology of Nitrogen and Sulfur Metabolism" (Bothe, H. and Trebst, A., eds) pp.233-243, Springer, Berlin, Heidelberg, New York.
Warburg, D. and Krippahl, G. (1955). *Z. Naturforsch.* 10b, 301-304.
Warburg, D. and Krippahl, G. (1960). *Z. Naturforsch.* 15b, 197-199.

GLYOXYLATE AND CYANIDE FORMATION

LARRY P. SOLOMONSON and ANDREA M. SPEHAR

Department of Biochemistry, University of South Florida, College of Medicine, Tampa, FL 33612, U.S.A.

I. INTRODUCTION

We have previously proposed a model for the regulation of nitrate assimilation in which CO_2 fixation and nitrate assimilation are coordinately regulated (Solomonson and Spehar, 1977). This model also provided a rationale for the possible regulation of nitrate reductase by cyanide *in vivo*. A key reaction in this regulatory scheme was the proposed reaction between hydroxylamine and glyoxylate to form glyoxylate oxime as an intermediate in the formation of cyanide utilized for the *in vivo* inactivation of nitrate reductase. We showed that crude extracts of *Chlorella* did indeed catalyze the formation of cyanide from glyoxylate and hydroxylamine (Solomonson and Spehar, 1977). This reaction required manganese and an additional low molecular weight factor. We subsequently found that ADP is a potent and specific effector for the formation of cyanide from glyoxylate and hydroxylamine in dialyzed extracts of *Chlorella* (Solomonson and Spehar, 1979). A combination of ADP and ATP was even more effective than ADP alone while AMP or ATP alone had no stimulatory effect. These results suggested that cyanide formation from glyoxylate and hydroxylamine may be regulated in part by adenylate energy charge.

In this communication we report on the presence of a similar ADP- and Mn-dependent enzyme system in preparations from spinach and further examine the reaction with respect to substrate and cofactor requirements.

II. COFACTOR AND SUBSTRATE REQUIREMENTS

As shown in Table I, ADP and Mn^{++} are both required for maximal rates of cyanide formation from glyoxylate and hydroxylamine catalyzed by crude spinach extracts. No significant formation of cyanide was observed in controls which contained no glyoxylate or hydroxylamine or in which heated extract was substituted for unheated spinach extract. These results are similar to those obtained previously

Table I Cofactor and substrate requirements

Condition[a]	units/mg protein[b]
Complete	31.2
+ heated extract	< 0.1
- glyoxylate	< 0.1
- NH_2OH	< 0.1
- $MnCl_2$	4.7
- ADP	< 0.1

[a]Conditions for assay of cyanide formation from glyoxylate and hydroxylamine were as described previously (Solomonson and Spehar, 1977, 1979) except that crude spinach extract was used as the enzyme. Spinach extract was prepared from 240 g of deveined spinach leaves which were suspended in 300 ml cold 10 mM potassium phosphate buffer, pH 7.5 (Buffer A), homogenized for 60 sec in a Waring blender and finally centrifuged for 10 min at 7,000 × g. The supernatant from this centrifugation was used as the enzyme source for these experiments. Heated extract was prepared by heating an aliquot of the crude extract in a boiling water bath for 2 min.

[b]One unit of enzyme activity is equal to one nmol of cyanide formed per hour under the conditions of the assay (Solomonson and Spehar, 1977, 1979). Protein was determined by the method of Lowry after precipitation and washing with cold 6% PCA to remove interfering substances.

with *Chlorella* extracts (Solomonson and Spehar, 1977, 1979). The level of activity per mg protein in fresh extracts is also comparable to that found in *Chlorella* extracts.

III. GLOXOYLATE OXIME FORMATION

We have previously shown that *Chlorella* extracts catalyze the formation of cyanide from chemically synthesized glyoxylate oxime in a reaction which is also stimulated by ADP (Solomonson and Spehar, 1979). These results were consistent with glyoxylate oxime being an intermediate in the formation of cyanide from glyoxylate and hydroxylamine. In order to determine whether the formation of glyoxylate oxime is a spontaneous reaction under the conditions of our assay for cyanide formation, we incubated equimolar amounts (30 mM) of glyoxylate and hydroxylamine in 60 mM HEPES-NaOH buffer (pH 7.5) at room temperature. The reactants, glyoxylate and hydroxylamine, were rapidly separated immediately after mixing and after 60 min incubation by passage of 0.8 ml of the above reaction mixture over a Pasteur pipet Dowex 50 (H^+) ion exchange column equilibrated with 60 mM HEPES-NaOH (pH 7.5). Glyoxylate and glyoxylate oxime are found in the flow-through fractions while hydroxylamine is retarded. To determine the extent of formation of glyoxylate oxime, we measured the appearance of glyoxylate oxime in the flow-through fractions and the disappearance of hydroxylamine in the appropriate retarded fractions relative to controls containing glyoxylate oxime alone or hydroxylamine alone. The concentration of glyoxylate oxime was determined from the absorbance of the dianionic species at 251 nm in 0.3 M carbonate buffer (pH 11.5) (Solomonson and Spehar, 1979). Glyoxylate oxime forms spontaneously under the latter conditions so it is essential to separate glyoxylate and hydroxylamine before assaying for glyoxylate oxime by the above method. Hydroxylamine was determined after oxidation to nitrite by the method of Hewitt and Nicholas (1964). The formation of glyoxylate oxime from glyoxylate and hydroxylamine was about 85% complete within one minute whether measured by appearance of glyoxylate oxime or by disappearance of hydroxylamine. The reaction was > 95% complete by 60 min. These results suggest that the formation of glyoxylate oxime is a non-enzymic reaction under the conditions of our assay for cyanide formation. The true substrate, therefore, for the enzyme-catalyzed formation of cyanide is probably glyoxylate oxime.

IV. AMMONIUM SULFATE FRACTIONATION

The enzyme system catalyzing the formation of cyanide was found in the supernatant fraction after high speed centrifugation to remove membrane particles. Initial attempts to further fractionate this activity with ammonium sulfate were unsuccessful due to an apparent loss of enzyme activity. This apparent loss was subsequently found to be due to inhibition of the enzyme by ammonium. Good recoveries were achieved after dialysis of the ammonium sulfate fractions to remove excess ammonium. As shown in Table II, the enzyme was largely recovered in the fraction sedimented between 40 and 50% ammonium sulfate saturation. These results indicate that ammonium sulfate fractionation may be used to partially purify this enzyme system and to separate it from other higher and lower molecular weight components.

Table II Ammonium sulfate fractionation of spinach extract

Fraction[(a)]	Total Units[(b)] 10^{-3}	% Recovery	units/mg protein	Fold-Purification
Extract	108	100	39.2	1.0
0-40% AS	34.9	32.3	36.0	0.9
40-50% AS	66.9	61.9	87.6	2.2
50-60% AS	3.5	3.2	15.8	0.4
40-50% AS plus 60 mM $(NH_4)_2SO_4$	-	-	8.2	-

[(a)] Spinach extract was prepared as described in the legend for Table I. Ammonium sulfate fractions were prepared by adding a saturated ammonium sulfate solution (pH 7.1) to the extract to give the desired percent saturation of ammonium sulfate. The indicated fractions were collected by centrifugation for 10 min at 7000 × g and were suspended to approximately 1/5 original volume with Buffer A. The fractions were dialyzed in 10 ml aliquots for 3-4 hours against 3.5 liters of Buffer A.

[(b)] Units of enzyme activity are as described for Table I.

V. ADENINE NUCLEOTIDE EFFECTS

The 40-50% ammonium sulfate fraction was used to test the effects of different adenine nucleotides and related analogues on the rate of cyanide formation from glyoxylate and hydroxylamine. As shown in Table III, neither AMP nor ATP alone were as effective as ADP alone. GDP, another purine nucleoside diphosphate, did not stimulate the rate of cyanide formation. The ADP analogue, α,β-methylene ADP, had no stimulatory effect by itself but inhibited the stimulatory effect of ADP. The ATP analogue, β,γ-methylene ATP also had no effect by itself but did give a slight stimulation in combination with ADP. The rate of cyanide formation in the presence of a combination of ATP and ADP was about four-fold higher than in the presence of ADP alone. Due to the presence of low levels of ATPase and ADPase activities in this enzyme preparation, it was not feasible to further evaluate the possible relationship between adenylate energy charge and the rate of cyanide formation.

Table III Adenine nucleotide effects

Addition[a]	Relative Rate of Cyanide Formation
None	< 1
AMP	< 1
ADP	100
ATP	27
ATP/ADP (3/1)	395
GDP	< 1
α,β-methylene ADP	< 1
β,γ-methylene ATP	< 1
ADP + α,β-methylene ADP	46
ADP + β,γ-methylene ATP	112

[a] Assay conditions were as described previously (Solomonson and Spehar, 1977, 1979) with the dialyzed 40-50% ammonium sulfate fraction of crude spinach extract as the enzyme. The total nucleotide concentration added in each case was 1 mM except in the two combinations of ADP with the methylene analogues of ADP and ATP in which each component was added at a concentration of 1 mM. The ratio of ATP/ADP indicated was determined by HPLC analysis of the reaction mixture after assay for cyanide formation (Solomonson and Spehar, 1979). An ATP-regenerating system (Solomonson and Spehar, 1979) was used to study the effect of ATP on the rate of cyanide formation. Individual components of the regenerating system had no effect on the rate of formation of cyanide either in the presence or absence of ADP. Activities are given relative to the rate of cyanide formation in the complete reaction mixture with ADP which is set at 100.

VI. VOLATILE PRODUCTS FROM [1-^{14}C] AND [2-^{14}C]-GLYOXYLATE

According to the proposed reaction sequence for the formationof cyanide from glyoxylate and hydroxylamine, the intermediate glyoxylate oxime is cleaved to form HCN and CO_2 as final reaction products. Both HCN and CO_2 are volatile under our assay conditions and can be collected in an alkali trap in a closed reaction system. To further test the

Table IV Relative rates of formation of cyanide and radioactive volatile products from [1-^{14}C]- and [2-^{14}C]-glyoxylate

Condition[(a)]	Cyanide Formed	[1-^{14}C]-Product	[2-^{14}C]-Product
Complete	100	670	110
- Enzyme	< 1	450	5
- NH_2OH	< 1	54	2
- ADP	< 1	740	6
- $MnCl_2$	6	120	13

[(a)] Assay conditions were as described previously (Solomonson and Spehar, 1977, 1979) with the dialyzed 40-50% ammonium sulfate fraction of spinach extract as the enzyme. [1-^{14}C] and [2-^{14}C]-Glyoxylate were prepared from [1-^{14}C]- and [2-^{14}C]-glycine, respectively, by incubation of the glycine radioisotopes with D-amino acid oxidase. The products were separated by ion exchange chromatography. The radiospecific activity of the [^{14}C]-glyoxylate was adjusted to 130 cpm/nmol with unlabelled glyoxylate. The final concentration of glyoxylate in the assay mixture was 30 mM. The amount of cyanide formed was determined as described previously. The amount of volatile [^{14}C]-product collected in the alkali trap of the Conway diffusion dishes was determined by liquid scintillation counting. The major volatile products are presumed to be CO_2 from [1-^{14}C]-glyxolate and HCN from [2-^{14}C]-glyoxylate in the presence of hydroxylamine. Activities are given relative to the rate of cyanide formation in the complete reaction mixture which is set at 100.

proposed reaction, we utilized [1-^{14}C]- and [2-^{14}C]-glyoxylate as substrates and measured the rate of volatile labelled products formed relative to the rate of cyanide formed as measured by our normal assay procedure. The expected volatile labelled products would be $^{14}CO_2$ and $H^{14}CN$ from [1-^{14}C]- and [2-^{14}C]-glyoxylate, respectively. According to the proposed reaction, the rates of cyanide formation and each of the volatile labelled products should be the same. The results of this experiment are shown in Table IV. The cofactor requirements and rate of formation of volatile radioactive products from [2-^{14}C]-glyoxylate are in quite good agreement with the rate of cyanide formed as determined by chemical methods (Solomonson and Spehar, 1977). The rate of formation of volatile radioactive product from [1-^{14}C]-glyoxylate, however, does not agree with the rate of cyanide formed. This can be attributed in part to the non-enzymic formation of CO_2 from glyoxylate and glyoxylate oxime and to a decarboxylase activity which is not dependent on ADP. It should be noted that in no case does the spontaneous or the enzyme-catalyzed formation of [^{14}C]-product represent more than 1% of the initial concentration of glyoxylate. The significance of these results is not clear at the present time. One possible interpretation is that cyanide is formed from glyoxylate oxime in a two-step reaction with CO_2 release preceding the ADP-dependent formation of cyanide. In view of the relative impurity of the enzyme system used in these experiments, however, such a conclusion would be premature at this time.

VII. CONCLUDING REMARKS

The results reported herein are in essential agreement with those reported earlier for *Chlorella* extracts indicating that the enzyme system catalyzing the formation of cyanide from glyoxylate and hydroxylamine is not unique to *Chlorella* cells but is present in higher plants as well. We have further shown that the formation of glyoxylate oxime from glyoxylate and hydroxylamine is a spontaneous chemical reaction under the conditions of our assay suggesting that glyoxylate oxime may be the true substrate for the reaction. Until more is known about the mechanism of the reaction, however, it is not possible to classify the enzyme system with certainty. It is not yet known, for example, whether one enzyme or a combination of enzymes is involved. These questions, as well as the precise role of adenine nucleotides in the reaction may be resolved upon further purification of the enzyme system.

These *in vitro* experiments together with earlier results (Solomonson and Spehar, 1977, 1979) suggest that glyoxylate oxime may be a possible precursor of cyanide utilized for the inactivation of nitrate reductase *in vivo*. Vennesland and coworkers have shown that cyanide can also be formed in good yield from certain amino acids such as D- or L-histidine in the presence of the appropriate amino acid oxidase supplemented with peroxidase or cytochrome *c* (Gewitz *et al.*, 1976, 1980; Pistorius *et al.*, 1977, 1979; Vennesland *et al.*, this volume). Furthermore, amino acid oxidases with specificity for these potential cyanide precursors have been isolated from algal cells (Pistorius and Voss, 1977, 1980). The relative importance of the glyoxylate system or amino acids such as histidine in the metabolic control of nitrate assimilation is not known at the present time. Knowledge accumulated to date through *in vitro* experiments will hopefully facilitate the design of *in vivo* experiments to resolve these questions in the future.

ACKNOWLEDGEMENTS

This research was supported by a grant (GM23407) from the National Institutes of Health.

REFERENCES

Gewitz, H.S., Pistorius, E.K., Voss, H. and Vennesland, B. (1976). *Planta* 131, 149-153.

Gewitz, H.S., Piefke, J., Langowska, K. and Vennesland, B. (1980). *Biochim. Biophys. Acta* 611, 11-26.

Hewitt, E.J. and Nicholas, D.J.D. (1964). *Modern Methods of Plant Analysis* 7, 67-172.

Pistorius, E.K. and Voss, H. (1977). *Biochim. Biophys. Acta* 481, 395-406.

Pistorius, E.K. and Voss, H. (1980). *Biochim. Biophys. Acta* 611, 227-240.

Pistorius, E.K., Gewitz, H.S., Voss, H. and Vennesland, B. (1977). *Biochim. Biophys. Acta* 481, 384-394.

Pistorius, E.K., Jetschmann, K., Voss, H. and Vennesland, B. (1979). *Biochim. Biophys. Acta* 585, 630-642.

Solomonson, L.P. and Spehar, A.M. (1977). *Nature* 265, 373-375.

Solomonson, L.P. and Spehar, A.M. (1979). *J. Biol. Chem.* 254, 2176-2179.

THE ROLE OF MYELOPEROXIDASE IN PHAGOCYTOSIS, WITH SPECIAL REGARD TO HCN FORMATION

TERESA STELMASZYŃSKA and JAN M. ZGLICZYŃSKI

Instytut Biochemii Lekarskiej, Akademia Medyczna, Kraków, Poland

Phagocytosis by polymorphonuclear leucocytes (PMNs) and all postphagocytic events occurring within the PMNs represent one of the lines of resistance of our body against invading microorganisms.

The term "phagocytosis" denotes the act of engulfment of bacteria. Postphagocytic events include: morphologic changes, a burst of leucocytic metabolic activity, and the killing and digestion of ingested microorganisms (for review see Klebanoff, 1975). The killing of microorganisms is accomplished by mechanisms which are in part independent of oxygen, and in part oxygen dependent. Myeloperoxidase (MPO) is an important component of the latter mechanism (Klebanoff, 1975).

I. GENERAL CHARACTERISTICS OF MYELOPEROXIDASE

Myeloperoxidase (MPO) belongs to the group of true peroxidases (donor: H_2O_2 oxidoreductase, E.C.1.11.1.7.). The enzyme is a two-heme protein with a molecular weight in the range of 135,000 - 150,000 (Ehrenberg and Agner, 1958; Schultz and Schmuckler, 1964; Odajima and Yamazaki, 1972). MPO is a cationic protein with pI > 10 (Agner, 1941) and possesses the most complex structure among the peroxidases (Harrison *et al.*, 1977).

MPO is present in mammalian PMNs and most probably in monocytes (Salmon *et al.*, 1970; Bos *et al.*, 1978). The concentration of MPO in human PMNs has been estimated to be about 5% of the dry weight of the cell (Schultz and Kaminker, 1962).

The distribution of the enzyme within the PMN depends on the physiological state of the cell. In resting PMNs, the MPO is entirely enclosed in azurophil granules (Dunn *et al.*, 1968; Bainton and Farquhar, 1968; Baggiolini *et al.*, 1969). During phagocytosis, degranulation occurs, and MPO is released into the phagocytic vacuole (Klebanoff, 1970). MPO discharged into the phagocytic vacuole accumulates on the bacterial surface (Klebanoff, 1970), thereby attaining a high local concentration and achieving intimate contact with the microorganisms. Indeed, the pre-coating of bacteria by purified MPO results in more efficient killing (Selvaraj *et al.*, 1978).

II. SOME CATALYTIC FUNCTIONS OF MYELOPEROXIDASE

Purified MPO preparations catalyse the oxidation of a wide variety of electron donors, such as phenols, aromatic amines, uric acid and halides (Cl^-, Br^- and I^-). As a rule, H_2O_2 acts as the electron accepting substrate.

From the physiological point of view, the peroxidation of Cl^- ions to HOCl appears to be of great interest (Agner, 1958, 1972; Zgliczyński *et al.*, 1971). Since chloride is present in abundance in the animal body and H_2O_2 is produced during phagocytosis by PMNs (Iyer *et al.*, 1961; Paul and Sbarra, 1968), it was reasonable to suspect the intracellular (intraphagosomal) formation of HOCl followed by subsequent chlorination reactions. We have, in fact, found that chlorination occurs in phagocytizing pMNs (Zgliczyński and Stelmaszyńska, 1975).

A. MYELOPEROXIDASE AS A CHLORINATING ENZYME

Enzymatic chlorination of biological compounds by the MPO-H_2O_2 - Cl^- system results in the formation of metabolically unusual products. It is not clear, as yet, which of the products are particularly active in the bactericidal action of PMNs.

Available data exists concerning the chlorination of amino compounds by the MPO - H_2O_2-Cl^- system (Zgliczyński *et al.*, 1971; Stelmaszyńska and Zgliczyński, 1978). These include the formation of *N*-mono- and *N*-dichloramines of amines, α-amino acids, dipeptides and a polypeptide (insulin). *N*-monochloramines of α-amino acids and of dipeptides decompose to ammonia and aldehydes or to *N*-(oxo-acyl)-amino acids, respectively. *N*-dichloramines yield nitriles.

N-dichloramines of glycine, of glycyl-amino acids and of a polypeptide with an *N*-terminal glycin (insulin) are of particular interest, since their decomposition (through cyanoformyl derivatives) yields HCN (Zgliczynski and Stelmaszyńska, 1979; Stelmaszyńska and Zgliczyński, 1978). This topic is the main subject of this review.

1. *Chlorination of glycine as a source of HCN*

The α-amino acids were the first physiological compounds with which enzymatic chlorination by human MPO was observed (Zgliczyński *et al.*, 1971).

$$H_2O_2 + Cl^- + \underset{\displaystyle COOH}{\overset{\displaystyle R}{\overset{|}{\underset{|}{HC}}}}\text{-}NH_3^+ \xrightarrow{MPO} \underset{\displaystyle COOH}{\overset{\displaystyle R}{\overset{|}{\underset{|}{HC}}}}\text{-}NH\text{-}Cl + 2\,H_2O \qquad (1)$$

The *N*-monochloroamino acids are unstable products and decompose to aldehydes, CO_2 and NH_3:

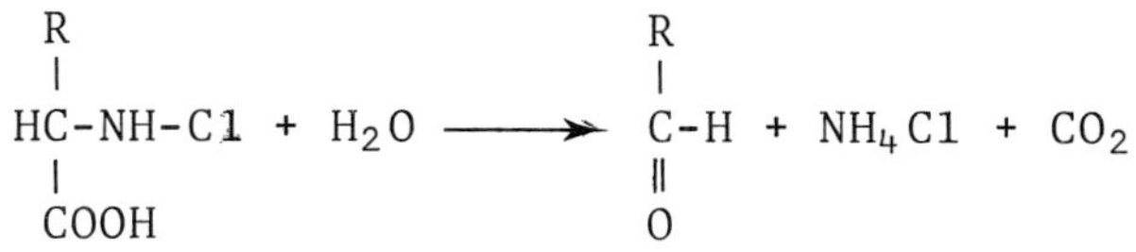

(2)

At lower pH values monochloramines undergo dismutation:

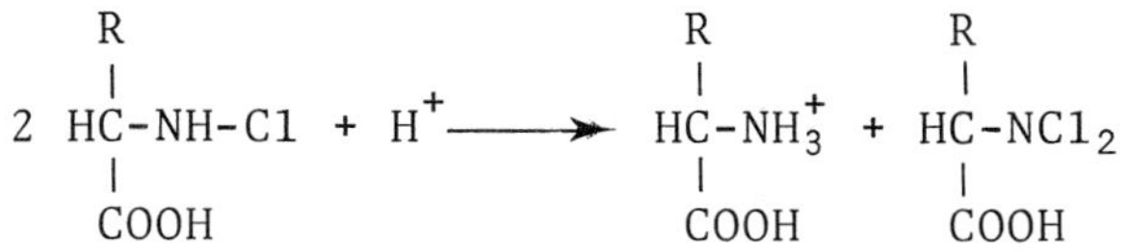

(3)

The *N*-dichloroamino acids yield the corresponding nitriles and CO_2 (Pereira *et al.*, 1973). In the particular case of *N*-dichloroglycine, HCN would be an expected product of degradation:

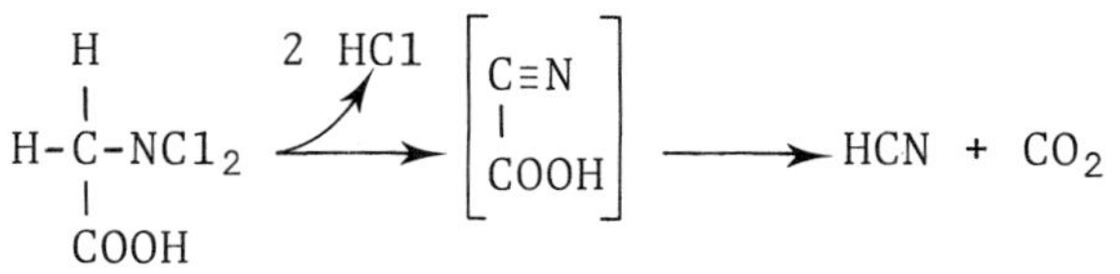

(4)

Actually, HCN is formed during the chlorination of glycine by the MPO-H_2O_2-Cl^- system, especially at lower pH values, when dichloroglycine is formed by reaction (3), (Table I).

To show that *N*-dichloroglycine is a precursor of HCN, the non-enzymatic synthesis of dichloroglycine was performed. Upon the addition of a two-fold excess of HOCl to glycine, dichloramine is formed with an absorption maximum at 305 nm (Fig. 1). It is an unstable compound with a half-life of 3.3, 2.8 and 1.6 minutes at pH 4.6, 5.8 and 6.6, respectively. HCN and ClCN are quantitatively recovered as degradation products (Fig. 1). Cyanogen chloride originates from a secondary reaction between HCN and the dichloramine:

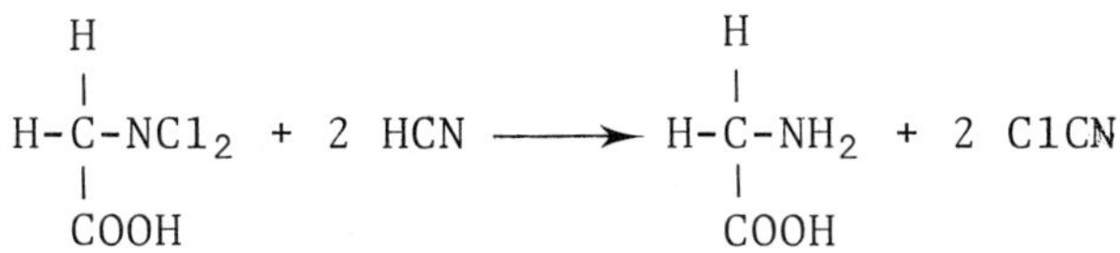

(5)

2. *Chlorination of glycyl-amino acids and an N-terminal glycyl polypeptide (insulin)*

The chlorination of dipeptides and polypeptides by the MPO-H_2O_2-Cl^- system results in formation of an *N*-terminal chloramino group (Stelmaszyńska and Zgliczyński, 1978).

Table I The products of glycine chlorination by the myeloperoxidase-H_2O_2-Cl^- system

pH	H_2O_2 (μmol)	H_2C-COOH | NHCl (μmol)	HCN (μmol)	ClCN (μmol)
5.7[(a)]	1.2	1.16	0	0
	2.4	2.2	0	0
	3.6	3.3	0	0
	4.8	4.0	0.05	0.1
	6.0	4.1	0	0.2
	7.2	4.2	0	0.25
4.8	1.4	0.7	0.08	0.12
	2.8	1.35	0.1	0.32
	4.2	1.95	0.05	0.63
	5.6	2.55	0.0	0.8
	7.2	2.8	0.0	1.07

[(a)]Concentration of products estimated after every fourth portion of H_2O_2.

The reaction mixture, 4 ml 50 mM phosphate/citrate buffer contained: 6 μmol glycine, 10 μg myeloperoxidase, 400 μmol NaCl: at pH 5.7, 7.2 μmol H_2O_2 added in 24 successive equal portions at 30-45 s intervals; at pH 4.8, 7 μmol H_2O_2 added in five successive equal portions at 2-3 min intervals (from Zgliczyński and Stelmaszyńska, 1979).

Since the chlorinated product of free glycine gives HCN and ClCN, similar products could be expected from chlorinated peptides and proteins. Indeed, chlorinated peptide has been shown to be a source of HCN, provided that an *N*-terminal glycyl residue is present (Stelmaszyńska and Zgliczyński, 1978). In contrast to glycine *N*-dichloramine, however, *N*-dichloropeptides are stable for hours. Moreover, the release of HCN and ClCN during the decomposition of *N*-dichloroglycyl-peptides at 37°C does not reflect the decrease of N-Cl bonds quantitatively (Fig. 2). Release of HCN is completed by heating at 70°C for 10 minutes. A two-step degradation of *N*-dichloroglycyl-peptide, with the formation of a cyanformyl derivative as a transient product is therefore proposed:

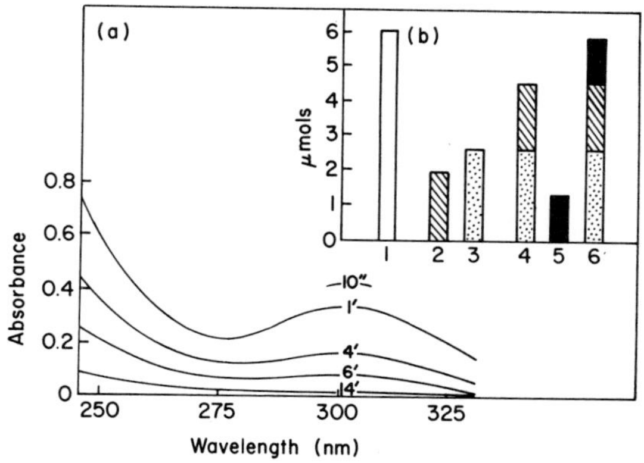

Fig. 1 Degradation of *N*-dichloroglycine.
(A) Time course of degradation: The absorption spectra of *N*-Cl_2-Gly at 10 sec, 1, 4, 6; 14 min after mixing of 6 μmoles of Gly, 12.2 μmoles of HOCl in 4 ml of 0.05 M phosphate-citrate buffer, pH 5.8.
(B) Final products of degradation: Bars - 1. - initial amount of *N*-Cl_2-Gly, 2. and 3. - HCN and ClCN, respectively, 4. - *N*-Cl_2-Gly yielding total HCN, 5. - *N*-Cl_2-Gly chlorinating HCN to ClCN, 6. - total amount of *N*-Cl_2-Gly yielding HCN and ClCN. HCN and ClCN are assayed according to Epstein (1947), for other experimental details see Zgliczyński and Stelmaszyńska (1979).

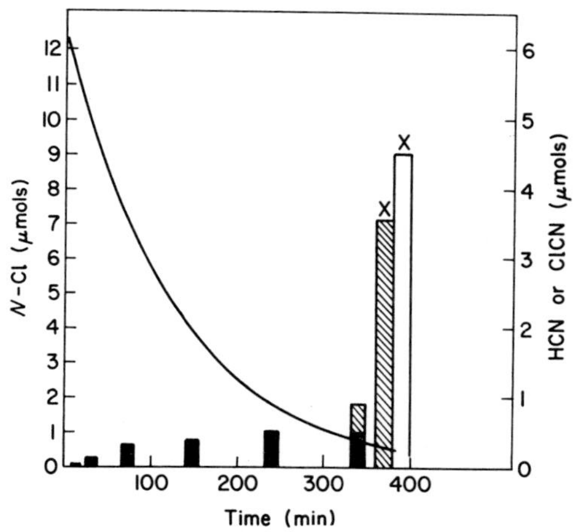

Fig. 2 Degradation of *N*-dichloro-glycyl-leucine.
N-Cl_2-Gly-Leu (6 μmoles) was incubated at 37°C, at pH 6.6, *N*-Cl ———, ClCN - filled bars, HCN - hatched bars, leucine - open bar, X - indicates HCN or leucine determined after heating at 70°C, for 10 min (from Stelmaszyńska and Zgliczyński, 1978).

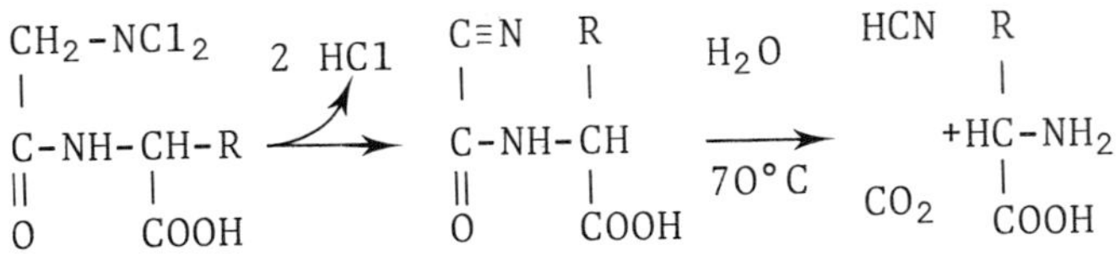

(6)

The chlorination of insulin which contains *N*-terminal glycine in chain A, resulted in the formation of *N*-dichloroglycine A1 and subsequent HCN formation, provided that over four-fold molar excess of HOCl, with respect to insulin, was added (Stelmaszyńska and Zgliczyński, 1978). This may be explained by the competition for HOCl between different protein residues, accessible to HOCl attack.

3. *HCN as an inhibitor and substrate of the MPO-H_2O_2-Cl^- system*

A surprising aspect of HCN accumulation during the MPO-mediated chlorination of glycine is the fact that HCN has no inhibitory effect on this reaction. HCN is well known as an inhibitor of heme-enzymes, and, in fact, binds to MPO with considerable affinity (for review see Odajima and Yamazaki, 1972; Zgliczyński and Stelmaszyńska, 1979).

In the presence of chloride, however, especially at acidic pHs, the binding of cyanide to peroxidases is strongly inhibited (Kimura and Yamazaki, 1978; Zgliczyński and Stelmaszyńska, 1979). Chloride and cyanide bind competitively to the active site of MPO, as shown by the dependence of HCN binding on the chloride concentration (Fig. 3A). The chloride binding is enhanced by a lowering of pH (Fig. 3B).

Therefore, cyanide is a rather poor inhibitor of the MPO-mediated chlorination at acidic pHs. Moreover, HCN, by virtue of chemical susceptibility to chlorination, may serve as a substrate for the MPO-H_2O_2-Cl^- system. The velocity of HCN chlorination to yield ClCN generally increases with the elevations of [Cl^-] and [H^+] , but depends in a more complex manner on H_2O_2 and HCN concentrations (Fig. 4).

III. HCN FORMATION DURING PHAGOCYTOSIS

In the light of the above results it is conceivable, that HCN is produced during phagocytosis, since chlorination in phagocytizing PMNs has been demonstrated (Zgliczyński and Stelmaszyńska, 1975), and the glycine-serine concentration in leucocytes is especially high (12 mM) (McMenamy *et al.*, 1960).

Indeed, preliminary experiments with surviving human PMNs, challenged with bacteria (*Staphylococcus epidermidis*) indicated that formation of HCN may be one of the phagocytosis markers (Table II). It should be pointed out that the bacteria themselves did not produce HCN, and, in samples with resting PMNs, only a trace of HCN could be

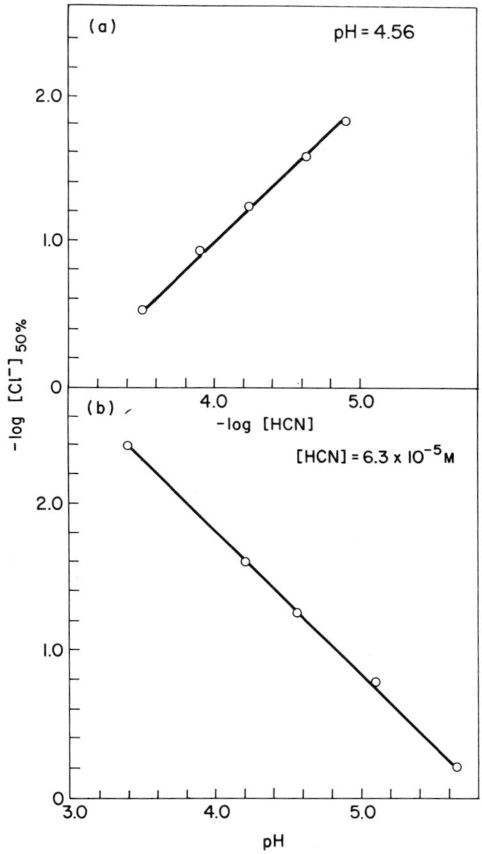

Fig. 3 The effect of cyanide concentration and pH on the $[Cl^-]_{50\%}$ values.
The $[Cl^-]_{50\%}$ values (the $[Cl^-]$ causing 50% saturation of MPO with Cl^-) are obtained from spectrophotometric titrations of 3.1 μM MPO-cyanide complex with NaCl:

A) at pH 4.56, in the presence of different cyanide concentrations.

B) in the presence of 63 μM cyanide, at different pH values. The slopes of both curves are 1.0 (for experimental details see Zgliczyński and Stelmaszyńska, 1979).

detected (Fig. 5). Thus, the postphagocytic events, namely the respiratory burst connected with H_2O_2 production, the MPO release into phagosomes and the pH decrease (for review see Klebanoff, 1975) are associated with HCN production.

The extent of HCN production by phagocytizing PMNs appears to be variable individually (Table II). Could this

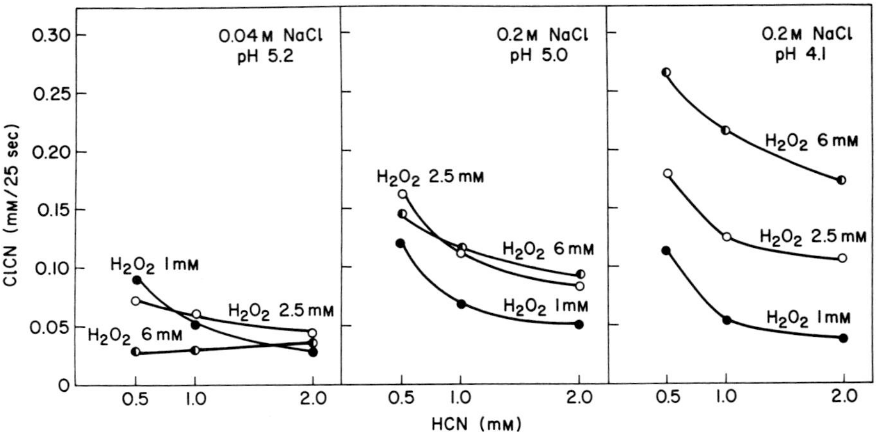

Fig. 4 The effect of HCN, H_2O_2, H^+ and Cl^- concentrations on ClCN formation.

The samples contained: 12 μg MPO, NaCl, HCN, H_2O_2 as indicated, in total volume of 1 ml of 0.05 M phosphate-citrate buffer. The reaction was started by the addition of H_2O_2, at 23°C. ClCN was assayed according to Epstein (1947), omitting the chloramine T addition.

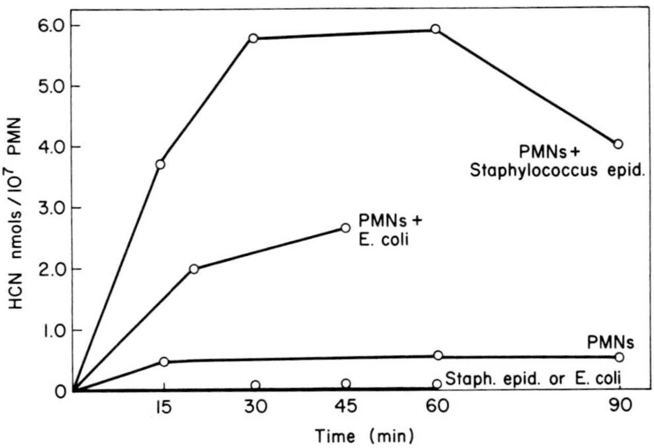

Fig. 5 Time course of HCN production during phagocytosis of *Staphylococcus epidermidis* and *Escherichia coli* by human PMNs.
Results from a typical experiment, with PMNs from one donor. Conditions as described under Table II (Stelmaszyńska, 1981, to be published).

Table II Production of HCN during phagocytosis of *Staphylococcus epidermidis* by human PMNs

No. of experiment	HCN (10^7 PMNs) 1^h		
	Blood donors		
	I	II	III
		nmoles	
1	3.2	4.0	1.75
2	5.9	2.0	2.8
3	3.6	5.2	1.5
4	4.2	5.6	-
5	3.7	4.9	-

Leucocytes were obtained from 3 healthy donors (blood A or B group) by agglutination of erythrocytes with O group plasma (Zgliczyński and Stelmaszyńska, 1975). PMNs ($1\text{-}2 \cdot 10^7$) were suspended in 1 ml of plasma diluted with 1 ml of 0.13 M NaCl + 10 mM glucose. Heat-killed bacteria suspended in 0.4 ml of plasma were added in Warburg vessels, at 37°C. HCN was collected (after acidification of the sample) in a central cup, containing 0.5 ml 0.1 M NaOH. The number of bacteria within the PMNs after 1^h of incubation, when monitored microscopically, was 30-50 per cell (Stelmaszyńska, 1981, to be published).

reflect the preactivation of blood donor PMNs by latent infection?

The quantities of HCN formed during phagocytosis depend also on the strain of bacteria used. The phagocytosis of *Staphylococcus epidermidis* results in about a doubling of the levels of HCN production, compared with those produced when *Escherichia coli* is engulfed (Fig. 5). One of the possible explanations may be the presence of penta-glycyl-seryl peptides in the peptidoglycan of *Staphylococcus epidermidis* cell walls (Tipper and Berman, 1969). The cell walls of *Escherichia coli* lack the glycyl-seryl structures.

In fact, the chlorination of *Staphylococcus epidermidis* (but not of *Escherichia coli*) by an isolated MPO-H_2O_2-Cl^- system yielded small amounts of HCN (Stelmaszyńska, to be published, 1981).

During the phagocytosis of *Escherichia coli* by PMNs, however, a production of HCN was also found. Thus, it may be supposed that free glycine or glycyl peptides coming from leucocytes and from the surrounding medium, as well as from the bacterial cell wall, may be a source of cyanide. Actually, the intraleucocytic concentration of glycine is high (McMenamy *et al.*, 1960).

Not only glycine but aromatic amino acids may also deliver HCN during phagocytosis. It has been found recently that the synergistic action of purified amino acid oxidase and peroxidase brings about HCN formation from aromatic amino acids (Gewitz *et al.*, 1980; see also Vennesland *et al.*, this volume). Finally, it is also known that cyanide may be formed during the peroxidase-mediated oxidation of thiocyanate (Sörbo and Ljunggren, 1958; Chung and Wood, 1970). Since all of these HCN-yielding reactions require the catalytic action of peroxidases, regardless of the substances, MPO is most probably responsible for HCN production during phagocytosis.

IV. SOME PHYSIOLOGICAL ASPECTS OF HCN PRODUCTION DURING PHAGOCYTOSIS

The biological significance of HCN formation during phagocytosis seems to be evident, if we take into account its possible bactericidal properties. The microbicidal ability would be satisfactorily explained by the poisoning of the bacterial respiratory chain, resulting from a local, temporary increase in HCN formed within the phagosome. Moreover, ClCN, the product of HCN chlorination by the MPO-H_2O_2-Cl^-system, could also be harmful to bacteria. An additional aspect of the biological role of HCN formation could be its possible regulatory effect on events in phagocytizing PMNs (Fig. 6).

The phagocytosis process as well as some postphagocytic events in PMNs are insensitive to HCN (Sbarra and Karnovsky, 1959). It has recently been reported that HCN even stimulates consumption of oxygen and the operation of the hexose monophosphate shunt during phagocytosis (DeChatelet *et al.*, 1977). Possible contribution of HCN to the metabolic events within phagocytizing PMNs is summarized in Fig. 6.

It has been shown, that HCN is excreted in trace amounts in the urine and the expired air of normal men (Boxer and Rickards, 1951; Boxer and Rickards, 1952). In the light of all mentioned findings it becomes tempting to speculate that the cyanide in our body originates, at least in part, from the defence processes continuously occurring in tissues.

ACKNOWLEDGEMENT

This work was supported by Grant II.1.2.11. from the Polish Academy of Sciences.

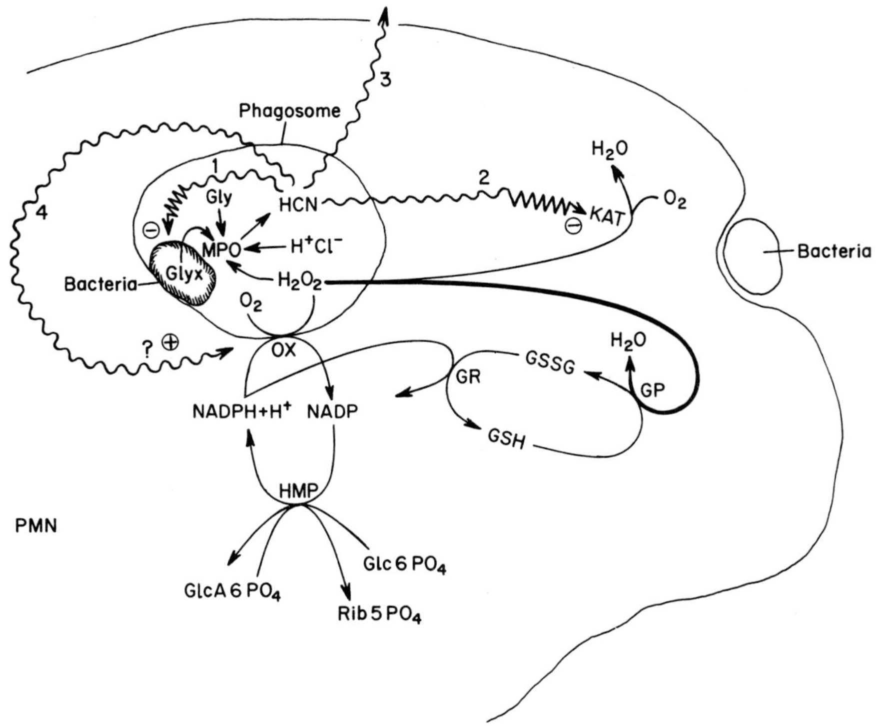

Fig. 6 Proposed contribution of HCN to the metabolic events within phagocytizing PMNs.
Upon contact of bacteria with PMN and subsequent formation of phagosome, a number of cyclic events are initiated: NADPH oxidase (OX) becomes activated, which results in H_2O_2 formation within phagosome (for review see Roos and Weening, 1979). Then the MPO-H_2O_2-Cl^- system can operate, and HCN is produced. HCN may act on bacterial heme-proteins (1), and/ or diffuse to cytosol and inhibit catalase (2), (CAT). Inhibition of catalase preserves H_2O_2 from degradation, H_2O_2, in turn, is required for generation of NADP via concerted action of glutathione reductase (GR) and glutathione peroxidase (GP) (Strauss *et al.*, 1969). NADP is the limiting factor for hexose monophosphate shunt (HMP). As a result of two HMP steps NADPH is formed and serves as a substrate for H_2O_2 generation (Iyer *et al.*, 1961). The possibility also exists that HCN directly stimulates oxidation of NADPH (4) (DeChatelet *et al.*, 1977).

REFERENCES

Agner, K. (1941). *Acta Physiol. Scand.* 2, (Suppl. VIII).

Agner, K. (1958). *Abstr. 4th Int. Congr. Biochem.* 5-58.

Agner, K. (1970). *In* "The Structure and Function of Oxidation-Reduction Enzymes" (Å. Åkeson, A. Ehrenberg, eds.). pp. 329-335, Pergamon Press, Elmsford, N.Y.

Baggiolini, M., Hirsch, J.G. and de Duve, C. (1969). *J. Cell. Biol.* 40, 529.

Bainton, D.F., Farquhar, M.G. (1968). *J. Cell. Biol.* 39, 299.

Bos, A., Wever, R. and Roos, D. (1978). *Biochim. Biophys. Acta* 525, 37-44.

Boxer, G.E. and Rickards, J.C. (1951). *Arch. Biochem. Biophys.* 30, 392-401.

Boxer, G.E. and Rickards, J.C. (1952). *Arch. Biochem. Biophys.* 39, 287-291.

Chung, J. and Wood, J. (1970). *Arch. Biochem. Biophys.* 141, 73-78.

DeChatelet, L.R., McPhail, L.C. and Shirley, P.S. (1977). *Blood* 49, 445-454.

Dunn, W.B., Hardin, J.H. and Spicer, S.S. (1968). *Blood* 32, 935.

Ehrenberg, A. and Agner, K. (1958). *Acta Chem. Scand.* 12, 95-100.

Epstein, J. (1947). *Anal. Chem.* 19, 272-274.

Gewitz, H.S., Piefke, J., Langowska, K. and Vennesland, B. (1980). *Biochim. Biophys. Acta* 611, 11-26.

Harrison, J.E., Pabalan, S. and Schultz, J. (1977). *Biochim. Biophys. Acta* 493, 247-259.

Iyer, G.Y., Islam, M.F. and Quastel, J.H. (1961). *Nature,* 192, 535-541.

Kimura, S. and Yamazaki, I. (1978). *Arch. Biochem. Biophys.* 189, 14-19.

Klebanoff, S.J. (1970). *In* "Biochemistry of the Phagocytic Process: Localization and the Role of Myeloperoxidase and the Mechanism of the Halogenation Reaction" (J. Schultz, ed.) 89-110, North-Holland Publ. Company, Amsterdam.

Klebanoff, S.J. (1975). *Seminars in Hematology XII,* 2, 117-142.

McMenamy, R.H., Lund, C.C., Neville, G.J. and Wallach, D.F.H. (1960). *J. Clin. Invest.* 39, 1675-1687.

Odajima, T., Yamazaki, I. (1972). *Biochim. Biophys. Acta* 284, 360-367.

Paul, B.B. and Sbarra, A.J. (1968). *Biochim. Biophys. Acta* 156, 168-178.

Pereira, W.E., Hoyano, Y., Summons, R.E., Bacon, V.A. and Duffield, A.M. (1973). *Biochim. Biophys. Acta* 313, 170-180.

Roos, D., Weening, R.S. (1979). *In* "Oxygen Free Radicals and Tissue Damage" (Ciba Foundation Symposium 65) pp. 225-248, Excerpta Medica, Amsterdam.

Salmon, S.E., Cline, M.J., Schultz, J. and Lehrer, R.I. (1970). *New Eng. J. Med.* 282, 250-254.

Sbarra, A.J. and Karnovsky, M.L. (1959). *J. Biol. Chem.* 234, 1355-1361.

Schultz, J. and Kaminker, K. (1962). *Arch. Biochem. Biophys.* 96, 465-467.

Schultz, J. and Schmuckler, H.W. (1964). *Biochemistry* 3, 1234-1238.

Selvaraj, R.J., Zgliczyński, J.M., Paul, B.B. and Sbarra, A.J. (1978). *J. Infect. Dis.* 137, 481-485.

Sörbo, B. and Ljunggren, J.G. (1958). *Acta Chem. Scand.* 12, 415-459.

Stelmaszyńska, T. and Zgliczyński, J.M. (1978). *Eur. J. Biochem.* 92, 301-308.

Strauss, R.R., Paul, B.B., Jacobs, A.A. and Sbarra, A.J. (1969). *Arch. Biochem. Biophys.* 135, 265-271.

Tipper, D.J. and Berman, M.F. (1969). *Biochemistry* 8, 2183-2191.

Zgliczyński, J.M., Stelmaszyńska, T., Domański, J., and Ostrowski, W. (1971). *Biochim. Biophys. Acta* 235, 419-424.

Zgliczyński, J.M. and Stelmaszyńska, T. (1975). Eur. *J. Biochem.* 56, 157-162.

Zgliczyński, J.M. and Stelmaszyńska, T. (1979). *Biochim. Biophys. Acta* 567, 309-314.

CYANIDE AND ARTHROPODS

SEAN S. DUFFEY

Department of Entomology,
College of Agricultural and Environmental Sciences,
University of California, Davis, California 95616, U.S.A.

I. INTRODUCTION

In contrast to the taxonomically widespread distribution of cyanogenesis in the plant kingdom (see Conn, 1979; Siegler, this volume), the production of HCN by animals is restricted, at this stage of our knowledge, to one phylum, the Arthropoda, out of about 31 (for taxonomic details refer to Barnes, 1980 and Meglitsch, 1967). Even within this phylum, composed of 11 extant classes (Borror and DeLong, 1971), the phenomenon is restricted to certain members of the classes Chilopoda (centipedes), Diplopoda (millipedes), and Insecta (insects). It seems unfitting to argue that this limited and skewed distribution of cyanogenesis has resulted from a continued susceptibility of animal tissues throughout evolutionary times to HCN poisoning. Many animal species at all levels of organization (protistans, poriferans, coelenterates, annelids, echinoderms, molluscans, and even vertebrates) produce or sequester natural products that are often much more toxic to susceptible foreign organisms than HCN (Duffey, 1980; Mebs, 1973, and Zlotkin 1973) (e.g. anabesine, batrachotoxin, benzoquinones, cardenolides, cobratoxin, murexine, nereistoxin, samarandine, tetrodotoxin). The producers or sequesterers obviously withstand their own toxins via a variety of physical and/or physiological means, and hence, in a teleological sense it would be reasonable to suppose that the evolution of adaptations for the biosynthesis of cyanogenic compounds would be possible. In view of the diversity of natural products (similar to those produced by plants) made by animals (see Duffey, 1977; Mebs, 1973; Rodriguez and Levin, 1976; Schildknecht, 1971; Zlotkin, 1973) this markedly narrow distribution of cyanogenic capabilities is striking.

Perhaps this apparent skewed distribution of cyanogenesis in the animal kingdom results from some inherent metabolic idiosyncrasy or is an indication that selection pressures that led to the evolution of cyanogenesis in centipedes and millipedes were not operative or relevant to most animals evolving in later geological periods. Supposedly, the millipedes and centipedes and some orders of insects evolved in the Silurian to Pennsylvanian periods (280-425 million years ago; compare Borror and DeLong, 1971, Ch. 7; Leppik, 1972; and Meglitsch, 1967, pp.927-39), well before angiosperms and many of the higher terrestrial animals.

Before this discussion turns in detail to cyanogenesis in arthropods, a few details will be given about the process in other animal groups. I am unaware of any multicellular animals, aside from arthropods, that produce HCN. There is a paucity of literature on the natural occurrence of oximes, nitriles, and other chemicals relatable to a metabolic sequence for cyanogenesis, suggesting that metabolism of $R'R''CH_2NH_2$ beyond the hydroxylamine is a rare event. Sponges in the family Vergonidae are noted for their metabolism of tyrosine to the nitrile aeroplysinin-1 and the cyclic oxime homoaerothionin (Fig. 1) (Cimino *et al.*, 1975,ab). Also, other derivatives of tyrosine, 4-hydroxyphenylpyruvic acid oxime and 3,5-dibromotyrosine, occur in these sponges, and are considered to be evidence that an oxime is an intermediate in the biosynthesis of the nitrile aeroplysinin-1 (Cimino *et al.*, 1975,ab). Sesquiterpenes and diterpenes substituted with formamide, isonitrile, or isothiocyanate groups have been isolated from some sponges. The co-occurrence of the formamide and the isonitrile have led to the postulate that the formamide is a precursor in the biogenesis of the isonitrile (see Iengo *et al.*, 1979). The sponge, *Axinella cannabina*, which produces the sesquiterpene axisonitrile-1 (Fig.1) and the corresponding amide axamide-1, was used to test this postulate by feeding the animal axamide-1-*formyl*-^{14}C. No radioactivity was subsequently found in axisonitrile-1 suggesting the nitrile is not synthesized via a formamide intermediate (Iengo *et al.*, 1979). Despite the presence of oximes and nitriles in sponges, no instances of cyanogenesis are known. In another peculiar instance, both *syn* and *anti*- phenylacetaldoxime have been found as testosterone dependent metabolites in the urine of male guinea pigs (Smith *et al.*, 1977). As far as I am aware this is the only report of aldoximes as natural products of mammals.

The bulk of the literature on cyanogenesis in the animal kingdom relates to certain taxa of arthropods. Consequently the remainder of this review will be limited to cyanogenesis in arthropods.

II. OCCURRENCE OF CYANIDE, CYANOGENIC GLYCOSIDES, AND RELATED COMPOUNDS IN ARTHROPODS

The Phylum Arthropoda consists of 11 extant classes in which there are approximately 1 million described species which comprise about three - quarters of the animal kingdom. In only 3 classes (Chilopoda, Diplopoda, and Insecta)

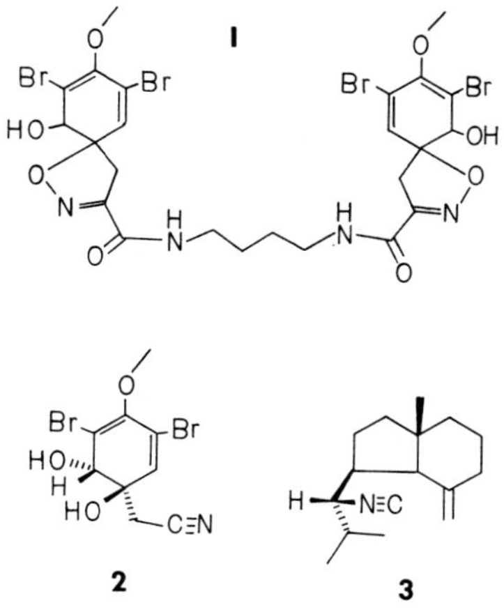

Fig. 1 Some natural products from sea sponges. 1 = Homoaerothionin; 2 = Aeroplysinin-1; 3 = Axisonitrile-1.

have cyanogenic species been described.

The chilopods or centipedes consist of approximately 3,000 species (Barnes, 1980) of which only 7 species are so far known to be cyanogenic, 6 geophilids and a scolopendrid (Table 1). The Insecta or insects comprise an extremely diversified group of about 750,000 species (Barnes, 1980) of which only 10 species are known to be cyanogenic, 3 beetles, 4 moths and 3 butterflies (Table 1). The most notorious producers of HCN, the diplopods or millipedes, comprise about 7,500 species (Barnes, 1980). Cyanogenesis in members of this class is known to occur only in one order of about 12, the Polydesmida (for taxonomic details see Barnes, 1980; Borror and DeLong, 1971; Chamberlin and Hoffman, 1958; Jeekel, 1970). All species of Polydesmida so far examined are cyanogenic, 46 out of about 2 to 3 thousand species (Table 1). Other taxa of diplopods contain species noted for their production of *p*-benzoquinones (Eisner, 1970), terpenoid alkaloids (Meinwald *et al.*, 1975), and quinazoline alkaloids (Meinwald *et al.*, 1966), but in no case is the production of any of these products coupled with cyanogenesis. With respect to cyanogenesis, the extremely distant taxonomic affinities between diplopods, chilopods, coleopterans, and lepidopterans points to the convergent evolution of the character rather than to atavism.

The production of HCN by polydesmoid millipedes was first described over 90 years ago (Guldensteeden-Egeling, 1882; Weber, 1882; and Wheeler, 1890). Guldensteeden-Egeling (1882) also showed that *Oxidus* (= *Fontaria paradesmus*) *gracilis* concomittantly produced benzaldehyde, but did not suggest that it resulted from the dissociation of mandelonitrile. In 1946 Pallares reported the presence of *p*-isopropylmandelonitrile glucoside (Fig. 2) in *Polydesmus*

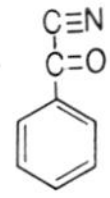

1

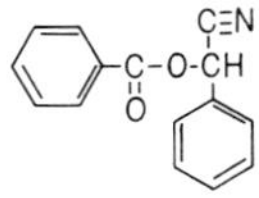

2

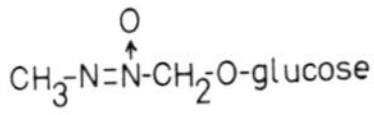

3

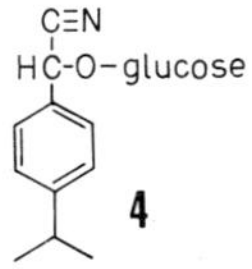

4

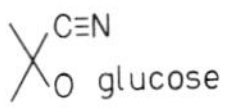

5

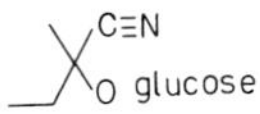

6

Fig. 2 Some natural products related to cyanogenesis in arthropods. 1 = Benzoyl cyanide; 2 = Mandelonitrile benzoate; 3 = Cycasin; 4 = *p*-Isopropylmandelonitrile glucoside; 5 = Linamarin; 6 = Lotaustralin

vicinus, a species which is probably synonomous with *Rhysodesmus vicinus* Sauss. (see Casnati *et al.*, 1963). In the 60's there was a rash of reports of chemicals associated with cyanogenesis in polydesmoids: mandelonitrile benzoate in *Orthomorpha coarctata* (Monteiro, 1961); a suspected mandelonitrile glucoside in *Pachydesmus crassicatus* (Blum and Woodring, 1962), and suspected mandelonitrile in *Apheloria corrugata* (Eisner *et al.*, 1963); D-(+)-mandelonitrile benzoate in *Polydesmus collaris collaris* (Casnati *et al.*, 1963) and *Gomphodesmus pavani* (Barbetta *et al.*, 1966); and D-(+)-mandelonitrile in *Gomphodesmus pavani* Barbetta *et al.*, 1966). (The determinations of configuration are based on sodium D-line rotations and are ambiguous). A few instances of cyanogenesis in other arthropods were found: in several zygaenid moths *Zygaena filipendulae*, *Z. lonicer*, *Z. trifolii* and *Procris geryon* (only HCN detected; Jones *et al.*, 1962); in three species of chrysomelid beetle larva, *Paropsis atomaria*, *Chrysophtharta variicollis*, and *C. amoena* (suspected mandelonitrile; Moore *et al.*, 1967); and in a geophilomorphid centipede *Pachymerium ferrugineium* (Schildkneckt *et al.*, 1968). To date only a small amount of additional data is available on cyanogenic arthropods (see Table I). The only new developments in identification of cyanogens and related products are the following: the isolation of R-mandelonitrile in

Harpaphe haydeniana (Duffey and Towers, 1978); the first report of the natural occurrence of benzoyl cyanide (Fig. 2) in a variety of polydesmoids and centipedes (Conner *et al.*, 1977; Duffey *et al.*, 1976; Jones *et al.*, 1976); the common occurrence of mandelonitrile benzoate (Fig. 2) in polydesmoids (Conner *et al.*, 1977; Duffey *et al.*, 1976); and most strikingly the presence of linamarin and lotaustralin (Fig. 2) in the moth *Zygaena filipendulae*, and the butterflies *Acraea eponina manjaca*, *A. natalica natalica*, and *A. terpsichore neobule* (Davis and Nahrstedt, 1979, and pers. commun.). Other minor reports of the co-occurrence of HCN and benzaldehyde in arthropods are listed in Table I.

In only two cases has the major cyanogenic chemical been unambiguously identified and quantified to account for the amount of HCN liberated. In the moth *Zygaena filipendulae* linamarin and lotaustralin total up to 2% of the wet weight of the freshly emerged gravid females (≈ 400 μg HCN/adult); these glucosides are primarily compartmentalized in the eggs (Davis and Nahrstedt, 1979), and hence absent from adult males (Davis and Nahrstedt, 1979; Jones *et al.*, 1962). This amount of these cyanogenic glucosides can account for the moths cyanogenic abilities; however, no work has yet been done to correlate the presence of these glucosides with β-glucosidase and α-hydroxynitrile lyase. In the polydesmoid *Harpaphe haydeniana*, R-mandelonitrile has been identified as the major cyanogen (Duffey *et al.*, 1974; Duffey and Towers, 1978). Each millipede contained about 0.2 μmoles (8 μg HCN) of mandelonitrile isolated as mandelic acid which was quantitatively comparable to 0.2 - 0.9 μmoles of HCN and benzaldehyde isolated per millipede (Duffey *et al.*, 1974). Each millipede also produced HCN and benzaldehyde in equimolar quantities. Additionally, pronounced α-hydroxynitrile lyase activity compared with miniscule β-glycosidase activity was demonstrated in an isolate from the paranota where the cyanogenic apparatus is housed. The presence of an α-hydroxynitrile lyase confirmed that most of the HCN formation in this millipede resulted from the dissociation of stored mandelonitrile.

Several other nitriles have been unambiguously identified as natural products of arthropods (see Table I): benzoyl cyanide in several species of centipedes (Jones *et al.*, 1976) and in a variety of species of polydesmoids (Conner *et al.*, 1977; Duffey *et al.*, 1976; Monteiro, 1961); and D(+)mandelonitrile from one species of millipede (Barbetta *et al.*, 1966). However, these studies did not prove that the cited product is the storage form of HCN and/or contributes significantly to HCN production.

For example, Pallares (1946) extracted 10 kg of live millipedes to isolate *p*-isopropylmandelonitrile glucoside from *Polydesmus vicinus*. Unfortunately, the occurrence of this rare natural product has not been reconfirmed, since Pallares' methods of identification were not definitive

Table I Some chemicals associated with cyanogenesis in arthropods.

ARTHROPODS[(a)]	COMPOUNDS									REFERENCE #
Class	HCN	ØCHO	R'R''CHO	MND	MNDBZ	ØCOCN	IMNDG	LL	OIL[c]	
Family										
Species										
CHILOPODA										
Geophilidae										
Geophilus cayugae	+	+				+				41
Geophilus vittatus	+	+		+		+				41
Pachymerium ferrugineum	+	+				+				56
Strigamia bothriopa	+	+				+				41
Strigamia chionophila	+	+				+				41
Strigamia icterica	+	+				+				41
Scolopendridae										
Asanada n. sp.	+									43
DIPLOPODA										
Astrodesmidae										
Astrodesmus laxus	+									28
Chelosodesmidae										
Caraibodesmus	+									20

Table I (continued)

	HCN	ØCHO	R'R''CHO	MND	MNDBZ	ØCOCN	IMNDG	LL	OIL[c]	REFERENCE #
Euryuridae										
Euryurus amycus Hoffman	+	+							+	20
Euryurus australis Bollman	+	+								25
Euruyrus leachii (Gray)	+	+							+	25,36
Euryurus maculatus (Koch)	+	+			+				+	22
Gomphodesmidae										
Gomphodesmus pavani Dem.	+	+		+	+					1
Nearctodesmidae										
Nearctodesmus cerasinus (Wood)	+	+							+	20
Paradoxosomatidae										
Orthomorpha coarctata (De Sauss.)	+	+			+					25,48
Oxidus gracilis Koch	+	+		+	+				+	4,22,25 27,34,59 61,62
Polydesmidae										
Polydesmus angustus Latzel	+	+							+	20
Polydesmus collaris collaris (Koch)	+	+			+					8
Pseudopolydesmus branneri (Bollman)	+	+							+	22,28

Table I (continued)

	HCN	ØCHO	R'R''CHO	MND	MNDBZ	ØCOCN	IMNDG	LL	OIL[c]	REFERENCE #
Pseudopolydesmus erasus (Loomis)	+	+			+				+	22
Pseudopolydesmus serratus Say	+	+		+	+	+			+	15, 28
Scytonotus insulanus	+	+							+	20
Xystodesmidae										
Apheloria coriacea (Koch)	+	+								60
Apheloria corrugata Wood	+	+		+		+			+	15,27,32
Apheloria kleinpeteri	+	+								28
Apheloria montana (Bollman)	+	+							+	
Apheloria trimaculata (Wood)	+	+		+		+			+	20,28
Boraria stricta (Brolemann)	+	+							+	20
Brachoria dentata Keeton	+	+							+	20
Brachoria sp.	+	+							+	20
Cherokia georgiana	+	+								27
Cherokia g. ducilla (Chamberlin)	+	+			+	+			+	22
Cherokia g. georgiana (Bollman)	+	+			+	+			+	22
Cherokia g. latassa Hoffman	+	+			+	+			+	22
Cleptoria rileyi (Bollman)	+	+			+	+			+	20,22
Cleptoria sp.	+	+							+	20
Dicellarius atlanta (Chamberlin)	+	+							+	20

Table I (continued)

	HCN	ØCHO	R'R''CHO	MND	MNDBZ	ØCOCN	IMNDG	LL	OIL[c]	REFERENCE #
Dixioria dactyligera Hoffman	+	+							+	20
Fontaria (=Polydesmus) *virginensis* Drury	+	+								62
Gylastethus monticollens Chamberlin	+	+							+	20
Harpaphe haydeniana (Wood)	+	+		+					+	23,24
Motyxia tiemanni Causey	+	+			+	+			+	22
Motyxia tularea (Chamberlin)	+	+			+	+			+	22
Motyxia sequoiae (Loomis & Davenport)	+	+			+	+			+	22
Nannaria sp.	+	+							+	20,27
Pachydemus crassicatus (Wood)	+	+								5
Paimokia sp.	+	+							+	22
Pleuroloma flavipes butleri (McNeill)	+									36
Pleuroloma sp.	+	+							+	20
Rhysodesmus (=Polydesmus) *vicinus* Sauss.	+	+[(b)]					+			50
Sigiria sp. nov.	+	+							+	20
Sigmoria nantahalae Hoffman	+	+			+	+			+	22

Table I (continued)

HCN = hydrogen cyanide; ØCHO = benzaldehyde; R'R"CHO = acetone and 2-butanone; MND = mandelonitrile: MNDBZ = mandelonitrile benzoate; ØCOCN = benzoyl cyanide; IMNDG = *p*-isopropylmandelonitrile glucoside; LL = linamarin and lotaustralin; OIL = presence of one large oil droplet in storage vestibule

[(a)] Author of species not cited unless indicated by researchers.

[(b)] Aldehyde is putatively cuminaldehyde.

[(c)] Presence of oil droplet determined by dissecting live specimens under binocular microscope (Duffey, unpublished data).

Table I (continued)

	HCN	ØCHO	R'R''CHO	MND	MNDBZ	ØCOCN	IMNDG	LL	OIL[c]	REFERENCE #
Stelgipus agrestis Loomis	+	+			+	+			+	22
INSECTA										
Chrysomelidae										
Chrysophtharta amoena	+	+								49
Chrysophtharta variicollis	+	+								49
Paropsis atomaria	+	+								49
Nymphalidae										
Acraea eponina manjaca	+		+					+		17
Acraea natalica natalica	+		+					+		17
Acraea terpsichore neobule	+		+					+		17
Zygaenidae										
Procris geryon (Heub.)	+									40
Zygaena filipendulae L.	+		+					+		16, 40
Zygaena lonicerae (von Schev.)	+									40
Zygaena trifolii (Esper.)	+									40

enough by modern standards to identify the cuminaldehydic moiety unambiguously. He dried the sample at 105°C for 2 hours prior to obtaining 0.9 gm of crystals from a defatted ethanolic extract. Under these conditions, mandelonitrile would decompose. Furthermore, no evidence was given that the millipede had the enzymatic capability to hydrolyze the glucoside. It consequently seems very unlikely that *Polydesmus vicinus* stores *p*-isopropylmandelonitrile glucoside as the major cyanogen.

In another study, Casnati *et al.*, (1963) isolated mandelonitrile benzoate from 9,000 specimens of *Polydesmus collaris collaris*.

They obtained "about 0.1 ml" of an "oily residue"; it is not possible to equate this amount of nitrile with total cyanogenic output. The extraction method used to obtain mandelonitrile benzoate involved washing an etheral extract with 5% NaOH; this would have decomposed any mandelonitrile if it were present. Also, Casnati *et al.*, (1963) offered no evidence that *Polydesmus collaris collaris* was capable of the enzymatic conversion of mandelonitrile benzoate to HCN, benzaldehyde and benzoic acid. Barbetta *et al.*, (1966) more convincingly isolated 50 mg of D(+)mandelonitrile from *Gomphodesmus pavani*. This suggested that mandelonitrile is the direct precursor of HCN and benzaldehyde, but did not provide any quantitative data on the total content of HCN of the millipedes.

Since the first mechanistic models of cyanogenesis in millipedes were proposed (Blum and Woodring, 1962; Eisner *et al.*, 1963; Woodring and Blum, 1963), it has been assumed that the ultimate cyanogen in arthropods is mandelonitrile and probably not a glycoside. This assumption is usually supported by giving chromatographic data for mandelonitrile isolated from a particular organism (Conner *et al.* 1977; Eisner *et al.*, 1963; Jones *et al.*, 1976). In many of these cases it is difficult to ascertain the factors contributing to cyanogenesis, because the cyanogenic secretions contain a mixture of HCN, benzaldehyde, mandelonitrile, mandelonitrile benzoate, benzoic acid, benzoyl cyanide, phenol, guaiacol, and fatty acids (Casnati *et al.*, 1963; Conner *et al.*, 1977; Duffey *et al.*, 1976; Jones *et al.*, 1976). If detailed information were available on the chemical content and enzymology of the cyanogenic secretions, more definitive statements could be made about the ultimate cyanogen(s). Most analyses of the cyanogenic secretions of arthropods show a predominance of benzaldehyde (along with HCN) over other products. These determinations range in sophistication from analyses of 2, 4-dinitrophenylhydrazine derivatives (e.g. Blum and Woodring, 1962; Eisner *et al.*, 1963; Moore, 1967) to identification by GLC-MS interfaces (Conner *et al.*, 1977; Duffey *et al.*, 1976; Jones *et al.*, 1976). In no case, other than that of cuminaldehyde (Pallares, 1946) and presumably acetone and 2-butanone from linamarin and lotaustralin respectively (Davis and Nahrstedt, 1979), has another aldehyde or ketone formed from the dissociation of a cyanogen been identified in the cyanogenic secretions of arthropods. The evidence points strongly towards mandelonitrile as the major cyanogen, particularly in millipedes. Benzoyl cyanide and mandelonitrile benzoate comprise individually up to 35% by weight of the secretion of various millipedes (Conner *et al.*, 1977; Duffey *et al.*, 1976), but there is no evidence for enzymes capable of degrading them.

In the light of Pallares' work on *p*-isopropylmandelonitrile glucoside, Woodring and Blum (1963) suggested that the precursor of cyanogenesis might be a glycoside of mandelonitrile stored within the lumen of the secretory storage gland (Fig. 4). They also speculated about the presence of a glucosidase and an α-hydroxynitrile lyase. The hypothetical cyanogenic glucoside was considered likely because of the presence of a mono- and disaccharide in the secreted cyanogenic fluid of the polydesmoid *Pachydesmus crassicatus* (Blum and Woodring, 1962). Similarly, Moore (1967) showed the presence of glucose in the secretions of the chrysomelid *Paropsis atomaria*, and suggested that mandelonitrile glucoside was formed at some stage of metabolism. In contrast, several investigators have failed to detect free sugars in the secretions of the millipede *Apheloria corrugata* (Eisner, H., *et al.*, 1963; Eisner *et al.*, 1963). Using radiotracers Duffey and Towers (1978) were able to isolate from *Harpaphe haydeniana* a bound form of mandelonitrile, similar in its chromatographic properties to prunasin and sambunigrin. An acetylated derivative failed, however, to crystallize to constant specific activity with prunasin tetraacetate, thus indicating that the bound form was not prunasin (millipede produces R-mandelonitrile). If a glucoside of mandelonitrile is present in *H. haydeniana* it occurs in miniscule quantities, because a highly purified isolate of 100 adults (~ 5 gm alive) analyzed by GLC (see Seigler, 1975 for methods) with a nitrogen specific-detector was shown to contain no detectable levels of any glycoside (Duffey, unpublished). The hypothetical polydesmoid-cyanogenic glucoside remains unknown. In fact, critical data are absent for the role of mandelonitrile in cyanogenesis in most arthropods.

Approximate values of the amount of HCN contained and/or liberated by various arthropods are presented in Table II.

Finally, a species of arctiid moth, *Seirarctia echo* contains cycasin (Teas, 1967), the glucoside of methylazoxymethanol (Fig. 2), classified as a pseudocyanogen (see Seigler, 1975). Cycasin is sequestered from the host plant, *Cycas*; following ingestion, the glucoside is hydrolyzed in the gut by the insect's and/or plant's enzymes, and the aglycone diffuses into the moth's tissues where a glucosyltransferase reconverts it to cycasin which remains dissolved in the insect's body fluids.

Table II Quantified cyanogenic capabilities of some arthropods

ORGANISM	μg HCN release at given time	Total μg of HCN per animal	Approximate body weight (gm)	Reference #
CENTIPEDES				
Asanada n. sp.	-	6.6	0.035	43
Pachymerium ferrugineum	-	2.2	-	56
MILLIPEDES				
Apheloria corrugata	0-600	-	0.4 - 1.4	29
Apheloria kleinpeteri	27	-	1.05	28
Apheloria trimaculata	16	-	0.769	28
Harpaphe haydeniana	-	~16	~0.25	24
Pseudopolydesmus branneri	32	-	0.199	28
MOTHS				
Zygaena filipendulae	200	370-460	0.066-0.299	16,40

III. THE BIOSYNTHESIS OF CYANIDE

The biosynthesis of HCN by arthropods has been little studied. The three published investigations (Duffey and Towers, 1978; Duffey *et al.*, 1974; and Towers *et al.*, 1972) to a large degree merely mirrored processes known to occur in plants. Basically, these studies demonstrate that two species of millipedes, *Oxidus gracilis* and *Harpaphe haydeniana*, have evolved a biosynthetic sequence for HCN production very similar to that known to occur in higher plants.

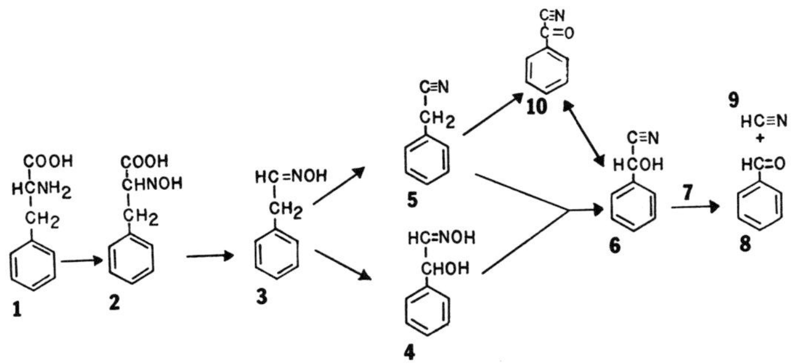

Fig. 3 Biosynthetic pathway for HCN and benzaldehyde in the polydesmoid millipede *Harpaphe haydeniana*. 1 = L-Phenylalanine; 2 = N-Hydroxyphenylalanine; 3 = Phenylacetaldoxime; 4 = α-Hydroxyphenylacetaldoxime; 5 = Phenylacetonitrile; 6 = Mandelonitrile; 7 = α-Hydroxynitrile lyase; 8 = Benzaldehyde; 9 = Hydrogen cyanide; 10 = Benzoyl cyanide

The first study with *Oxidus gracilis* (Towers *et al.*, 1972) showed that dietary ^{14}C-D, L-phenylalanine, depending on which carbons contained ^{14}C, could be specifically incorporated in HCN and/or benzaldehyde, as had been shown for prunasin (Ben-Yehoshua and Conn, 1964; see also Conn, 1973). These encouraging results led to a more detailed investigation of the metabolic sequence in *Harpaphe haydeniana* (Duffey *et al.*, 1974). In this case, the use of specifically labelled ^{14}C- and ^{3}H-precursors showed that the metabolic sequence from the amino acid phenylalanine to HCN and benzaldehyde was as depicted in Fig. 3 (the sequence 1 through 9).

The enzymatic oxidation of phenylacetonitrile to mandelonitrile is stereospecific as evidenced by the isolation of non-racemic mandelonitrile from several millipedes; R- from *H. haydeniana* (Duffey and Towers, 1978), D(+) from *Gomphodesmus pavani* (Barbetta *et al.*, 1966), and D(+) from *Polydesmus collaris collaris* (Casnati *et al.*, 1963). No work has been done to see if the enzymes involved in mandelonitrile biosynthesis are a channeled system like that found for dhurrin production by sorghum (see Conn, 1979). The presence of benzoyl cyanide suggests that it may result from dehydrogenation of mandelonitrile or oxidation of phenylacetonitrile (Fig. 3)(Jones *et al.*, 1976). *Cherokia georgiana* is able to convert ^{14}C-phenylacetonitrile into benzoyl cyanide (Duffey, unpublished data). It was not determined if mandelonitrile was an efficient precursor.

Undoubtedly mandelonitrile benzoate arises from the acylation of mandelonitrile. The cyanogenic secretions of many polydesmoid millipedes that contain benzoyl cyanide and mandelonitrile benzoate also usually contain significant quantities of benzoic acid (Conner *et al.*, 1977; Duffey *et al.*, 1976). Jones *et al.*, (1976) hypothesized that the benzoic acid arose from hydrolysis of benzoyl cyanide. This remains unproven. Barbetta *et al.* (1966) suggested that the existence of small amounts of mandelonitrile benzoate in the secretions of *Gomphodesmus pavani* was an artefact arising from esterification of mandelonitrile by benzoic acid during the isolation procedures. This is not the case since freshly collected secretions of several Appalachian species of millipedes contain copious quantities of this ester (Duffey *et al.*, 1976).

Additionally, evidence for the presence of small pools of phenylacetaldoxime and phenylacetonitrile in *H. haydeniana* (Duffey and Towers, 1978) further substantiated the proposed pathway (Fig. 3). Also, because this millipede stores R-mandelonitrile in its cyanogenic glands it was relatively easy to isolate microgram quantities of it in a (non-)radioactive form (Duffey *et al.*, 1974; Duffey and Towers, 1978). When *H. haydeniana* was given ^{14}C-labelled glucose or phenylacetonitrile, it was possible to isolate a bound form of mandelonitrile which behaved like a glucoside of mandelonitrile in its chromatographic mobility and its sensitivity to emulsin (Duffey and Towers, 1978). The identity of this material was not established.

In concordance with the sequence of cyanogenesis in certain plants, the cyanogenic glands of *H. haydeniana* were shown to contain both β-glucosidase and α-hydroxynitrile lyase activity. The β-glucosidase was able to hydrolyse both prunasin and sambunigrin rapidly, but taxiphyllin only very slowly. The rates of hydrolysis of these substrates cannot account for the rapid release of HCN by the live millipede (about a microgram of HCN when disturbed). However, the cyanogenic gland was also shown to contain an α-hydroxynitrile lyase with sufficient activity to account for the *in vivo* production of HCN (Duffey and Towers, 1978). This lyase could also dissociate *p*-hydroxymandelonitrile. The presence of this lyase in the reaction chamber is consistent with the storage of mandelonitrile as the precursor of HCN and benzaldehyde production; this millipede would be unable effectively to utilize a glucoside of mandelonitrile as a storage product. There are also other limitations to the use of a cyanogenic glucoside by millipedes; these limitations will be discussed later.

It is worth pointing out that an obvious but salient difference between millipedes and certain plants in their

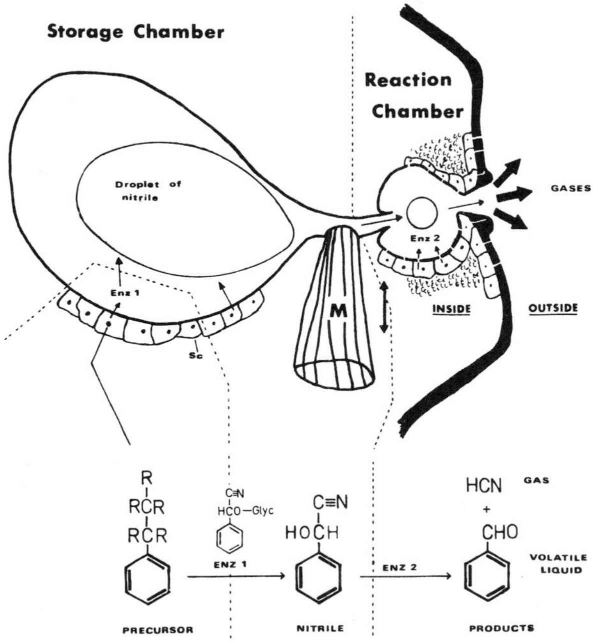

Fig. 4 Diagram of the relationship between metabolic events and morphological structures of the cyanogenic gland of *Harpaphe haydeniana*.
Precursor = most likely exogenously derived phenylalanine; ENZ 1 = β-glucosidase either in secretory cells (Sc) or lumen of storage chamber; ENZ 2 = α-hydroxynitrile lyase stored in reaction chamber; M = muscle to control entry of nitrile into reaction chamber; NITRILE = R-mandelonitrile stored as large droplet.

utilization of mandelonitrile as a labile precursor for HCN. Consider again *H. haydeniana* as the model system of Fig. 4. Herein *H. haydeniana* utilizes an exogenous source of phenylalanine, and within the walls of the secretory cells of the storage chamber converts it to mandelonitrile (Duffey and Towers, 1978). The next step is hypothetical, but perhaps as in plants, mandelonitrile is converted to a glycoside. This may facilitate transport through the cell to the boundary between the secretory cells and the lumen of the storage chamber. In contrast to the plant system (sorghum as the model) which stores the glycoside in the vacuoles of the epidermis, spatially separated from the glucosidase and lyase in the mesophyll (see Conn, 1979), the millipede stores mandelonitrile in the storage chamber physically isolated from the more distally located reaction chamber in which resides the α-hydroxynitrile lyase

(Fig. 4, ENZ 2). More detailed biochemical work on the putative glycoside's role in deposition of mandelonitrile in the storage chamber is needed. In fact, no information is avilable as to how *H. haydeniana* deposits and stabilizes the droplet of mandelonitrile within the storage chamber. Mandelonitrile is definitely not stored as an aqueous emulsion as stated by Eisner *et al.*, (1963). A survey of 33 species of live millipedes (Table I, OIL) indicated that they all contained a large oily droplet occupying nearly the total volume of each storage chamber (Duffey, unpublished data). It may be reasonable to conjecture that the putative millipede-glycoside is secreted intact into the lumen of the storage chamber where β-glucosidase (Fig. 4, ENZ 2) hydrolyzes it to the nitrile. The lyase probably originates in the secretory cells surrounding the reaction chamber. Pores through the cuticle of the reaction chamber probably permit the enzyme to be secreted into the lumen of the chamber (Fig. 4).

All the evidence indicates that cyanogenesis in other arthropods is the result of *de novo* biosynthesis of cyanogens within that species rather than of sequestration of the cyanogen from exogenous sources. It has been speculated that certain unpalatable species of butterflies may sequester cyanogens from certain species of cyanogenic plants (e.g. certain nymphalid butterflies feeding on aristolochiaceous plants; see Brower and Brower, 1964; Erlich and Raven, 1964; Rothschild, 1972). This has never been confirmed, and Jones *et al.*, (1962) and Davis and Nahrstedt (1979) have provided evidence that the presence of linamarin and lotaustralin in zygaenid moths is the result of *de novo* synthesis. Likewise, Moore (1967) has demonstrated that chrysomelid beetle larvae did not sequester their cyanogen from eucalypts.

IV. THE MECHANISMS OF CYANOGENESIS

The mechanism of cyanogenesis is best described in polydesmoid millipedes. This will be dealt with in detail first, and then compared with cyanogenesis in zygaenid moths, and a scolopendrid centipede. *H. haydeniana* will be used as the model system for cyanogenesis in polydesmoid millipedes. This system is similar to that proposed by Eisner for *Apehloria corrugata* (Eisner, 1970; Eisner *et al.*, 1963) and by Blum and Woodring for *Pachydesmus crassicatus* (Blum and Woodring, 1962; Woodring and Blum, 1963), except that more definitive data will be supplied.

H. haydeniana is a glossy black millipede (35 mm × 4.5 mm) with highly contrasting bright yellow paranota (= phalanges), suggestive of warning coloration. As in most polydesmoid millipedes, each multicellular cyanogenic gland is situated in the distal portion of a phalange (Fig. 5), actually in the metazonite of the diplosegment. The majority of the dipolosegments, 20 in polydesmoids, have prominent bilateral phalanges, but not all the segments bear the paired cyanogenic glands. In most polydesmoids there are 9 pairs of cyanogenic glands situated bilaterally along the length of the animal in diplosegments V, VII, IX, X, XII, XV, XVI, XVII, and XVIII.

As depicted in Fig. 5, the cyanogenic gland is composed of two chambers, a large thin-walled and flexible storage chamber (SC) approximately 1 mm × 0.4 mm connected by a neck (NK) to a thicker walled and more rigid reniform reaction chamber (RC) approximately 160 microns in diameter. Just prior to the junction of the reaction chamber and the storage chamber there is a muscle (M) attached to the neck; this muscle controls the occlusion of the neck by the self-sprung restriction (O). Note also that the neck of the storage chamber inserts itself as a nozzle (NZ) approximately half-way into the reaction chamber and ends in an unblocked orifice. Directly in front of the nozzle (30 - 40 microns in diameter), and of the same diameter, is the pore canal leading directly to the unblocked external pore of the reaction chamber. The pore (Pp) has a slight collar which raises the edge of the pore above the surrounding external pit (see pictures B + C, Fig. 5).

A survey of the gross morphology of the cyanogenic glands of approximately 100 species of polydesmoid millipedes from 10 families indicated that the two-chambered apparatus is the basic plan, with minor modifications in the shape and size of the reaction chamber and the storage chamber, and the position of the external pore. These structural variations were mostly associated with space limitations within the phalange of variously sized species of millipedes (Duffey, unpublished data). From this basis it is reasonable to consider *H. haydeniana* a representative millipede species for describing the mechanism of HCN formation.

The process of cyanogenesis happens as follows. When *H. haydeniana* is alarmed it quickly rolls into a spiral with the head at the center of the spiral. In doing this the millipede falls on its side exposing a lateral set of 9 cyanogenic glands (actually the external pore) facing upwards. Further tactile stimulation of the millipede induces it to increase the hydrostatic pressure of its haemolymph, to contract the muscle attached to the neck of the storage chamber, and to squeeze an aliquot of mandelonitrile through the reaction chamber into the pore canal leading to the exterior (see sequence 1-4 in Fig. 6). At this point the muscle relaxes, loosing the constriction to sever the aliquot of mandelonitrile from the droplet in the storage chamber. This severance may impart an additional velocity to the severed aliquot, ejecting it to the exterior under its own kinetic energy. The imparted velocity serves to eject it, largely intact, to the exterior of the millipede where the previously expelled hydroxynitrile lyase (see sequence 2, Fig. 6) degrades the nitrile rapidly. The salient feature here is that the bulk of HCN production occurs outside the millipede.

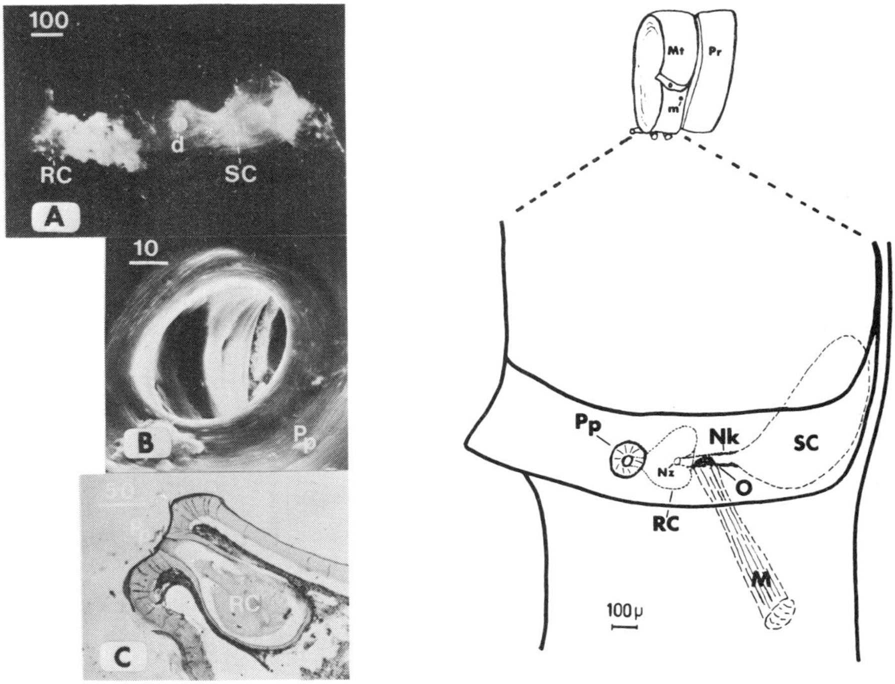

Fig. 5 Gross features of the cyanogenic gland of *Harpaphe haydeniana*. d = Droplet of mandelonitrile in storage chamber fragmented during excision of entire gland. M = Muscle controlling restriction between two chambers; Mt = Metazonite or posterior portion of diplosegment; Nk = Neck connecting the storage chamber to the reaction chamber; Nz - Nozzle intruding into centre of reaction chamber; O = Occlusion in neck of storage chamber; Pp = Pore and pit area of external portion of gland; Pr = Prozonite, or anterior portion of diplosegment. RC = Reaction chamber; SC = Storage chamber.

Diagram shows situation of cyanogenic gland within the phalange of the metazonite: Picture A demonstrates the presence of droplets of mandelonitrile, badly fragmented during excision of the whole gland, within the storage chamber. The reaction chamber can also be seen to the left: Picture B is an SEM of the external pore of the cyanogenic gland. Looking into the pore, one can see the beginning of the reaction chamber: Picture C shows a longitudinal section of the reaction chamber leading to the pore canal and the external pore. The pit is also clearly shown. The numbers above the white horizonal bars indicate the scale in microns.

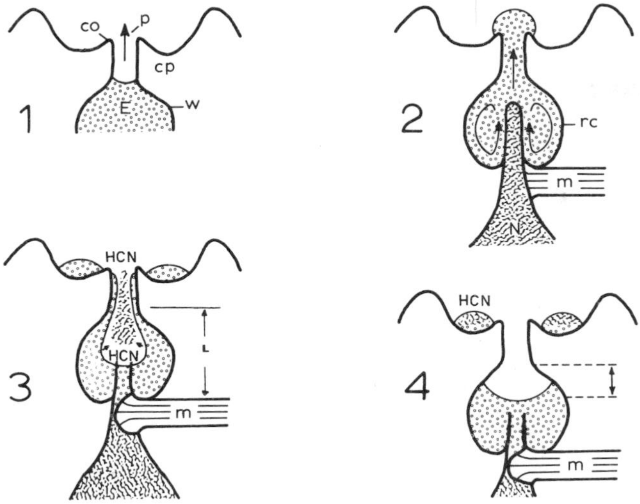

Fig. 6 Diagrammatic representation of sequence of HCN production. co = collar; cp = pore canal; E = enzyme solution in reaction chamber; L = length of reaction chamber; M = muscle; N = plug of nitrile; rc = reaction chamber; w = walls of reaction chamber.
1/ Reaction chamber at rest with fluid forming meniscus near beginning of pore canal. 2/ Displacement of fluid from reaction chamber to exterior because of entry of plug of nitrile. 3/ Plug of nitrile in reaction chamber. 4/ Plug of nitrile expelled; loss of fluid from reaction chamber about 20%.

Hydrostatic pressure in the haemocoele is definitely involved in the expulsion of mandelonitrile into the reaction chamber, for if one carefully excises the terminal diplosegment of anaesthesized millipedes and permits them to return to normal, the millipede is incapable of increasing hydrostatic pressure in its haemocoele and hence incapable of producing HCN. *H. haydeniana* is capable of "firing" individual cyanogenic glands depending on where the millipede is stimulated physically. Most millipedes, e.g. *H. haydeniana*, *Cherokia georgiana* sbspp., *Sigmoria nantahalae*, and *Oxidus gracilis* secrete the cyanogenic fluid in an oozing fashion. In contrast, *Cleptoria rileyi* can squirt jets of cyanogenic fluid from several of its glands simultaneously up to a distance of several centimeters. In essence, this is like rapidly squeezing a tube of toothpaste. The above millipedes can also repeatedly "fire" glands singly or in unison, but usually repetitive physical stimulation inhibits "firing".

The phenomenon described above demands a more detailed examination in order to appreciate how a millipede like

H. haydeniana is elegantly designed biochemically and physically to be a microcyanogenic apparatus. It is easiest to start with the details concerning the storage vestibule and work sequentially through the process outlined previously.

The flexible storage chamber, shaped like a round-bottom Erlenmeyer flask, is usually full of a large oily droplet. Remnants of such a droplet in *H. haydeniana* are shown in Fig. 5, A; the droplet is fragile and it fragments during excision of the glandular apparatus. In good dissections the single large droplet is observed to be held, presumably by capillary action, at the neck; whereas, the droplet does not wet the walls of the rest of the chamber. This places the beginning of the droplet adjacent to the constriction so that it is ready to be extruded into the reaction chamber. The significant feature of the droplet is that it is much more stable than an emulsion, probably giving a significantly longer half-life to the pool of labile mandelonitrile, and hence reducing the rate of metabolism required to keep that pool at the level of operational mass. In many millipedes the oil droplet is not composed of pure mandelonitrile. Carefully excised storage chambers of *Cherokia georgiana*, *Cleptoria rileyi*, and *Sigmoria nantahalae* reveal, upon analysis by GLC, significant proportions (up to 30% of the total) of benzoic acid, benzoyl cyanide, and mandelonitrile benzoate (Duffey, unpublished data). It is possible that an admixture of these chemicals with mandelonitrile helps to stabilize the droplet. Other workers have identified fatty acids and their esters in the defensive secretions of polydesmoids (Casnati *et al.*, 1963; Conners *et al.*, 1977) besides some of the above components; perhaps these fatty acids and derivatives serve to stabilize the droplet.

The droplet of mandelonitrile, with or without admixtures, has certain physical properties that lend themselves to the employed mechanism of cyanogenesis. The droplet is approximately 8 times more viscous than water, has half the surface tension of water, and is immiscible with water. Thus, when the droplet is placed under pressure during expulsion into the reaction chamber it will tend to behave as a solid or bullet. The size of the bullet will of course be determined by the rate of expulsion from the chamber as well as by the time the muscle remains contracted. Assume that the bullet acquires the following dimensions: the distance from the beginning of the reaction chamber where the muscle ends to the beginning of the pore canal [the distance marked L in Fig. 6, (3)]. When a bullet of these dimensions is expelled, under a possible pressure of one to several atmospheres, it will be directed by the nozzle towards the pore canal. Under these physical conditions the bullet will behave, as mentioned, somewhat like a solid (a liquid undergoing laminar flow much like water through a hose), and because it is viscous and immiscible with the aqueous contents of the reaction chamber, the bullet will resist distortion and remain integral. The projection of the nozzle into the centre of the reaction chamber probably aids in maintaining the rigidity of the bullet during its outward progress.

Some details about the content of the reaction chamber are needed to appreciate the fate of the in-coming bullet of mandelonitrile. The reaction chamber is filled up to the beginning of the pore canal [(Fig. 6, (1)] with an aqueous solution of α-hydroxynitrile lyase at pH 4 (in *Cherokia georgiana georgiana*, *Cleptoria rileyi*, *Harpaphe haydeniana*, *Oxidus gracilis*, and *Sigmoria nantahalae*; Duffey *et al.*, 1976). In several species of millipedes, *Oxidus gracilis*, *Pseudopolydesmus erasus*, and *Euryurus maculatus* the fluid also contains phenol and guaiacol (Duffey, unpublished data). Also, formic, acetic and isovaleric acids have been reported in the cyanogenic secretions of polydesmoids (Conner *et al.*, 1977; Casnati, 1963); it is possible these are actually in the reaction chamber and provide the acidity. At pH 4 the dissociation of mandelonitrile is very slow compared to the rate of dissociation catalyzed by the hydroxynitrile lyase, which coincidentally has a very distinct pH optimum of 4 (Duffey and Towers, 1978).

Thus, when a bullet of mandelonitrile is accelerated from rest into the reaction chamber, as depicted in Fig. 6, (1-4), it coincidentally displaces a small volume of reaction chamber fluid to the external pit. It is conjectured that when the muscle relaxes, the constriction (like half a coil of a spring) snaps shut, adding additional momentum to the outwardly bound bullet. The force of this momentum is sufficient to overcome retarding forces such as viscous drag, gravity, and atmospheric pressure, and hence permit the bullet to continue outward once continuity with mandelonitrile in the storage chamber is broken. As the bullet passes through the reaction chamber HCN and benzaldehyde will be rapidly evolved at the interface between the enzyme in water and the bullet. The hydrogen cyanide will likely instantaneously dissolve in the water; thus, the pressure contributed by HCN and benzaldehyde vapors will be negligible compared to the expulsion force of momentum. Also, as the bullet passes through the reaction chamber undergoing laminar flow it will induce the water to undergo directional flow (sequence 2); once the bullet is severed by the muscle this directional flow will also facilitate expulsion of the bullet by providing additional momentum as well as by physically guiding the bullet to the pore canal. After the bullet has left the reaction chamber, it will be deposited in the pit where it turbulently interacts with the hydroxynitrile lyase creating an external well of cyanogenesis.

This type of mechanism would not be operable if mandelonitrile were held as an emulsion in the storage chamber, for an aqueous emulsion, unless very viscous, would mix with the contents of the reaction chamber. Considering the high solubility of HCN in water, the degree of external cyanogenesis would be limited by the rate of diffusion of HCN through the pore canal into the air. Ridding the reaction chamber of the benzaldehyde would also be problematical in such a system. The beauty of the bullet-system is that minimal amounts of HCN and benzaldehyde remain in the reaction chamber.

Figure 6,(4) implies that about 20% of the volume of the reaction chamber is lost during cyanogenesis. This process can be readily visualized in small semitranslucent polydesmoids like *Scytonotus insulanus*, *Polydesmus angustus*, *Pseudopolydesmus erasus*, *Oxidus gracilis*, and *Euryurus maculatus*, by observing them immersed in water under a binocular dissecting microscope. In rapidly decapitated millipedes the meniscus was observed to be in the position shown in Fig. 6, (1); whereas, in alarmed specimens after cyanogenesis and decapitation, the meniscus was observed to be positioned much further down the chamber as shown in Fig. 6, (4). Incidentally, the angle at which the gland fires is irrelevant because the surface tension of the aqueous fluid is great enough always to keep the meniscus fixed. Rotation of the fluid by gravity is impossible. This facilitates the correct operation of the gland.

The reaction chamber fluid of *Cherokia georgiana georgiana*, which is a copious producer of benzoyl cyanide and mandelonitrile benzoate as well as of HCN and benzaldehyde, does not have any enzyme present capable of degrading either benzoyl cyanide or mandelonitrile benzoate. Those chemicals merely pass to the exterior unaltered.

With the type of cyanogenic mechanism just described, one can perhaps appreciate that reliance of cyanogenic glycoside as the storage product would not be feasible. A glycoside could not be concentrated in aqueous or organic solvents to the same degree as the nearly neat liquid nitrile. If the organism were to store a concentrated aqueous solution of a glycoside the solution would have to be very viscous in order to function like the bullet of mandelonitrile during the process of expulsion, that is to exhibit laminar flow and low miscibility. The reaction chamber would require an additional enzyme, a very active glycosidase, and also make cyanogenesis a two-step enzymatic process with the likelihood of being less efficient at rapid and copious HCN production. If a miscible solution of a glycoside were injected into the reaction chamber, the consequence would be similar to that arising from the injection of an emulsion of mandelonitrile - the bulk of cyanogenesis would occur ineffectually inside the reaction chamber. The bullet-system more effectively prevents the loss of enzyme from the reaction chamber.

Why does the evidence to date indicate that all millipedes that utilize this type of cyanogenic apparatus rely on mandelonitrile? Why don't they rely on acetone cyanohydrin and/or 2-butanone cyanohydrin? The answer may be very simple; these aliphatic hydroxynitriles have much greater water solubilities than mandelonitrile, and hence may be too miscible with water to be utilized effectively. Perhaps, also because of their greater water solubility, it is much more difficult to get them to form an oil droplet similar to those observed for mandelonitrile.

The occurrence of linamarin and lotaustralin, the glycosides of acetone cyanohydrin and 2-butanone cyanohydrin respectively, in the zygaenid moth *Zygaena filipendulae* (Davis and Nahrstedt, 1979) may seem to contradict the previous statements concerning the necessity for mandelonitrile as the cyanogen in polydesmoid millipedes. In fact, the zygaenids do not have cyanogenic glands. Their cyanogens appear to be in the body fluids or tissues generally (Jones *et al.*, 1962); crushing the insect liberates HCN. The mechanism of spatial separation of these glucosides from the glucosidase and a putative nitrile lyase is unknown. In terms of the mechanism of cyanogenesis used by the zygaenids, a very water soluble, non-labile, non-toxic storage product is essential. Linamarin and lotaustralin seem ideally suited for this purpose.

A system of cyanogenesis even less explored than that of the zygaenids is the one used by the scolopendrid centipede *Asanada* n. sp. in which a multitude of unicellular glands, each with a single pore opening to the external cuticle, are spread all over the body from segment two to the second from last segment (Maschwitz *et al.*, 1979). The pores are present at a density of about 300 per segment. There are two different types of cellular glands lying adjacently; on release of an unknown cyanogenic precursor, the contents of the two glands apparently mix. Proteins are detectable in the secretion, but it is not known whether these proteins are catalytic enzymes for cyanogenesis, or whether one gland produces the cyanogen and the other gland produces the enzyme(s).

V. DETOXICATION MECHANISMS

As pointed out earlier, one of the adaptive features of cyanogenesis in polydesmoid millipedes is that the majority of evolution of HCN and benzaldehyde occurs externally, for the most part on the tip of the phalanges somewhat separated from the ventrally located spiracles. It has not been determined how much HCN and benzaldehyde are absorbed or inhaled during cyanogenesis, but for the sake of argument we can assume that a millipede must contend with some level of contamination by these potentially toxic agents. What metabolic adaptations does such an organism have, to metabolize HCN and benzaldehyde?

Both *Oxidus gracilis* and *Harpaphe haydeniana* are able to convert HCN to β-cyanoalanine, asparagine, and thiocyanate (Fig. 7). The conversion of HCN to SCN is the predominant reaction (Duffey and Blum, 1977; Duffey and Towers, 1978). No further work has been done to locate any sulfur transferases or β-cyanoalanine synthetase,

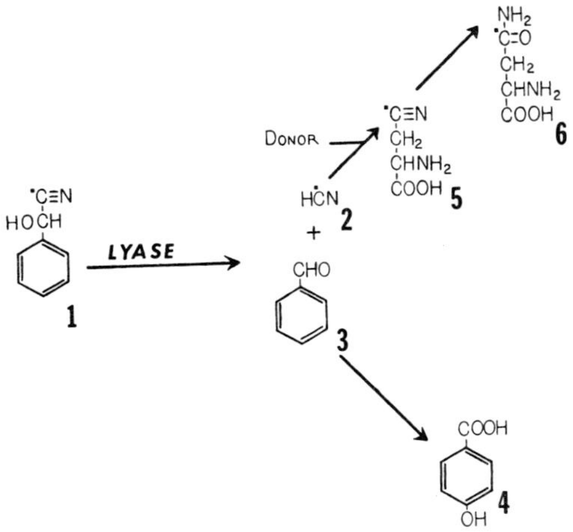

Fig. 7 Metabolism of HCN and benzaldehyde by *Harpaphe haydeniana*. 1/ Mandelonitrile; 2/ Hydrogen cyanide; 3/ Benzaldehyde; 4/ *p*-Hydroxybenzoic acid; 5/ β-Cyanoalanine; 6/ Asparagine.

nor has any definitive study been done to prove that these metabolic systems confer resistance to HCN. Non-cyanogenic arthropods also have the ability to convert HCN into β-cyanoalanine, asparagine, and aspartic acid, as well as SCN. Larvae of the noctuid moths *Heliothis zea* and *Spodoptera exigua*, and adults of the lygaeid bug *Oncopeltus fasciatus* possess this ability, but still are at least a 100-fold more sensitive to HCN vapours than cyanogenic polydesmoid millipedes (Duffey, unpublished data). Jones *et al*., (1962) found that the cyanogenic larvae of the zygaenid moths, Z. *filipendulae* and Z. *lonicerae* did not contain rhodanese; whereas, only some of these moths' endoparasites (flies and wasps) contained rhodanese. Yet Parsons and Rothschild (1964) demonstrated that *Zygaena filipenduale*, Z. *lonicerae*, and a bufferfly *Polyommatus icarus* had rhodanese. The exact role of rhodanese remains unclear, but probably partly relatable to the ability of the moths and butterflies to feed upon cyanogenic plants (Jones, 1972).

It would be interesting to determine if the conversion of HCN to β-cyanoalanine is the result of bacterial contaminants or symbiotes within these arthropods. Arthropod tissues are often rampant with pseudomonads. Several polydesmoid millipedes were shown to have an undetermined species of *Salmonella* living in the reaction chamber of the cyanogenic gland (Duffey and Blum, 1977). Perhaps such an organism provides the β-cyanoalanine synthetase? In retrospect, it really needs to be confirmed that some symbiotic microorganism residing within the secretory cells of the storage chamber is not the producer of mandelonitrile.

Non-cyanogenic arthropods that are resistant to HCN have been known for years. It has been posulated that strains of California red scale, *Aeonidiella aurantii*, a homopteran insect, are resistant to HCN because of the presence of "metal-free autoxidizable respiratory enzymes, possibly of the flavoprotein type" (Yust and Sheldon, 1952). The susceptible strains possessed a metal containing enzyme which was inactivated by CN^-. In the cyanogenic millipedes, *Euryurus leachii*, and *Pleuroloma flavipes butleri*, Hall *et al.*, (1971) found that HCN penetrated the millipedes' bodies, and that the greater degree of resistance as compared to 2 sensitive species of cockroaches could be attributed in the millipedes to either an excess of cytochrome oxidase or a resistant terminal oxidase; their results did not permit them to distinguish between the two.

H. haydeniana and *Oxidus gracilis* also metabolize inhaled benzaldehyde to *p*-hydroxybenzoic acid (Duffey *et al.* 1976; Duffey and Towers, 1978). (Fig. 7). Whether or not this represents a major mechanism of detoxication has not been determined.

VI. BIOLOGICAL ROLE(S) OF CYANOGENESIS

The virtue of cyanogenesis in millipedes as an anti-predator device has been extolled for years (Eisner, 1961, 1970; Eisner and Eisner, 1965; Eisner and Meinwald, 1966). Usually, the evidence for the defensive excellence of HCN and benzaldehyde is acquired by observing in the laboratory the reaction of suspected natural and artificial predators, (such as birds, lizards, kangaroo rats, and predacious arthropods) when millipedes are included in their diet. The results of these confrontations are usually dramatic, the predator being quickly deterred from feeding by the cyanogenic secretion. This provides grounds for suspecting that such a defensive system operates in the field, and that perhaps selection pressure from predators was one of the contributing factors that led to the evolution of the primeval millipedes' cyanogenic abilities. However, if one takes a cold look at the data (Duffey, 1977), there is no evidence from field studies of natural populations to support or refute the supposition. Gathering such evidence is more easily said than done, as exemplified by Jones' (1972) persistent and model work on the genetics of cyanogenesis in *Trifolium* and *Lotus*.

To be purposely absurd about the limited data on the defensive function of HCN-production by millipedes, it is well documented that certain phengodid beetle larvae are voracious predators of both cyanogenic and benzoquinone producing millipedes (see Duffey *et al.*, 1976); hence, one could argue that cyanogenesis is not a defence against predators. Cloudsley-Thomson (1968) reports that starlings and toads consistently eat millipedes. Obviously, a balanced and much more strongly evidenced documentation of the defensive role of cyanogenesis against predators is required. Research has emphasized the short term behavioral modifications induced in predators when they attempt to eat a cyanogenic arthropod. Perhaps the long-term and potentially more insidious effects of chronic exposure to chemicals such as benzoyl cyanide and mandelonitrile benzoate are more important for regulating the interaction between populations of prey and predators.

It might even be reasonable to consider that cyanogenesis as well as the production of cyanophoric chemicals (mandelonotrile benzoate and benzoyl cyanide) function to keep the cuticle of the litter-dwelling millipede aseptic. This hypothesis is weakly supported by evidence that benzoic acid, benzoyl cyanide, mandelonitrile benzoate, phenol and guaiacol have the ability to inhibit significantly spore germination and radial growth of several types of soil-dwelling fungi (*Cladosporium*, *Penicillium*, and *Trichoderma*) at a concentration of 1×10^{-4} M (Duffey, Roncadori, Blum, unpublished data). The presence of phenol, guaiacol and/or benzoic acid in the reaction chamber fluid might also prevent rampant growth of undesirable microorganisms (Duffey *et al.*, 1976).

VII. CONCLUSIONS

Our knowledge of the bases and roles of cyanogenesis in arthropods is very limited. A great opportunity exists for a detailed analysis of the comparative biochemistry of cyanogenesis, to obtain a more complete comprehension of biological functions of HCN in a diverse array of organisms. Unfortunately, studies on cyanogenesis in arthropods have been heavily polarized towards the descriptive aspects of chemistry with the interpretations of the biological function(s) of cyanogenesis being dictated by teleological explanations of what the chemicals should do rather than by what organisms do, as observed *via* natural history, morphology, ecology, genetics, and toxicology, as examples of fields lending themselves to interdisciplinary reasoning.

ACKNOWLEDGEMENTS

I thank the European Molecular Biology Organisation and the University of California, Davis, for travel funds permitting attendance at the conference. I also thank E. E. Conn and B. Vennesland for helpful critical comments.

REFERENCES

1. Barbetta, M., Casnati, G. and Pavan, M. (1966). *Mem. Soc. Entomol. Ital.* 45, 169-76.
2. Barnes, R.D. (1980). *In:* "Invertebrate Zoology", 4th ed., Saunders College, Philadelphia. 1089 pp.
3. Ben-Yoshua, S. and Conn, E.E. (1964). *Plant Physiol.* 39, 331-333.

4. Blum, M.S., MacConnell, J.G., Brand, J.M., Duffield, R.M. and Fales, H.M. (1973). *Ann. Entomol. Soc. Amer.* 65, 235.
5. Blum, M.S. and Woodring, J.P. (1962). *Science* 138, 512-513.
6. Borror, D.J. and DeLong, D.M. (1971). *In:* "An Introduction to the Study of Insects," 3rd ed., Holt, Rinehart and Winston, New York. 812 pp.
7. Brower, L.P. and Brower, J.V.Z. (1964). *Zoologica* 49, 137-159.
8. Casnati, G., Nencini, G., Quilico, A., Pavan, M., Ricca, A. and Salvatori, T. (1963). *Experientia* 19, 409-411.
9. Chamberlin, R.V. and Hoffman, R.L. (1958). *U.S. Nat. Mus. Bull. (Smithson Instit.)* 212, 1-236.
10. Cimino, G., De Stefano, S. and Minale, L. (1975a). *Experientia* 31, 757.
11. Cimino, G., De Stafano, S., Minale, L. and Sodano, G. (1975b). *Comp. Biochem. Physiol.* 50B, 279-285.
12. Cloudsley-Thompson, J.L. (1958). *In:* "Spiders, Scorpions, Centipedes, and Mites", Pergamon Press, New York. 228 pp.
13. Conn, E.E. (1979). *In:* "Herbivores: Their Interaction with Plant Secondary Metabolites", eds. G.A. Rosenthal and D.H. Janzen. Chpt. 10: 387-412. Academic Press, New York.
14. Conn, E.E. (1973). *Biochem. Soc. Symp.* 38, 277-302.
15. Connor, W.E., Jones, T.H., Eisner, T. and Meinwald, J. (1977). *Experientia* 33, 206-207.
16. Davis, R.H. and Narhstedt, A. (1979). *Comp. Biochem. Physiol.* 64, 395-397.
17. Davis, R.H. and Nahrstedt, A. (1979). Pers. commun.
18. Duffey, S.S. (1980). *Ann. Rev. Entomol.* 25, 447-477.
19. Duffey, S.S. (1977). *Proc. XV Int. Congr. Entomol. Wash. D.C. Aug. 1976.* 15, 323-394.
20. Duffey, S.S. (1980). Unpublished data.
21. Duffey, S.S. and Blum, M.S. (1977). *Insect Biochem.* 7, 57-65.
22. Duffey, S.S., Blum, M.S., Fales, H.M., Evans. S.L., Roncadori, R.W., Tiemann, D.L. and Nakagawa, Y. (1977). *J. Chem. Ecol.* 3, 101-113.
23. Duffey. S.S. and Towers, G.H.N. (1978). *Can. J. Zool.* 56, 7-16.
24. Duffey, S.S., Underhill, E.W. and Towers, G.H.N. (1974). *Comp. Biochem. Physiol.* 47B, 753-766.
25. Duffield, R.M., Blum, M.S. and Brand, J.M. (1974). *Ann. Entomol. Soc. Amer.* 67, 821-822.
26. Ehrlich, P.R. and Raven, P.H. (1964). *Evolution* 18, 586-608.
27. Eisner, H.E., Eisner, T. and Hurst, J.J. (1963). *Chem. Ind.* 124-125.
28. Eisner, H.E., Wood, W.F. and Eisner, T. (1975). *Psyche* 82, 20-23.
29. Eisner, T. (1970). *In:* "Chemical Ecology", Eds. E. Sondheimer and J.B. Simeone, Chpt. 8, 157-217. Academic Press, New York.
30. Eisner, T. (1961). *Ann. Rev. Entomol.* 7, 107-136.
31. Eisner, T., Eisner, H.E. (1965). *Nat. History* 74(3), 30-35.
32. Eisner, T., Eisner, H.E., Hurst, J.J., Kafatos, F.C. and Meinwald, J. (1963). *Science* 139, 1218-1220.
33. Eisner, T. and Meinwald, J. (1966). *Science* 153, 1341-1350.
34. Guldensteeden-Egeling, C. (1882). *Arch. Gesamte Physiol. Munchen Tierre (Pflugers)* 28, 576-579.
35. Hall, F.R., Hollingworth, R.M. and Shankland, D.L. (1971). *Comp. Biochem. Physiol.* 38B, 723-737.
36. Hall, F.R., Hollingworth, R.M. and Shankland, D.L. (1969). *Entomol. News* 80, 277-282.

37. Iengo, A., Santacroce, C. and Sodano, G. (1979). *Experientia* 35, 10-11.
38. Jeekel, C.A.W. (1970). Monograph. Nederl. Entomol. Vereniging, No.5: 1-412.
39. Jones, D.A. (1972). *In:* "Phytochemical Ecology", Ed. J.B. Harbone. Chpt. 7, 103-124. Academic Press, New York.
40. Jones, D.A., Parsons, J. and Rothschild, M. (1962). *Nature*, 193, 52-53.
41. Jones. T.H., Conner, W.E., Meinwald, J., Eisner, H.E. and Eisner, T. (1976). *J. Chem. Ecol.* 2, 421-429.
42. Leppik, E.E. (1972). *In:* "Evolutionary Biology", Vol. 5, eds. T. Dobzhansky, W.C. Hecht, and W.C. Steere. Chpt. 3, 49-85.
43. Maschwitz, U., Lauschke, U. and Wurmli, M. (1979). *J. Chem. Ecol.* 5, 901-907.
44. Mebs, D. (1973). *Experientia* 29, 1328-1334.
45. Meglitsch, P.A. (1967). *In:* "Invertebrate Zoology", Oxford University Press, London. 961 pp.
46. Meinwald, J., Smolanoff, J., McPhail, A.T., Miller, R.W., Eisner, T. and Hicks, K. (1975). *Tetra. Let.* 26, 2367-2370.
47. Meinwald, Y.C., Meinwald, J. and Eisner, T. (1966). *Science* 154, 390-391.
48. Monteiro, H.J. (1961). *Anais Assoc. Brazil Quim.* 20, 29-31.
49. Moore, B.P. (1967). *J. Austral. Entomol. Soc.* 6, 36-38.
50. Pallares, E.S. (1946). *Linn. Arch. Biochem. Biophys.* 9, 105-108.
51. Parsons, J.A. and Rothschild, M. (1964). *Entomol. Gaz.* 15, 58-59.
52. Rodriguez, E. and Levin, D.A. (1976). *In:* "Biochemical Interactions Between Plants and Insects", Rec. Adv. Phytochem. Vol. 10, eds., J.W. Wallace and R.L. Mansell. Chpt. 5, 214-270. Plenum, New York.
53. Rothschild, M. (1972). *In:* "Ecological Genetics and Evolution", ed. H.F. van Emden. Chpt. 10, 59-83. Blackwell Scientific Publ. Oxford.
54. Seigler, D.S. (1975). *Phytochem.* 14, 9-29.
55. Schildknecht, H. (1971). *Endeavour.* 30, 136-141.
56. Schildknecht, H., Maschwitz, U. and Krauss, D. (1968). *Naturwissen.* 55, 230.
57, Smith, A.B. III, Bryne, K.J. and Beauchamp, G.K. (1977). *J. Chem. Ecol.* 3, 309-319.
58. Teas, H.J. (1967). *Biochem. Biophys. Res. Commun.* 26, 686-690.
59. Towers, G.H.N., Duffey, S.S. and Seigel, S.M. (1972). *Can. J. Zool.* 50, 1047-1050.
60. Weatherston, J. and Gardiner, E.J. (1973). *Can. Entomol.* 105, 1375-1376.
61. Weber, M. (1882). *Arch. Mikrosk. Anat.* 21, 468-475.
62. Wheeler, W.M. (1890). *Psyche* 5, 422.
63. Woodring, J.P. and Blum, M.S. (1963). *Ann. Entomol. Soc. Amer.* 56, 448-453.
64. Yust, H.R. and Sheldon, F.F. (1952). *Ann. Entomol. Soc. Amer.* 45, 220-228.
65. Zlotkin, E. (1973). *Experientia* 29, 1453-1588.

BACTERIAL CYANIDE-RESISTANT RESPIRATION: A REVIEW

MICHÈLE-FRANCE HENRY

Laboratoire de Biochimie (CNRS-ER 235 et INSERM U.191), Département de Recherche Fondamentale, Centre d'Etudes Nucléaires, 85X, 38041 Grenoble cedex, France

I. INTRODUCTION

Bacterial respiratory systems often present similarities with that of mitochondria. They are membrane-bound and exhibit energy conservation through coupling of the respiratory chain redox reactions to ATP synthesis. Perhaps one of the major characteristics of bacterial systems is the wide range of redox carriers which may have an oxidase function (namely cytochromes of the *a*, *b*, *c* and *d* type). Combination of up to four of these terminal redox carriers is not an uncommon feature in bacterial membranes, and has been shown in different species (for very fully documented accounts of bacterial systems see: Gel'man *et al.*, 1967 and 1975; White and Sinclair, 1971; Lemberg and Barrett, 1973; Jurtshuk *et al.*, 1975; Jones, 1977; Haddock and Jones, 1977).

A consequence of the plurality of terminal oxidases and their simultaneous occurrence within the bacterial plasma membrane is the development of branched alternate routes for electron flux, and a decrease in their relative sensitivity to respiratory inhibitors, especially to cyanide.

Although the literature contains a massive amount of data on the capacity of some eukaryotic organisms to exhibit active respiration even in the presence of cyanide (for reviews see Lloyd, 1974; Henry and Nyns, 1975; Solomos, 1977), little attention has been paid to cyanide-resistance in prokaryotes. This survey therefore presents a more general review of bacterial cyanide-insensitive branched respiratory chains and considers some reasons for their adaptive synthesis, their possible physiological role in bacterial metabolism and their energy conservation efficiency.

II. DISTRIBUTION OF CYANIDE-RESISTANCE AMONG BACTERIAL SYSTEMS

The presence of respiration tolerant to concentrations of cyanide adequate to inhibit the cytochrome *c* oxidase of mammalian systems is not restricted to mitochondria of higher plants or eukaryotic microorganisms. It has also been observed in various prokaryotes, as can be seen from Table I. Cyanide-sensitivity varies widely among prokaryotes. For example, respiration of *Anacystis nidulans* or *Proteus vulgaris* is highly cyanide-sensitive, whereas respiration of *Pseudomonas aeruginosa* or *Achromobacter* is hardly inhibited by cyanide. It should be noted that Table I is restricted to bacterial respiratory systems which resemble that of mitochondria. No mention is made of peroxidases and oxygenases that are insensitive to cyanide, such as the "old yellow enzyme" (Atmungsferment) already reported by Warburg and Christian some fifty years ago (1932a, b).

III. APPEARANCE OF A CYANIDE-RESISTANT RESPIRATION

Variations in the composition of the electron transport chain, especially amongst the terminal oxidases, often results in a general loss of sensitivity to respiratory inhibitors. These changes are caused mainly by replacement of one (or more) redox carrier by another or by the addition or deletion of specific carriers. These differences in respiratory chain composition generally occur in response to environmental changes. Alterations of the growth conditions, in particular with respect to the nature of the terminal electron acceptor, are usually accompanied by changes at the level of the terminal oxidases. This can be exemplified by the replacement of cytochrome oxidase aa_3 by nitrite reductase in species such as *Paracoccus denitrificans* (Newton, 1969) upon shifting from aerobic respiration to anaerobiosis with nitrate as the terminal electron acceptor.

Cyanide-insensitive respiration can occur under natural conditions, by mutation of photosynthetic bacteria (Marrs and Gest, 1973) or upon changing the nitrogen or the carbon source in the growth medium (van Verseveld and Stouthamer, 1978). Cyanide-insensitivity can also be induced during growth under conditions which promote cyanide evolution (Niven *et al.*, 1975), or upon addition of cyanide to the culture medium (Mizushima and Arima, 1960a; Mizushima *et al.*, 1959, 1960; McFeters *et al.*, 1970; Ashcroft and Haddock, 1975; Henry and Vignais, 1979). Cyanide insensitivity has also been observed when the culture reaches the stationary phase of growth (Trutko *et al.*, 1979) or when the availability of oxygen is greatly diminished (Linton *et al.*, 1976).

Table I Cyanide-resistant respiration in several prokaryotes

Species	Substrates	Cyanide Concentration (mM)	Cyanide % inhibition	References
Acetobacter suboxydans (P)[a]	NADH	0.75	65	Daniel, 1970
Achromobacter Strain 7 (P)	NADH	1.00	33	Mizushima and Arima, 1960
Achromobacter Strain D (C)	Succinate	0.05	0	Arima and Oka, 1965
Aerobacter aerogenes	Pyruvate	0.1	50	Tissieres, 1957
Aerobacter cloacae (P)	NADH	1.0	0	Mizushima *et al.*, 1959
Anacystis nidulans (P)	NADH	0.5	80	Peschek, 1980
Azotobacter vinelandii (P)	NADH	0.04	0	Jones and Redfearn, 1967
Bacillus cereus (C)	Endogenous	1.0	40	McFeters *et al.*, 1970
Beneckea natriegens (P)	Succinate	1.0	50	Weston *et al.*, 1974
Chromobacterium violaceum (P)	NADH	4.0	50	Niven *et al.*, 1975
Corynebacterium diphteriae	Succinate	2.5	50-60	Pappenheimer *et al.*, 1962
Escherichia coli C-1 (P)	NADH	0.5	50	Ashcroft and Haddock, 1975
Hydrogenomonas H-20 (E)	H_2	0.3	62	Bongers, 1967
Kurthia zopfii (P)	NADH	{0.7 {∞	{50 {70	Knowles *et al.*, 1978
Micrococcus lysodeikticus (P)	NADH	1.2	17	Ishikawa and Lehninger, 1962
Mycobacterium phlei (P)	NADH	3	55	Asano and Brodie, 1964
Myxococcus xanthus (P)	NADH	1	34	Dworkin and Niederpruem, 1964
Neisseria gonorrhoeae (P)	NADH	0.094	74	Kenimer and Lapp, 1978
Paracoccus denitrificans (P)	NADH	0.5	70	Henry and Vignais, 1979
Paracoccus denitrificans	H_2	0.1	0	Porte and Vignais, 1980
Pasteurella tularensis (P)	NADH	6	76	Robinson and Mills, 1961
Proteus vulgaris (P)	NADH	3.3	84	Feldman and O'Kane, 1960
Pseudomonas aeruginosa (P)	NADH	1	20-30	Trutko *et al.*, 1979
Pseudomonas ovalis Chester (P)	Malate	1	50-80	Francis *et al.*, 1963
Rhodopseudomonas capsulata St. Louis (P)	NADH	0.1	30	Baccarini-Melandri *et al.*, 1973
Staphylococcus aureus (P)	NADH	1	60	Taber and Morrison, 1964
Veillonella alcalescens (P)	NADH	1	70	de Vries *et al.*, 1978

(a) Symbols used: C = whole cells; E = cell-free extract; P = particulate fraction.

The next two sections will place particular emphasis on various aspects of the appearance of cyanide-resistance in bacteria.

A. NATURAL OCCURRENCE OF CYANIDE-RESISTANT RESPIRATION

Cyanide has been widely used to establish the presence of terminal oxidases. Monitoring its inhibitory effects on oxygen uptake occasionally permits the detection of a residual cyanide-resistant respiration. It has been found that several bacteria possess, under natural conditions, branched pathways of electron transport to oxygen, one branch being less sensitive to cyanide than the other (White and Sinclair, 1971). The marine bacterium *Beneckea natriegens* (Weston *et al.*, 1974) or wild types of the photosynthetic bacteria *Rhodopseudomonas capsulata* (Baccarini-Melandri *et al.*, 1973; Paul *et al.*, 1979) and *Rhodopseudomonas palustris* (King and Drews, 1975) display terminal branching of their respiratory systems. In most cases where terminal branching and cyanide-resistance occur, this insensitivity develops as an adaptive mechanism to environmental conditions.

1. Presence of Cyanide in the Environment

In some bacteria, the appearance of a respiration tolerant to cyanide may have an ecological origin. Indeed, many plants and fungi, but only a few bacteria, appear to be cyanogenic and to release significant amounts of cyanide into the soil (Knowles, 1976).

Some pseudomonads and *Chromobacterium violaceum* produce cyanide during their life cycle, depending on the growth conditions (Niven *et al.*, Knowles, 1976). In the latter organism, cyanide production was stimulated when 2 mM glycine and 0.5 mM L-methionine were included in the growth medium; it was found that up to 1.8 mM cyanide could be formed (Niven *et al.*, 1975). Ascorbate-TMPD oxidase activity was depressed in a particulate fraction isolated from cells producing high levels of cyanide, whereas NADH and succinate oxidase activities proved to be very resistant to cyanide inhibition.

The cyanobacterium *A. nidulans* excreted some cyanide when histidine was present in the medium (Vennesland *et al.*, this volume), but the respiratory system of this organism has not yet been described under these particular growth conditions.

Another source of cyanide in the environment comes from the release of cyanide-containing waste waters by several industries, causing great damage to living organisms and altering natural ecosystems. Cyanide pollution can also be related to the presence of increasing amounts of organic nitrogen compounds appearing during decomposition of organic matter.

2. *Changes in Oxygen Tension*

The concentration of oxygen in the growth environment can cause drastic effects on the qualitative and quantitative composition of bacterial electron transport systems. Oxygen deficiency often results in an increased synthesis of the alternative oxidases *o* or *d* which will in part replace cytochrome oxidase aa_3 (see the review of Jurtshuk *et al.*, 1975). The effects of changes in dissolved oxygen tensions were studied in some bacteria and will be discussed in more detail below.

One hypothesis for the presence of cyanide-resistant respiration in some bacteria under natural conditions is that it is a relic of an ancestral respiratory system that evolved in response to a change in the composition of the earth's atmosphere from anaerobic to aerobic but which still contained much cyanide (see Oro and Lazcano-Aranja, this volume).

B. INDUCTION OF CYANIDE-RESISTANT RESPIRATION

1. *Addition of cyanide to the culture medium*

In a number of cases it has been observed that the presence of respiratory chain inhibitors during growth resulted in marked modifications amongst the terminal oxidases together with the appearance of respiration that was more or less tolerant to cyanide. In *Achromobacter* strain 7, the oxidation of glucose, succinate or fumarate was cyanide-sensitive unless 1 mM KCN was added to the culture medium. Under the latter conditions, the inhibition of respiration by 1 mM cyanide was only 20-30% of the control (Mizushima and Arima, 1960a). Another strain of *Achromobacter*, which required isoleucine and adenine to grow, exhibited respiration that was totally insensitive to 50 μM cyanide when grown under vigorous aeration in a broth supplemented with 1 mM KCN. Cells grown in the absence of inhibitor were 100% inhibited by 50 μM cyanide (Arima and Oka, 1965). Skowronski and Strobel (1969) were able to grow a soil isolate of *Bacillus pumilus* in the presence of 0.1 M cyanide. The rate of respiration of the cells grown in the presence of cyanide was half the rate of control cells. A strain of *Bacillus cereus*, the respiration of which was 70% inhibited by 1 mM cyanide, displayed a slightly decreased rate of respiration when 1 mM cyanide was added to the culture medium. This respiration was only 40% sensitive to 1 mM cyanide (McFeters *et al.*, 1970). *Escherichia coli* strain C-1, was able to grow aerobically with D-xylose as carbon source, in the presence of cyanide. At concentrations below 1 mM, KCN had little effect on the growth rate, but caused a lag in the onset of growth and decreased the final cell yield (Ashcroft and Haddock, 1975). Growth in the presence of cyanide did not affect NADH oxidase activity in membrane preparations, but considerably lowered its sensitivity towards cyanide; to reach 50% inhibition 500 μM cyanide was required instead of 75 μM (Ashcroft and Haddock, 1975). In a similar fashion, *P. denitrificans* could carry out aerobic growth in the presence of cyanide concentrations lower than 100 μM. Up to 300 μM cyanide was tolerated by the cells, but during a period of 40 h no growth was observed. Eventually growth began even though cyanide was still present in the culture medium (Henry and Vignais, 1979). A concentration of 2 mM KCN was required to bring about 95% inhibition of NADH oxidase activity in membrane particles isolated from cells grown in the presence of 0.3 M KCN, whereas 100 μM KCN were sufficient to block oxygen uptake completely when the cells had been grown in a cyanide-free medium (Henry and Vignais, 1979). Mizushima *et al.*, (1959) also reported adaptation of *Aerobacter cloacae* to growth in the presence of cyanide.

2. *Effect of Mutation*

Isolation of mutants lacking a terminal oxidase or defective in an electron carrier required to drive the electron flow to an alternative acceptor has proved to be a useful tool for the study of bacterial energetics.

Membranes from the St. Louis strain of the purple nonsulfur photosynthetic bacterium *R. capsulata*, grown aerobically in the dark, showed a biphasic dependency of NADH oxidation upon KCN concentrations. This observation led Baccarini-Melandri *et al.*, (1973) to suggest the presence of two different sites of action of the inhibitor and to propose a model for a branched respiratory chain in this organism. Using a genetic approach, Marrs and Gest (1973) isolated mutants defective in one of the two cyanide-sensitive sites. These mutants, called M6 and M7, were subjected to a careful study by La Monica and Marrs (1976) and Zannoni *et al.*, (1976, 1978). Mutant M7 lacked the cytochrome oxidase activity associated with the high potential cytochrome b_{413} (E'_0 = +413 mV) (Zannoni *et al.*, 1976). This mutant showed only one inhibition constant for cyanide.

3. *Effect of Aeration*

As already mentioned, changes in the availability of molecular oxygen during growth can impair the electron transfer properties of bacterial cells. A reduced oxygen concentration in the growth medium often leads to an increased synthesis of cytochrome components, especially the terminal oxidase (Sinclair and White, 1970). This applies to *E. coli* (Moss, 1952), *P. denitrificans* (Sapshead and Wimpeney, 1970), *Haemophilus parainfluenzae* (White, 1963), *Achromobacter* (Arima and Oka, 1965) and *Klebsiella aerogenes* (Harrison, 1973b). As an example, Rice and Hempfling (1978) observed that cytochrome *o* was the only oxidase when *E. coli B* was grown under high dissolved oxygen tensions. However, when growth rates were decreased by oxygen limitation, the bacteria responded by a *de novo* synthesis of cytochromes a_1 and *d* and by an enhancement in b_1 and *o* content. Unfortunately, sensitivity of respiration to cyanide by oxygen-limited cultures was not assayed; probably a loss in sensitivity to cyanide would have been observed since cytochrome *d* is relatively resistant to cyanide (Kauffman and van Gelder, 1973; Pudek and Bragg, 1974).

These changes in the redox carrier pattern reflect attempts by the bacteria to overcome significant decreases in respiration rates. The synthesis of components which may have higher turnover numbers or greater affinities for oxygen will enable the cells to utilize the limited supply of oxidant as effectively as possible.

Ackrell and Jones (1971) noted that growth of the obligate aerobe *Azotobacter vinelandii* in the presence of excess oxygen depressed the level of cytochromes *a* and *o* while enhancing the synthesis of cytochrome *d*.

4. *Effect of Carbon Source*

Another environmental factor that can affect the formation and composition of bacterial electron transport systems is the carbon source used for growth.

In *P. denitrificans*, when methanol was used as the sole carbon and energy source, respiration on endogenous substrates proceeded through a branched electron transfer pathway and displayed a biphasic inhibition towards cyanide (van Verseveld and Stouthamer, 1978). The authors suggested on the basis of the results so far obtained, that a cytochrome *o* and an *a*-type cytochrome could both act as terminal oxidases. Electron transport *via* the *a*-type cytochrome was more sensitive to KCN than the other pathway *via* cytochrome *o*.

Similarly, cell-free extracts derived from autotrophically-grown cells (H_2-CO_2-O_2-grown) of *P. denitrificans* were partly devoid of cytochrome oxidase aa_3 while an *o*-type cytochrome was induced and was assumed to play the role of the terminal oxidase when H_2 was the electron donor. A concomitant resistance to cyanide was observed (Porte and Vignais, 1980).

5. *Effect of the Culture Age*

The growth phase at which the cells are harvested can also determine the levels and the nature of the cytochromes formed, particularly of the terminal oxidases. In some instances, changes in cytochrome content during the different growth phases can be attributed to a decrease in oxygen tension of the culture, especially when it reaches the stationary phase (Sinclair and White, 1970).

In *P. aeruginosa*, Trutko and his co-workers (1979) observed that cells reaching the stationary phase of growth developed respiration that was resistant to cyanide. The decrease in sensitivity to cyanide occurred without accumulation of this inhibitor in the growth medium and in the absence of oxygen-limitation. NADH oxidase activity of a particulate fraction was inhibited by 70% by 1 mM cyanide when the cells were harvested in the exponential phase of growth, whereas the inhibition was only 20-30% when the membranes were isolated from cells at stationary phase. In *E. coli*, Pudek and Bragg (1974) observed that particles prepared from cells harvested in the stationary phase of growth were less sensitive to cyanide than when the cells were collected in the logarithmic phase. The insensitivity to cyanide increased as the concentration of cytochrome *d* increased relative to cytochrome *o*.

Transition from vegetative cells of *Myxococcus xanthus* to microcysts also led to the appearance of respiration tolerant to cyanide. NADH oxidase activity in particles from vegetative cells was 69% inhibited by 1 mM cyanide, while an inhibition of only 34% was observed in microcysts under similar conditions (Dworkin and Niederpruem, 1964).

IV. MOLECULAR APPROACHES TO CYANIDE-RESISTANT RESPIRATION

A. NATURE OF THE ELECTRON DONOR

The insensitivity of respiration to cyanide depends primarily on the point of entry of the electrons into the respiratory chain. In *Neisseria gonorrhoeae*, a cyanide-insensitive electron transport pathway favored NADH oxidation, whereas a cyanide-sensitive pathway preferentially carried the electron flow from succinate. However, since the inhibition by cyanide was not complete with either substrate, both must have had access to the two branches of the respiratory system (Kenimer and Lapp, 1978). The marine bacterium, *B. natriegens* possesses a branched respiratory chain to O_2. Unlike eukaryotic organisms, branching occurs after the site of action of antimycin A. Inhibitor studies indicated that ascorbate-TMPD oxidation was almost completely inhibited by 1 μM cyanide, while oxidation of NADH, succinate, and D(-) and L(+) lactate required cyanide concentrations close to 10 mM for full inhibition (Weston *et al.*, 1974). These observations indicate that respiration with ascorbate-TMPD proceeded only through the cyanide-sensitive electron transport pathway.

Cyanide-resistance also depended on the nature of the electron donor in *P. denitrificans*. In membrane particles prepared from autotrophically-grown cells, electron transport from NADH and succinate proceeded through both pathways of the branched respiratory system, whereas H_2 donated its electrons only to the branch that was less sensitive to cyanide (Porte and Vignais, 1980).

In *A. nidulans* a different situation occurred. When the cells were grown under conditions which induced hydrogenase, H_2 and ascorbate-TMPD oxidations were fully sensitive to 0.5 mM cyanide. However, nearly 20% residual respiration remained in the presence of cyanide when either NADH, NADPH or succinate were the substrates being oxidized (Peschek, 1980).

There are several reports in the literature of other cases where the two pathways of a branched respiratory system can be distinguished by the substances used as electron donors. In *Kurthia zopfii* (Knowles *et al.*, 1978), *R. palustris* (King and Drews, 1975), *C. violaceum* (Niven *et al.*, 1975) and *A. vinelandii* (Jones and Redfearn, 1967), NADH and succinate oxidase activities were only weakly inhibited by cyanide, while ascorbate-TMPD or ascorbate-DCIP oxidations were highly sensitive to cyanide.

B. INSENSITIVITY TO OTHER INHIBITORS

In a number of cases, listed in Table II, whenever respiration appeared rather insensitive to cyanide it also proved insensitive to other inhibitors such as azide, antimycin A or HQNO. However, respiration was usually sensitive to CO.

Contrary to the situation found in cyanide-insensitive mitochondria (Henry and Nyns, 1975), the alternative respiratory pathways of bacteria are not inhibited by hydroxamic acid derivatives. Only one exception has been found so far. The cyanobacterium *A. nidulans* exhibited respiration in the presence of 0.5 mM cyanide which amounted to nearly 20% of the total respiration rate measured in the absence of inhibitor, when either NADPH or succinate were oxidized. This residual oxygen uptake could be further inhibited by about 50% upon addition of either 1 nM *m*-chlorobenzhydroxamic acid or salicylhydroxamic acid (Peschek, 1980). In *A. nidulans* the cyanide-insensitive respiration also proved to be very sensitive (63 to 75%) to 80 μM bathophenanthrolin. According to Peschek, inhibition was related to the lipophilic nature of the inhibitor, more lipophilic agents being better inhibitors of cyanide-resistant oxygen uptake.

C. PRESENCE OR ABSENCE OF COUPLED ATP PRODUCTION DURING CYANIDE-RESISTANT RESPIRATION

In studying bacterial energetics it is important to know whether the cyanide-insensitive respiratory pathway is coupled to energy conservation. Difficulties have been encountered in measuring oxidative phosphorylation in bacterial cells or in bacterial membranes. Bacterial membranes are devoid of an adenine nucleotide translocase and therefore a direct assay of ADP/O ratios (Chance and Williams, 1956) is not possible. In the chemiosmotic hypothesis for oxidative phosphorylation proposed by Mitchell (1966), respiration-linked proton translocation reflects the number of energy coupling sites. Nevertheless, the stoichio-

Table II Effect of respiratory chain inhibitors on oxidase activities of cyanide-resistant prokaryotes

Species	Substrates	Cyanide		Antimycin		N_3^-		HQNO		References
		Concentration (nM)	Inhibition %	Concentration	Inhibition %	Concentration (nM)	Inhibition %	Concentration	Inhibition	
Acetobacter suboxydans	NADH	0.75	65	50 μM	55	0.5	10	50 μM	60	Daniel, 1970
Achromobacter	Succinate	0.05	0			0.25	46			Arima and Oka, 1965
Azotobacter vinelandii	NADH	0.04	0			4	0			Jones and Redfearn, 1967
	Succinate	0.04	30			4	25			Jones and Redfearn, 1967
Chromobacterium violaceum	NADH	3.9	50			87	50			Niven *et al.*, 1975
	Succinate	2.3	50			87	50			Niven *et al.*, 1975
Hydrogenomonas H-20	H_2	0.3	72	40 μg/ml	3	0.1	0	1.4μg/ml	65	Bongers, 1967
Micrococcus lysodeikticus	NADH	1.2	17			1.25	0			Ishikawa and Lehninger, 1962
Neisseria gonorrhoeae	NADH	0.094	74	40 μM	53					Kenimer and Lapp, 1978
	Succinate	0.031	80	45.5μM	55					Kenimer and Lapp, 1978
	Malate	0.059	78	42.8μM	44					Kenimer and Lapp, 1978
Paracoccus denitrificans	NADH	0.1	70	10 μM	70			1 mM	40	Henry and Vignais, 1979
Pseudomonas aeruginosa	NADH	1	30					27 μM	60	Trutko *et al.*, 1979
	Malate	1	30					27 μM	35	Trutko *et al.*, 1979
Rhodopseudomonas palustris	NADH	0.1	54	0.1 mM	78	1	63	0.1 mM	25	King and Drews, 1975
	Succinate	0.1	52	0.1 mM	40	1	65	0.1 mM	12	King and Drews, 1975
Veillonella alcalescens	Lactate	5	44	25 μM	54	50	25	70 μM	90	de Vries *et al.*, 1978

metry of H^+ translocated per redox segment has been a subject of controversy and has been recently questioned (Brand *et al.*, 1976). A stoichiometry of 3 and even 4 H^+ translocated per energy transduction site has been determined in mitochondria.

Before the important work of Scholes and Mitchell (1970) on the bacterium *P. denitrificans*, little was known about energy transduction in bacteria. Meyer and Jones (1973) and more recently Jones *et al.* (1977, 1978) made an interesting survey of oxidative phosphorylation and respiration-linked proton translocation in bacteria containing different cytochrome oxidases. The efficiency of bacterial respiratory-chain energy conservation greatly depended on the cytochrome composition and on the nature of the terminal limb of the electron transport chain. In bacteria such as *Bacillus megaterium*, *E. coli*, *Klebsiella pneumoniae*, *Arthrobacter globiformis* or *Aerobacter punctata* which either lacked cytochrome *c* or contained a respiratory pathway terminated by cytochrome *d* $\rightarrow H^+/O$ ratios lower than 4 were measured. Values of nearly 6 were found when cytochrome *c* donated its electrons to either cytochrome oxidase aa_3 or cytochrome *o* (Jones *et al.*, 1975, 1978).

Since resistance to cyanide was not demonstrated for those species containing cytochrome *d* as terminal oxidase, it is not possible to relate the presence of an alternative, cyanide-resistant respiratory pathway unambiguously to a loss in energy conservation efficiency. On the other hand, it was suggested that H_2 oxidation catalyzed by the cyanide-resistant respiratory pathway via cytochrome *o* in *P. denitrificans* was indeed coupled to energy transduction (Porte and Vignais, 1980).

With the observations obtained so far, it appears likely that electron transfer via the cytochrome $b \rightarrow d$ segment is not associated with proton ejection (Jones *et al.*, 1978). More results should be gathered before clearcut conclusions can be drawn.

V. SELECTED CASES OF CYANIDE-RESISTANCE

A. ACHROMOBACTER

Achromobacter, a soil bacterium, is able to grow in a cyanide-containing medium where it forms a respiratory system resistant to this inhibitor. The mechanism of cyanide-resistance in this organism was studied by Arima and his colleagues (Mizushima and Arima, 1960a, b and c; Mizushima *et al.*, 1960; Arima and Oka, 1965; Oka and Arima, 1965).

Addition of 1 mM cyanide to the aerobic culture medium did not significantly inhibit the final growth yield, though a prolonged lag period was observed before the onset of growth. This lack of inhibitory effect of cyanide could be ascribed to an adaption to growth in the presence of the inhibitor. The reason for the eventual initiation of growth was not the disappearance of the inhibitor from the medium since it was demonstrated that during the exponential phase of growth cyanide was not degraded (Mizushima and Arima, 1960a).

Respiration of the adapted cells was only slightly affected by 1 mM cyanide (20 to 30% inhibition), whereas respiration of non-adapted cells was fully inhibited by the same cyanide concentration (Mizushima and Arima, 1960a). In a later report (Oka and Arima, 1965), the authors indicated that cyanide-resistant cells required 200 times more cyanide (i.e. 2 mM KCN instead of 10 μM) than non-adapted cells to be inhibited by 50%. No strong differences were found in the particulate fractions isolated from adapted and non-adapted cells concerning succinate oxidase and NADH oxidase activities (Mizushima and Arima, 1960a).

The reversibility of the adaptation indicated that this phenomenon was not the result of a mutation. When cells adapted to cyanide were transferred to a cyanide-free culture medium, respiration again became as sensitive to cyanide as that of non-adapted cells after growth for 7 or 8 generations, (Mizushima and Arima, 1960a). Such an adaptation to cyanide could also be induced in resting cells (Mizushima and Arima, 1960b) or in cells grown microaerobically under very low oxygen pressure (7 l air/min instead of 200 l air/min for aerobic growth) (Mizushima *et al.*, 1960). Chloramphenicol, at a concentration of 10 μM, almost completely prevented the appearance of the cyanide-insensitive respiration in resting cells, suggesting the involvement of protein synthesis in the process (Mizushima and Arima, 1960b). Mizushima and Arima (1960b) also studied the effects of amino acids and of the nature of the carbon source (glucose or succinate) on the appearance of cyanide-resistant oxygen uptake in resting cells. When the induction medium was deprived of amino acids or glucose, no cyanide-insensitive respiration could be elicited, even in the presence of cyanide. However, glucose, at a concentration of 20 mM proved effective for the adaptation to cyanide, whereas succinate did not. Casamino acids (0.2%) either alone, or together with glucose substantially increased the adaptation (Mizushima and Arima, 1960b). These observations indicated an energy requirement to drive adaptive synthesis of the alternative, cyanide-resistant respiratory pathway.

Arima and his colleagues observed a close relationship bewteen the growth phase, the amount of cytochrome formed and resistance of respiration to cyanide. During the exponential phase of aerobic growth, cells contained mainly cytochromes b_1 and *o*. Upon reaching the stationary phase or during growth under reduced aeration, cytochromes a_1 and *d* were induced. The appearance of the latter two cytochromes was parallel to a nearly two-fold increase of cytochrome b_1 and a 40% decrease in cytochrome *o* content. A similar situation was observed when growth was carried out in the presence of 1 mM cyanide. No *c*-type cytochrome could be detected under any of the growth conditions (Arima and Oka, 1965).

When cells grown aerobically in the presence of cyanide were transferred to a cyanide-free aerobic growth medium, the cytochrome pattern returned to the initial situation present during highly aerated growth. Cytochromes a_1 and d vanished, and the cytochrome o remained at nearly the same level (Arima and Oka, 1965).

To identify the cyanide-resistant oxidase, Arima and Oka (1965) studied the oxidation-reduction level of the cytochromes in cell-free extracts of *Achromobacter* strain D, a double auxotrophic mutant of strain 7 used in the previous studies. In the aerobic steady-state, when the reduction of the cytochromes was assayed in the presence of succinate and 0.5 mM cyanide, cytochrome d was not completely reduced and could be reoxidized by slight aeration. Vigorous aeration was required to partly reoxidise cytochrome b_1 while cytochrome a_1 always remained reduced. No mention was made of the role of cytochrome o which was also present in cyanide-resistant cells.

To define more accurately the individual roles of the different potential oxidases (a_1, o, d) in a system where more than one oxidase was present, Oka and Arima (1965) used the photochemical technique devised by Castor and Chance (1959) and based on the relief by light of CO-inhibition of respiration. The experiments were also conducted on cyanide-sensitive cells where cytochrome o functioned as the only oxidase (Arima and Oka, 1965). To discriminate between cytochrome o and d as terminal oxidases, the authors used blue and red filters at appropriate wavelengths, so that CO-inhibited cells would be illuminated with light absorbed by one pigment only. In the absence of cyanide, photodissociation of CO-inhibition in adapted cells occurred with light transmitted by both filters, whereas upon addition of cyanide only red light restored the activity. Blue light was able to relieve CO-inhibition in cyanide-sensitive cells containing only cytochrome o as the terminal electron carrier.

On the basis of kinetic analysis, redox steady state measurements and photochemical action spectra, the authors concluded that the electron transfer pathway from cytochrome b_1 to d was cyanide-resistant. Cytochrome a_1 appeared to be a cyanide-sensitive electron carrier, while cytochrome d could be considered as the cyanide-resistant oxidase able to mediate electron flow from succinate to oxygen, even at high cyanide concentrations (Fig. 1).

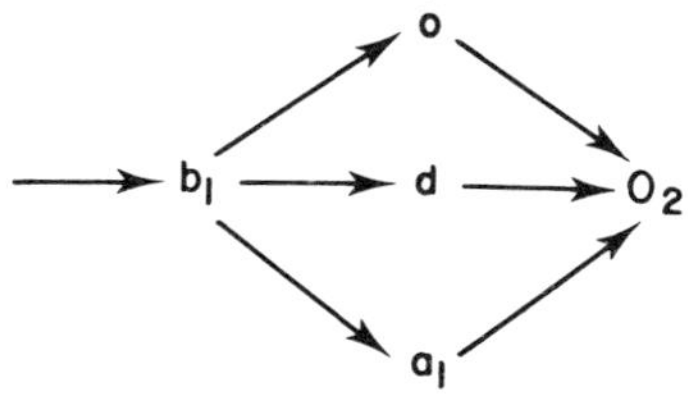

Fig. 1 Schematic representation of the cytochrome chain of *Achromobacter* grown in the presence of 1 mM KCN (after Arima and Oka, 1965).

B. AZOTOBACTER VINELANDII

The respiratory system of *A. vinelandii* consists of a complex set of redox carriers (Jones and Redfearn, 1966) among which cytochromes a_1, d and possibly o may act as terminal oxidases (Jones and Redfearn, 1967). The electron transport system of *A. vinelandii* is the most extensively studied bacterial branched respiratory system (for references see the reviews of Jurtshuk *et al.*, 1975 and of Haddock and Jones, 1977). It is not relevant to this paper to discuss in detail the characteristics of this interesting respiratory system; only some of the properties of the cyanide-insensitive pathway will be reported.

A particulate preparation isolated from cells grown aerobically on N_2 as sole nitrogen source actively oxidized NADH, succinate and ascorbate-DCIP. Low concentrations of cyanide (40 μM) or azide (4 mM) failed to or only partially inhibited NADH and succinate oxidases, but almost completely blocked ascorbate-DCIP oxidoreductase activity. A concentration of 2 mM cyanide was required to inhibit the oxidases fully (Jones and Redfearn, 1967).

Action spectra used to determine the relief of CO-inhibition in whole cells of *A. vinelandii* oxidizing endogenous substrates indicated an important contribution of cytochrome d relative to a_1 and o. When respiratory particles oxidized NADH, a strong inhibition by CO was observed which could be relieved by high intensity white light, or to a much lesser extent by red light but not by blue light. A concentration of 50 μM KCN neither inhibited NADH oxidase nor did it change the restoration by light of CO-inhibition (Jones and Redfearn, 1967).

These results, pointing to the role of cytochrome d as the major terminal oxidase in *A. vinelandii* particles, were strengthened by aerobic steady-state reduction experiments. The inability of low concentrations of cyanide or azide to increase the reduction of cytochrome b_1 significantly suggested that the cytochrome $b_1 \rightarrow d$ segment of the respiratory chain was able to carry most of the electron flow from NADH to O_2. The other pathway, sensitive to low concentrations of cyanide and azide, contained cytochromes $c_4 + c_5$ and o or a_1 as the terminal oxidases. The electrons from ascorbate were donated at the level of the *c*-type cytochromes, c_4 and c_5 (Jones and Redfearn, 1967). Recently, Kauffman and van Gelder (1974) provided kinetic and spectroscopic evidence confirming the role of cytochrome *d* as the major terminal oxidase.

As in other bacterial systems no respiration-driven energy transduction could be demonstrated for the cytochrome $b \rightarrow d$ segment of *A. vinelandii*, whereas the terminal branch, consisting of cytochromes $c_4 + c_5$ to *o*, a_1, indeed exhibited energy coupling (Ackrell and Jones, 1971a). Proton translocation experiments (Downs and Jones, 1975) confirmed these observations.

A. vinelandii is a nitrogen-fixing, obligate aerobe. It is well known that nitrogenase is readily inactivated by molecular oxygen (Drozd and Postgate, 1970). Therefore the organism is faced with the paradox of maintaining an active nitrogenase while carrying out respiration-driven energy conservation. Ackrell and Jones (1971b) studied the effects of oxygen concentrations on the cytochrome composition of the branched respiratory system of *A. vinelandii*. Under highly aerated growth conditions, the electron flow proceeded mainly through the cyanide-insensitive pathway and was also associated with a loss of energy coupling at site I. However, oxygen limitation was accompanied by a 9- to 13-fold increase in activity of the minor, cyanide-sensitive respiratory pathway and a great enhancement in phosphorylation efficiency. From these observations the authors proposed a mechanism for protection of nitrogenase (Fig. 2).

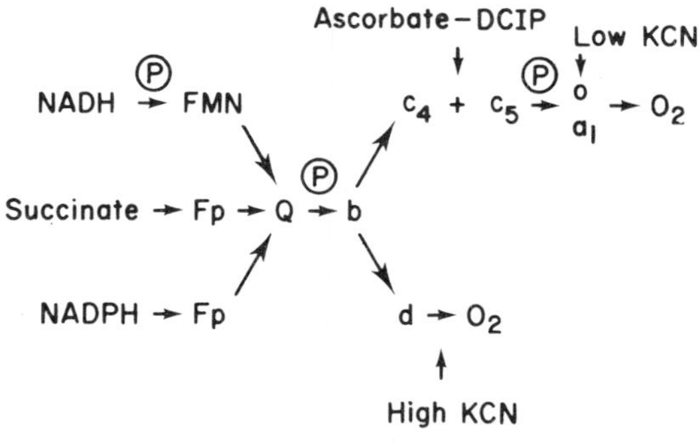

Fig. 2 Respiratory system of *A. vinelandii* modified after Jones and Redfearn (1967) and Downs and Jones (1975). The arrows indicate the routes of electron transfer. Ⓟ represents the approximate sites of energy transduction.

C. BENECKEA NATRIEGENS

The marine bacterium *B. natriegens*, previously *Pseudomonas natriegens* (Payne *et al.*, 1961), contains a complex respiratory chain with a large number of cytochromes able to bind CO (a_1, *d*, *o*, and *c*) which are potentially terminal oxidases. The respiratory system of this organism has been extensively studied (Weston and Knowles, 1973, 1974; Weston *et al.*, 1974; Linton *et al.*, 1975, 1976).

A particulate fraction, isolated from cells grown under high aeration, actively oxidized NADH, succinate and L(+) and D(-) lactate. Ascorbate-TMPD was oxidased at a 7-12 times greater rate than the other substrates. Inhibitor studies indicated a biphasic titration curve of cyanide for all oxidases tested except for ascorbate-TMPD oxidase which was almost fully inhibited by 1 μM cyanide. The NADH, succinate, D(-) and L(+) lactate oxidases each exhibited two apparent K_i values for cyanide of about 5 μM and 2 mM, the two sites titrated being separated by a "plateau" region at about 50% inhibition. These oxidases were also very resistant to azide and sulphide. These results suggest that two respiratory pathways from physiological substrates to oxygen operate in particles of *B. natriegens*, while the artificial substrate ascorbate-TMPD is oxidized only via the cyanide-sensitive route of electron flow (Weston *et al.*, 1974). Such a biphasic response to cyanide could not be demonstrated with whole cells. However, the degree of inhibition by cyanide greatly depended on the respiration rate of the cells, as all the cells tested were always cyanide-sensitive at high respiration rates (Linton *et al.*, 1976). The latter authors also suggested that the occurrence of a branched respiratory system in membrane particles may not absolutely indicate its presence *in vivo*. Therefore, according to Linton *et al.*, (1976), it seems unlikely that a cyanide-insensitive respiratory pathway will function as the major route of electron flow *in vivo*.

In contrast, Weston *et al.*, (1974) observed with isolated particles that as the oxidase capacity increased the degree of inhibition by cyanide in the plateau region decreased. They suggested that the ascorbate-TMPD pathway accepted the electron flow more easily, while the excess of reducing equivalents passed through the cyanide-insensitive pathway.

The cyanide-resistant respiratory pathway was found to have an affinity for molecular oxygen 3.5 times higher than the cyanide-sensitive one (3 μM against 10.6 μM O_2, respectively) (Weston *et al.*, 1976). This greater affinity for O_2 may be related to the presence of cytochrome *d* as a major oxidase in *B. natriegens* (determined by action spectra), though it was barely detectable by adsorption difference spectra (Weston and Knowles, 1974).

D. CHROMOBACTERIUM VIOLACEUM

C. violaceum is able to form up to 1.8 mM cyanide by the start of the stationary phase when grown on a complex medium containing glycine and L-methionine (Niven *et al.*, 1975; Collins *et al.*, 1980). When growth was carried out on a minimal medium, only 30 μM cyanide was produced (Niven *et al.*, 1975). Some properties of the respiratory system of this bacterium were studied by Niven *et al.* (1975) under conditions where the organism produced either high or low amounts of cyanide.

Membrane particles, isolated from cells grown on both complex and minimal medium, oxidized NADH and succinate at high rates, although a 3- to 6-fold greater activity for these two substrates was found in particles from the complex medium. These latter particles were unable to oxidize ascorbate-TMPD unlike particles derived from cells evolving low amounts of cyanide.

NADH and succinate oxidase activities in particles from cells grown on the complex medium were weakly inhibited by cyanide, azide and CO. Total inhibition could only be reached at infinite concentrations of cyanide. The inhibition titration curves for these inhibitors proved monophasic in contrast to those obtained with particles isolated from cells grown on a minimal medium. In the latter particles, the two phases were separated by a plateau region where no further inhibition was observed. For 50% inhibition of the two phases, 4 μM and about 2 mM cyanide were required, respectively. Ascorbate-TPMD oxidation in particles grown on minimal medium was highly sensitive to cyanide, with a K_i of 4 μM, and proved to be monophasic (Niven *et al.*, 1975).

Once again, these results suggest the presence of a branched respiratory system in particles from cultures evolving low amounts of cyanide, whereas only the alternative, cyanide-resistant branch would be present in particles from cells grown in the complex medium. This system resembles in many respects that of the marine bacterium *B. natriegens*.

Low temperature absorption difference spectra of the particulate fraction of cells grown on complex medium indicated the presence of cytochromes a_1, d, o and of a CO-binding c-type cytochrome. Cytochromes a_1 and d were virtually absent when the cells were grown under conditions producing low amounts of cyanide. The exact role of the different cytochromes as potential terminal oxidases could not be ascertained accurately. Therefore the nature of the terminal, cyanide-resistant oxidase of *C. vidaceum* remains unknown (Niven *et al.*, 1975).

E. PARACOCCUS DENITRIFICANS

P. denitrificans can grow aerobically in the presence of up to 300 μM cyanide (Henry and Vignais, 1979). Membrane particles isolated from cells grown in the presence of 300 μM cyanide exhibited biphasic curves for inhibition by cyanide of NADH oxidase activity and an incomplete inhibition by antimycin A, suggesting a branched respiratory system. One branch is sensitive to low concentrations of KCN (K_i = 5.10^{-5}M) whereas the second branch is sensitive to much higher KCN concentrations (70% inhibition of total oxygen uptake at 5.10^{-4}M KCN). An inhibition of 95% was reached with 1 - 2 mM KCN.

Membrane fractions isolated from aerobically-grown *P. denitrificans* contained the usual set of cytochromes *b*, *c* and cytochrome oxidase *aa*$_3$. Growth in the presence of cyanide was accompanied by the appearance of a CO-binding b-type cytochrome, usually referred to as cytochrome *o* (Castor and Chance, 1959), by the appearance of cytochrome *d* and a sharp decrease in cytochrome oxidase *aa*$_3$ content, which was almost absent. Cytochrome *d* may play the role of the cyanide-resistant oxidase since blocking cytochrome oxidase *aa*$_3$ during growth also enhanced by about 10-fold the affinity of the alternative respiratory pathway for molecular oxygen (Henry and Vignais, 1979).

A similar situation occurred when the bacterium was grown autotrophically on H_2 as the source of reducing equivalents, CO_2 and O_2 (H_2:CO_2:O_2, 7/1/2, by vol.). Titration by KCN of NADH oxidase activity in membrane preparations proved to be biphasic. The two sites titrated by KCN indicated K_i values of 10^{-5}M and 1 mM (Porte and Vignais, 1980). In these membranes H_2 oxidation showed a monophasic dependence on KCN concentration and was sensitive only to high cyanide concentrations. It seems likely that a branched respiratory system operates in these membranes with electrons from H_2 going only to the more cyanide-resistant oxidase. As H_2 oxidation also proved to be insensitive to rotenone and resistant to antimycine A, it was proposed that the branching point occurred after the rotenone- and before the antimycine A-sensitive sites, as already suggested by van Verseveld and Stouthamer (1978) for methanol-grown *P. denitrificans* (Fig. 3).

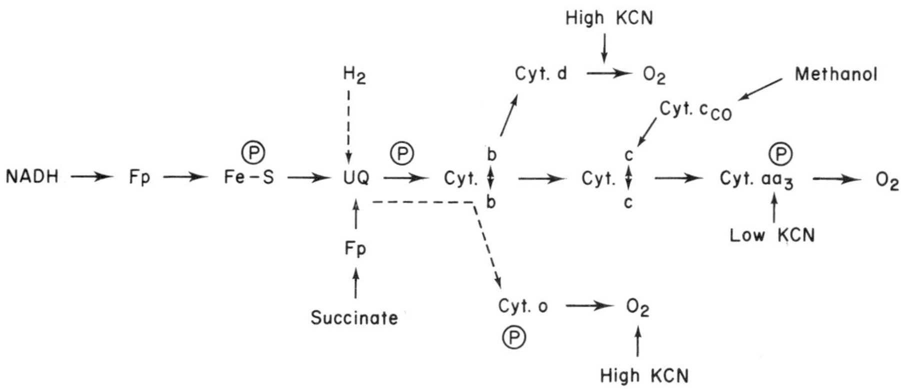

Fig. 3 Proposed respiratory system in *P. denitrificans*. The arrows indicate the pathways of electron flow, the broken arrow represents the way of H_2 oxidation, and (P) refers to the presumed coupling sites. The scheme is modified from van Verseveld and Stouthamer (1978); Henry and Vignais (1979); Porte and Vignais (1980).

Respiration-driven proton translocation studies suggested that the second pathway from H_2 to oxygen might be coupled to ATP synthesis. An $\rightarrow H^+/O$ ratio of 6 with H_2 was observed, suggesting the presence of two coupling sites. Endogenous substrates gave $\rightarrow H^+/O \simeq 9$ (Porte and Vignais, 1980).

A particulate fraction of cells of *P. denitrificans* grown on $H_2:CO_2:O_2$ contained high amounts of cytochrome *o* and only traces of cytochrome oxidase aa_3. Cytochrome *d* could not be detected in this fraction (Porte and Vignais, 1980). The authors suggested a possible role for cytochrome *o* as a terminal oxidase although no kinetic evidence could be obtained by Lawford *et al.* (1976) to ascribe such a role for cytochrome *o* in *P. denitrificans*.

VI. PHYSIOLOGICAL IMPORTANCE OF THE CYANIDE-RESISTANT RESPIRATION

Many organisms are resistant or can become resistant to cyanide by degrading it to non-toxic products. However, the reason for the adaptive built-up of a respiratory chain resistant to cyanide, involving the synthesis of new components is not known.

In plant mitochondria cyanide-insensitive respiration appears in mature tissues or in tissues which have been wounded. In thermogenic tissues like araceae it is concomitant with the increase in respiration associated with heat production (for reviews see Henry and Nyns, 1975; Solomos, 1977).

Cyanide-resistance has also been found during respiratory burst in polymorphonuclear leukocytes during phagocytosis. This increase in oxygen consumption seems to be mediated by a membrane-bound, though non-mitochondrial, NAD(P)H oxidase system, and results in the production of large amounts of superoxide anions and hydrogen peroxide (Karnovsky, 1973; Klebanoff, 1975; Babior, 1978; Stelmaszyñska and Zgliczyñski, this book).

In *A. vinelandii* the two branches of the respiratory system have different phosphorylation efficiencies (Ackrell and Jones, 1971b; Downs and Jones, 1975) and could be used differentially by the organism as a mechanism to protect its nitrogenase from the deleterious effects of O_2 (Ackrell and Jones, 1971b). Indeed, during growth at an high oxygen concentration, the electron flow would preferentially proceed through the non-phosphorylating, cytochrome *d* pathway. Under oxygen deprivation conditions, when protection of the nitrogen-fixing apparatus is not required, the cyanide-sensitive respiratory pathway would predominate (Ackrell and Jones, 1971b).

In several bacterial species (see above), the induction of cytochrome *d* and sometimes a_1 at low oxygen tensions may again reflect attempts by the organism to overcome oxygen deprivation by maintaining high respiration rates with cytochromes having higher turnover numbers and greater affinities for molecular oxygen. This mechanism could operate at the expense of energy conservation.

ACKNOWLEDGEMENTS

I am deeply indebted to Dr P.M. Vignais (Grenoble, France) for her critical review of the manuscript, and to Ms J. Bournet for manuscript preparation.

REFERENCES

Ackrell, B.A.C. and Jones, C.W. (1971a). *Eur. J. Biochem.* 20, 22-28.
Ackrell, B.A.C. and Jones, C.W. (1971b). *Eur. J. Biochem.* 20, 29-35.
Arima, K. and Oka, T. (1965). *J. Bacteriol.* 90, 734-743.
Asano, A. and Brodie, A. (1964). *J. Biol. Chem.* 239, 4280-4291.
Ashcroft, J.R. and Haddock, B.A. (1975). *Biochem. J.* 148, 349-352.
Babior, B.M. (1978). *N. Engl. J. Med.* 298, 659-668.
Baccarini-Melandri, A., Zannoni, D. and Melandri, B.A. (1973). *Biochim. Biophys. Acta* 314, 298-311.
Bongers, L. (1967). *J. Bacteriol.* 93, 1615-1623.
Brand, M.D., Reynafarje, B. and Lehninger, A.L. (1976). *J. Biol. Chem.* 251, 5670-5679.
Castor, L.N. and Chance, B. (1959). *J. Biol. Chem.* 234, 1587-1592.
Chance, B. and Williams, G.R. (1956). *Adv. Enzymol.* 17, 65-134.
Collins, P.A., Rodgers, P.B. and Knowles, C.J. (1980). *J. Gen. Microbiol.* 117, 73-80.
Daniel, R.M. (1970). *Biochem. Biophys. Acta* 216, 328-341.
de Vries, W., Donkers, C., Boellard, M. and Stouthamer, A.H. (1978). *Arch. Microbiol.* 119, 167-174.
Drozd, J. and Postgate, J.R. (1970). *J. Gen. Microbiol.* 63, 63-73.
Dworkin, M. and Niederpruem, D.J. (1964). *J. Bacteriol.* 87, 316-322.
Feldman, W. and O'Kane, D. (1960). *J. Bacteriol.* 80, 218-224.
Francis, M.J.O., Hughes, D.E., Kornberg, H.L. and Phizackerley, P.J. R. (1963). *Biochem. J.* 89, 430-438.
Gel'man, N.S., Lukoyanova, M.A. and Ostrovskii, D.N. (1967). *In* "Respiration and Phosphorylation in Bacteria" pp.71-159. Plenum Press, New York and London.
Gel'man, N.S., Lukoyanova, M.A., and Ostrovskii, D.N. (1975). *Biomembranes Vol.6*, pp. 129-209, Plenum Press, New York and London.
Haddock, B.A. and Jones, C.W. (1977). *Bacteriol. Rev.* 41, 47-99.
Harrison, D.E.F. (1973). *Biochim. Biophys. Acta* 275, 83-92.
Henry, M.-F. and Nyns, E.J. (1975). *Sub-Cell. Biochem.* 4, 1-65.
Henry, M.-F. and Vignais, P.M. (1979). *FEBS Lett.* 100, 41-46.
Ishikawa, S. and Lehninger, A.L. (1962). *J. Biol. Chem.* 237, 2401-2408.
Jones, C.W. (1977). *In* "Microbial Energetics" (B.A. Haddock and W.A. Hamilton, eds.). pp.23-59. Cambridge University Press, Cambridge.
Jones, C.W., Brice, J.M., Downs, A.J. and Drozd, J.W. (1975). *Eur. J. Biochem.* 52, 265-271.
Jones, C.W., Brice, J.M., and Edwards, C. (1978). *In* "Functions of Alternative Terminal Oxidases" (H. Degn, D. Lloyd and G.C. Hill, eds) Vol. 49, pp.89-97, 11th FEBS meeting, Copenhagen 1977, Perga-

mon Press.
Jones, C.W. and Redfearn, E.R. (1966). *Biochim. Biophys. Acta,* 113, 467-481.
Jones, C.W. and Redfearn, E.R. (1967). *Biochim. Biophys. Acta,* 143, 340-353.
Jurtshuk, P., Jr., Mueller, T.J. and Acord, W.C. (1975). *C.R.C. Critical Reviews in Microbiology* 3, 399-468.
Karnovsky, M.L. (1973). *Fed. Am. Soc. Exp. Biol.* 32, 1527-1533.
Kauffman, H.F. and van Gelder, B.F. (1973). *Biochim. Biophys. Acta,* 314, 276-283.
Kauffman, H.F. and van Gelder, B.F. (1974). *Biochim. Biophys. Acta,* 333, 218-227.
Kenimer, E.A. and Lapp, D.F. (1978). *J. Bacteriol.* 134, 537-545.
King, M.T. and Drews, G. (1975). *Arch. Microbiol.* 102, 219-231.
Klebanoff, S.J. (1975). *Semin. Hematol.* 12, 117-142.
Knowles, C.J. (1976). *Bacteriol. Rev.* 40, 652-680.
Knowles, C.J., Collins, P.A. and Niven, D.F. (1978). *In* "Functions of Alternative Terminal Oxidases" (H. Degn, D. Lloyd and G.C. Hill, eds). 11th FEBS Meeting, Copenhagen 1977, Vol. 49, pp.123-132, Pergamon Press.
La Monica, R.F. and Marrs, B.L. (1976). *Biochim. Biophys. Acta,* 423, 431-439.
Lawford, H.G., Cox, J.C., Garland, P.B. and Haddock, B.A. (1976). *FEBS Lett.* 64, 369-374.
Lemberg, R. and Barrett, J. (1973). *In* "Cytochromes", pp.217-326. Academic Press, New York.
Linton, J.D., Harrison, D.E.F. and Bull, A.T. (1975). *J. Gen. Microbiol.,* 90, 237-246.
Linton, J.D., Harrison, D.E.F. and Bull, A.T. (1976). *FEBS Letters,* 64, 358-363.
Lloyd, D. (1974).*In* "The Mitochondria of Microorganisms", pp.137-158, Academic Press, London, New York and San Francisco.
Marrs, B. and Gest, H. (1973). *J. Bacteriol.* 114, 1045-1051.
McFeters, G.A., Wilson, D.F. and Strobel, G.A. (1970). *Can. J. Microbiol.,* 16, 1221-1226.
Meyer, D.J. and Jones, C.W. (1973). *Eur. J. Biochem.,* 36, 144-151.
Mitchell, P. (1966). *Biolog. Rev.,* 41, 445-502.
Mizushima, S. and Arima, K. (1960a). *J. Biochem.,* 47, 351-360.
Mizushima, S. and Arima, K. (1960b). *J. Biochem.,* 47, 600-607.
Mizushima, S. and Arima, K. (1960c). *J. Biochem.,* 47, 837-845.
Mizushima, S., Nakano, M. and Sakaguchi, K.I. (1959). *J. Biochem.* 46, 373-381.
Mizushima, S., Oka, T. and Arima, K. (1960). *J. Biochem.,* 48, 205-213.
Moss, F.J. (1952). *Austral. J. Exper. Biol. Med. Sci.,* 30, 531.
Newton, N. (1969). *Biochim. Biophys. Acta,* 185, 316-331.
Niven, D.F., Collins, P.A. and Knowles, C.J. (1975). *J. Gen. Microbiol.,* 90, 271-285.
Oka, T. and Arima, K. (1965). *J. Bacteriol.,* 90, 744-747.
Paul, F., Colbeau, A., and Vignais, P.M. (1979). *FEBS Lett.* 106, 29-33.
Pappenheimer, A., Howland, J. and Miller, P. (1962). *Biochim. Biophys. Acta,* 64, 229-0000.
Payne, W.J., Eagon, R.G. and Williams, A.K. (1961), *Antonie van Leeu-*

wenhoek, 27, 152-160.
Peschek, G.A. (1980). *Arch. Microbiol.*, 125, 123-131.
Porte, F. and Vignais, P.M. (1980). *Arch. Microbiol.*, 121, 1-10.
Pudek, M.R. and Bragg, P.D. (1974). *Arch. Biochem. Biophys.* 164, 682-693.
Rice, C.W., and Hempfling, W.P. (1978). *J. Bacteriol.*, 134, 115-124.
Robinson, D.A. and Mills, R.C. (1961). *Biochim. Biophys. Acta*, 48, 77-84..
Sapshead, L.M. and Wimpenny, J.W.T. (1972). *Biochim. Biophys. Acta*, 267, 388-397.
Scholes, P.B. and Mitchell, P. (1970). *J. Bioenergetics*, 1, 309-323.
Sinclair, P.R. and White, D.C. (1970). *J. Bacteriol.*, 101, 365-372.
Skowronski, B. and Strobel, G.A. (1969). *Can. J. Microbiol.*, 15, 93-98.
Solomos, T. (1977). *Ann. Rev. Plant Physiol.*, 28, 279-297.
Taber, H.W. and Morrison, M. (1964). *Arch. Biochem. Biophys.*, 105, 367-379.
Tissieres, A. (1951). *Biochem. J.*, 50, 279.
Trutko, S.M., Golovchenko, N.P. and Akimento, V.K. (1979). *Biokhimiya*, 44, 720-728.
van Verseveld, A.W. and Stouthamer, A.H. (1978). *Arch. Microbiol.*, 118, 13-20.
Warburg, O. and Christian, W. (1932a). *Naturwissenschaften*, 20, 688.
Warburg, O. and Christian, W. (1932b). *Biochem. Z.*, 254, 438-458.
Weston, J.A. and Knowles, C.J. (1973). *Biochem. Biophys. Acta*, 305, 11-18.
Weston, J.A. and Knowles, C.J. (1974). *Biochim. Biophys. Acta*, 333, 228-236.
Weston, J.A. Collins, P.A. and Knowles, C.J. (1974). *Biochim. Biophys. Acta*, 368, 148-157.
White, D.C. (1963). *J. Biol. Chem.*, 238, 3757-3761.
White, D.C. and Sinclair, P.R. (1971). *In* "Advances in Microbial Physiology" (A.H. Rose and J.F. Wilkinson, eds) Vol. 5, pp.173-211, Academic Press, New York.
Zannoni, D., Melandri, B.A. and Baccarini-Melandri, A. (1976). *Biochim. Biophys. Acta*, 423, 413-430.
Zannoni, D., Melandri, B.A. and Baccarini-Melandri, A. (1978). *In:* "Functions of Alternative Terminal Oxidases" (H. Degn, D. Lloyd and G.C. Hill, eds) Vol. 49, pp.169-171, 11th FEBS Meeting, Copenhagen 1977, Pergamon Press.

ABBREVIATIONS USED

DCIP : 2,6-dichlorophenolindophenol

HQNO : 2-n-heptyl-4-hydroxyquinoleine-N-oxide

TMPD : N,N,N',N'-etramethyl-1,4-phenylenediamine dihydrochloride.

CYANIDE-RESISTANT RESPIRATION IN EUKARYOTIC CELLS

J. M. PALMER

Department of Botany, Imperial College, University of London

I. INTRODUCTION

The process of cellular respiration is normally considered to be characterized by the degradation of carbohydrates and fats with the concomitant reduction of pyridine nucleotide and flavin coenzymes. These coenzymes are then oxidized by the electron transport chain and the energy released is coupled to the synthesis of ATP. The process of cellular respiration in the mammalian cell is inhibited by cyanide which is known to interact with cytochrome a_3, which acts as the terminal oxidase. Thus this review will deal only with the processes of electron transport responsible for the reoxidation of NADH and reduced flavoproteins. Most of our detailed knowledge of the operation of the electron transport chain is derived from studies using mammalian tissue in which the oxidation of the coenzymes is achieved by a series of flavoproteins, iron-sulphur proteins, ubiquinone, cytochromes and copper ions. The study of this process has been facilitated because the electron transport chain can be isolated in the mitochrondrial fraction and because the redox state of the individual components can be readily detected using spectroscopic techniques. The mammalian system is susceptible to inhibition at three specific points; cyanide, azide or carbon monoxide inhibit electron flux through the terminal oxidase, antimycin A prevents electron flux between cytochrome *b* and cytochrome *c*, and rotenone or piericidin A inhibit electron transfer through the iron-sulphur components of the NADH dehydrogenase. These three sites of inhibition correspond closely with the three sites of ATP synthesis during oxidative phosphorylation.

While these inhibitors are capable of causing at least 95% inhibition of oxidation in mitochondria isolated from mammalian cells it has been frequently reported that all three classes of inhibitors are less effective in preventing electron transport in mitochondria obtained from other types of eukaryotic tissue, notably protozoa, microorganisms, such as yeast and *Neurospora crassa*, and higher plants. The phenomenon of cyanide- and antimycin A- resistant respiration, the subject of this review, has been widely recognized whilst the phenomenon of rotenone resistance, which is equally widespread, has attracted less interest. Many papers have been written on the subject of cyanide-resistant respiration and there can be no doubt that some of the reports have caused confusion because of the failure to appreciate possible artifacts when using intact tissue rather than purified mitochondria oxidizing a defined substrate. One major advance in our understanding of the nature of cyanide-resistant respiration has been the discovery that the pathway can be inhibited by substituted benzhydroxamates (salicylhydroxamic acid; SHAM) (Schonbaum *et al.*, 1971). This has led to a large number of publications claiming to show that the cyanide-resistant, SHAM-sensitive, alternative oxidase has a role in a variety of intact tissue (Lambers and Van de Dijk, 1979). The precise interpretation of this data is confusing on two counts. Firstly, the hydroxamates inhibit enzymatic processes other than the alternative oxidase, such as peroxidases (Schonbaum, 1973) and polyphenol oxidases (Rich *et al.*, 1978). Secondly, when using intact tissue, care must be taken not to confuse cyanide-resistant oxygen uptake, due to enzymes such as lipoxygenase (Parrish and Leopold, 1978), which would not count as respiration, with the activity of a true alternative oxidase participating in the respiratory process.

The other artifact that needs to be evaluated is to what extent a low level of cyanide-resistant oxygen uptake, particularly when giving rise to hydrogen peroxide, represents a natural process or whether it is induced by the assay treatment. Thus inhibition by cyanide could cause a component of the respiratory chain to become very reduced and liable to auto-oxidation, which may be prevented in the more oxidized state in which it normally exists. Another danger with microorganisms, such as some of the protozoa that live in low oxygen tensions, is that assay in the elevated oxygen concentrations characteristic of air-saturated aqueous medium may cause the auto-oxidation of intermediates not normally prone to this process. Elevated oxygen concentrations have been observed to stimulate the auto-oxidation of reduced ubiquinone in mammalian mitochondria (Boveris *et al.*, 1976). Thus, although the presence of a cyanide-resistant, SHAM-sensitive oxygen consumption may be evidence for the existence of an alternative respiratory chain, care must be exercised in the interpretation of the data.

A. OCCURRENCE AND CHARACTERISTIC OF CYANIDE-RESISTANT OXIDASES

The occurrence of the phenomenon of cyanide-resistant oxygen uptake in eukaryotic cells is widespread (Henry and Nyns, 1975) and has been reported from animals, microorganisms and plants. However, it has only been investigated extensively in certain classes of protozoa, microorganisms, such as yeasts and *Neurospora crassa*, and higher plants. The available literature suggests that the oxidase present in yeasts, *N. crassa* and higher plants has many features in common while that described in protozoa, characterized by the trypanosomes and *Ascaris*, appears substantially different.

B. THE OXIDASE PRESENT IN TRYPANOSOMES

The literature concerning the oxidases in these organisms is extensive and relatively confusing since there seems to be a high degree of variability between different species of trypanosomes and the oxidase present is very dependent on the culture conditions. The systems present in *Trypanosoma brucei* (Hill, 1977) or *T. mega* (Kronick and Hill, 1974) have been extensively characterized.

In their life cycle trypanosomes exist in two forms. One is found in the blood stream of the mammalian host and referred to as the bloodstream form. The other form is found in the insect vector. When the trypanosome is grown in culture it has many of the characteristics of the form in the insect vector. The respiratory systems present in the bloodstream and culture forms have been extensively studied.

In the bloodstream form the development of the mitochondria appears to be incomplete and the cells do not contain a functional Krebs cycle or any cytochrome system. The cells derive their energy from glycolysis which produces large amounts of pyruvate and the resulting NADH is reoxidized by oxygen (Bowman and Flynn, 1976). The oxidation of the NADH is achieved indirectly through the combined activity of an NAD^+-linked α-glycerol-3-phosphate dehydrogenase and an α-glycerol-3-phosphate oxidase. These two enzymes catalyse the cyanide-resistant oxidation of NADH which is not coupled to the synthesis of ATP. There is general agreement that the glycerol-3-phosphate dehydrogenase is located in the microbody fraction (Bowman and Flynn, 1976; Opperdoes and Borst, 1976). Data concerning the subcellular location of the α-glycerol-3-phosphate oxidase are not so clear. It has been generally believed to be located in the microbody fraction (Bowman and Flynn, 1976); however, since the cells do not have fully developed mitochondria it is not easy to distinguish this organelle during the fractionation procedure. Opperdoes and Borst (1976) have shown that in *T. brucei* the glycerol-3-phosphate oxidase resides in a fraction rich in oligomycin-sensitive ATPase and conclude that it is in the promitochondria.

The nature of the oxidase remains unsolved. The oxidase is relatively specific for glycerol-3-phosphate which is oxidized 20 times faster than other hydrogen donors. The oxidation of glycerol-3-phosphate to dihydroxyacetone phosphate can occur in the presence of electron acceptors such as phenazine methosulphate or molecular oxygen. No precise information is available concerning the nature of the prosthetic groups involved although FAD, iron-sulphur proteins and copper have been considered as possible intermediates (Hill, 1976). The product formed by the oxidase appears to be water and the oxidase is inhibited by hydroxamates and stimulated by bovine serum albumin. The K_m for oxygen is relatively high (2.1 μM), thus the affinity for oxygen is considerably lower than that of the cytochrome oxidase which has a K_m for O_2 in the region of 0.1 μM (Hill, 1977).

When the trypanosomes are grown in culture their respiratory systems alter and there is the rapid appearance of functional mitochondria with an active Krebs cycle and functional respiratory chain containing cytochromes *a*, *b* and *c* (Hill, 1977; Ray and Cross, 1972). The level of ubiquinone 9 also increases by a factor of 4-fold during this process (Bowman and Flynn, 1976). In this condition the respiratory system becomes relatively sensitive to cyanide, although the reports in the literature are very variable concerning the level of cyanide resistance (Hill, 1972; Ray and Cross, 1972). The characteristics of the cyanide-resistant oxidase in the mitochondria of the culture form are less well defined. It appears to exist in the mitochondria and work alongside a functional cytochrome oxidase (Hill, 1977); differs from the α-glycerol-3-phosphate oxidase by having a greater affinity for oxygen (K_m for O_2 is 0.1 μM) and is capable of oxidizing a variety of substrates including succinate and NADH. It differs from the system in higher plants, because, although resistant to cyanide and azide, it is sensitive to CO (Ray and Cross, 1972). The sensitivity of this oxidase to SHAM seems variable although Hill (1977) reports the existence of two cyanide-resistant oxidases, one sensitive and one resistant to inhibition by hydroxamates.

Consideration of the nature of the oxidase has centred around the observation that mitochondria from the culture form of trypanosomes contain, (in addition to cytochrome a_3), a CO-binding pigment, which has a major absorption band at 419 nm and looks very similar to cytochrome *o* which acts as a cyanide-resistant terminal oxidase in prokaryotic cells (Kusel and Storey, 1973). Kusel and Storey (1973) point out that other haemoproteins such as peroxidase will bind CO and produce a spectrum similar to cytochrome *o*.They emphasize that it is necessary to show that the action spectrum for the photo-reversal of CO inhibition has a peak at 420 nm before a functional cytochrome *o* can be identified. Kunsel and Storey (1973) showed that the CO-binding pigment in *Crithidia fasciculata* originally reported as being cytochrome *o* (Hill, 1972) played no role as the terminal oxidase. In contrast the CO-binding pigment with an absorption maximum at 420 nm in *T. brucei* and *T. mega* does appear to play a small role in bringing about cyanide-resistant respiration, because about 10% of the original rate of oxygen consumption can be recovered by using 420 nm light to reverse the CO-induced inhibition (Kronick and Hill, 1974). Thus the possibility that cytochrome *o*, an oxidase characteristic of prokaryotic cells, may play a role in eukaryotic cells as an alternative oxidase remains; however, more data are necessary to confirm this possibility.

The situation concerning the role of cytochrome *o* in mediating respiration in the trypanosomes is made additionally complicated by observations with a similar respiratory system found in *Ascaris lumbricoides* (Kikuchi *et al.*, 1959; Kikuchi and Ban, 1961; Cheah and Chance, 1970). This organism can catalyse cyanide-resistant respiration and contains large amounts of a CO-binding pigment which was initially thought to be cytochrome *o* (Cheah, 1972). However, spectral studies of Cheah and Chance (1970) have shown that the action spectrum for the reversal of CO inhibition does not confirm that cytochrome *o* plays an active role in the respiratory system. The role of this second CO-binding pigment in *Ascaris* is not fully understood although it is interesting to note that it can be oxidized by fumarate (Cheah, 1972). *Ascaris* cells contain an interesting system that can oxidize NADH by reducing fumarate to succinate, this system being able to synthesize ATP at the first coupling site of oxidative phosphorylation. Therefore it appears that the second CO-binding pigment may play a role in this anaerobic, cyanide-resistant respiration. Hayashi and Terada (1973) have also studied the cyanide-resistant respiratory system in *Ascaris* and have concluded that it may be mediated by a flavoprotein oxidase that produces hydrogen peroxide and the peroxide is reduced to water using cytochrome *c* peroxidase, this latter protein forming a CO derivative with a spectrum that could be confused with cytochrome *o*.

C. THE OXIDASE ASSOCIATED WITH OTHER MICRO-ORGANISMS AND HIGHER PLANTS

The situation in these tissues is simpler than that discussed for the trypanosomes. In all cases the oxidase is located in the mitochondria and frequently co-exists with cytochrome *c* oxidase. Little is really known about the nature of the oxidase but there is a large measure of agreement that the oxidase is similar in yeast, *Euglena*, *Neurospora* and higher plants. The development of our ideas concerning the nature of this cyanide-resistant oxidase is well described by Bendall and Bonner (1971), Henry and Nyns (1975) and Solomos (1977). It is therefore unnecessary to recount redudant theories and only the current ideas will feature in this review. The oxidase is capable of oxidizing all endogenous coenzymes and is completely insensitive to inhibition by cyanide, azide or carbon monoxide. The insensitivity to CO clearly distinguishes this oxidase from that in the culture form of the trypanosomes.

The cyanide-resistant respiration is also insensitive to antimycin A, proving that if the oxidase branches from the main respiratory chain it must occur before cytochrome *b*. Spectral study of the cytochromes in higher plant mitochondria show that cytochrome oxidase is the only CO-binding pigment present and there is no evidence that any cytochrome is involved in the operation of the cyanide-resistant oxidase. One of the problems encountered in studying the operation of this oxidase is that spectral analysis of the components involved is difficult and does not provide definite answers. The best attempt at spectral analysis is that by Storey (1976) in which it appears that in mitochondria treated with CO to prevent the turnover of cytochrome a_3, evidence could be obtained that the ubiquinone and a proportion of the flavin were oxidized by a SHAM-sensitive oxidase. This data has led to suggestions that a flavoprotein may be involved in mediating electron flux from the main pathway to the cyanide-resistant oxidase (Solomos, 1977). It seems unlikely that the terminal oxidase is a simple flavoprotein because the oxidase has a relatively low K_m for O_2 (10 μM) which is far too low for most flavoproteins (Solomos, 1977). The end product of the cyanide-resistant oxidase appears to be water (Huq and Palmer, 1978a; Rich and Bonner, 1978) rather than hydrogen peroxide which would be expected from flavoprotein oxidases (Bendall and Bonner, 1971).

There is increasing evidence that ubiquinone is involved in supplying electrons to the oxidase. The most convincing evidence comes from those studies in which the removal of endogenous quinone prevents cyanide-resistant oxygen uptake and re-incorporation of native quinone or quinone analogues reactivates the oxidase (Hanssens *et al.*, 1977; Huq and Palmer, 1978b). Rich and Moore (1976) have proposed a theoretical scheme based on the ubiquinone cycle which suggests that the cyanide-resistant oxidase directly oxidizes the ubiquinol. Rich and Bonner (1977) have even suggested that the alternative oxidase is simply a pool of rapidly auto-oxidizable quinone which can readily accept electrons from the main pool of ubiquinone associated with the succinic dehydrogenase. The main objection to this theory is that the end product of the auto-oxidation of quinones is normally accepted to be superoxide or peroxide (Boveris *et al.*, 1976). It is also clear that recent attempts to isolate the alternative oxidase (Huq and Palmer, 1978a; Rich, 1978) have succeeded in obtaining a protein fraction that can catalyse the oxidation of quinols. This suggests the presence of a terminal oxidase that is responsible for the oxidation of the quinol rather than direct autooxidation.

Another theory that has received much attention is the possibility that an iron-sulphur protein is closely associated with the cyanide-resistant oxidase. This theory has arisen because of the frequent observation that iron chelators such as orthophenanthroline, potassium thiocyanate and SHAM all inhibit the alternative oxidase (Bendall and Bonner, 1971). Palmer (1976) has pointed out that these chelators are not capable of extracting the iron from functional iron-sulphur proteins and has shown (Palmer, 1972) that the results obtained using thiocyanate are not consistent with the direct inhibition of the alternative oxidase by this compound. A systematic investigation of the iron-sulphur proteins of *Arum* mitochondria (Cammack and Palmer, 1977) failed to identify any unique iron-sulphur protein which could be attributed to the cyanide-resistant oxidase. The cyanide-resistant, SHAM-sensitive duroquinol oxidase isolated by Huq and Palmer (1978a) as a candidate for the oxidase does not contain any iron-sulphur protein. Therefore there is no experimental proof that iron-sulphur proteins play any direct role in mediation of electron flux through the cyanide-resistant oxidase. At present we have little precise information concerning the nature of the alternative oxidase except that it is dependent on the presence of ubiquinone. Two attempts have been made to isolate the oxidase, both from mitochondria of *Arum maculatum* (Huq and Palmer, 1978a; Rich, 1978). Huq and Palmer (1978a) have isolated a duroquinol oxidase resistant to inhibition by cyanide, which distinguishes it from normal polyphenol oxidases. The preparation is sensitive to SHAM which makes it a potential candidate for the cyanide-resistant oxidase, although this can only be finally proved by careful re-incorporation experiments. Unfortunately, although this approach is potentially valuable and is possibly the best method of solving the nature of the oxidase it has not yielded impressive results. The oxidase appears to be a protein that oxidizes low molecular weight quinols to form water. The preparation is characterized by a high catalase activity, which is completely prevented by cyanide, and water is always identified as the end product. The only possible redox components identified in the preparation are a flavoprotein and copper ions. The redox behaviour of these compounds is difficult to measure and their role in the redox process awaits clarification.

D. RELATIONSHIP BETWEEN THE CYANIDE-RESISTANT OXIDASE AND THE NORMAL RESPIRATORY CHAIN

The problem discussed in this section applies only to systems which have both a fully developed respiratory chain and a cyanide-resistant oxidase, and has only been extensively investigated in higher plants and *N. crassa*.

The first possibility that has been considered is that the oxidase is actually a modified component of the normal respiratory chain that can be auto-oxidized by oxygen. The major candidate for this role has been a component of the succinate dehydrogenase (Lyr and Schewe, 1975; Sharpless and Butow, 1970). However, this is difficult to accept because endogenous NADH is an excellent substrate to supply electrons to the cyanide-resistant oxidase. Studies by

Moore *et al.*, (1976) showed that the high potential iron-sulphur protein (centre S-3), together with a free radical of ubiquinone were closely related to the operation of the cyanide-resistant oxidase in higher plant tissue. Rich and Bonner (1977) argue that the S-3 centre has the thermodynamic properties to be a candidate for the oxidase. They were able to show however, that the S-3 centre could be removed by washing sub-mitochondrial particles at pH 9.9 and the treated preparation could still oxidize NADH in a cyanide-insensitive manner when the pH was returned to 7.0. Thus it seems unlikely that any component of the normal succinate dehydrogenase fulfils the role of the cyanide-resistant dehydrogenase.

The evidence currently favours the view that the cyanide-resistant oxidase is a redox component different from those normally attributed to the conventional respiratory chain. It is therefore necessary to decide whether the cyanide-resistant oxidase represents the terminal component of a branch from the conventional chain or whether it is the last member of a parallel redox chain. This is a very fundamental problem because the answer is central in ressolving issues of regulation and metabolic significance. Most reviewers of this subject (Henry and Nyns, 1975; Solomos, 1977) consider that the cyanide-resistant pathway is a branch of the normal respiratory chain, arising at the level of ubiquinone. There can be no doubt that this is frequently the case especially when the presence of the cyanide-resistant oxidase has been induced by growth in the presence of respiratory inhibitors such as antimycin A (Kawakita, 1971), or by specific mutation as in the *poky* mutants of *N. crassa* (Edwards, 1977) or suppression of mitochondrial protein biosynthesis by chloramphenicol (von Jagow and Klingenberg, 1972). Thus when the oxidase is induced in response to an impaired operation of the cytochrome a, a_3 system the experimental data favour the view that the oxidase acts as a branch from ubiquinone. The electrons appear to traverse the rotenone-sensitive components of the NADH dehydrogenase and produce ATP at the first site of oxidative phosphorylation before being diverted to the alternative oxidase (Slayman, 1977).

The situation may be different in higher plant mitochondria. In this tissue the cyanide-resistant oxidase is frequently found to be a constitutive enzyme, present through the life of the tissue and not being induced by any specific environmental factor. Plant mitochondria also contain a very much more complex NADH dehydrogenase system than the microorganisms (Palmer and Colman, 1974) and little attention has been paid to which NADH dehydrogenase feeds electrons to the alternative oxidase. It is generally believed that even in higher plant mitochondria electrons are usually supplied to the alternative oxidase primarily by the rotenone-sensitive NADH dehydrogenase. However, there are no reports, to my knowledge, that show that rotenone will cause an inhibition of respiration if added after cyanide or antimycin A. Thus the rotenone-resistant dehydrogenase, which by-passes the first site of oxidative phosphorylation, has sufficient capacity to cause full activity of the alternative oxidase. It is certain that if the energy charge (Bomsel and Pradet, 1968) is lowered by adding ADP and the function of cytochrome a_3 impaired by adding cyanide then electrons do pass through the rotenone-sensitive step and give rise to phosphorylation at site I (Solomos, 1977). It is important to consider whether this represents the normal pathway by which electrons reach the cyanide-resistant oxidase or whether it may be an artifact that becomes possible under these particular, *in vitro*, assay conditions. There is no real evidence to suggest that the *in vivo* energy charge of plant tissue is really very low or that there is any natural inhibitor to impair the cytochrome oxidase. Therefore, what can be demonstrated to happen in an oxygen electrode may not happen *in vivo*. One observation that questions a simple branched pathway is that in most plant mitochondria (with the exception of skunk cabbage and *Arum maculatum*, both of which produce heat as a result of the activity of the oxidase), the oxidation of external NADH can only be achieved by the cytochrome oxidase and exogenous NADH cannot supply electrons to the cyanide-resistant oxidase (Tomlinson and Moreland, 1975; Solomos, 1977; Huq and Palmer, 1978b). Since it is normally assumed that ubiquinone is involved in electron flux between exogenous NADH and oxygen it is difficult to interpret this data without assuming the existence of two pools of quinone, one specifically involved in donating electrons to cytochrome *c* and the other able to communicate with both cytochrome *c* and the alternative oxidase. There are reports in the literature that the quinone may not act as an homogenous pool (Huq and Palmer, 1978b; Storey, 1976). Therefore the presence of inhibitor-resistant NADH dehydrogenases and oxidases and multiple pools of ubiquinone make it possible to argue that, in plant tissue, the alternative oxidase may well be the terminal oxidase of a parallel and alternate respiratory chain. If this turns out to be the case there is strong evidence to show that both respiratory chains exist in the same mitochondrion. One factor favouring parallel chains is the observation by Cammack and Palmer (1973) that the induction of the cyanide-resistant oxidase in potato tuber tissue was accompanied by an equal increase in the activity of the piericidin A-resistant NADH dehydrogenase.

One of the points of major interest concerning the relationship of the alternative oxidase with the conventional chain is how it influences the efficiency of oxidative phosphorylation. There is no real doubt that there is no ATP synthesis coupled to the oxidation of ubiquinone by the cyanide-resistant oxidase (Passam and Palmer, 1972; Moore, 1977). Thus the oxidation of succinate by the alternative oxidase never leads to ATP synthesis while the oxidation of endogenous NADH can lead to one mole of ATP production if the system is branched or no ATP if parallel chains exist.

E. CONTROL OF ELECTRON FLUX THROUGH THE CYANIDE-RESISTANT OXIDASE

In the absence of detailed knowledge concerning the components involved in the pathway or the rate limiting step, it is difficult to reach definite conclusions on the precise control mechanisms. The only information available comes from studies on higher plant mitochondria where the problem is most complex because both cytochrome oxidase and the alternative oxidase co-exist in the same organelle and neither is necessarily rate-limiting. The studies of Chance and Hackett (1959) showed that in skunk cabbage mitochondria supplied with plentiful ADP (i.e. State 3, Chance and Williams, 1955) the efficiency of ATP synthesis was high and the cytochrome oxidase mediated most of the oxidation. When the ADP had been converted to ATP (State 4) the rate of respiration continued in the absence of ATP synthesis. It was clear that under these conditions electron transport had been diverted via the cyanide-resistant, non-phosphorylating oxidase. Studies of Schonbaum *et al.* (1971) confirmed this conclusion when they showed that the addition of hydroxamates markedly improved the respiratory control ratio (i.e. rate in State 3 ÷ rate in State 4) which occurred because the hydroxamate-sensitive pathway played a greater role under State 4 conditions than under State 3 conditions.

Bahr and Bonner (1973a, 1973b) carried out a detailed investigation into the possible methods of regulation of the two oxidase systems and reached the conclusion that priority was given to supplying electrons to the cytochrome oxidase and when this demand was satisfied the excess electrons were supplied to the alternative oxidase. They suggested that regulation of this type could be achieved by the redox poise of the component at the branch point between the normal chain and the alternative oxidase. If electron flux through the cytochrome oxidase is impaired this component will become very reduced and capable of donating electrons to the alternative oxidase. This scheme adequately explains the regulation of a branched oxidase providing it is accepted that there is a natural system for impairing electron flux through the cytochrome oxidase. However, the evidence that the energy charge of an intact cell can rise sufficiently high to impose respiratory control is lacking and there are grounds to question whether control mechanisms based on attaining State 4 *in vivo* are metabolically meaningful. The control mechanisms suggested by Bahr and Bonner (1973a, 1973b) would not adequately explain regulation if the systems were organized as parallel chains.

In micro-organisms such as *Euglena* (Sharpless and Butow, 1970) or *Moniliella tomentosa* (Vanderleyden *et al.*, 1979) the cyanide-resistant oxidase is markedly stimulated by AMP and this could be a potential control mechanism. AMP has no effect on the cyanide-resistant oxidase in *Arum* mitochondria (Palmer, unpublished data) and this represents a major difference between the oxidase in microorganisms and in higher plants.

F. METABOLIC SIGNIFICANCE OF CYANIDE-RESISTANT RESPIRATION

There seems to be a good case for arguing that the metabolic importance of the alternative oxidase is significantly different in microorganisms, where it frequently arises in response to the prevention of the proper function of cytochrome oxidase, from that in higher plants where it often co-exists with a fully functional cytochrome a_3.

The role of the oxidase in microorganisms seems almost certainly to provide a means for the re-oxidation of coenzymes primarily to provide ATP for cellular processes. When the cyanide-resistant oxidase mediates electron transport the synthesis of ATP is less efficient and occurs at the substrate level and at the first site of oxidative phosphorylation.

The role of the oxidase in plant tissue, where the oxidase is found in conjunction with a fully functional cytochrome oxidase that has more capacity than is needed to mediate all cellular respiration, is less apparent. It seems unlikely that its major role is energy production since cytochrome oxidase would be the preferred oxidase. Therefore the only viable alternative is to suggest that in plant tissue the role of the alternative oxidase is to oxidize and adjust the redox poise of the coenzymes without the synthesis of ATP. At first sight this would appear to be an unreasonable proposal. However, it is possible to imagine that the energy charge of a leaf cell could be kept high by the process of photosynthesis while the continual supply of carbon skeletons produced by the activity of the Krebs cycle is necessary for continued biosynthesis. Under these conditions it is necessary to reoxidize the NADH to maintain the continued operation of the Krebs cycle. In non-photosynthetic tissue, which often contains the alternative oxidase, the argument is more difficult to sustain. However, if there is a high rate of carbon metabolism the rate of substrate level phosphorylation may be sufficient to maintain the energy charge. If the role of the alternative oxidase in higher plant tissue is to modulate the redox state of the pyridine nucleotides independently of the energy charge of the adenylate nucleotides then it would be preferable to by-pass all three sites of oxidative phosphorylation as would be expected if both oxidases represented the terminal components of parallel respiratory chains.

REFERENCES

Bahr, J.T. and Bonner, W.D. (1973a). *J. Biol. Chem.* 248, 3441-3445.

Bahr, J.T. and Bonner, W.D. (1973b). *J. Biol. Chem.* 248, 3446-3450.

Bendall, D.S. and Bonner, W.D. (1971). *Plant Physiol.* 47, 236-245.

Bomsel, J-L. and Pradet, A. (1968). *Biochim. Biophys. Acta* 162, 230-242.

Boveris, A., Cadenas, E. and Stoppani, A.O.M. (1976). *Biochem. J.* 156, 435-444.

Bowman, I.B.R. and Flynn, I.W. (1976). *In* "Biology of the Kinetoplastida" (W.H.R. Lumsden and D.A. Evans, eds.) Vol. 1, pp. 435-476. Academic Press, London.

Cammack, R. and Palmer, J.M. (1973). *Ann. N.Y. Acad. Sci.* 222, 816-823.

Cammack, R. and Palmer, J.M. (1977). *Biochem. J.* 166, 347-355.

Chance, B. and Hackett, D.P. (1959). *Plant Physiol.* 34, 33-49.

Chance, B. and Williams, G.R. (1955). *J. Biol. Chem.* 217, 383-393.

Cheah, K.S. (1972). *In* "Comparative Biochemistry of Parasites" (H.van den Bossche, ed.) pp.417-432. Academic Press, New York.

Cheah, K.S. and Chance, B. (1970). *Biochim. Biophys. Acta* 223, 55-60.

Edwards, D.L. (1977). *In* "Functions of Alternative Terminal Oxidases" (H. Degn, D. Lloyd and G.C. Hill, eds) pp. 21-29. Pergamon Press, Oxford.

Hanssens, L., Verachtert, H. and van Jagow, G. (1977). *In* "Functions of Alternative Terminal Oxidases" (H. Degn, D. Lloyd, and G.C. Hill, eds) pp. 47-53. Pergamon Press, Oxford.

Hayashi, E. and Terada, M. (1973). *J. Parasitology (Japan)* 22, 1-22.

Henry, M.-F. and Nyns, E.J. (1975). *Sub-Cell. Biochem.* 4, 1-65.

Hill, G.C. (1972). *In* "Comparative Biochemistry of Parasites" (H. van den Bossche, ed.) pp. 395-416. Academic Press, New York.

Hill, G.C. (1976). *In* "Biochemistry of Parasites and Host-Parasite Relationships" (H. van den Bossche, ed.) pp. 31-50. North Holland Publ. Co., Amsterdam.

Hill, G.C. (1977). *In* "Functions of Alternative Terminal Oxidases" (H. Degn, D. Lloyd and G.C. Hill, eds) pp. 67-77. Pergamon Press, Oxford.

Huq, S. and Palmer, J.M. (1978a). *FEBS Lett.* 95, 217-220.

Huq, S. and Palmer, J.M. (1978b). *In* "Plant Mitochondria" (G. Ducet and C. Lance, eds) pp. 225-232. Elsevier/North Holland Biomedical Press, Amsterdam.

Kawakita, M. (1971). *J. Biochem. Tokyo* 69, 35-42.

Kikuchi, G. and Ban, S. (1961). *Biochim. Biophys. Acta* 51, 387-389.

Kikuchi, G., Ramirez, J. and Guzman Barron, E.S. (1959). *Biochim. Biophys. Acta* 36, 335-342.

Kronick, P. and Hill, G.C. (1974). *Biochim. Biophys. Acta* 368, 173-180.

Kusel, J.P. and Storey, B.T. (1973). *Biochim. Biophys. Acta* 314, 164-177.

Lambers, H. and van de Dijk, S.J. (1979). *Physiol. Plant.* 45, 235-239

Lyr, H. and Schewe, T. (1975). *Acta biol. med. germ.* 34, 1631-1641.

Moore, A.L. (1977). *In* "Functions of Alternative Terminal Oxidases" (H. Degn, D. Lloyd and G.C. Hill, eds) pp.141-148. Pergamon Press, Oxford.

Moore, A.L., Rich, P.R., Bonner, W.D. and Ingledew, W.J. (1976). *Biochem. Biophys. Res. Commun.* 72, 1099-1107.

Opperdoes, F.R. and Borst, P. (1976). *In* "Biochemistry of Parasites and Host-Parasite Relationships" (H. van den Bossche, ed.) pp.509-517. North Holland Publishing Co., Amsterdam.

Palmer, J.M. (1972). *Phytochemistry* 11, 2957-2961.

Palmer, J.M. (1976). *Ann. Rev. Plant Physiol.* 27, 133-157.

Palmer, J.M. and Coleman, J.O.D. (1974). *In* "Horizons in Biochemistry and Biophysics" (E. Quagliariello, F. Palmieri and T. P. Singer, eds). Vol. 1, pp. 220-260. Addison-Wesley, Massachussets.

Parrish, D.J. and Leopold, A.C. (1978). *Plant Physiol.* 62, 470-472.

Passam, H.C. and Palmer, J.M. (1972). *J. Exp. Bot.* 23, 366-374.

Ray, S.K. and Cross, G.A.M. (1972). *Nature New Biol.* 237, 174-175.

Rich, P.R. (1978). *FEBS Lett.* 96, 252-256.

Rich, P.R. and Bonner, W.D. (1977). *In* "Functions of Alternative Terminal Oxidases" (H. Degn, D. Lloyd and G.C. Hill, eds) pp.149-158. Pergamon Press, Oxford.

Rich, P.R. and Bonner, W.D. (1978). *Arch. Biochem. Biophys.* 188, 206-213.

Rich, P.R. and Moore, A.L. (1976). *FEBS Lett.* 65, 339-344.

Rich, P.R., Wiegand, N.K., Blum, H., Moore, A.L. and Bonner, W.D. (1978). *Biochim. Biophys. Acta* 525, 325-337.

Schonbaum, G.R. (1973). *J. Biol. Chem.* 248, 502-511.

Schonbaum, G.R., Bonner, W.D., Storey, B.T. and Bahr, J.T. (1971). *Plant Physiol.* 47, 124-128.

Sharpless, T.K. and Butow, R.A. (1970). *J. Biol. Chem.* 245, 58-70.

Slayman, C.W. (1977). *In* "Functions of Alternative Terminal Oxidases" (H. Degn, D. Lloyd, and G.C. Hill, eds) pp. 159-168. Pergamon Press, Oxford.

Solomos, T. (1977). *Ann. Rev. Plant Physiol.* 28, 279-297.

Storey, B.T. (1976). *Plant Physiol.* 58, 521-525.

Tomlinson, P.F. and Moreland, D.E. (1975). *Plant Physiol.* 55, 365-369.

Vanderleyden, J., Kurth, J. and Verachtert, H. (1979). *Biochem. J.* 182, 437-443.

Von Jagow, G. and Klingenberg, M. (1972). *FEBS Lett.* 24, 278-282.

ISOLATION AND CHARACTERIZATION OF THE CYANIDE-RESISTANT OXIDASE FROM THE SPADICES OF *ARUM MACULATUM*

J. M. PALMER and S. HUQ[†]

Department of Botany, Imperial College, London
[†]*Present address: Department of Botany, University of Dacca, Dacca, Bangladesh*

I. INTRODUCTION

The nature of the cyanide resistant oxidase associated with plant respiration has been the subject of much speculation for many years. The early studies of James and Beevers (1950) using slices of the spadix of *Arum maculatum* showed that the oxidase appeared to have a rather high K_m for oxygen and led them to propose that it may be a flavoprotein. Modern measurements now suggest that the K_m for oxygen is much lower than that estimated by James and Beevers (Solomos, 1977) whose measurements may have been complicated by problems associated with the diffusion of oxygen into the slices of tissue. Later work by James and Elliot (1955) and Hackett (1957) showed that the cyanide resistant respiration was located in the mitochondrion and subsequent studies into the nature of this oxidase have concentrated on this subcellular organelle. Chance and Hackett (1959) working with mitochondria isolated from the spadix of skunk cabbage, *Sympolocarpus foetidus*, found that cytochrome *c* was not completely reduced in the presence of cyanide and suggested that cyanide resistant oxidation was caused by the incomplete inhibition of cytochrome oxidase by cyanide. This theory was discounted by the observation that, in skunk cabbage mitochondria, the oxidation of ascorbate plus 2,3,5,6-tetramethyldiaminobenzene (DAD), which can only supply electrons to cytochrome oxidase, is almost completely inhibited by cyanide, whilst the oxidation of succinate remains unaffected by addition of this inhibitor (Bendall and Bonner, 1971). Much evidence was also obtained to indicate that at least one of the cytochrome *b* components may play a role in mediating cyanide resistant oxidation (Bendall and Hill, 1956; Chance and Hackett, 1969; Lundegårdh, 1960). All these authors showed that cytochrome *b* remained partially oxidised in the presence of cyanide. However, more recent studies (Storey and Bahr, 1969; Bendall and Bonner, 1971) showed that while the *b* type cytochromes remained oxidized in the presence of cyanide they became completely reduced in the presence of antimycin A, which inhibits electron flux between cytochromes *b* and *c* but does not inhibit cyanide-resistant oxidation. Thus cytochrome *b* does not appear to have a role in mediating electron flow to the cyanide-resistant oxidase. Erecinska and Storey (1970) obtained spectral evidence that flavoproteins may be involved in the process of cyanide-resistant oxidation. Storey (1976) showed that about 20% of the total flavoprotein may be involved in this pathway and determined the midpoint redox potential of this component to be +20 mV.

Non-haem iron-sulphur proteins have been implicated in the cyanide-resistant pathway, based on the observation that hydroxamic acids (Schonbaum *et al.*, 1971) and other chelators (Bonner *et al.*, 1967) are capable of inhibiting the cyanide-resistant pathway. Lyr and Schewe (1975) suggested that the high potential iron-sulphur centre, S-3, associated with succinic dehydrogenase may itself be auto-oxidized and thus act as the oxidase. Rich and Bonner (1978) showed that alkaline pH treatment removed the S-3 component but did not affect the cyanide-resistant oxidation of NADH. Thus S-3 does not appear to be the oxidase. Careful studies using electron paramagnetic resonance techniques (Cammack and Palmer, 1977) found no evidence for a unique iron-sulphur centre that could be attributed to the oxidase.

While evidence has been accumulating to show that the cytochromes are not involved in mediating electron flux to the cyanide-resistant oxidase there has been increasing evidence that a proportion of the ubiquinone pool does appear to play an active role. Storey (1976) used spectrophotometric techniques to show that ubiquinone remained oxidized in the presence of carbon monoxide and became reduced in the presence of hydroxamic acids. Moore *et al.* (1976) showed the presence of a split electron paramagnetic resonance signal centred around g = 1.98 which they attributed to an interaction between a high potential iron-sulphur centre, probably S-3 of succinic dehydrogenase, and two semiquinones which appeared to be related to the operation of the cyanide-resistant pathway. Rich and Moore (1976) proposed on theoretical grounds that ubiquinone represents one of the components close to the cyanide-resistant oxidase. Huq and Palmer (1978) showed that extraction of the ubiquinone resulted in an inhibition of cyanide-resistant oxidation. Rich and Bonner (1977) proposed that the cyanide-resistant oxidation may be caused by the auto-oxidation of one of the quinone components in the mitochondrial membrane system. However, this seems unlikely because the product of auto-oxidation of quinones is accepted to be either superoxide or peroxide while the end product of cyanide-resistant respiration appears to be water (Huq and Palmer, 1978a; Rich and Bonner, 1978). Therefore it is to be anticipated that some form of quinol oxidase may be present to mediate cyanide-resistant oxidation. This paper describes data obtained from experiments designed to solubilise, purify and characterise a cyanide-resistant, hydroxamic acid sensitive oxidase from mitochondria isolated from the spadix of *Arum maculatum* which is known to contain very high levels of the cyanide-resistant oxidase.

II. MATERIALS AND METHODS

A. MATERIALS

Arum maculatum inflorescences were collected from locations in north Kent. Salicylhydroxamic acid was obtained from Aldrich Chemical Co. Ltd., duroquinol from K and K Chemicals Inc. and DE23 anion exchange cellulose from Whatman Ltd. Lubrol was a generous gift from ICI Ltd.

B. MITOCHONDRIAL PREPARATION

The sterile portion of the spadix was removed and the mitochondria isolated using the method described by Cammack and Palmer (1977). After preparation they were stored at 77° K before extraction of the oxidase.

C. ISOLATION OF THE OXIDASE

The mitochondrial preparations contained approximately 40 mg protein/ml and were diluted to 10 mg protein/ml using 10 mM phosphate buffer (pH 7.5). A typical preparation would use 800 mg of protein. After dilution a solution of 10% (w/v) lubrol would be added such that the final concentration of lubrol was 0.5% (w/v) and the mixture stirred for 10 min. The solution was then centrifuged at 100,000 *g* for 1 hour. The insoluble material formed a pellet and the supernatant had a clearly distinguishable denser layer just above the pellet which comprised about 20% of the total volume. This lower layer was removed with a Pasteur pipette and discarded along with the pellet. The remainder of the supernatant was then applied to a column (4 cm^2 x 30 cm) of DE23 cellulose pre-equilibrated with 10 mM potassium phosphate buffer (pH 7.5) containing 0.5% lubrol. The detergent was present in all the subsequent buffers used in conjunction with the column. Once the oxidase had been bound to the DE23 cellulose the column was washed with 10 mM potassium phosphate (pH 7.5) until no further protein was eluted. The oxidase was then removed using 100 mM potassium phosphate (pH 7.5). All the oxidase could be removed in 60 ml of buffer. This preparation was then diluted to 600 ml by adding distilled water and applied to a second DE23 column. After extensive washing with 10 mM potassium phosphate buffer the oxidase was eluted using 200 ml of phosphate gradient between 10-100 mM. The oxidase was eluted in a 50 ml volume near the centre of the gradient. All operations were carried out at 4°C.

D. OXYGEN UPTAKE

The uptake of oxygen was measured polarographically using a Clark-type oxygen electrode. The reaction medium was 0.3 M sucrose, 10 mM N-((trishydroxymethyl)methyl)-2-aminoethanesulphonic acid, 5 mM KH_2PO_4 and 5 mM $MgCl_2$ at pH 7.2. *Other methods* were described by Huq and Palmer (1978, 1978b).

III. RESULTS

When separating complexes of the respiratory chain it is necessary to have suitable assay systems available to determine the success of the procedures. Therefore, before isolating the cyanide-resistant oxidase a suitable electron donor to determine its activity must be available. Since the extraction of ubiquinone had been found to inhibit the cyanide-resistant oxidase (Huq and Palmer, 1978) it was decided to test short chain quinols as potential electron donors. Duroquinol (tetramethylquinol) was found to be oxidized as rapidly as any natural substrate and in *Arum* mitochondria the oxygen uptake was resistant to cyanide and antimycin A while it was sensitive to benzhydroxamates. Data presented in Table I compare the rate of oxidation of NADH and duroquinol by lyophilized *Arum* mitochondria before and after the extraction of the natural quinone using pentane. It is apparent that both NADH and duroquinol were oxidized at the same velocity before quinone depletion; however, the removal of quinone prevented

Table I Oxidation of NADH and durohydroquinol by lyophilized (control) and quinone-depleted, lyophilized *Arum* mitochondria. (Rates are nmoles O_2 used per min per mg lyophilized mitochondria.)

	Control		Quinone-depleted	
	Control	+ 1 mM SHAM	Control	+ 1 mM SHAM
NADH	112	18	10	10
Durohydroquinone	112	10	115	6

the oxidation of NADH but had no significant effect on the rate of oxidation of duroquinol. In all cases the rate of oxidation was sensitive to inhibition by 1 mM salicylhydroxamic acid. Thus it can be concluded that duroquinol can donate electrons directly to the cyanide-resistant oxidase without involving the pool of natural quinone.

All quinols, especially those with short isoprenoid chains and a reasonable degree of water solubility are prone to auto-oxidation. However, the rate of duroquinol oxidase was found to be directly proportional to the concentration of mitochondria added and the data presented in Fig. 1 show that the relationship between the rate of oxygen uptake and duroquinol concentration was that predicted from Michaelis Menton kinetics, confirming that the oxidation of the duroquinol was mediated by an enzymic process and was not occurring as the result of simple non-catalysed auto-oxidation. Other experiments showed that duroquinol could also act as a donor to the cyanide-resistant oxidase in mitochondria extracted from cassava (*Manihot esculenta*) and sweet potato *(Ipomea batatas)*.

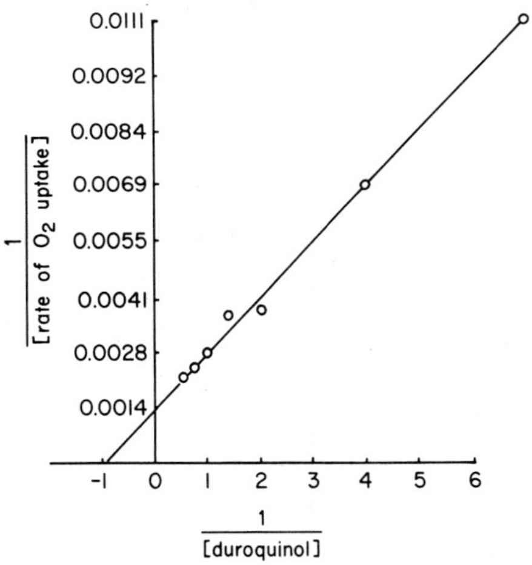

Fig. 1 Lineweaver-Burke plot of duroquinol concentration against rate of oxygen uptake.
The rate of oxygen uptake was measured using an oxygen electrode as described in the methods. The duroquinol concentration used in the calculations was expressed as mmol/litre. The rate of oxygen uptake was expressed as nmol O_2/min/mg protein. The graph shows the K_m for duroquinol is 1 mM and the V_m obtained was 720 nmol O_2/min/mg protein.

Attempts were then undertaken to solubilise from the *Arum* mitochondria a duroquinol oxidase which would be a potential candidate for the cyanide-resistant oxidase. Treatment with a variety of detergents was tested with respect to their ability to remove a duroquinol oxidase from the membrane and separate it from the cytochrome oxidase, which was assayed using a mixture of ascorbate and tetramethylphenelenediamine as an electron donor. The non-ionic detergent, Lubrol, was found to be the most effective in this process, resulting in a high degree of solubilisation of the duroquinol oxidase whilst leaving most of the cytochrome oxidase in the membrane pellet or the lower layer of the supernatant. The *Arum* mitochondria were prepared, as described in the methods, in a solution containing 40 mg protein per ml; this was diluted to 10 mg protein per ml with 10 mM potassium phosphate buffer, pH 7.5, then lubrol was added to a final concentration of 0.5% (w/v) and the mixture stirred for 10 minutes at 4°C. The solubilised preparation was then subjected to centrifugation at 100,000 *g* for one hour and the resulting pellet and dense layer of the supernatant was discarded (see materials and methods), since it was found to contain the bulk of the cytochrome oxidase as well as some of the cyanide-resistant oxidase. The upper layer of the supernatant contained most of the benzhydroxamate sensitive oxidase and was retained for further purification, which was achieved by ion exchange chromatography on DE23 cellulose as described in the section on materials and methods.

The results obtained are presented in Table II and represent the percentage obtained in each fraction using the level characteristic of intact mitochondria as 100%. The specific activity of the salicylhydroxamic acid sensitive duroquinol oxidase, which is related to the degree of purity, was found to be equivalent to 303 nmoles of oxygen used per min per mg protein in the original mitochondria and 542 nmoles of oxygen used per min per mg protein in the eluate from the second DE23 column. Further attempts to purify the preparation were unsuccessful and resulted in a decrease in the specific activity of the oxidase. Therefore attempts were made to characterise the components present in the preparation. Polyacrylamide electrophoresis in the presence of sodium dodecyl sulphate showed the presence of at least 5 main polypeptides together with several lesser contaminants (over 140 bands can be recognized in the original mitochondria). It is therefore not possible to assume that the oxidase has been completely purified. Optical analysis shows the presence of a chromophore with three absorption peaks at 421, 447 and 477 nm, respectively. The addition of sodium dithionite results in little alteration of the spectra although a small amount of bleaching occurs at 421 nm, which would be consistent with the presence of a flavoprotein. Fluorescence spectrophotometry shows (Fig. 2) that in freshly prepared and highly active oxidase there is virtually no fluorescence. However, the enzyme is rapidly denatured at temperatures above 5°C and this loss of activity is closely correlated to the development of a powerful fluorescence at 520 nm, indicating the presence of a flavoprotein which, in the active preparations has its fluoresc-

Table II Fractionation of *Arum* mitochondria and purification of the cyanide-resistant oxidase. (Figures are % of values originally present in the untreated mitochondria).

	Cyanide-resistant oxidase	Cytochrome oxidase	Cytochrome *b*
Mitochondria	100	100	100
Supernatant after lubrol (0.5% w/v)	65	1.5	14
After first treatment with DEAE	50	0	0.1
After second treatment with DEAE	40	0	0

ence strongly quenched.

The purified oxidase was subjected to electron spin resonance analysis which failed to show the presence of any detectable signal at $g = 1.94$, $g = 2.0$ or $g = 6.0$, indicating that it did not contain any large amounts of iron-sulphur protein, ubiquinone or manganese. Careful analysis for metals using neutron activation or plasma induced atomic emission (Table III) showed the presence of detectable quantities of copper which, by the use of suitable control treatments, seems to be present in association with the oxidase protein. With the amounts of oxidase available for analysis strictly limited, the levels of metal remained close to the minimum level detectable and further data are needed before the role of copper in this oxidase can be confirmed. If all the main bands detected in the SDS-polyacrylamide electrophoresis are subunits of the oxidase then there is only sufficient copper for 1 mole of metal per mole of enzyme, but if several of the polypeptides are finally recognised as contaminants then there may be more than one mole of metal per mole of enzyme.

IV. DISCUSSION

A method of isolating the cyanide-resistant oxidase from *Arum maculatum* spadix mitochondria has been developed. The final preparation contained approximately 40% of the cyanide-resistant, benzhydroxamate sensitive, duroquinol oxidase present in the intact mitochondria, with an increase of 18-fold in specific activity. The enzyme was stable if stored at 77° K but it was unstable at temperature above 5°C. Half the activity was lost if the preparation was stored at 20°C for one hour.

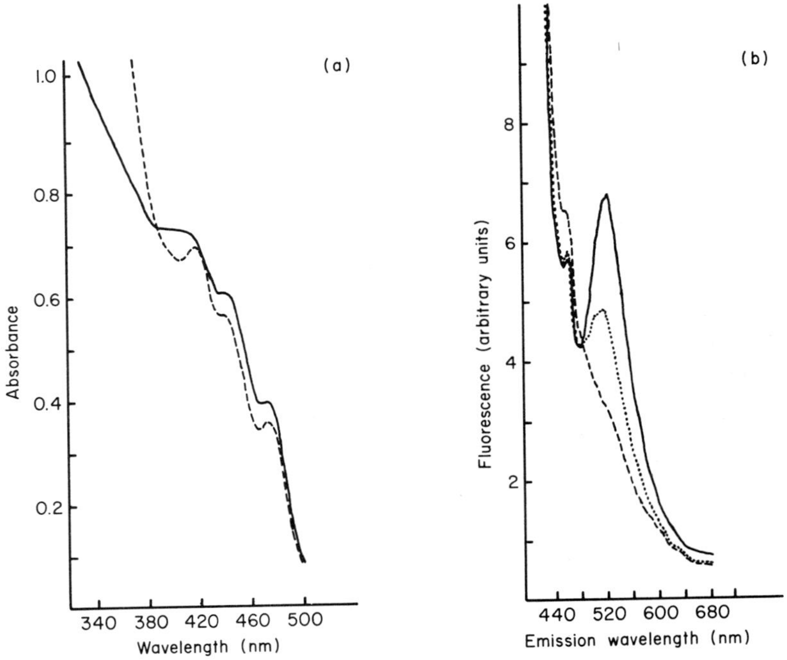

Fig. 2 The spectra shown in (a) are those of the purified oxidase as prepared (solid line) and plus sodium dithionite (broken line). Both spectra were run against a reagent blank. The spectra shown in (b) are the fluorescence emission spectra. The activation was achieved at 400 nm. The dotted line was the spectrum obtained with freshly prepared oxidase, the solid line was the fluorescence present after 2 hours at 20°C and the broken line was the spectrum obtained when dithionite was added after 2 hours at 20°C.

Table III Metal content of the purified oxidase.

Technique	Metal (µg/mg protein)		
	Cu	Zn	Mn
Plasma atomic emission	0.22	0.00	-
Neutron activation	0.37	-	0.001

The evidence presented in this paper favours the view that the oxidation of the duroquinol is mediated by a catalyst rather than being the result of non-catalyzed auto-oxidation of the water soluble quinol. This view was reinforced by the observation that water, rather than hydrogen peroxide which is the product of auto-oxidation, was the product of the oxidase reaction.

Efforts to establish the redox active prosthetic groups within the oxidase have been only partially successful. The most highly purified preparation contains a flavoprotein with an extensively quenched fluorescence spectrum and small amounts of copper. It has not been possible to establish whether either of these two types of redox centres are involved in the operation of the oxidase. However, when dealing with an oxidase that forms water, where four electrons have to be supplied to oxygen before the product is released, it is desirable to have a protein with more than one redox centre. The experimental observation that the fluorescence of the flavin is quenched and the copper has no detectable electron paramagnetic resonance spectrum (Huq and Palmer, 1978b) makes it very difficult to establish whether either of these components undergoes a redox change during the oxidase reaction.

ACKNOWLEDGEMENTS

This study was supported by grants from the Tropical Products Institute, the Science Research Council, The Royal Society and the Central Research Fund, University of London. S. Huq acknowledges the receipt of a studentship from the Tropical Products Institute.

REFERENCES

Bendall, D.S. and Bonner, W.D. (1971). *Plant Physiol.* 47, 236-245.
Bendall, D.S. and Hill, R. (1956). *New Phytol.* 55, 206-212.
Bonner, W.D., Bendall, D.S. and Plesnicar, M. (1967). *Proc. Fedn. Am. Socs.* 26, 731.
Cammack, R. and Palmer, J.M. (1977). *Biochem. J.* 166, 347-355.
Chance, B. and Hackett, D.P. (1959). *Plant Physiol.* 34, 33-49.
Erecinska, M. and Storey, B.T. (1970). *Plant Physiol.* 46, 618-624.
Hackett, D.P. (1957). *J. Exp. Bot.* 8, 27-32.
Huq, S. and Palmer, J.M. (1978). *In* "Plant Mitochondria" (G. Ducet and C. Lance, eds) pp. 225-232. Elsevier/North Holland Biomedical Press, Amsterdam.
Huq, S. and Palmer, J.M. (1978a). *Plant Sci. Lett.* 11, 351-358.
Huq, S. and Palmer, J.M. (1978b). *FEBS Lett.* 95, 217-220.
James, W.O. and Beevers, H. (1950). *New Phytol.* 49, 353-374.
James, W.O. and Elliot, D.C. (1955). *Nature,* 175, 89.
Lundegårdh, H. (1960). *In* "Encyclopedia of Plant Physiology" (W. Rhuland, ed.) pp. 311-364. Springer-Verlag, Berlin.
Lyr, H. and Schewe, T. (1975). *Acta biol. med. germ.* 34, 1631-1641.
Moore, A.L., Rich, P.R. and Bonner, W.D. (1976). *Biochem. Biophys. Res. Commun.* 72, 1099-1107.

Rich, P.R. and Bonner, W.D. (1977). *In* "Functions of Alternative Terminal Oxidases" (H. Degn, D. Lloyd and G.C. Hill, eds) pp. 149-158 Pergamon Press, Oxford.
Rich, P.R. and Bonner, W.D. (1978). *Biochim. Biophys. Acta* 501, 381-395.
Rich, P.R. and Moore, A.L. (1976). *FEBS Lett.* 65, 339-344.
Schonbaum, G.R., Bonner, W.D., Storey, B.T. and Bahr, J.T. (1971). *Plant Physiol.* 47, 124-128.
Solomos, T. (1977). *Ann. Rev. Plant Physiol.* 28, 279-297.
Storey, B.T. (1976). *Plant Physiol.* 58, 521-525.
Storey, B.T. and Bahr, J.T. (1969). *Plant Physiol.* 44, 115-125.

METHODS OF LIBERATING AND ESTIMATING HYDROCYANIC ACID FROM CYANOGENIC PLANT MATERIAL

ADOLF NAHRSTEDT*, NORBERT ERB**
and HANS-DIETMAR ZINSMEISTER**

**Institut für Pharmazeutische Biologie der Technischen Universität, D-3300 Braunschweig, F.R.G.*

***Fachbereich Botanik der Universität des Saarlandes, D-6600 Saarbrücken, F.R.G.*

I. INTRODUCTION

As a result of the intensive interest by workers in the fields of waste chemistry, food chemistry, toxicology, drug chemistry, phytochemistry, and biochemistry there exist many procedures for quantitative estimation of prussic acid. In every case quantitative estimation needs three steps:

(1) liberation of hydrocyanic acid from plant material or other objects
(2) isolation and concentration of the liberated HCN into a trap in order to remove interfering substances
(3) estimation of the isolated acid normally using the chemical reactivity or physical behaviour of the cyanide ion.

Since the concentration of free prussic acid or of compounds from which cyanide is liberated are normally low in biological materials phytochemists and biochemists are interested in methods that allow concentration and determination of low levels of cyanide. In the following overview useful methods but also problems of liberation, isolation and estimation of cyanide from biological material are summarised especially regarding cyanogenic glycosides. Special summaries on these problems are given by Seifert (1955) and Zitnak (1973), the latter discussing intensively the many procedures for liberation and isolation of free or bound HCN. Therefore, the newer literature of phytochemical interest is mainly considered. Additionally, our own experiences, particularly regarding low content plant material, are dealt with.

II. LIBERATION OF HCN FROM CYANOGENIC GLYCOSIDES

The preparation of the plant material in order to avoid loss of cyanogenic compounds either by enzymic degradation or due to the instability of some of them is discussed by Nahrstedt (this volume).

The most deficient step of the quantitative analysis of hydrocyanic acid is the liberation and isolation of hydrocyanic acid bound in cyanogenic glycosides of plant materials or foodstuffs. For estimation of hydrocyanic acid it is very important that the plant material is ground. The finer the particles the better the yield of hydrocyanic acid (Rosenthaler, 1932; Lüdtke, 1952). Generally there are few basic methods for liberating prussic acid from cyanogenic glycosides. These are (i) enzymatic hydrolysis, (ii) acid hydrolysis, and (iii) combined enzymatic and acid hydrolysis. In the case of estimation of free HCN from biological material the procedure starts with its isolation as described under Section III.

A. ENZYMATIC HYDROLYSIS

Enzymatic hydrolysis can be done in a so-called autoenzymatic version by the action of the plants own β-glucosidases (e.g. Lüdtke, 1952; Vetter and Haraszti, 1977; Hunt and Taylor, 1976; Schröder 1977) or by adding external β-glucosidase preparations (Akazawa *et al.*, 1960; Nahrstedt, 1970; Egli, 1977). In the use of enzymatic methods, some conditions, such as specific temperature and pH-values, have generally to be fulfilled (Seifert, 1955; Butler *et al.*, 1965; Hanssen and Sturm, 1967; Haisman and Knight, 1967; Hösel and Nahrstedt, 1975; Cooke *et al.*, 1978; see also W. Hösel, this volume). The yield of hydrocyanic acid can be strikingly diminished by blocking the β-glucosidases by heavy metals (Larnen, 1960) or pesticides such as captan or lindane (Wegler, 1970). Thus, when caryopses of *Zea mays* had been treated by the pesticide captan, HCN was detected only when the pesticide has been removed by repeated washing with ethanol (Zinsmeister *et al.*, 1980). Blocking by heavy metals can be prevented by ethylenediaminetetraacetic acid (EDTA) (Nahrstedt, 1970, 1971).

The use of the autoenzymatic method is restricted, since the activity of suitable β-glucosidases varies strikingly from plant to plant and there are some species which do not contain enzymes capable of cleaving cyanogenic glycosides (Dilleman, 1958; Zechner, 1966; Jones, 1972) so the addition of these enzymes to plant homogenates is preferable. Zitnak (1973) recommends a two step hydrolysis with endogenous and added enzymes. Using plant material with unknown cyanogenic glycosides it is necessary to test different β-glucosidase preparations for their influence on the yield of hydrocyanic acid (e.g. Secor *et al.*, 1977). Although most naturally occurring cyanogenic glycosides are cleaved by emulsion there are some which cannot be degraded completely by this enzyme (see also the contribution of Nahrstedt, this volume, IV D, and literature cited there for crude preparations of different β-glucosidases). The fermentation time is dependent on the amount of glycoside, the activity and/or specificity of the enzyme used (Hösel and Nahrstedt, 1975; Tjon Sie Fat, 1977). It is also recommended that a surplus of enzyme is always used (Zinsmeister *et al.*, 1980). To avoid too long a fermentation time, which may lower the yield (Lüdtke, 1952; Pulss 1962), the quantity of plant material should be kept as small as possible. Before use the activity of an enzyme preparation must always have been proven. Standard conditions for enzymatic hydrolysis are pH 5-6, temperature 35-40°C, incubation time of 4-8 hours and an air stream as the vehicle. In some cases a new enzyme portion is added some hours after the initial hydrolysis.

B. ACID HYDROLYSIS

Some authors report the cleavage of cyanoglycosides by dilute acids (e.g. Gondwe, 1974; Wokes and Willimot, 1951). Pulss (1962) however reported lower yields of hydrocyanic acid using this method, which he attributed to a secondary fixation of liberated hydrocyanic acid in the plant homogenate. Hanssen and Sturm (1967) who obtained similar results suggested that there was a stabilization of cyanohydrin at low pH-values (< 3.5). It is also known that cyanogenic glycosides are hydrolysed in the presence of strong acids to the corresponding α-hydroxy carbonic acid and ammonium salt (e.g. Eyjólfsson, 1970). On the other hand higher hydrocyanic acid contents sometimes have been measured by acidic hydrolysis (Lehmann and Zinsmeister, 1979).

C. COMBINED ENZYMATIC AND ACID HYDROLYSIS

Several authors (Rosenthaler, 1932; Winkler, 1951; Seifert, 1955; Wood, 1965) described a combined method using enzymatic hydrolysis followed by an acid hydrolysis. However, Hanssen and Sturm (1967) found lower hydrocyanic acid values than with an exclusively enzymatic hydrolysis. Considering the different results reported, enzymatic hydrolysis with added enzymes should be preferred.

III. ISOLATION OF HCN

Two methods have been mainly used to isolate the liberated hydrocyanic acid, namely aeration (Lüdtke, 1952; Seifert, 1955; Akazawa *et al.*, 1960; Wood, 1965; Nahrstedt, 1971; Vetter and Haraszti, 1977) and distillation (Wokes and Willimot, 1951; Lüdtke, 1952; Seifert, 1955; Luh and Pinochet, 1959; Pulss, 1962; Hanssen and Sturm, 1967; Gondwe, 1974; Bates and Buick, 1976; Schröder, 1977). The hydrocyanic acid isolated by means of aeration and distillation is trapped in an alkaline receiving solution such as sodium hydroxide (Seifert, 1955 and others), sodium carbonate (Wood, 1966) or directly in alkaline picrate solution (Gillingham, *et al.*, 1969; Radin, 1972; Vetter and Haraszti, 1977). Goulden *et al.*, (1972) found during trace analysis that HCN was distilled from a solution but not quantitatively absorbed in the trap. They developed an absorption column through which the absorbing NaOH was recirculated by a pump, thus obtaining 100% recovery. Blaedel *et al.*, (1971) and Cooke (1978) estimated hydrocyanic acid directly in the hydrolysate. Some workers isolated HCN simply by diffusion in a closed system like the Conway chamber (Feldstein and Klendshoj, 1954; Møller and Conn, 1979) or a Warburg vessel (Gewitz *et al.*, 1976; Dziewanowska *et al.*, 1979) from one compartment containing the sample into another containing the alkaline trap.

A. AERATION METHOD

This method is based on the isolation of the liberated hydrocyanic acid by a stream of air or nitrogen. A design of an apparatus for this method is given by Seifert (1955), and by Kröller (1965). For quick isolation of small amounts of HCN, Wissing (this volume) has also reported a method. In contrast to the distillation method the aeration method is also suitable for larger quantities of plant material, which is important for investigating those species that contain only very small amounts of hydrocyanic acid. The yield of hydrocyanic acid however is dependent on parameters such as the size of the apparatus, the velocity of the gas stream, the kind of plant material, the temperature, the fermentation time, and on the rate of stirring (Seifert, 1955; Pulss, 1962; Zinsmeister *et al.*, 1980; Wissing, this volume). Pulss (1962) additionally recommends use of nitrogen as the gas stream, but in our experience it is not necessary, if enzymatic hydrolysis at a temperature of no more than 45°C is used. Whereas the HCN from KCN-solutions can be transferred to the trap under optimal conditions with relative small losses (about 10%), they increase up to 70% in the presence of plant material (Pulss, 1962; Zinsmeister *et al.*, 1980).

B. DISTILLATION METHOD

The design of an apparatus for the distillation method is given by Hanssen and Sturm (1967). A disadvantage of this method is that it increases the turbidity of the trap solution, which may often hinder the following photometric estimation, especially where the amount of hydrocyanic acid is very low.

Distillation of liberated hydrocyanic acid is impossible with large quantities of homogenized plant material. Additionally coloration of the trap solution is observed. In the presence of plant material there are also large losses of the hydrocyanic acid formed.

IV. CRITICAL REMARKS ON LIBERATION AND ISOLATION

In view of all the difficulties described above it is clear that at this time no reliable and really quantitative method is available for estimating hydrocyanic acid directly from plant homogenates. There are too many possible sources of errors which cannot be completely excluded. Thus Rosenthaler (1932) warns against overheating the plant material during distillation since hydrocyanic acid may be formed. Nahrstedt (1971) found that a homogenate of cherry leaves released hydrocyanic acid with repeated fermentation- and distillation-steps for up to 104 hours, each step yielding about the same amount of cyanide (Fig. 1). Obviously *de novo* production of hydrocyanic acid occ-

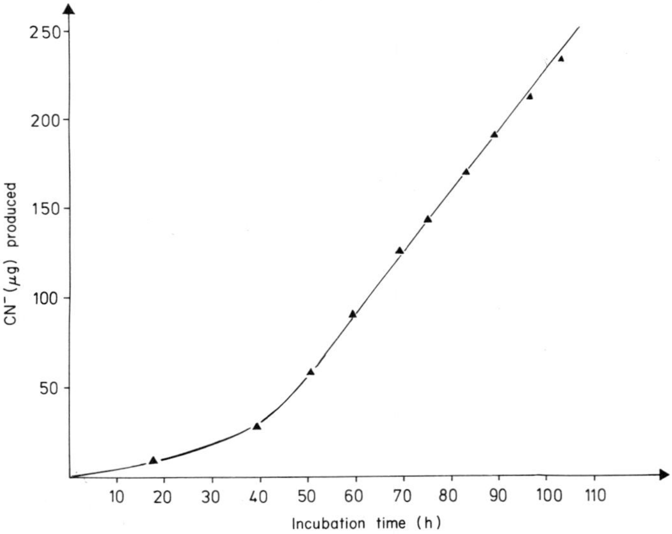

Fig. 1 Continuous production of HCN (measured by the method of Kröller, 1965, and Guilbault and Kramer, 1966) from homogenized cherry leaves. The incubation mixture was boiled for one hour before every new incubation step (▲) and 50 mg of a crude emulsin preparation was added (Nahrstedt, 1971).

urred in each step. Continuous production of HCN was also observed from a pulp of fruits of *Sambucus nigra* without boiling the incubation mixture (Nahrstedt, unpublished). Again, formation of prussic acid arose from the action of a pectinase preparation, an enzyme which occurs in plants and microorganisms (Nahrstedt, 1971). Pistorius *et al.*, (1977) and Pistorius and Voss (1977) showed the generation of hydrocyanic acid from various amino acids by oxidases supplemented with peroxidase or metals.

Mitchell and Hamilton (1929) mentioned the oxidation of glycine by chloramine to HCN. Lehmann and Zinsmeister (1979) observed HCN-production from various amino acids under oxidative conditions.

Lower yields of HCN may be due, for example, to addition of hydrocyanic acid to glucose, to pyruvate or oxalacetate or other compounds with carbonyl groups, to form cyanohydrins (Hackett, 1960; Kröller, 1968; Kröller and Krull, 1972). Volatile aldehydes can distill into the alkaline receiving solution and lead to a conversion of hydrocyanic acid to secondary and tertiary amino acids (Migrdichian, 1947). These losses may be prevented by adding semicarbazide-dihydrochloride to the plant homogenate (Nahrstedt, 1971; Table 1).

Table I Recovery of HCN from samples containing crotonaldehyde after isolation by a nitrogen stream when semicarbazide-dihydrochloride was present or absent (Nahrstedt, 1971).

No.	cyanide added [μg]	croton-aldehyde [μg]	semicarbazide ·2 HCl [mg]	cyanide recovered [μg]
1	10.0	100	-	9.8
2	10.0	1000	-	6.9
3	10.0	2000	-	3.2
4	10.0	1000	200	10.2
5	10.0	2000	500	9.8

However, recovery experiments in which KCN solutions were added to plant homogenates indicated that losses of HCN during analysis seem to occur more often and to be more significant than a secondary artificial production of HCN. Accurate results using the aeration or the distillation method according to Nahrstedt (1970, 1971) and Hanssen and Sturm (1967) respectively are obtained only if the cyanogenic compounds are extracted and isolated in a fairly pure state (containing minimal quantities of amino acids, proteins, carbohydrates and lipophilic substances). For serial HCN assays, however, this method needs too much expenditure of time and chemicals, especially when used with large quantities of plant material. Also one runs into the danger of losing some of the cyanogenic glycoside during isolation; this may lead to a high percentage error mainly when there are only small amounts of cyanogenic glycosides present (Zinsmeister *et al.*, 1980).

Classical aeration and distillation methods (with plant homogenates) are, however, suitable for a relatively quick evaluation of hydrocyanic acid content in cases where approximate values are sufficient. In every case, control of the applied method is necessary by addition of a known amount of KCN or of pure cyanogenic glycosides (compare Pulss, 1962).

V. ESTIMATION OF HCN

Again there are many methods available for measuring the isolated cyanide in the alkaline trap. Spectrophotometric methods are most important for quantitative cyanide estimation because they are sensitive, uncomplicated and practicable in many laboratories. Comparative overviews are given by e.g. Brockelt and Pohloudek-Fabini (1958), Bark (1962) and Zitnak (1973). An important method is based upon the König reaction (König, 1905) which was introduced in order to form dyestuffs: cyanogen halogenides formed by treatment of cyanide with bromine or chlorine are reacted with pyridine to form glutaconic aldehyde which is then coupled with primary amines or compounds with active methylene groups (e.g. Schwarzenbach and Weber, 1942; Epstein, 1947; Nahrstedt, 1977). This reaction was used by Aldridge, (1944, 1945) for cyanide quantification and he introduced benzidine as the amine, which forms a red colour. The first variation to increase sensitivity was described by Nusbaum and Skupeko (1951) who also discussed the specificity of the method. Kröller (1965) has changed some reagents in order to prolong their stability. Bark and Higson (1964a, 1964b) investigated many aromatic amines and substituted the carcinogenic benzidine with *p*-phenylendiamine. Since this compound is reported to be strongly allergenic, Nahrstedt (1977) introduced anthranilic acid as a coupling compound in the procedure of Kröller (1965). The method allows estimation of cyanide down to 0.04 μg/ml. Another non-carcinogenic amine is tetramethylbenzidine which has not yet been tested in this reaction.

Other modifications of the König reaction for cyanide assay use the reactive methylene hydrogens of pyrazolone to obtain a blue dye (Epstein, 1947). However, the reagents are rather unstable (Brockelt and Pohloudek-Fabini, 1958). Modifications of the method are reported by Baar (1966), Cooke *et al.*, (1978), and Jaulmes and Mestres (1960), who also discuss sources of errors and how to avoid them, and by Wissing (this volume).

Use of another coupling compound, barbituric acid, was proposed by Asmus and Garschagen (1953). This procedure was improved by Lambert *et al.*, (1975), who introduced stable reagents and increased the sensitivity to 0.01 μg/ml. Recently the Merck company (Darmstadt) has introduced a special kit (Spectroquant CN) for determination of HCN in water. This procedure uses N,N-dimethylbarbituric acid as the coupling compound.

In a sensitive and specific method with *p*-nitrobenzaldehyde and *o*-dinitrobenzene, cyanide acts as a catalytic component in forming the highly coloured purple dianion of *o*-nitrophenyl hydroxylamine in alkaline solution (Guilbault and Kramer, 1966). In view of its high sensitivity, the reagents have to be absolutely free from cyanide. Wawschinek *et al.*, (1968) applied this method to the determination of HCN in blood and organ homogenates with a detection limit of 0.01 μg/ml. Another modification of this method has a sensitivity of 0.005 μg/ml cyanide in the test solution of which a reaction volume of 0.1 ml (0.5 ng cyanide absolute) can be employed (Gewitz *et al.*, 1976). Since cyanide catalyses the development of the colour the sensitivity may be increased by prolonging the reaction time.

Another simple method was developed by Baumeister and Schievelbein (1971) using the relatively stable binding of cyanide to the oxidized form of haemoglobin. The absorbance of the complex is measured at 422 nm. The sensitivity is 0.1 μg per 0.5 ml used in the assay but the haemoglobin reagent is not stable for more than two days.

The picrate test (Mirande, 1909) which is used normally for qualitative tests is sometimes applied for quantification. There are many false positive results arising from this test (Larsen, 1978; Larsen and Sørensen, in preparation; Nahrstedt, 1981). The picrate test has been used as a diffusion technique, involving absorption of HCN on the picrate paper and elution of the dye formed for spectrophotometric estimation (e.g. Hunt and Taylor, 1976; Cooper-Driver *et al.*, 1977). Lambert and Manzo (1968) estimated cyanide by reaction with phenanthroline with a sensitivity of 1 μg/ml; Pranitis and Stolman formed tetracyanonickelate from cyanide and $NiCl_2$ (sensitivity 0.5 μg/ml). Very recently Morgan and Way (1980) have developed a fluorimetric determination of cyanide in biological fluids, with pyridoxal.

Cyanogen bromide and cyanogen chloride formed from cyanide and bromine water or chloramine T, respectively, have been estimated by gas chromatography down to 0.01 μg/ml (e.g. Nota and Palombari, 1973; Valentour *et al.*, 1974; Brunnemann *et al.*, 1977). For analysis in the picogram range a nitrogen selective detector is necessary (Donike, 1973). Voltametric titration of cyanide in the range 40-200 ppb is described by Harzdorf and Dorn (1977), and determination with cyanide-selective membrane electrodes down to c.25 ng/ml has been performed by, for example, Frant *et al.*, (1972) and Egekeze and Oehme (1979). In a special case, β-glucosidase was immobilised in a polymer gel layer coupled to a cyanide-sensing membrane electrode in order to analyse small samples of amygdalin (Llenado and Rechnitz, 1971). By means of a polarographic differential pulse technique 1.5 μg/25 ml cyanide was measured by Wisser (1977); and HCN was determinated in the ppb range using atomic absorption spectrometry by Jungreis and Ain (1977).

REFERENCES

Akazawa, T., Milianich, P. and Conn, E.E. (1960). *Plant Physiol.* 35, 535-538.

Aldridge, W.N. (1944). *Analyst* 69, 262-265.

Aldridge, W.N. (1945). *Analyst* 70, 474.

Asmus, E. and Garschagen, H. (1953). *Fresenius' Z. Anal. Chem.* 138, 414.

Baar, S. (1966). *Analyst* 91, 268.

Bates, B.L. and Buick, D.R. (1976). *J. AOAC* 59, 1390-1395.

Bark, L.S. (1962). *Ind. Chemist,* 525.

Bark, L.S. and Higson, H.G. (1964a). *Talanta* 11, 471-479, etc.

Bark, L.S. and Higson, H.G. (1964b). *Talanta* 11, 621-631.

Baumeister, R. and Schievelbein, H. (1971). *Z. Anal. Chem.* 225, 362-363.

Blaedel, W.I., Easty, D.B., Anderson, R. and Farrell, T.R. (1971). *Anal. Chem.* 43, 890-894.

Brockelt, G. and Pohloudek-Fabini, R. (1958). *Pharmazie* 13, 737.

Brunnemann, K., Yu, L. and Hoffmann, D. (1977). *J. Anal. Toxicol.* 1, 38-42.

Butler, G.W., Bailey, R.W. and Kennedy, L.D. (1965). *Phytochemistry* 4, 369-381.

Cooke, R.D. (1978). *J. Sci. Food Agric.* 29, 345-352.

Cooke, R.D. Blake, G.G. and Battershill, J.M. (1978). *Photochemistry* 17, 381-383.

Cooper-Driver, G., Finch, S., Swain, T. and Bernays, E. (1977). *Biochem. Syst. Ecol.* 5, 177-183.

Dillemann, G. (1958). *In* "Handbuch der Pflanzenphysiologie" (W. Ruhland, ed.) Vol. VIII, p. 1050. Springer, Berlin.

Donike, M. (1973). *Z. Naturforsch.* 28b, 533.

Dziewanowska, K., Niedzwiedz, I. and Lewak, S. (1979). *Physiol. Veg.* 17, 681-686.

Egekeze, J.O. and Oehme, F.W. (1979). *J. anal. Toxocol.* 3, 119.

Egli, K.L. (1977). *J. AOAC* 60, 954-956.

Epstein, J. (1947). *Anal. Chem.* 19, 272-274.

Eyjólfsson, R. (1970). *In* "Fortschritte der Chemie organischer Naturstoffe" (W. Herz, H. Grisebach and A.I. Scott, eds), Vol.28, p.74, Springer, Wien, New York.

Feldstein, D. and Klendshoj, N.C. (1954). *J. Lab. chi. Med.* 44, 166-170.

Frant, M.S., Ross, J.W. and Riseman, J.H. (1972). *Anal. Chem.* 44, 2227.

Gewitz, H.S., Pistorius, E.K., Voss, H., Vennesland, B. (1976). *Planta (Berl.)* 131, 145-148.

Gillingham, J.T., Shirer, N.N. and Page, N.R. (1969). *Agronom. J.* 61, 716-718.

Gondwe, A.T.D. (1974). *East African Agr. and For. J.* 40, 161-167.

Gondwe, A.T.D., Seigler, D.S. and Dunn, J.E. (1978). *Phytochemistry* 17, 271-274.

Goulden, P.D., Afghan, B.K. and Brooksbank, D. (1972). *Anal. Chem.* 44, 1845-1849.

Guilbault, G.G. and Kramer, D.N. (1966). *Anal. Chem.* 38, 834-836.

Hackett, D.P. (1960). *In* "Handbuch der Pflanzenphysiologie" (W. Ruhland, ed), Vol. XII#2, p.30. Springer Verlag, Berlin.

Haismann, D.R. and Knight, D.J. (1967). *Biochem. J.* 103, 528-534.
Hanssen, E. and Sturm, W. (1967). *Z. Lebensm. Unters. Forsch.* 134, 69-80.
Harzdorf, C. and Dorn, L. (1977). *Z. Anal. Chem.* 284, 189-192.
Hösel, W. and Nahrstedt, A. (1975). *Hoppe-Seylers Z. physiol. Chem.* 356, 1265-1275.
Hunt, B.J. and Taylor, A.O. (1976). *N.Z. J. Exp. Agric.* 4, 191-194.
Jaulmes, P. and Mestres, R. (1960). *Ann. Falsif. Expert. Chim.* 53, 455-468.
Jones, D.A. (1972). *In* "Phytochemical Ecology" (J.B. Harborne, ed.) p.113. Academic Press, London, New York.
Jungreis, E. and Ain, F. (1977). *Anal. Chim. Act.* 88, 191.
König, W. (1905). *Z. angew. Chem.* 18, 115.
Kröller, E. (1965). *Z. Lebensmittel-Unters. Forsch.* 127, 130-136.
Kröller, E. (1968). *Z. Lebensm. Unters. Forsch.* 136, 321 pp.
Kröller, E., Krull, L. (1972). *Z. Lebensmittel Unters. Forsch.* 148, 16-18.
Lambert, J.L. and Manzo, D.J. (1968). *Anal. Chem.* 40, 1354.
Lambert, J.L., Ramasamy, J. and Paukstelis, J.V. (1975). *Anal. Chem.* 47, 916-918.
Larnen, J. (1960). *In* "The Enzymes" (P.D. Boyer, H. Lardy, K. Myrbäck, eds) Vol. 4, pp.375. Academic Press, London.
Larsen, L.M. (1978). Paper presented at the EMBO-Workshop on Cyanide Metabolism, Canterbury, August 14-18).
Lehmann, G. and Zinsmeister, H.D. (1979). *Z. Lebensm. Unters. Forsch.* 169, 357-358.
Lehmann, G., Zinsmeister, H.D., Erb, N., and Neunhoeffer, O. (1979). *Z. Ernährungswiss.* 18, 16-22.
Llenado, R.A. and Rechnitz, G.A. (1971). *Anal. Chem.* 43, 1457-1461.
Lüdtke, M. (1952). *Biochem. Z.* 322, 310-319.
Luh, B.S. and Pinochet, F. (1959). *Food Res.* 24, 423-427.
Migrdichian, V. (1947). Chemistry of Organic Cyanogen Compounds. Reinhold Publ. Corp., New York.
Mirande, M. (1909). *C. R. Acad. Sci.* 149, 140.
Mitchell, H.H. and Hamilton, T.S. (1929). The Biochemistry of the Amino Acids. The Chemical Catalog Comp., New York.
Møller, L. and Conn, E.E. (1979). *J. Biol. Chem.* 254, 8575-8583.
Morgan, R.L. and Way, J.L. (1980), *Anal. Toxicol.* 4, 78.
Nahrstedt, A. (1970). *Phytochemistry* 9, 2085-2089.
Nahrstedt, A. (1971). Dissertation Univ. Freiburg.
Nahrstedt, A. (1972). *Phytochemistry* 11, 3121-3126.
Nahrstedt, A. (1976). *Z. Naturforsch.* 31c, 397-400.
Nahrstedt, A. (1977). *Deutsch. Apoth. Z.* 117, 1357-1359.
Nahrstedt, A. (1981). *Photochemistry* 19, 2757-2758.
Nota, G. and Palombari, R. (1973). *J. Chromatogr.* 84, 37-41.
Nusbaum, I. and Skupeko, P. (1951). *Sew. Ind. Wastes* 23, 875-879.
Pistorius, E.K. and Voss, H. (1977). *Biochem. Biophys. Acta* 481, 395-406.
Pistorius, E.K. and Gewitz, H.S., Voss, H. and Vennesland, B. (1977) *Biochem. Biophys. Acta* 481, 384-394.
Pranitis, P.A.F. and Stolman, A. (1977). *J. Forensic Sci.* 22, 443-445.
Pulss, G. (1962). *Z. Anal. Chem.* 190, 402-409.
Radin, J.W. (1972). *Crop. Sci.* 12, 609-611.

Rosenthaler, L. (1932). *In* "Handbuch fur Pflanzenanalyse" (G. Klein, ed.) Vol. III/2, p.1042. Springer Verlag, Wien.
Schröder, V.N. (1977). Soil and Crop. Sci. Florida Proc. 36, 195-197.
Schwarzenbach, G. and Weber, R. (1942). *Helv. Chim. Act.* 25, 1628.
Secor, J.B., Conn, E.E., Dunn, J.E. and Seigler, D.S. (1976). *Phytochem.* 15, 1703-1706.
Seifert, P. (1955). *In* "Moderne Methoden der Pflanzenanlyse" (K. Paech, M.V. Tracey, eds) Vol. IV, p.676-688, Springer Verlag, Berlin, Göttingen, Heidelberg.
Tjon Sie Fat, L. (1977). *Proc. Koninkl. Nederl. Akad. wetensch.* 80C, 227-237.
Valentour, J.C., Aggarwal, V. and Sunshine, I. (1974). *Anal. Chem.* 46, 924.
Vetter, J. and Haraszti, E. (1977). *Act. Agr. Acad. Sci. Hung.* 26, 15-22.
Wawschinek, O., Paletta, B. and Beyer, W. (1967). *Arch. Toxokol.* 23, 52.
Wegler, R. (1970). Chemie der Pflanzenschutz- und Schädlingsbekämpfungsmittel, Vol.2, pp. 108-109, Springer, Berlin, Heidelberg, New York.
Winkler, W.O. (1951). *J. AOAC,* 34, 541.
Wisser, K. (1977). *Z. anal. Chem.* 286, 351-354.
Wokes, F. and Willimot, S.G. (1951). *J. Pharm. Pharmacol.* 3, 905-917.
Wood, T. (1965). *J. Sci. Food Agric.* 16, 300-305.
Wood, T. (1966). *J. Sci. Food Agric.* 17, 85-90.
Zechner, L. (1966). *In* "Die Rohstoffe des Pflanzenreichs" (J. v. Wiesner, ed.) 5th edn. Lieferung 5; p.66 J. Cramer, Weinheim.
Zinsmeister, H.D., Erb, N. and Lehmann, G. (1982). In prep.
Zitnak, A. (1973). *In* "Chronic Cassava Toxicity" (B. Nestel and R. McIntyre eds), p.89-96, Intern. Development Research Centre, Ottawa.

A SMALL SCALE HCN TRANSFER TECHNIQUE FOR THE RAPID ASSAY OF ENZYMATIC HCN FORMATION

F. WISSING

Department of Biochemistry,
The Royal Dental College, DK-8000 Aarhus C, Denmark

There has always been much interest in the assay of cyanide and several reviews have been written on this topic (Seifert, 1954; Bark, 1962; Bark and Higson, 1963; Harada and Nyusu, 1978; Williams, 1979). The quantitative methods most commonly used are (a) silver nitrate titration, which requires at least 1 μmole of HCN, and (b) the colorimetric methods of Epstein (1947) or Lambert *et al.* (1975) with sensitivities down to 1 nmole of HCN.

The principle of HCN determination presented here is based upon the Epstein method and involves the distillation of cyanide from 2 ml of a cyanide-producing enzyme solution into a 1 ml trap of 0.1 M NaOH. A relatively strong flow of air is used, with the enzyme solution stirred maximally. Every 4 min the NaOH is changed for a fresh solution, and HCN collected in the previous tube is assayed. A brief description of this method has been published earlier (Wissing, 1974), but a more detailed presentation was found necessary as some of the experimental conditions are critical in order to obtain reproducibility and a good recovery of cyanide.

The apparatus, which can be used under aerobic as well as under anaerobic conditions, is shown schematically in Fig. 1. The reaction chamber consists of a round-bottomed glass test tube (inner diameter 15 mm, overall height 80 mm) with a 14 mm ground glass conical socket joint. A glass mantle is fused to the test tube for the purpose of thermostating by water circulation. The glass mantle is not fused onto the bottom of the test tube to prevent the possibility of changing the shape of its round bottom. It is important that there is fast and smooth running stirring with a small magnetic bar in the test tube. An actual example of stirring is shown in Fig. 2, in which a 2 ml enzyme solution was stirred such that the solution was forced cylindrically up the vertical face of the vessel with a nearly laminar flow. It is necessary to stir rapidly to obtain a reproducible rate of distillation of cyanide.

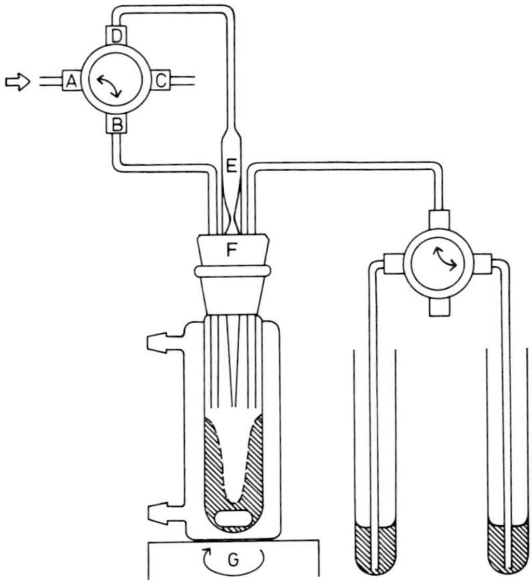

Fig. 1 Apparatus for measuring cyanide production in enzyme solutions or bacterial suspensions. Air or nitrogen is passed through the reaction chamber via a microvalve in position A-B and is further distributed by another microvalve to either one of two test tubes containing NaOH for the collection of cyanide. With the microvalve in position A-D the pipette E can be emptied during the experiment. In position C-D the pipette can be filled before the experiment. The reaction chamber is closed with a rubber stopper (F). The suspension is stirred by a magnetic stirring device (G).

A rubber stopper fitting the reaction chamber has three apertures: one for a gas-inlet tube, one for a gas-outlet tube, and one for a 100 µl constriction pipette, which serves as a substrate reservoir. Before air or nitrogen is passed into the reaction chamber, the flow rate (420 ml/min) is measured by a flow rate meter and frequently checked during the experiment. The air is distributed through a three-way valve (LV-3 valve, Pharmacia Fine Chemicals, Sweden) so that its flow can be directed either through the inlet tube, or for emptying purposes through the constriction pipette. Figure 2 shows how the substrate is pressed up over the constriction so that there is no risk of early substrate addition. The outlet tube is connected to another three-way valve, leading the gas flow to either one of two 10 x 100 mm test tubes, each containing 1 ml of 0.1 M NaOH for collection of cyanide. They are changed every 4 minutes. To prevent too much bubbling their rims are lightly smeared with silicone grease.

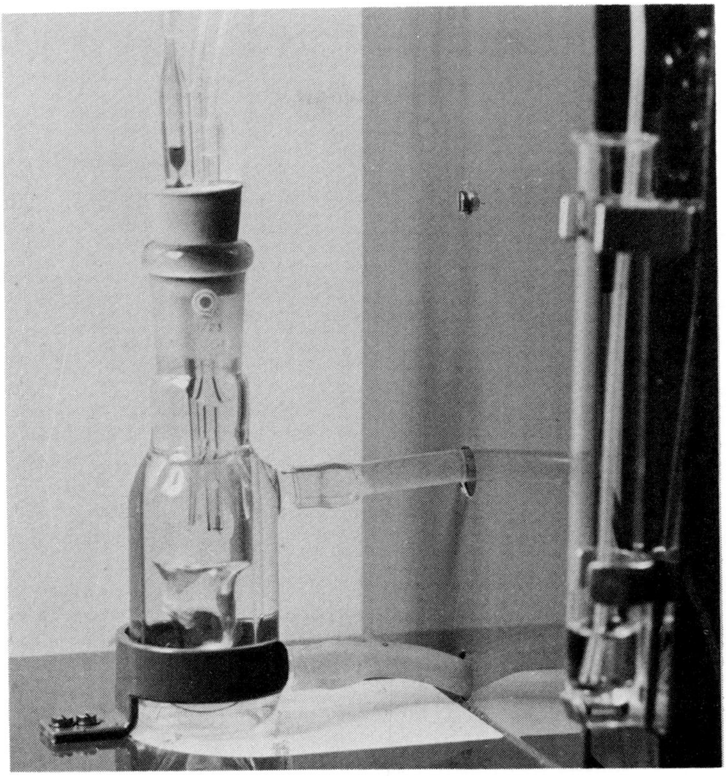

Fig. 2 The reaction chamber with an enzyme solution being stirred. Note the position of substrate in the constriction pipette under experimental conditions.

The air supply is first passed through a gas-reduction valve, an empty trap, a trap with 5 N NaOH and a water trap. It then passes through a flow meter and a small water trap, kept at the same temperature as the thermostating bath, to avoid volume changes in the enzyme solution during long running experiments. The flow meter was obtained from A/S Mobro Instruments, DK-3460 Birkeroed, Denmark. It has the following specifications: type: 10A3135N, tube: FP-1/8-20-P-3/37, scale: 100% = 2190 cm^3/min, air: 20°C and 0.2 ato. If the air is obtained from a reciprocating pump, it is also passed through two 1-litre Erlenmeyer flasks in order to steady the flow.

By use of this method, linear standard curves for known amounts of cyanide can be obtained in the range of 2-40 nmoles of cyanide. Figure 3 shows that only a little deviation occurs between the two standard curves made by determining the cyanide either directly in 0.1 M NaOH or aft-

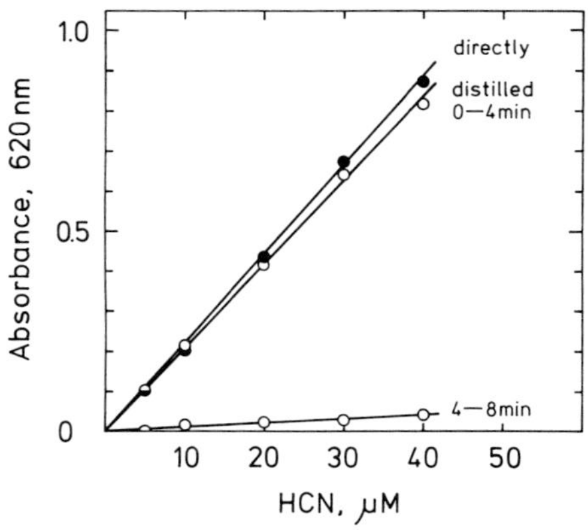

Fig. 3 Standard curves for HCN determination with the Epstein method. Directly in 0.1 M NaOH (●) and via the aeration apparatus with 4 minutes of distillation and further 4 minutes of distillation of the same sample (○). The HCN was distilled from TRIS-HCl buffer (0.1 M, pH = 8.2) into 0.1 M NaOH.

ter it has been distilled from TRIS-HCl buffer (0.1 M, pH 8.2) into NaOH. Identical results were obtained with pyrophosphate or orthophosphate buffers. Figure 3 also shows that only negligible amounts of HCN are recovered during a further 4 minutes period of distillation.

Practical details of the Epstein assay are described by Boxer and Rickards (1951). However, interference of the Epstein assay has been observed with NH_4^+ ions when $(NH_4)_2SO_4$-precipitated enzymes are tested. A pink colour appears which also shows light absorption at 625 nm, the wavelength used in the Epstein assay. The respective absorption spectra are shown in Figure 4. The following modification, where the NaOH with the collected HCN is only neutralized to pH 8, before the addition of chloramine T, eliminates the development of the pink colour. NaH_2PO_4 (200 µl, 0.5 M) and chloramine T (100 µl, 1% w/v) are added successively to the test tubes. They are closed and their contents mixed thoroughly. After standing for 1 minute, 3 ml of pyrazolone reagent (see below) is added and the solution mixed. After standing for 45 minutes at room temperature the absorption of the sample is read at 625 nm. The pyrazolone reagent is made by dissolving 20 mg bis-(1-phenyl-3-methyl-5-pyrazolone) in 20 ml pyridine and then adding 100 ml of saturated, filtered solution of 1-phenyl-3-methyl-5-pyrazolone in water. The pyrazolone and bis-pyrazolone are from Fluka, Switzerland and British Drug House, England, respectively.

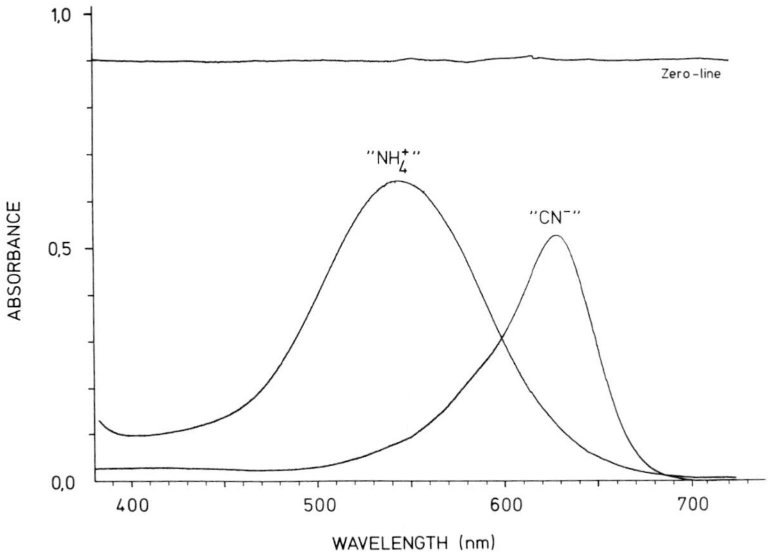

Fig. 4 Absorption spectra of the normal blue coloured compound ("CN^-") and the NH_4^+ ion induced pink coloured compound ("NH_4^+") formed by the Epstein assay. The two curves are obtained from assays made on 20 nmoles of CN^- or 20 µmoles of NH_4^+ respectively.

REFERENCES

Bark, L.S. (1962). *The Industrial Chemist.* 38, 525-528.
Bark, L.S. and Higson, H.G. (1963). *The Analyst* 88, 751-760.
Boxer, G.E. and Rickards, J.C. (1951). *Arch. Biochem.* 30, 372-381.
Epstein, J. (1947). *Anal. Chem.* 19, 272-274.
Harada, H. and Nyusu, T. (1978). *Kagaku Kogyo Shiryo* 13, 2, 40-45.
Lambert, J.L., Ramasamy, J. and Paukstelis, J.V. (1975). *Anal. Chem.* 47, 916-918.
Seifert, P. (1954). *Moderne Methoden der Pflanzenanalyse* 4, 676-688.
Williams, W.J. (1979) "Handbook of Anion Determination", Butterworths, England.
Wissing, F. (1974). *J. Bacteriol.* 117, 1289-1294.

DIFFERENT ORIGINS OF CYANIDE CONTAMINATION IN SMALL RIVERS

HILDEGARD KRUTZ

Institute for Water Research, Dortmund, F.R.G.

The following study aims at a description of the occurrence of cyanides (free and combined) in small rivers and brooks of North-West Germany. The investigated area (Fig. 1) encloses parts of the industrial zone of the Lower Rhine and Aachen in the north, agricultural areas of the loess zone, and the forest, pastures and meadows of the Northern Eifel mountains in the south.

I. METHODS

Water samples were taken every fortnight to determine the concentration of total cyanide. They were analysed by colorimetry, with the pyridine-pyrazolone reagent (Ludzack *et al.* 1954). A detection limit of 0.1 μg/l was reached by additional extraction of the polymethine pigment with *n*-butanol. This was necessary to measure the low concentrations in the natural waters.

As a screening of cyanide concentration only may be insufficient to permit interpretation of the data, other parameters determining the water quality were observed simultaneously. Suspended matter, organic carbon, the degree of oxygen demand, the pH, conductivity, heavy metals and nutrient concentrations were taken from a study with synchronous measurements by Symader, Thomas and Richartz under the direction of Hermann (1978).

For the explanation of the spatial variances 35 factors were chosen to describe the nature of the 30 catchment areas. Those factors were geological, geomorphological and pedological variables, such as rocks, relief, type of soil, and meterological and hydrological parameters such as precipitation and runoff. Account was also taken of the social and economic structure of the catchment areas: population density, type and capacity of factories and sewage effluents, etc.

The results of the study were based upon the evaluation of correlation coefficient matrices which were calculated individually for each of the 30 streams. The correlation coefficients were grouped by a multivariate statistical

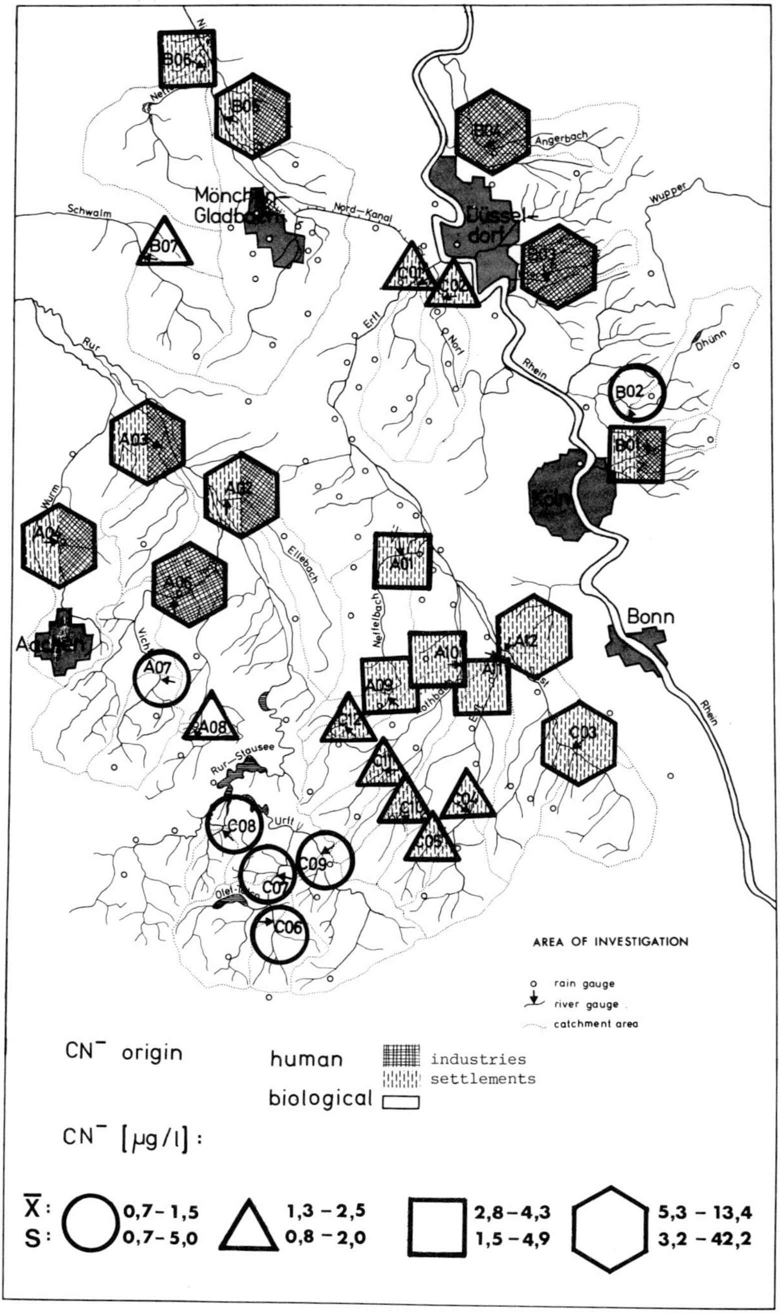

Fig. 1 Cluster analysis of cyanide contaminations.

method which is known as principal component analysis and based upon computer programs (Veldman, 1967). Another statistical method applied was cluster analysis as proposed by Ward (1963). This method was used to classify cyanide values into groups with a high degree of similarity in their temporal variances.

II. SPATIAL AND TEMPORAL VARIANCE

One of the results was the correlation between the level of cyanide contamination and the population density (correlation coefficient r = 0.6) or the existence of steel and galvanic industries (r = 0.6) in the catchment areas.

Rivers which are polluted by peak discharges from galvanic industries showed cyanide concentrations with high means ($\bar{x}$) and high standard deviations (s). Concentrations up to 200 µg/l occurred (Fig. 1). As expected, the occurrence of higher cyanide levels is coupled to high concentrations of heavy metals in water.

Cyanide concentrations in rural watersheds with smaller settlements are not coupled with seasonal changes. Their mean value is about 3 µg/l. In these waters cyanides are not of industrial origin. Which parameter is correlated with cyanide depends on the ecological system. In some streams cyanide is connected with phosphate or with sodium, both of which indicate domestic sewage influences. Meganathan and Castric (1977) pointed to a relation between the HCN-production by *Pseudomonas aeruginosa* and the phosphate range of 1.0 to 10.0 mM.

In the case of a very high content of green algae, correlations to the growth phase of algae in spring and to the decomposition of organic matter in autumn were found (Fig. 2).

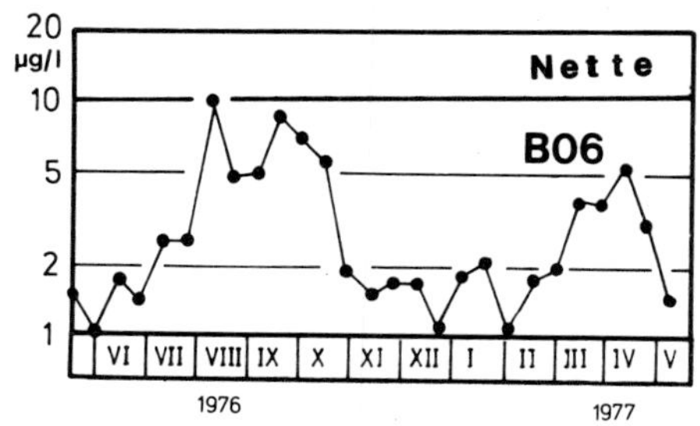

Fig. 2 River Nette

Fairly polluted natural waters have cyanide contents between 0.7 and 2.1 µg/l which are strongly dependent on seasonal changes.

In some streams of the Eifel mountains, higher cyanide values correlate significantly to phosphate (r = 0.6), but in these cases phosphate is derived from fertilisers.

The following example illustrates the complex interactions of parameters internal to the water body on one hand

and parameters influencing the water body from the outside on the other hand.

III. AN EXAMPLE: THE WEHEBACH BROOK

The Wehebach, a brook in the Northern Eifel National Park, belongs to a group of waters with a maximum cyanide content in winter. Others have their maximum in summer. This catchment area is only 2.5 km^2. The area is covered by forest (52%) (*Luzula fagetum* - Jahn (1972)) and by pastures (42%).

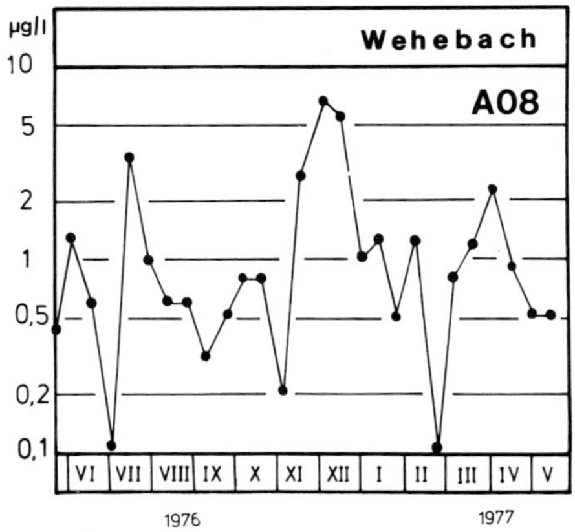

Fig. 3 Wehebach Brook

Low concentrations of cyanide were found in spring and late summer (0.5 µg/l) (Fig. 3). A minimum occurred at mid summer, coupled to a high water temperature (25°C). Evaporation at elevated temperatures may explain the low cyanide concentrations in summer. One occurrence of high cyanide concentration in July coincided with low temperatures due to antecedent heavy rainfall. Elevated concentrations of manganese, nickel, zinc, iron, potassium, sodium and phosphate were observed together with a relatively high conductivity. As phosphate indicates soil erosion processes in this area (Symader 1976), this event may be explained by an input of cyanide from outside the water body.

When the cyanide contents are calculated in loads, that is mass transfer per unit of time, the difference between the summer loads with 0.2 g CN^-/day and the winter maximum with 6 g CN^-/day is even more significant. The question arises, where this load of 6 g CN^-/day in winter comes from.

In a water sample taken in winter with a cyanide concentration of 0.8 µg/l, 8 µg/l of amino acids was found by column chromatography, including phenylalanine, leucine, isoleucine, tyrosine, histidine and glycine. These amino acids are known precursors for the production of cyanogenic glycosides and cyanide by plants, bacteria and algae, and point to a biological source of HCN (Conn, 1973; Gewitz *et al.*, 1976; Wissing, 1975).

An input of cyanide from the atmosphere must also be taken into account. Snow contains approximately 0.8 μg/l of cyanides in this area.

A transport of cyanides from outside into the water body hence cannot be excluded. Cyanide belongs to the substances which are relatively mobile in soil (Fuller, 1977).

Plant sociological surveys (Schwickerath, 1944; Jahn, 1972) showed that at least nine higher plants containing cyanogenic glycosides are associated with the type of forest in this area, especially *Pteridium aquilinum* and *Dryopteris filiximas*.

Another source of cyanide is sediment erosion. The brook bed consists of coarse stones with scattered sediment areas. The sediment fraction with a particle diameter less than 1 mm contains about 0.2 mg/kg of total cyanide, only a small amount of it being easily set free (0.04 mg/kg). The ratio in the water body is just the opposite: the major part is easily set free. The total organic matter in the sediment is about 15%, which shows that the transport of organic substances *via* sediment erosion must also be taken into account. Our own investigations proved that the rising content of organic matter in sediments was accompanied by an enrichment of cyanide in the sediment (Richartz *et al.*, 1978; Krutz, 1979).

Not only cyanides, but also other parameters are subject to transport phenomena. Discriminant analysis was used to detect statistical similarities between cyanide and other parameters. Discriminant analysis is a multivariate statistical method which uses a group of variables to obtain maximum separation between different groups of cyanide range. (Miller, 1962; Decoursey, 1973; Herrmann, 1974). In this case 4 ranges of cyanide concentrations are applied:

Range of groups:	CN^- (μg/l)
1:	< 0.6
2:	0.7 - 1.3
3:	1.4 - 3.2
4:	3.3 - 6.5

One combination of steering variables is the potassium concentration of the solution, the turbidity (measured as the extinction at 420 nm) and the discharge at the time of sampling. High concentrations of potassium in autumn and winter from leaching of fallen leaves (Gosz *et al.*, 1973) are significantly correlated to cyanide (r = 0.7). The very low pH (down to 4.3) may be due to an increasing input of humic acids formed by decomposition of organic carbon material such as fallen leaves (Symader, 1976), coordinated with a higher turbidity and a higher discharge, corresponding to the maximum of precipitation in winter. For the Wehebach brook, these variables are independent, which is quite unusual.

The following discriminant function was computed and explains with a level of 0.01 significance about 80% of the total variance:

$$T = 0.050\ (K)^{1/2} - 0.4305\ (TR)^{-1/2} - 0.9012\ (Q)^{1/3}$$

T = discriminant score
K = potassium concentration in the water solution (mg/l)
TR = turbidity (extinction at 420 nm)
Q = run-off at the time of sampling (m^3/s)

Reproducing the measured cyanide concentrations with the steering variables, (that means assigning an individual observation to that group with the smallest sum of squared deviations between the group means and the discriminant score), 67% of the cyanide values are assigned to the correct groups of the cyanide range whereas others fall into neighbour groups. For further details see Krutz (1979).

IV. CONCLUSIONS

With various forms of multivariate statistical evaluations it was shown that cyanide concentrations in small rivers have different origins. Galvanic industries are a direct anthropogenic source. Rivers with a higher content of phosphate and potassium from a constant input of domestic sewage have only a low variation in cyanide concentrations during the year. The reason is probably a bacterial production of HCN. Brooks receiving a relatively high contribution of biologically active inflows due to their small size show an extreme seasonal change in the cyanide content with its maximum in winter. Possible reasons are: a production by microorganisms in the water body, cyanide formation outside by plants and microorganisms with a subsequent transport into the river, and a cyanide input from the atmosphere. Potassium, precipitation and run-off, the steering variables of the discriminant function to determine the cyanide range, point to the three sources mentioned above.

REFERENCES

Conn, E.E. (1973). *Biochem. Soc. Symp.* 38, 227-302.

Decousey, D. (1973). *Water Resources Research*, 9, 93-102.

Fuller, H.W. (1977). *In:* "Movement of Selected Metals, Asbestos and Cyanide in Soil: Applications to Waste Disposal Problems", Arizona Univ. Tucson; US Environ. Protect. Agency Contract Nr. 68-03-0208.

Gewitz, H.S., Pistorius, E.K., Voss, H. and Vennesland, B. (1976).

Planta (Berl.) 131, 149-153.
Gosz, J.R., Likens, G.E. and Bormann, F.H. (1973). *New Hampshire; Ecological Monographs*, 43, 173-191.
Herrmann, R. (1974). *Catena*, 1, 367-385.
Herrmann, R. (1978). *In:* "Mathematical prediction modelling of chemical interactions between solution, suspended matter and sediment in water", Deutsche Forschungsgemeinschaft, Bonn, He 482/8.
Jahn, G. (1972). Forstliche Wuchsraumgliederung und waldbauliche Rahmenplanung in der Nordeifel; Dissertationes Botanicae 16, Verlag J. Cramer
Krutz, M. (1975). Grundlagen eines rationellen Verfahrens zur Analyse ninhydrinpositiver Substanzen in Oberflächengewässern. Veröff. der Hydrolog. Abt. der Dortmunder Stadtwerke AG und des Instituts für Wasserforschung GmbH, 20, Dortmund.
Krutz, H. (1979). Cyanverbindungen in Fleissgewässern - eine mathematische Beschreibung ihres raumzeitlichen Verhaltens und ihrer Wechselwirkungen zwischen Wasserkörper und Sediment- Veröff. des Instituts für Wasserforschung GmbH Dortmund in der Hydrol. Abt. der Dortmunder Stadtwerke AG, 28, Dortmund.
Ludzack, F.J., Moore, W.A. and Ruchhoft, C.C. (1954). *Analytical Chemistry* 26, 11, 1784-1792.
Meganathan, R. and Castric, P.A. (1977). *Arch. Microbiol.* 114, 51-54.
Miller, G. (1962). *Statistical Prediction by Discriminant Analysis; Meteor. Monographs*, 4, 1-50.
Richartz, H. and Herrmann, H. (1978). *Vom Wasser* 51, 47-54.
Rump, H.H., Symader, W. and Herrmann, R. (1976). *Catena*, 3, 1-16.
Schwickerath, M. (1944). "Das hohe Venn und seine Randgebiete; Pflanzensoziologie", Vol.6, Verlag G. Fischer, Jena.
Seigler, D.S. (1977). *The Naturally Occurring Cyanogenic Glycosides; Progress in Phytochemistry*, 4, 83-120, Pergammon Press, Oxford.
Symader, W. (1976). Multivariate Nährstoffundersuchungen zu Vorhersagezwecken in Fliessgewässern am Nordrand der Eifel; *In:* "Mathematische Vorhersagemodelle zur Gewässergüte, I." Kölner Georg. Arbeiten, 34.
Veldman, D. (1967). Fortran Programming for the Behavioural Sciences, Holt, Rinehart and Winston, New York.
Ward, J.H. (1963). *American Statistical Assoc. J.* 58, 236-244.
Wissing, F. (1975). *J. Bacteriology*, 121,2, 695-699.

ECOTOXICOLOGY OF CYANIDES IN FRESHWATER

GÉRARD LEDUC

Department of Biological Sciences, Concordia University, Montréal, Quebec, Canada

I. INTRODUCTION

Cyanide is a widespread chemical found in surface waters originating not only from direct industrial wastes but often from biological sources. The various industries responsible for cyanide pollution include the petrochemical, mining, metal electroplating, photographic, steel and coke manufacturing industries. The biological sources of cyanide in water are numerous. Several bacteria, fungi and algae produce cyanide (HCN) as part of their nitrogen metabolism. There are also many terrestrial plants that contain cyanogenic glucosides that release free HCN when their cellular structure is disrupted. When cyanogenic plant material decomposes near streams or falls in the water, it may become a significant source of cyanide in the water.

Given the right physical and chemical water conditions, appreciable amounts of free cyanide may be produced as a metabolic product of bacteria, fungi, and algae and/or from the bacterial decompositon of cyanogenic plant detritus. These phenomena have long been recognised and they may contribute to mortality of fish during dense algal bloom. However, the causes and effects of low sublethal concentrations of free cyanide from biochemical origins have received only little attention and deserve much more.

A. TERMINOLOGY

In aquatic toxicology, the chemical terminology of cyanides has often been confusing if not erroneous due to the different forms under which the chemicals exist. A knowledge of the various species of cyanide is essential to the understanding of toxicological properties and to the logical formulation of water quality objectives.

The chemical forms of cyanides vary primarily according to their source but also in response to environmental chemicals and physical and biological factors. The generic names used to describe cyanide are: free cyanide, cyanide ion, cyanide salt, complex cyanides and total cyanide.

Free cyanide describes molecular HCN from any source, existing independently or part of an equilibrium reaction in the gaseous or dissolved state. The chemical names for HCN are: *hydrogen cyanide, hydrocyanic acid, cyanhydric acid*. The older technical literature has also used the name of *Prussic acid*.

HCN, a weak acid, will dissociate into H^+ and CN^- ions. *Cyanide ion* refers to the anion (CN^-) derived from hydrocyanic acid in solution. This cyanide ion species, CN^-, is also referred to as *free cyanide ion*.

Most of the cyanide used in industrial processes is in the form of technical *cyanide salts;* these are alkali salts such as potassium (KCN), sodium (NaCN) or calcium cyanide ($Ca(CN)_2$), all of which are soluble in water. There are also several other cyanide salts of alkali, alkaline earth or heavy metals, of varying degrees of solubility. These are simple cyanides that ionize in water to release cyanide ion (Eqn. 1) which, depending on pH, will hydrolyze to form *hydrocyanic acid* (Eqn. 2):

$$NaCN \rightleftarrows Na^+ + CN^- \tag{1}$$

$$CN^- + HOH \rightleftarrows HCN + OH^- \tag{2}$$

HCN is a weak acid with a dissociation constant of $K_d = 7.2 \times 10^{-10}$ at 25°. As can be seen from Equation (2) a larger fraction of the cyanide will be present as CN^- at high pH whereas acidification will reverse the equilibrium. From the dissociation constant it can be calculated that at pH 7 about 99% of the cyanide is in the form of HCN while at pH 9.3 equal quantities of HCN and CN^- exist (Smith, 1976).

Since HCN is extremely soluble in water, acidification of dilute solutions of cyanide salts will not initiate any greater escape of HCN than normally occurs at the air-water interface. However, acidification of concentrated solutions will promote the formation of HCN with the ensuing escape of the gas phase above the solution.

Transition metals such as iron, nickel, cobalt, copper, zinc or silver form "ligand" bonds with cyanide to create *cyanide complexes* with quite different chemical and toxicological properties from the simple cyanides. In solution, these complexes form metallo-cyanide ions which can dissociate to yield further metal and cyanide ions. This is illustrated by the nickelocyanide complex in Equation (3).

$$[Ni(CN)_4]^{-2} \rightleftarrows NI^{++} + 4CN^- \tag{3}$$

The term *total cyanide*, which is often encountered in the literature on the quality of water, includes all cyanide-containing compounds such as simple and complex cyanides, cyanoglycosides and free cyanide. It is a measure of the free cyanide present in solution after release by acidification or digestion. Free cyanide (HCN) is the toxic form and the only biologically meaningful expression of cyanide toxicity.

II. TOXICITY TO FISH

At high concentrations, free cyanide rapidly kills aerobic organisms. The lethal toxicity of cyanide is, however, subject to several modifying factors related to the chemical state of the toxicant and/or the metabolic conditions of the organisms. The toxicity of cyanide to fish has long been established and it is generally agreed that the lethal level to various species of fish is in the range of 30 to 150 μg/l as HCN (Doudoroff, 1976).

Once in the general circulation, cyanide rapidly inhibits the electron transport chain of vital organs such as the heart, brain and the breathing apparatus. Fish rapidly show signs of distress, increase ventilation, come to the surface, gulp for air, swim frantically in circles with their snout out of the water. They later lose control and swim violently against the bottom or the sides of aquaria; in a lake or stream, fish are often seen swimming up onto the beach. Finally, they enter into convulsions and tremors, sink to the bottom and die with widely extended opercula.

Some harmful effects have been shown on fish at sublethal concentrations as low as 5 μg/l HCN. Information on the effects of cyanide on aquatic organisms other than fish is virtually non-existent.

Two important physiological functions are affected by cyanide poisoning: the respiratory chain by CN^- and the function of the thyroid gland by SCN^- resulting from detoxication by rhodanese. This enzyme is present in such large quantities in tissues that it is believed that the limiting factor in the conversion of HCN to SCN^- is mobilization and supply of sulfur. Given that rhodanese is present in fish and that the thyroid gland of fish function much the same way as in mammals, there are all reasons to believe that fish could develop goiter under chronic cyanide exposure as has been observed in humans (Bourdoux *et al.* 1978).

The results of various chronic toxicity tests of cyanide on fish carried out in our laboratory together with information from other sources are summarized in Fig. 1, which is a composite graph that illustrates in general the effects of cyanide at lethal and sublethal levels.

We have shown that cyanide could markedly reduce the performance of several physiological functions of fish tested in the laboratory, but it is difficult to arrive at an overall significant judgement as to the toxicity of cy-

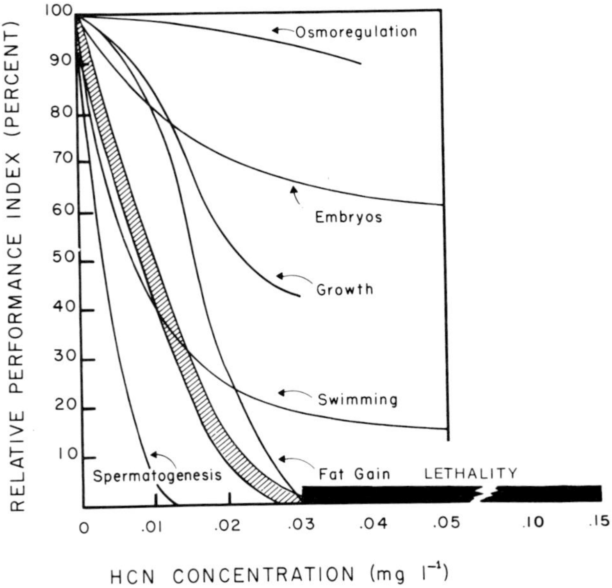

Fig. 1 Relative performance of fish measured on various physiological responses to long-term exposure to sublethal concentrations of cyanide. The sources of information for the different parameters are as follows: osmoregulation, Leduc and Chan (1975); Embryos, Leduc (1978); growth, Dixon and Leduc (1981); swimming, Neil (1957), Broderius, (1970), Speyer (1975); fat gain, Dixon and Leduc, (1981); spermatogenesis, Ruby *et al.*, (1979). The hatched tracing is a generalized estimate of the effects of cyanide on the overall performance or Relative Performance Index.

anide to fish unless one can synthesize various responses into one. Not all of the functions tested are of equal importance nor were they equally affected by cyanide. In an attempt to arrive at an overall evaluation of the chronic toxicity of cyanide, the approach taken by Warren *et al.* (1973) was followed. It consists in drawing on the same graph experimentally obtained relative performance curves plotted against test concentrations while giving a value of 100 to the controls. Performance curves have been plotted in Fig. 1 and a Relative Performance Index curve was then drawn, trying, to the best of our judgement, to integrate in one line (heavy trait) a generalized response curve to cyanide. The Relative Performance Index curve suggests a 50% reduction of total performance at 10 μg/l, and further suggests that even though fish could survive indefinitely at 30 μg/l HCN in the laboratory, the different physiological requirements necessary to survive in nature could not be met.

It is interesting to note that this concentration of 30 μg/l coincides exactly with the lower portion of the range of lethal concentrations of cyanide measured and reported by different authors. This range of 30 to 150 μg/l includes the lethal thresholds and median tolerance concentrations for most cold and warm water freshwater fishes. The concentration of 30 μg/l would then appear to coincide with the *incipient lethal concentration*, i.e. the concentration that cannot be tolerated indefinitely and ultimately causing death.

III. CYANIDE IN RIVER WATERS

Independent studies in Germany (Krutz, 1979) and in Canada (PPWB, 1978) have concluded that significant amounts of free cyanide occurring in streams of rural and wilderness areas is related to the size of the watershed and seasonal run-off. Krutz (1979) found mean annual values of about 3 μg/l (total cyanide) in rural watersheds as compared with 20 μg/l in industrial areas. In small watersheds covered with grasslands and forests but with no settlement, cyanide averaged between 0.7 to 2 μg/l with peak concentrations of approximately 5 μg/l occurring in the fall and winter seasons during the decomposition of fallen leaves. Larger rivers showed a different pattern in which cyanide was low in the winter due to dilution by high run-off but peaked in the summer as a result of production by plants.

The survey carried out in Canada (PPWB, 1978) from 1974 to 1977 looked at 11 rivers located in western and central parts of the country and included about 50 physical and chemical parameters. Although the data have not been systematically analysed as well as those obtained by Krutz (1979), several points are obvious. The water quality objective of 0.01 mg/l total cyanide is often exceeded by concentrations reaching 30 to 60 μg/l (total cyanide). The values vary considerably but seem related to discharge rates. In the small rivers (1,000 to 5,000 cubic feet/sec peaks of cyanide were more frequently observed in fall and winter during minimal run-off. In some rivers, pulses occurred in the spring and summer but before or after the annual spring peak run-off. In medium size rivers (5,000 to 25,000 cfs) the same relation seems to hold whereas in the larger rivers (15,000 to 75,000 cfs) the peak cyanide levels occurred during and/or after the May/June peak run-off. The latter observation agrees with the work done in Germany (Krutz, 1979).

It is important to point out that in these two studies, the cyanide levels were reported as total cyanide and not free cyanide. However, except for waters subjected to industrial discharges, where most of the total cyanide would exist as the less toxic metallo-complexes, it is reasonable to assume that total cyanide in wilderness and rural areas would represent free HCN measured as such.

These two reports of the biological/biochemical occurrence of cyanide in German and in Canadian waters raise two questions. First, how important is the human factor? Second, what are the effects on the biota?

In answer to the first question, the human influence is obvious in industrial cyanide pollution but the origin of cyanide in wilderness and rural watershed needs investigation. Answers to the second question as regards the effects (harmful, harmless or beneficial) of these sporadic changes in level of cyanide on stream-dwelling organisms in rural and wilderness areas vary depending on one's points of view.

Given the occasional high levels of cyanide (30 to 60 μg/l HCN) reported in Canadian streams by PPWB (1978) and the almost constant low levels (5 μg/l HCN) reported by PPWB and Krutz, how can fish populations survive in these streams?

The bulk of the literature on the aquatic toxicology of cyanide comes from tests carried out in the laboratory at fixed concentrations (for the duration of the tests) on fish that have never been subjected to cyanide. These three test conditions are obviously highly unrealistic compared to the natural environment.

Notwithstanding the difference between "wild" and "laboratory" fish, acclimation through continuous exposure to low levels of cyanide could enhance their resistance to potentially lethal concentrations (Doudoroff, 1976 p.48). On the other hand, low levels of cyanide which are harmful when applied constantly may well be harmless under seasonal variations which allow the organism to recover and/or to set up detoxification mechanisms. There is indeed laboratory evidence from our studies that fish eventually overcome growth retardation during chronic cyanide poisoning (Leduc, 1966; Dixon and Leduc, 1981).

Unless these questions of adaptive resistance to lethal levels of cyanide and/or the long term effects of discontinuous sublethal concentrations are verified, at least in the laboratory, it becomes very difficult to assess the effects of these seasonal pulses of cyanide on the biota. The simultaneous variation of other important environmental parameters such as oxygen, pH, and temperature also deserve attention.

One can ask whether low seasonal variations on the levels of cyanide might be beneficial. Given the high biological reactivity of cyanide and its seasonal appearance in natural (wilderness) watersheds, it appears unlikely that this chemical would have had no evolutionary influence on aquatic organisms. Low levels of cyanide, through its effects on the respiratory chain or indirectly as thiocyanate through the thyroid gland, could have a profound influence on some physiological functions of ecological significance yet to be discovered.

VI. CONCLUSIONS

We have seen earlier that cyanide is often present in river waters at levels which are known to be toxic under laboratory conditions. In view of the naturally occurring levels of cyanide, the assumption that extremely low levels of cyanide must be maintained at all times in order to protect aquatic life is not entirely defensible. However, we still maintain that cyanide levels in receiving waters should not exceed 5 μg/l in order to protect fish population from harmful sublethal effects. To protect fish population from acute lethal conditions cyanide levels should never exceed 30 μg/l as HCN.

These recommendations are based on laboratory evidence and do not take into consideration possible effects on organisms other than fish. Nor do they take into account the role of various modifying factors of toxicity that prevail in nature such as varying temperature, current, size of animals, water chemistry, adaptation, etc.

There is indeed growing evidence from our studies and from other sources that the toxicity of cyanide is profoundly influenced by variations in the metabolic rate of fish which in turn is affected by size, temperature, and activity (Kovacs, 1979; McCracken and Leduc, 1980). There is also evidence that low concentrations of cyanide can actually promote faster growth of fish (Negelski, 1973; McCracken and Leduc, 1980). Given the widespread occurrence of cyanide contamination of ground and surface waters research should be extended to explore the following problems:

(1) the sensitivity of benthic and planktonic organisms to cyanide;
(2) the role of current, size and temperature variations on the toxicity of cyanide to freshwater organisms;
(3) the natural occurrence of cyanide in wilderness and rural watersheds;
(4) the toxicity of cyanide to marine organisms to anticipate the effects of cyanide discharges at sea.

Information on the effects of cyanide on marine organisms is virtually non-existent.

REFERENCES

Bourdoux, P., Delange, F., Gérard, M., Mafuta, M., Hanson, A. and Ermans, A.M. (1978). Evidence that cassava ingestion increases thiocyanate formation: A possible etiologic factor in endemic goiter. *J. Clin. Endoc. and Meta.* 46, 613-621.

Broderius, S.J. (1979). Determination of molecular hydrocyanic acid in water and studies of the chemistry and toxicity to fish of the nickelocyanide complex. M.S. Thesis. Oregon State University, Corvallis. 93pp.

Dixon, D.G. and Leduc, G. (1981). Chronic cyanide poisoning of rainbow trout and its effect on growth, respiration and liver histopathology, *Arch. Environ. Toxicol.* 10, 117-131.

Doudoroff, P. (1976). Toxicity to fish of cyanides and related compounds; a review. Ecol. Res. Ser. EPA 600/3-76-038. Office of Res. and Devel., Environ. Res. Lab., U.S. Environmental Protection Agency, Duluth, Minn. vi + 154 pp.

Kovacs, T.G. (1979). The effect of temperature on cyanide toxicity to rainbow trout (*Salmo gairdneri*); Part I: acute toxicity, Part II: sublethal toxicity. M.S. Thesis. Concordia University, Montreal, 66 pp.

Krutz, H. (1979). Cyanverbindungen in Fliessgewässern - eine mathematische Beschreibung ihres raumzeitlichen Verhaltens und ihrer Wechselwirkungen zwischen Wasserkörper und Sediment - Veröff. des Instituts für Wasserforschung GmbH Dortmund und der Hydrol. Abt. der Dortmunder Stadtwerke AG, 28 Dortmund.

Leduc, G. (1966). Some physiological and biochemical responses of fish to chronic poisoning by cyanide. Ph.D. Thesis. Oregon State Univ., Corvallis, 146 pp.

Leduc, G. and Chan, K.S. (1975). The effects of chronic cyanide poisoning on the tolerance of rainbow trout to varying salinity. *In* "Water Pollution Research in Canada", (T.C. Hutchinson, ed), vol. X, pp.118-125.

Leduc, G. (1978). Deleterious effects of cyanide on early life stages of Atlantic salmon (*Salmo salar*). *J. Fish. Res. Bd. Can.* 35, 166-174.

McCracken, I.R. and Leduc, G. (1980). The allometric growth response of exercised rainbow trout (*Salmo gairdneri*) to cyanide poisoning. Aquatic Toxicology, ASTM, STP 107, Philadelphia, pp.303-320.

Negilsky, D.S. (1973). Individual and combined effects of cyanide, pentachlorophenol and zinc on junvenile chinook salmon and invertebrates in model stream communities. M.S. Thesis. Oregon State University, Corvallis, 80 pp.

Neil, J.H. (1957). Some effects of potassium cyanide on speckled trout *Salvelinus fontinalis*. Pp. 74-96 *in* Papers presented at the 4th Ontario Industrial Waste Conference, Honey Harbor, Ontario. Waste and Poll. Advisory Comm., Ontario Water Resources Comm., Toronto. 156 pp.

PPWB (Prairie Provinces Water Board). (1978). Interprovincial river water quality data at PPWB monitoring stations. April 1974 to December 31, 1977, Regina, Sask.

Ruby, S.M., Dixon, D.G. and Leduc, G. (1979). Inhibition of spermatogenesis in rainbow trout during chronic cyanide poisoning. *Arch. Environm. Contam. Toxicol.* 8, 533-544.

Speyer, M.R. (1975). Some effects of chronic combined arsenic and cyanide poisoning on the physiology of rainbow trout. M.Sc. Thesis. Sir George Williams Campus, Concordia University, Montreal. 76 pp.

Smith, N.B. (1976). Sources and treatment of cyanides in iron and steel industry wastewaters. *Dechema-monographien-cisti.* 80, 159-177.

THE GENETIC CONTROL OF PLANT CYANOGENESIS

MONICA A. HUGHES

Department of Genetics, Ridley Building, The University, Newcastle upon Tyne NE1 7RU, England

I. THE GENETIC CONTROL OF PLANT CYANIDE PRODUCTION

All the cyanogenic plant species, which have been investigated in any detail, show variation in the amount of hydrogen cyanide (HCN) produced. This may reflect either variation in the amount of cyanoglucoside in the tissue examined or variation in the activity of a hydrolytic enzyme.

Variation has been reported within individual plants depending on the type of tissue tested, the size and age of the plant and the cultural conditions. Sinha and Nair (1968) show that the rind of cassava tubers may contain three times the amount of cyanoglucoside of the cortex tissue. Rogers and Frykolm (1937) report an increase in the cyanogenic reaction, as measured with the picrate test, with increasing size of white clover plants. A quantitative measurement of cyanoglucoside content shows that decreasing the cultural temperature from 27°C to 19°C increases the cyanoglucoside content of white clover leaves from the same plant by 50% (Hughes, unpublished).

Environmental differences will also produce variation between individual plants. In 21 day old flax (*Linum usitatissimum L.*) seedlings, changing the light intensity from 1,000 to 2,500 foot candles, doubles the cyanoglucoside content of the shoots (Trione, 1960). There are also reports (Nass, 1972) of inherited variation between plants in hydrocyanic acid production. This variation is due to differences in the genotype of plants. Trione (1960) reports 400 ppm HCN in seedling shoots of the flax variety Punjab 47 and 130 ppm HCN in shoots of the variety Rio, when both varieties were grown in a uniform environment. Interaction between the genotype and the environment is another source of variation in cyanide production between plants.

In some species of plants the variation is discrete in that populations may contain plants which are cyanogenic and plants which produce no detectable HCN (acyanogenic plants). These polymorphic species include *Trifolium repens L* (Williams, 1939), *Lotus tenuis* Waldst. and Kit.

(Dawson, 1941) and *Lotus corniculatus L* (Dawson, 1941). Recently Fikenscher and Hegnauer (1977) have reported a number of other species that are polymorphic for cyanogenesis. These include *Taxus baccata L.*, two *Achillea* species and three *Campanula* species. Amongst the cyanogenic plants of these species there is continuous inherited variation in the amount of cyanide produced (Corkill, 1942; Dawson, 1941) and this variation is also found in those species which are not polymorphic.

Most of the studies on the variation in cyanide production by non-polymorphic species have been made in *Sorghum* species. *Sorghum sudanese* (Piper) Stapf. (sudan grass) and *Sorghum bicolor* (L.) Moench (grain sorghum) both produce dhurrin which is broken down by a β-glucosidase and an oxynitrilase to give *p*-hydroxybenzaldehyde and hydrocyanic acid. Authors differ in their conclusions about the number of genes involved and about the dominance relationships of the alleles of these genes. Snyder (1950) concluded that one gene determined high versus low HCN production in sudangrass, with low-HCN-production dominant. Barnett and Caviness (1968) showed that in grain sorghum x sudangrass hybrids the inheritance of HCN production was multigenic with high-HCN-production dominant. Estimates of heritability have been made in grain sorghum using plants up to 18 days old (Eck *et al.*, 1975). The measurement of narrow sense heritability (ratio of additive genetic variance to total phenotypic variance) decreased as plants aged, indicating little likelihood that significant changes in the HCN content of older hybrid plants could be made by selecting their parents on the basis of the HCN content of the seedling. On the other hand, the estimate of broad sense heritability (ratio of total genetic variance to phenotypic variance) was high for all ages indicating that significant genetic advance from selection among pure lines or hybrids could still be expected. Broad sense heritability includes variance due to dominance.

The basic genetic details of the inheritance of the cyanogenic character in *Trifolium repens* (white clover) were elucidated by Corkill (1942). White clover produces two related glucosides, linamarin and lotaustralin, and HCN is released when these are hydrolysed by a β-glucosidase, since the aglycones are unstable. There is no evidence for an oxynitrilase in white clover. The inheritance of cyanogenesis is diploid in white clover. Plants which possess at least one functional allele of a gene, designated *Ac*, produce both glucosides, and plants with two non-functional alleles (*ac ac*) produce no measurable glucoside. Similarly, white clover plants with at least one functional allele of a gene designated *Li*, produce the β-glucosidase (linamarase) and plants with two non-functional alleles (*li li*) and have no measurable linamarase activity. The gene *Li* segregates independently, and is probably on a different chromosome, from the gene *Ac*. Only plants with at least one functional allele of both genes are cyanogenic and contain both the cyanoglucosides and linamarase in their leaf tissue. However, the presence of either enzyme or glucoside in an acyanogenic plant may be shown by adding the appropriate extract to the tested leaf tissue (Table I).

Table 1 Picrate test (Guignard, 1906) for hydrocyanic acid production by *Trifolium repens* L.

Genotype	Test: leaf + glucoside	Test: leaf + linamarase	Phenotype
Li Li Ac Ac	+	+	cyanogenic
Li li Ac ac	+	+	cyanogenic
li li Ac Ac	-	+	acyanogenic
li li Ac ac	-	+	acyanogenic
Li Li ac ac	+	-	acyanogenic
Li li ac ac	+	-	acyanogenic
li li ac ac	-	-	acyanogenic

(+) = HCN release; (-) = no HCN release

The inheritance of cyanogenesis has also been studied in the polymorphic species *Lotus corniculatus*. *L. corniculatus* produces linamarin and lotaustralin and, similar to *Trifolium repens*, four phenotypes can be recognised (Jones 1977). The original study was made by Dawson (1941), who only recognised two phenotypes, cyanogenic and acyanogenic. It would appear from his data that he was studying the segregation of alleles of a single gene and since absence of either the glucoside or the hydrolytic enzyme gives rise to the acyanogenic phenotype we cannot know whether he was looking at the segregation of a gene controlling enzyme production or glucoside production. Dawson's data fit a pattern of tetrasomic inheritance and this was confirmed by Bansal (1966). However, the genetic data for the cyanogenic polymorphism in *Lotus corniculatus* is not as satisfactory as that for white clover and more work should be done with this species.

Within the limits of resolution possible in white clover genetic studies the units *Ac* and *Li* have been considered as single genes. A number of studies have been aimed at providing information about the nature of these genetic units. Table II (Maher and Hughes, 1973) shows the level of β-glucosidase and β-galactosidase activity in a number of plants. Plants with the genotype *li li* have no activity against the natural substrate, linamarin, and have low activity against the synthetic substrates *p*-nitrophenyl-β-D-glucoside and *p*-nitrophenyl-β-D-galactoside.

Table II Specific activities of crude leaf extracts of white clover plants

Plant	Genotype[b]	Mean Specific Activity[a] (± SE) against the Substrates		
		Linamarin-Lotaustralin	*p*-Nitrophenyl β-D-glucoside	*p*-Nitrophenyl β-D-galactoside
CS	Li Li	2.58 ± 0.23	3.44 ± 0.16	2.07 ± 0.10
C2	Li Li	2.35 ± 0.16	3.55 ± 0.18	1.94 ± 0.08
C3	Li li	0.60 ± 0.02	1.18 ± 0.03	0.65 ± 0.04
C4	Li li	0.93 ± 0.04	1.60 ± 0.01	0.86 ± 0.03
C5	Li li	0.64 ± 0.04	1.14 ± 0.04	0.64 ± 0.02
C7	Li li	1.20 ± 0.06	1.99 ± 0.06	1.07 ± 0.04
C11	Li li	0.20 ± 0.01	0.57 ± 0.02	0.37 ± 0.03
C14	Li li	1.31 ± 0.03	2.21 ± 0.03	1.26 ± 0.05
D4	li li	0	0.16 ± 0.01	0.19 ± 0.003
D9	li li	0	0.31 ± 0.01	0.21 ± 0.01

[a] micromoles substrate hydrolysed per mg of protein in 10 min.

[b] all plants *ac ac*.

The absence of enzyme inhibitors in these *li li* plants can easily be shown by experiments where leaf extracts are mixed. The heterozygous plants *Li li* have levels of activity intermediate between the homozygotes *li li* and *Li Li*. Thus although the *Li* allele is scored as dominant with the picrate test, the level of β-glucosidase activity in the plant depends on the number of *Li* alleles present. A similar result can be seen when the *Ac* allele is studied in relation to the quantity of the two cyanoglucosides produced in the leaf (Table III, Hughes, unpublished data). That is, the amount of cyanoglucoside per mg soluble leaf protein is related to the number of functional *Ac* alleles present.

Table III Cyanoglucoside content of crude leaf extracts of white clover plants

Plant	Genotype[(b)]	Cyanoglucoside content[(a)]
84B	Ac Ac	0.310
6B	Ac Ac	0.377
20B	Ac Ac	0.230
45B	Ac Ac	0.321
44B	Ac Ac	0.394
5B	Ac Ac	0.307
71B	Ac Ac	0.358
204B	Ac ac	0.156
197B	Ac ac	0.183
83B	Ac ac	0.170
85B	Ac ac	0.158
226B	Ac ac	0.051
261B	Ac ac	0.170
90B	ac ac	0
4D	ac ac	0
9D	ac ac	0
242D	ac ac	0

[(a)] micromoles of cyanoglucoside per mg soluble protein

[(b)] all plants *li li*.

If the *li* allele is not responsible for the production of an inhibitor, we may consider two possible alternatives for the nature of the *Li* gene. Firstly, it may be the site specifying the structure of linamarase or secondly, it may represent a site which controls the synthesis of the enzyme. Our first approach was to look for immunological evidence for the structural gene hypothesis. Table IV (Hughes and Maher, 1973) shows levels of enzyme activity and levels of β-glycosidase antigen in a number

Table IV Adsorption of β-glucosidase antibodies with crude leaf extracts of various strains of white clover

Plant	Genotype	Units of enzyme activity in extract[a]	Units of antibody adsorbed[b]
CS	Li Li	62.6	59.0
EDT36	li li	6.8	12.0
EDT5	li li	0.4	10.0
L50	li li	4.6	7.3
L44	li li	3.3	5.9
L35	li li	5.0	7.5
L34	li li	1.1	15.8
DWW1	li li	8.3	10.8
DWW2	li li	4.4	10.0
DWW3	li li	3.1	9.3
DWW4	li li	2.7	9.0
S18436	li li	6.1	9.0
S18427	li li	3.4	4.6
S18414	li li	2.4	5.0

[a] mμmoles of *p*-nitrophenyl β-D-glucoside hydrolysed in 10 min.

[b] Increase in activity over control in which the serum was pre-incubated with buffer.

of plants containing only *li li* alleles compared with the levels of enzyme activity and antigen in a *Li Li* plant. If the *li* allele represents a mutation in a structural gene then we might find a particular *li* allele which represents a mutation which has altered the enzyme active site but not changed its immunological properties. Such mutants have been characterised in a number of microorganisms. The figures in Table IV however show that the level of antigen in each *li li* plant is equivalent to the level of enzyme activity. In other words there was no evidence for a structurally altered enzyme protein in any of these plants and the data thus provides no evidence for or against a structural *Li* gene.

This work illustrates one major problem in the analysis of the nature of the genes controlling the white clover cyanogenic polymorphism. The plants shown in Table IV were selected from a wide range of commercial varieties in an attempt to screen a number of independent *li* producing mutations, but since the *li* alleles have come from natural populations and not been produced in the laboratory we cannot know how many independent mutations there are. In other words all the plants in Table IV may contain the same mutation. Further all the *li* alleles must have been subject to selection and may not represent a single mutation.

A second approach was to look for a plant containing linamarase with a different physical property and study the segregation of this property together with the segregation of *Li*/*li* alleles in test cross progeny. If all the *Li* progeny have an enzyme with this abnormal physical property one can say that the *Li* locus or a closely linked site is responsible for the enzyme structure. Conversely if the presence of high enzyme activity (*Li* progeny) and the abnormal physical property segregate we can say that the *Li* locus does not specify the enzyme structure. No physically abnormal linamarase has been found in white clover but Table II shows one plant (C11) which has a very low level of enzyme activity apparently caused by the production of small amounts of enzyme. This plant, which was heterozygous (*Li li*), was crossed to a homozygous *li li* plant and the progeny segregating for *Li*/*li* were tested for levels of enzyme activity (Maher and Hughes, 1973). Table V shows linamarase activity in *Li li* progeny of C11 compared with the activity of *Li li* progeny from two plants having normal amounts of enzyme. The figures show that the *Li* allele and low linamarase activity are inherited together and this suggests that the gene *Li* controls the amount of enzyme produced by leaf tissue.

This conclusion has been supported by later work which shows that at least two *li li* plants produce no linamarase protein. The cyanogenic β-glucosidase in white clover represents about 5% of the total protein in a crude buffer extract of leaf acetone powder. By following linamarase activity, I have purified the enzyme by molecular exclus-

Table V Specific activities of crude extracts of the progeny from crosses involving white clover plants C7, C11 and C14

Parents	Genotype of progeny[b]	No. of progeny analysed	Mean specific activity[a] (± SE) against		
			Linamarin-Lotaustralin	*p*-nitrophenyl β-D-glucoside	*p*-nitrophenyl β-D-galactoside
C7 x D4	Li li	20	1.52 ± 0.05	2.23 ± 0.06	1.35 ± 0.04
	li li	20	0	0.27 ± 0.01	0.18 ± 0.01
C11 x D4	Li li	18	0.22 ± 0.01	0.51 ± 0.03	0.32 ± 0.002
	li li	10	0	0.15 ± 0.01	0.17 ± 0.01
C14 x D4	Li li	16	1.22 ± 0.05	1.84 ± 0.06	1.08 ± 0.04
	li li	9	0	0.24 ± 0.02	0.17 ± 0.02

[a] Micromoles substrate hydrolysed per mg protein in 10 min.

[b] All plants *ac ac*.

ion chromatography on Sephadex G200, followed by ion exchange chromatography on CM cellulose. The product exhibited one major protein and one minor protein on SDS acrylamide gel electrophoresis (Hughes, unpublished). In fact the major band was converted into the minor band on freezing and thawing the sample. The major band is visible in SDS acrylamide gels of crude extracts and of semi-purified preparations from plants which contain the *Li* allele and linamarase activity, and is absent from plants with no linamarase activity and only nonfunctional *li* alleles (Fig. 1, Hughes, unpublished data). Plant C11, which has low linamarase activity also has a reduced band after electrophoresis on SDS acrylamide gel.

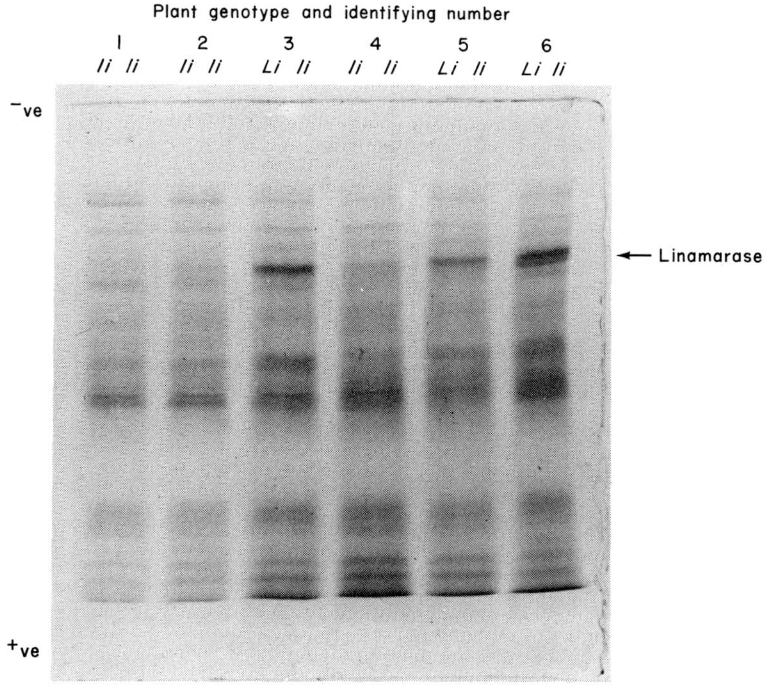

Fig. 1 SDS Acrylamide gel electrophoresis of semi-purified leaf extracts from white clover. Plants from a segregating backcross progeny produced by crossing CS (*Li Li*) and D9 (*li li*) then backcrossing a F1 heterozygote (*Li li*) on to D9 (*li li*). Plants 3, 5 and 6 had linamarase activity in their leaves and gave a positive picrate reaction when tested with a glucoside test solution. Plants 1, 2 and 4 were picrate negative in this test and had no linamarase activity. The plant extracts were produced by molecular exclusion chromatography (Sephadex G200 in 0.2 M tris maleate pH 5.6) of an acetone powder buffer extract. The same column fractions taken for each plant extract, and each pressure dialysed (Diaflo XM50 ultraflo filter) to reduce the volume. A 10% SDS acrylamide gel was run in trisglycine buffer pH 8.6 and stained with Coomasie blue.

The function of the locus *Ac*, controlling cyanoglucoside production, has been investigated in a study (Hughes and Conn, 1976) designed to determine which step in the biosynthesis of linamarin and lotaustralin is affected by this gene. When ^{14}C-valine is fed to cyanoglucoside positive (S100) white clover plants, the ^{14}C is incorporated into linamarin. No synthesis of ^{14}C-linamarin occurs in ^{14}C-valine-fed cyanoglucoside-negative (DWW) plants. Table VI shows the incorporation of ^{14}C from labelled isobutyraldoxime into linamarin. About 2.5% of the aldoxime was converted into linamarin in the cyanoglucoside positive S100 plants whilst no ^{14}C-linamarin was found in the cyanoglucoside negative DWW plants. In other words some step

Table VI Incorporation of ^{14}C-isobutyradloxime into linamarin in white clover

Plant	Cyanoglucoside Content[(a)]	U-^{14}C isobutyraldoxime administered (μCi)	Converted to linamarin (%)
S100-1	2.60	0.90	2.4
S100-1	2.60	0.90	2.5
S100-10	2.44	0.90	2.0
S100-10	2.44	0.90	2.6
DWW-1	0	0.90	0
DWW-1	0	0.90	0
DWW-3	0	0.90	0
DWW-3	0	0.90	0

[(a)] Micromoles per 100 mg fresh weight, first expanded leaf.

after isobutyraldoxime is missing in the cyanoglucoside negative plants. Table VII shows the results of an experiment in which ^{14}C-valine was fed to the two phenotypes in the presence of cold isobutyraldoxime, which traps the ^{14}C if the isobutyraldoxime is a biosynthetic intermediate in the plant. In cyanoglucoside-positive (S100) plants, about 0.5% of the radioactivity was trapped as isobutyraldoxime but no radioactivity was found in this fraction in the cyanoglucoside negative (DWW) plants. This demonstrates that some step before isobutyraldoxime is missing in the DWW plants. The conclusion of these feeding experiments must be that in these plants, at least two steps in the cyanoglucoside biosynthetic pathway are missing.

If two of the enzyme activities involved in the biosynthesis of linamarin and lotaustralin are missing in *ac ac* plants, then there are several possible hypotheses for the nature of this genetic unit. The locus may specify the structure of two separate enzyme polypeptides or it may control the synthesis of the whole biosynthetic pathway (or at least several steps in the pathway). An alternative

Table VII Incorporation of ^{14}C-valine into linamarin in white clover shoots treated with isobutyraldoxime

Plant	Cyanoglucoside content[a]	Fresh Weight (g)	Isobutyraldoxime administered (μmoles)	U-^{14}C-valine administered (μCi)	% converted to linamarin	% trapped as isobutyraldoxime
S100-1	2.60	1.5	43.2	3.68	2.9	0.3
S100-10	2.44	0.6	21.6	1.84	3.5	0.7
DWW-1	0	1.3	43.2	3.68	0	0
DWW-3	0	0.7	21.6	1.84	0	0

[a] Micromoles per 100 mg fresh weight, first expanded leaf.

hypothesis arises from the demonstration by McFarlane *et al.* (1975) that, in sorghum, a microsomal fraction catalyses the synthesis of *p*-hydroxymandelonitrile *in vitro*. If cyanoglucoside biosynthesis in white clover involves a membrane bound or particulate system, then it is possible that the loss or alteration of a single polypeptide, essential to the functional integrity of the system, would lead to the lack of more than one step in the cyanoglucoside biosynthetic pathway. In this case the *Ac* locus may represent the structural gene for a single protein.

A long-term study of several aspects of the inheritance of different levels of cyanoglucoside synthesis in white clover has been carried out (Hughes, unpublished). A number of *Ac Ac li li* plants were selected which contained different amounts of cyanoglucoside in their leaves. These plants were crossed to the same acyanogenic *ac ac li li* plant (D4). The heterozygous *Ac ac li li* progeny from each cross were again backcrossed to the *ac ac li li* plant (D4) to produce several second backcross progenies which segregate for the alleles of *Ac*. A number of second generation backcross *Ac ac li li* heterozygotes from each original parent were further backcrossed to D4 to produce the third backcross generation, and the crossing programme was repeated to produce a fourth and fifth backcross generation. In each generation the functional *Ac* allele has been selected and crossed on to a single recurring *ac ac* plant.

In an inbreeding species this procedure can be expected to produce lines in which different *Ac* alleles have been crossed into the same genetic background. White clover however is an outbreeding species, with a gametophytic incompatability system and two features of the breeding system mean that isogenic lines different only in the *Ac* allele cannot be produced in this way. Firstly, the incompatability system means that at each generation one S allele from the cyanoglucoside positive parent is selected as well as the *Ac* allele. Secondly, white clover plants are heterozygous at many loci and there will therefore be segregation for the heterozygous genes of D4 at each generation.

Despite this, the data from these crosses illustrate that the amount of cyanoglucoside produced by plants containing functional *Ac* alleles is inherited. Figure 2 shows the cyanoglucoside content of the first generation *Ac ac* plants plotted against the mean cyanoglucoside content of their second generation *Ac ac* progeny. A clear relationship between the level of cyanoglucoside in the parent (1st generation) and the mean level in the progeny (2nd generation) can be seen in this figure. The 1st generation plants shown in Fig. 2 were derived from 3 homozygous *Ac Ac* plants; plant 750 had a high level, plant 296 had a low level and plant 272 had an intermediate level of cyanoglucosides. Figure 2 also shows that the mean 1st generation cyanoglucoside content for 296 is lower than the mean for the offspring of 750. The 1st generation progeny of the plant 272 which was intermediate, show segregation for high *versus* low cyanoglucoside content. Further the "high" 1st generation plants gave rise to "high" second generation offspring and *vice versa* for the "low" plants.

This figure shows that the amount of cyanoglucoside produced by *Ac* containing plants is inherited. This figure also provides some evidence that the level of cyanoglucoside produced may be partly determined by the *Ac* allele itself since the simplest interpretation of the results of plant 272 is that it contained two functional *Ac* alleles, one determining high levels of production (Ac^{high}), the other low (Ac^{low}) and thus had an intermediate glucoside content. Each heterozygous 1st generation offspring will inherit just one allele, either Ac^{high} or Ac^{low}, which will be passed into the 2nd generation progeny giving the pattern of segregation seen in Fig. 2.

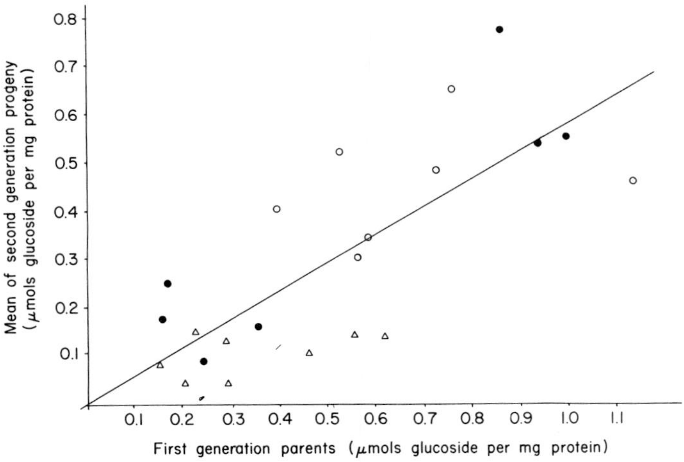

Fig. 2 A comparison of the cyanoglucoside content of white clover leaves from heterozygous first generation parents and their heterozygous second generation backcross progeny. All plants are *Ac ac li li*, progeny of 296 = △ , progeny of 750 = ○, progeny of 272 = ● , line of best fit = y = 0.579 x, correlation coefficient (r) = 0.78.

The conclusion that there are different *Ac* alleles is supported by the fact that differences between the progeny of 750 and 296 are maintained in the 5th backcross generation and analysis of variance shows that they are significant at the 0.005 level (750 mean = 0.166 μmoles glucoside/mg protein, 296 mean = 0.053 μmoles glucoside/mg protein). Although the 5th generation plants are by no means isogenic the variation in glucoside content, between plants with the same *Ac* allele, has decreased compared with the 2nd generation. Following the inbreeding of the crossing programme, all plants show a general reduction in the glucoside content which is restored on outcrossing the fourth generation.

REFERENCES

Bansal, R.D. (1966). Studies on procedures for combining clones of Birdsfoot Trefoil, *Lotus corniculatus* L. Ph.D. Thesis. Cornell University, U.S.A.

Barnett, R.D. and Caviness, C.E. (1968). *Crop Sci.* 8, 89-91.

Corkill, L. (1942). *N.Z.J. Sci. Technol. (Ser. B)*. 23, 178-193.

Dawson, C.D.R. (1941). *J. Genetics* 42, 49-72.

Eck, H.V., Gilmore, E.C., Ferguson, D.B. and Wilson, G.C. (1975). *Crop Sci.* 15, 421-424.

Fikenscher, L.H. and Hegnauer, R. (1977). *Pharm. Weekbl. Ned.* 112, 11-14.

Guiguard, M.L. (1906). *Compt. Rend.* 142, 545-553.

Hughes, M.A. and Maher, E.P. (1973). *Biochem. Genet.* 8, 1-12.

Hughes, M.A. and Conn, E.E. (1976). *Phytochemistry* 15, 697-701.

Jones, D.A. (1977). *Heredity* 39, 27-44.

Maher, E.P. and Hughes, M.A. (1973). *Biochem. Genet.* 8, 13-26.

McFarlane, I.J., Lees, E.M. and Conn, E.E. (1975). *J. Biol. Chem.* 250, 4708-4713.

Nass, H.G. (1972). *Crop Sci.* 12, 503-506.

Rogers, C.F. and Frykolm, O.C. (1937). *J. Agr. Res.* 55, 533-537.

Sinha, S.K. and Nair, T.V.R. (1968). *Indian J. Agri. Sci.* 38, 958-963.

Snyder, F.B. (1950). Inheritance and association of hydrocyanic acid potential, disease reactions and other characters in sudangrass. Ph.D. Thesis. University of Wisconsin, Madison, U.S.A.

CYANIDE AND COEVOLUTION

DAVID A. JONES

Unit of Genetics, University of Hull, Hull HU6 7RX, England

I. INTRODUCTION

For a long time entomologists have puzzled over how female insects choose the plants on which to lay their eggs. Early casual observations suggested that females littered their eggs over vegetation in a haphazard way, some laying clusters of eggs, others like the Northern Eggar moth (*Lasiocampa quercus callunae* (Palmer)) dropping their eggs as they fly. That there was some understanding of food plant preferences is evident from the names *Pieris brassicae* (L.), *Strymonidia pruni* (L.) and *Aglais urticae* (L.), but even then it was thought that the larvae which survived were those hatching from eggs fortuitously laid on the correct food plant.

Careful observations showed that although a female butterfly may settle on plants of many different species during the course of a day she lays her eggs on only a few species or, indeed, on only one species of plant. By rearing the larvae found on a particular plant species it is easy to compile a list of food plant preferences for most of the lepidoptera.

How do these female insects know which is the right plant? The relation between the insect, the odour of the food plant and plant chemistry was first pointed out by Verschaffelt (1910) when studying the relationship between the *Pieris* genus of butterflies and the mustard-oil glycosides (glucosinolates) produced by their *Brassica* L. food plants. Dethier (1937, 1941) later showed the relationship between *Danaus plexippus* (L.) and the odour produced by *Asclepias* L. species and between *Papilio* (L.) species and various Umbelliferae.

Painter (1936, 1951) meanwhile had been considering the resistance of plants to insect attack, arguing that plants could gain protection by developing defence mechanisms that would interfere with the utilisation of their tissues as food by insects.

These two approaches were combined, tentatively by Dethier (1954) and more forcefully by Fraenkel (1959), who argued that "the examples cited of insects specific to plants of the families Umbelliferae, Leguminosae, Solanaceae, Moraceae and Gramineae clearly demonstrated the function of secondary substances in these plants as means of repelling or attracting insects". Taking this further, Ehrlich and Raven (1964) developed the concept of coevolution (a term borrowed subconsciously (?) from Mode (1958)) as follows:

The fortuitous production of secondary compounds by some plants has been favoured because it makes them less palatable to their original herbivores. Some of these herbivores have, by chance, coevolved methods of detoxifying or sequestering the plant defence compounds. Such an animal is placed at an enormous selective advantage because it escapes from the competitive situation pertaining on plants not so protected that are being eaten by other phytophagous species. There is, in consequence, very strong selection for any mechanism that enables the coevolved herbivore to detect the protected plant. The suggestions are that the mechanisms involved are partly visual and partly olfactory (e.g. Gilbert, 1975; Rothschild and Schoonhoven, 1977; Chew, 1977).

Although an eminently reasonable hypothesis it is extremely difficult in practice to demonstrate that a particular secondary compound in a plant has a defensive function. The difficulty has been explained by Jones (1971) as follows: If a plant is monomorphic for a secondary compound, how do you know that a putative herbivore could and would eat that plant if the secondary compound were not present? If the plant is polymorphic for the production of the secondary compound and herbivores preferentially eat the forms lacking the secondary substance or, alternatively, if the degree of herbivory is related negatively to the concentration of the secondary compound then we will have proved beyond reasonable doubt that the secondary substance does have a protective function.

II. CYANOGENESIS AND PLANT DEFENCE

The suggestion that cyanogenesis may have a protective function was first suggested by Stahl (1888) and hinted at by Corkill (1952) and by Daday (1955), but the first clear demonstration was by Jones (1962) who found that some mollusc species preferentially ate the acyanogenic form when offered a choice between cyanogenic and acyanogenic *Lotus corniculatus* L. Furthermore, there was a negative correlation between the amount of HCN released by cyanogenic plants (from linamarin and lotaustralin) and the quantity of the plant consumed. Angseesing and Angseesing (1973) subsequently demonstrated selective grazing of the acyanogenic form of *Trifolium repens* L. in a semi-natural situation outside the laboratory.

Woodhead and Bernays (1978) found a correlation between the concentration of HCN released when *Sorghum bicolor* (L). Moench (grain sorghum) is bitten by *Locusta migrator-*

ia(L.) and the unpalatability of individual sorghum plants to the locust. During this work they showed that it was not the cyanoglucoside itself (dhurrin) which was the deterrent. Mallmaire (1949) has suggested that because of the resistance of cassava, *Manihot esculenta* Crantz, to the migratory locust, cassava production became popular in many areas of Africa. Perhaps it is cyanogenesis which is the basis of this resistance. Other experiments with the African grasshopper *Zonocerus variegatus* (L.) and cassava *M. esculenta* led Bernays *et al.* (1977) to the conclusion that the grasshopper is normally deterred from eating cassava by the production of relatively large amounts of HCN (from linamarin). They are also convinced that the rate of release of the HCN is important.

Another example of the protective function of cyanogenesis is in the bracken fern *Pteridium aquilinum* (L.) Kuhn. In Richmond Park, Surrey, England, most of the individuals contain both prunasin and the corresponding β-glucosidase and so are cyanogenic. In some patches of plants the proportions of the acyanogenic form could be as high as 98% and Cooper-Driver and Swain (1976) found that the fronds in these areas were heavily grazed by deer and by sheep. Further examination revealed that where there was a proportion nearer to equality of the two types of plant, only fronds from the acyanogenic form were eaten. This selection of acyanogenic bracken by sheep is very puzzling because sheep show no preference for acyanogenic as opposed to cyanogenic white clover, *Trifolium repens* (Corkill, 1952), tolerating a daily intake equivalent of 15-50mg HCN/kg (Coop and Blakley, 1949).

There is a negative correlation between the number of species of insect found on bracken and the HCN content of the fronds (Lawton, 1976) and so it appears that cyanogenesis may be acting as a deterrent. The complication is that the young croziers and fronds contain a higher concentration of prunasin than old fronds, the measurable HCN produced by any particular plant declining from mid-May to mid-October. Lawton (1978) has argued that it may not be the decline in the HCN content of the fronds that allows more insect species to exploit the bracken, but rather it is the increase in the number of microhabitats available, resulting from the change in the architecture of the plant as it matures. Although this interpretation is of great interest to ecologists, the relevant question in the context of the present article is why bracken is able to dispense with one of its defensive substances as it matures.

Bracken is not the only plant to behave in this way. Eck *et al.* (1975) found that the concentration of available HCN in 10 day-old seedlings of *Sorghum bicolor* was much higher than in 14 and 18 day-old seedlings, although there were great differences between the cultivars tested. Exactly the same pattern was found with flax, *Linum usitatissimum* L. (Trione, 1960). It may be that selection has favoured the protection of the juvenile stages of *P.*

aquilinum, *S. bicolor* and *L. usitatissimum*, but there comes a point during the development of the plant at which the 'cost' of losing plant material by herbivory ceases to exceed the 'capital expenditure' necessary to maintain the protection. At this stage the protective mechanism is effectively redundant and may be lost.

Similarly, the evergreen chaparral shrub *Heteromeles* (syn. *Photinia* Lindl.) *arbutifolia* M. Roem. has a high concentration of the cyanoglucoside prunasin in young leaves in the spring when herbivore pressure is high. The cyanoglucoside concentration falls as summer progresses and this corresponds with a decline in herbivore pressure and also with reduced availability of nitrogen. In the autumn, however, there is a resurgence of cyanoglucoside synthesis and Dement and Mooney (1974) suggest that this may be related to the increase in herbivore pressure on *H. arbutifolia* known to occur at that time of the year (Swan, 1952).

III. CYANIDE AND COEVOLUTION

I have argued elsewhere (Jones, 1979) that because plants and animals require a source of small quantities of cyanide for primary metabolism, and also a means of detoxifying excess cyanide, the evolution of cyanogenesis as a 'macro' phenomenon is readily understandable in terms of a change in the regulation of the biosynthetic pathways involved. On the other hand, so many species which are not cyanogenic are capable of metabolizing exogenous HCN that it appears likely that HCN commonly occurs in plants and in animals and needs to be detoxified. Consequently, changes in the regulation of the synthesis of the existing enzymes involved in cyanide metabolism would enable animals to graze cyanogenic plants or predate (or parasitise) cyanogenic animals.

Thus, given that cyanogenesis does have a defensive function in some plants, an ability to detoxify or be in some other way tolerant of HCN must be the coevolutionary response of would-be herbivores or parasites of cyanogenic plants. With *Lotus corniculatus*, for instance, there are now numerous examples. The larvae of the Common Blue butterfly *Polyommatus icarus* (Rott.) and the weevil *Hypera plantaginis* (Degeer) detoxify HCN using rhodanese (Parsons and Rothschild, 1964). The leaf-spotting pathogen, *Stemphylium loti* Graham uses an HCN induced formamide hydro-lyase that converts HCN to formamide (H $CONH_2$) (Fry and Millar, 1972). Fry and Evans (1977) have shown this to be a general characteristic of fungal pathogens of cyanogenic plants (see also Fry and Myers, this volume).

Perhaps the longest chain is *Lotus corniculatus*, *Zygaena filipendulae* (L.) *Apanteles zygaeranum* (Marshall) and *Mesochorus temporalis* (Thompson). *L. corniculatus* is a cyanogenic species, the larvae of *Z. filipendulae* graze *L. corniculatus* and are also cyanogenic, *A. zygaenarum* is an internal parasite of *Zygaena* species and can detoxify HCN, whereas *M. temporalis* is an endoparasite of *A. zygaenarum* and contains neither cyanogenic substances nor detoxifying enzymes (Jones *et al.*, 1962). Cyanogenesis in *Z. filipendulae* is now known to be based on the cyanoglucosides linamarin and lotaustralin (Davis and Nahrstedt, 1979).

It should be clear from these few examples that we would expect a herbivore or indeed any parasite of a cyanogenic plant to be capable of metabolizing the HCN produced, but frequently the actual mechanism is not known. Trione (1960), for example, found no correlation between the resistance to flax rust (*Fusarium oxysporum lini* (Bolley) Snyder et Hansen) and the HCN content of the flax plant (*Linum usitatissimum*), but offered no explanation. So much research has been done with cassava (Nestel and Cock, 1976) that Bellotti and van Schoonhoven (1978) were surprised how little is known about the insect pests of this plant. There appear to be no reports on the mechanism of resistance by the pests to the HCN produced when cassava is eaten. Similarly, Rehr *et al.*, (1973) found that *Spodoptera (Prodenia) eridania* (Cramer), the polyphagous Southern Armyworm, tolerates HCN although they admit that they do not know the mechanism involved.

Scriber (1978) also used the Southern Armyworm for feeding trials with cyanogenic plants, but did not investigate the mechanism of tolerance. He demonstrated that there were no differences between larvae fed on cyanogenic and acyanogenic *Lotus corniculatus* with respect to their consumption rate, assimilation efficiency, nitrogen or caloric utilisation efficiencies or in their growth rate. He did detect a poorer performance of larvae fed on 20-week-old plants as opposed to those fed on 4-week-old plants, but this was independent of cyanogenesis. There is a possibility, however, that this work suffers from an unconscious error because Scriber reports that he used larvae from a culture of *S. eridania* maintained on *Phaseolus vulgaris* L. (kidney-beans). The problem is that *P. vulgaris* is a cyanogenic species (Nayer and Fraenkel, 1963). Thus the strain he used in his experiments may already have been conditioned to, or even been selected for, eating cyanogenic plants. Certainly there is evidence that *S. eridania* eats cassava under cultivation (Corseuil, 1955) and that the cyanogenic *Phaseolus lunatus* L. (syn. *P. limensis* Macfad.) is a preferred food plant of the Southern Armyworm in captivity (Soo Hoo and Fraenkel, 1966).

The genus *Acacia* L. is particularly interesting because it seems that some species may have lost their cyanogenic ability and adopted an alternative method of defence. Rehr *et al.*, (1973) found that whereas the majority of the *Acacia* species they tested were cyanogenic (acacipetalin, Seigler *et al.*, 1978), those grouped in the broad category of "Ant-acacias" were not. The ants (*Pseudomyrmex* Latreille species) live in the enlarged spines of the plant and protect the foliage of their host. When ants are removed from ant-acacia plants defoliation by a broad spectrum of insect species follows. There was, however, one cyanogenic ant-acacia, *A. chiapensis*, and the array of insects able to feed on this plant when the ants were removed was much smaller. Thus coevolution between ants and acacias may have resulted in some acacias foregoing cyanogenesis for protection by ants. Alternatively, cyanogenesis may have evolved in those species of *Acacia* which were unable to strike-up a coevolutionary symbiotic relationship with ants.

It does seem, however, that ant-acacias can be at a severe disadvantage compared with their cyanogenic relatives under certain circumstances. The white-faced monkey *Cebus capucinus* preys intensively on the obligate acacia ant *Pseudomyrmex belti*. The monkeys tear branches and thorns off the acacias in their attempts to obtain the ants and the damage is often so severe that it results in the death of the plant (Freese, 1976).

Earlier in this essay I discussed the criteria to be used for determining whether a putative defence compound does indeed have that role in nature. There are two other advantages in studying plants polymorphic for cyanogenesis. In those regions of the world where the cyanogenic form is rare, the coevolutionary process in the herbivores may be at a more primitive stage than elsewhere. Secondly, we can ask why these plant species are polymorphic and not monomorphic for cyanogenesis and go on to study the advantages or disadvantages to an individual plant of being cyanogenic. During pursuit of the second problem it has been found that some plants are capable of changing their phenotype from cyanogenic to acyanogenic (in a sense that is biologically meaningful) or *vice versa* in response to environmental changes, particularly to temperature (Ellis *et al.*, 1977). This could pose some severe problems for the coevolving species and it would not be surprising to find that plants polymorphic for cyanogenesis are grazed by herbivores showing polymorphism for tolerance or resistance to HCN.

This article is not self-contained and should be read in conjunction with others in this volume, especially those of S. S. Duffy, W. E. Fry and J. M. Palmer.

ACKNOWLEDGEMENTS

I am grateful to the European Molecular Biology Organisation for the opportunity to take part and to contribute to the Workshop on Cyanide Metabolism. The financial support of the SERC and the NERC is acknowledged with thanks.

REFERENCES

Angseesing, J. P. A. and Angseesing, W. J. (1973). *Heredity* 31, 276-282.

Bellotti, A. and van Schoonhoven, A. (1978). *Ann. Rev. Entomol.* 23, 39-67,

Bernays, E.A., Chapman, R.F., Leather, E.M., McCaffery, A.R. and Modder, W.W.D. (1977). *Bull. Ent. Res.* 67, 391-404.

Chew, F.S. (1977). *Evolution* 31, 568-579.

Coop, I.E. and Blakley, R.L. (1949). *N.Z. J. Sci. Tech.* 30A, 277-291.

Cooper-Driver, G.A. and Swain, T. (1976). *Nature*, 260, 604.

Corkill, L. (1952). *N.Z. J. Sci. Tech.* 35A, 1-16.

Corseuil, E. (1955). *Bol. Campo.* 11, 3-7.

Daday, H. (1955). *J. Britt. Grassland Soc.* 10, 266-274.

Davis, R.H. and Nahrstedt, A. (1979). *Comp. Biochem. Physiol.* 64B, 395-397.

Dement, W.A. and Mooney, H.A. (1974). *Oecologia* 15, 65-76.

Dethier, V.G. (1937). *Biol. Bull.* 72, 7-23.

Dethier, V.G. (1941). *Amer. Nat.* 75, 61-73.

Dethier, V.G. (1954). *Evolution* 8, 33-54.

Eck, H.V., Gilmore, E.C., Ferguson, D.B. and Wilson, G.C. (1975). *Crop Science* 15, 421-424.

Ehrlich, P.R. and Raven, P.H. (1964). *Evolution* 18, 586-608.

Ellis, W.M., Keymer, R.J. and Jones, D.A. (1977). *Heredity* 38, 339-347.

Fraenkel, G.S. (1959). *Science* 129, 1466-1470.

Freese, C.H. (1976). *Biotropica* 8, 278-281.

Fry, W.E. and Evans, P.H. (1977). *Phytopathology* 67, 1001-1006.

Fry, W.E. and Millar, R.L. (1972). *Arch. Biochem. Biophys.* 151, 468-474.

Gilbert, L.E. (1975). *In* "Coevolution of Animals and Plants" (L. E. Gilbert and P. H. Raven, eds), pp. 210-240. University of Texas Press, Austin and London.

Jones, D.A. (1962). *Nature* 193, 1109-1110.

Jones, D.A. (1971). *Science* 173, 945.

Jones, D.A. (1979). *Amer. Nat.* 113, 445-451.

Jones, D.A., Parsons, J. and Rothschild, M. (1962). *Nature* 193, 52-53.

Lawton, J.H. (1976). *Bot. J. Linn. Soc.* 73, 187-216.

Lawton, J.H. (1978). *In* "Diversity of Insect Faunas" (L.A. Mound and N. Waloff, eds), pp.105-125. Blackwell Scientific Publications, Oxford.

Mallmaire, A. (1949). *Cong. Manoic Plantes Féculentes Trop. Inst. Colonial Marseilles*, pp.72-73.

Mode, C.J. (1958). *Evolution* 12, 158-165.

Nayer, J.K. and Fraenkel, G.S. (1963). *Ann. Ent. Soc. Amer.* 56, 174-178.

Nestel, B. and Cock, J. (1976). Cassava - The Development of an International Research Network. *Int. Dev. Res. Cent.* Ottawa, Canada. IDRC-059e 70pp.

Painter, R.H. (1936). *Amer. Nat.* 70, 547-566.

Painter, R.H. (1951). "Insect Resistance in Crop Plants". Macmillan Co., New York.

Parsons, J. and Rothschild, M. (1964). *Ent. Gaz.* 15, 58-59.

Rehr, S.S., Feeny, P.P. and Janzen, D.H. (1973). *J. Anim. Ecol.* 43, 405-416.

Rothschild, M. and Schoonhoven, L.M. (1977). *Nature* 266, 352-356.

Scriber, J.M. (1978). *Oecologia* 34, 143-155.

Seigler, D.S., Dunn, J.E., Conn, E.E. and Holstein, G.L. (1978). *Phytochemistry* 17, 445-446.

Soo Hoo, C.F. and Fraenkel, G. (1966). *J. Insect Physiol.* 12, 693-709.

Stahl, E. (1888). *Jena. Z. Naturw.* 22, 557-684.

Swan, L.H. (1952). The ecology of arthropods associated with *Photinia arbutifolia*. Ph.D. thesis Stamford University, California.

Trione, E.J. (1960). *Phytopathology* 50, 482-486.

Verschaffelt, E. (1910). *Proc. K. ned. Akad. Wet.* 13, 536-542.

Woodhead, S. and Bernays, E.A. (1978). *Entomologia exp. appl.* 24, 123-144.

THE ROLE OF HCN AND ITS DERIVATIVES IN PREBIOTIC EVOLUTION

J. ORÓ* and A. LAZCANO-ARAUJO**

**Departments of Biophysical Sciences and Chemistry, University of Houston, Houston, Texas 77004, U.S.A.*

***Instituto de Astronomia, Universidad Nacional Autonoma de Mexico Mexico 20, D. F., Mexico*

> ... nothing could be clearer than the possibility that cyanogen compounds might be formed at a time when the Earth was partly or wholly in an incandescent state. Life arose from fire, and its foundations were laid at the time when the Earth was a fiery incandescent globe... If one thinks of the immeasurable long period of time during which the Earth's surface was cooling at an exceedingly slow rate, cyanogen and its compounds had plenty of time and opportunity to follow their great tendency to transformation and polymerization, and by the addition of oxygen and, later, also of water and salts to change to a labile protein, which constitutes living matter...
>
> E. Pflüger, 1885.

I. INTRODUCTION

The question of the nature and the origins of life is one of the most fundamental inquiries that man has been concerned with, since he began to ask about his own existence and that of the world around him. Although the idea of spontaneous generation of micoorganisms was developed following Leeuwenhoek's pioneering observation of bacteria, it was not until the eighteenth and nineteenth centuries that Lamarck and other scientists proposed that such a process lay at the very foundations of the ladder of life. The classical developments of evolutionary theory by Darwin and Wallace were to reinforce the view that the origin of life was one of the most fundamental events of biological evolution. Ironically, in 1858, the same year that the *Origin of Species* appeared in England, Louis Pasteur was initiating the long series of experiments which would lead him to demolish the ill-founded hypothesis of the spontaneous origin of microorganisms.

To most scientists, Pasteur's experiments demonstrated the uselessness of inquiring into the origin of living systems. Some of them suggested that life had no origin at all, while others, like von Helmholtz (1871) and Arrhenius (1912) proposed an extraterrestrial origin for life on Earth, a view that simply transfers the problem to other worlds, places and processes, without solving it.

The German biologist E. Pflüger was among the few nineteenth century scientists who attempted to explain the origin of life as the result of an evolutionary process that took place in the early stages of the Earth's formation. Led by the well-known exothermic condensation of hydrogen cyanide and by the results of chemical elementary analysis that demonstrated the abundance of carbon, nitrogen and hydrogen in living matter, Pflüger (1875) suggested that life was the result of a continual series of small explosions occurring in proteins, which he considered alive, and which had originated from HCN in the hot, fiery environment of the early Earth.

Pflüger views were further developed by the Spanish chemist J. R. Carracido (1920) who attempted to explain the origin of at least some amino acids and proteins from hydrogen cyanide (Fernandez, 1964; Sanchez-Moscoso, 1971), and by the Mexican naturalist A. Herrera, who after lifelong efforts to explain the origin of protoplasm by natural causes (Beltran, 1978; Del Rio, 1978) proposed in 1942 the so-called sulphocyanic theory of the origin of life (Herrera, 1942), attempting to get some insight into the appearance of life from artifacts formed by ammonium thiocyanate and formaline.

However, the later development of biochemistry was to show that Pflüger and his followers had oversimplified the question of the nature and origin of life, which certainly does not depend on a single compound. It was the pioneering work of A. I. Oparin (1924) and J. B. S. Haldane (1928) that provided the theoretical and preliminary basis for the scientific study of the origin of life. The detection of the cyanogen and CH radicals in cometary spectra, the presence of hydrocarbons in carbonaceous meteorites, and the abiotic formation of hydrocarbons by hydrolysis of metallic carbides, led Oparin (1924) to propose that the first life forms which appeared on the Earth were the result of a long series of chemical syntheses and processes of self-organization which took place in the reducing environment of the primitive Earth. Similar views suggested independently by J. B. S. Haldane (1928) led to the formulation of the hypothesis of chemical evolution as a necessary preamble to the appearance of life. This view, which is solidly based on the contemporary biochemical knowledge of molecular processes essential to life, is strongly substantiated by laboratory work, done in the past three decades, which has demonstrated that practically all the biochemical compounds essential to life can be synthesized from simple molecules under plausible primitive Earth conditions.

Recent radioastronomical observations have shown that HCN is a very abundant cosmic molecule, and the above experiments have demonstrated that HCN plays a crucial role in primordial organic synthesis, being the prebiotic precursor of the most important molecules, such as the amino acids, and the purines, specifically, adenine and guanine. What is remarkable about these observations is that HCN is toxic to the majority of living organisms. In spite of this, it appears to have been, paradoxically, one of the most important precursors for the prebiotic generation of the key molecules of life.

II. INTERSTELLAR ORGANIC MOLECULES

Although the existence of simple diatomic chemical species (CN, CH, C_2, CO, NH) in the atmosphere of the Sun and other relatively cool stars had been known for some time, the first most interesting simple substance observed in interstellar space were the methylidyne radical (CH), the cyanogen radical (CN) and the methylidyne ion (CH^+), which were discovered in the 1937-1941 period by observation of their sharp absorption lines superimposed on the optical spectra of hot O-type stars (Adams, 1943). Later compilations of elementary cosmic abundances (Suess and Urey, 1956; Cameron, 1959) were to show that with the exception of the noble gases He and Ne, six of the most abundant elements in the Universe (H, C, N, O, S, P) were precisely the major constituent elements of living systems. It was therefore logical to conclude (Oró, 1963a) that the molecules formed from these elements should be the most abundant compounds in the Universe, and that the prevailing chemistry in the cosmos should be organic cosmochemistry.

This conclusion was confirmed several years later when the first simple organic molecule, formaldehyde, was detected in the interstellar space by radioastronomy (Snyder *et al.*, 1969). This was followed quickly in the following year by the radiotelescopic detection in interstellar clouds of carbon monoxide, the cyanogen radical, hydrogen cyanide and cyanoacetylene. Since then, a large number of organic compounds, as well as inorganic molecules of biological relevance, have been observed in the Milky Way and in other galaxies by microwave spectroscopy (Oró, 1972; Turner, 1980). These molecules range in complexity from simple diatomic ones to cyanooligoacetylenes (HC_3N, HC_5N, HC_7N, HC_9N) and related compounds like cyanamide (NH_2CN), methyl cyanide (CH_3CN), vinyl cyanide (CH_2CHCN) and others. A number of mechanisms suggested for the formation of these organic molecules may be found in Turner (1980).

However, one of the most remarkable surprises which emerged from the radioastronomical observations of the gas and dust clouds of our Galaxy was that just those molecules that had been used previously in prebiotic organic synthesis were found among the identified interstellar molecules. These unique molecules, plus phosphine which has only been detected so far in Jupiter, can be regarded as the prebiological precursors of essentially all the biochemical compounds present in living systems, and are listed in Table I. It should be noted, however, that the

Table 1 Biochemical monomers and properties which can be derived from interstellar molecules

	Interstellar Molecules	Formulae	Biochemical Monomers and Properties
1.	Hydrogen	H_2	Reducing Agent, Protonation
2.	Water	H_2O	Universal Solvent, Hydroxylation
3.	Ammonia	NH_3	Base Catalysis Amination
4.	Carbon monoxide	$CO(H_2)$	Hydrocarbons and Acids
5.	Formaldehyde	CH_2O	Monosaccharides (ribose) and Glycerol
	Acetaldehyde	CH_3CHO	Deoxypentoses (deoxyribose)
	Aldehydes (HCN)	RCHO	Amino Acids
6.	Thioformaldehyde	CH_2S	Cysteine and Methionine
7.	Hydrogen cyanide	HCN	Purines (adenine, guanine) and Amino Acids
8.	Cyanacetylene	HC_3N	Pyrimidines (cytosine, uracil, thymine)
9.	Cyanamide	H_2NCN	Polypeptides, Polynucleotides and Lipids
10.	Phosphine (Jupiter)	PH_3	Phosphates and Polyphosphates

From Oró *et al.*, 1978b. With the exception of phosphine (PH_3) which has been detected in Jupiter, all the other molecules have been detected in interstellar clouds. With the exception of the monosaccharides and some of the lipids the prebiotic formation of most of the biochemical compounds (amino acids, purines, pyrimidines, etc.) requires the participation of HCN or its derivatives.

search for interstellar pyrimidine, pyridine (Simon and Simon, 1973) and glycine (Brown *et al.*, 1979) has yielded negative results so far, probably due to the highly reducing conditions of the interstellar environment, which would inhibit further chemical evolution. Nevertheless, the wide distribution of HCN and its many derivatives in space not only points to the universal importance of HCN and to its key role in cosmic organic synthesis, but can also be considered an essential part of the very first stage of the evolutionary processes that led to the emergence of life on Earth (Oparin, 1972).

III. SOLAR SYSTEM CYANOGEN COMPOUNDS

Since the pioneering analytical work on carbonaceous meteorites by Thenard, Berzelius, Wholer, Berthelot and other chemists from the last century (Nagy, 1975) and the spectroscopic observations of the Sun, planets and comets, it is known that there are organic compounds in these many parts of the solar system. Some recent observations indicate that a large group of asteroids, minor planets of the asteroidal belt, are considered to be the parent bodies from which the carbonaceous chondrites are derived. However, the only bodies in the solar system in which R-CN type molecules have been observed are in the Sun, in whose spectrum the cyanogen radical is an easily detectable feature, and the comets. On the Earth itself, HCN is primarily a by-product of biological activity. It remains to be seen whether the thiocyanate which has recently been found in deep ocean trenches is of primeval origin or not (Ingmanson *et al.*, 1980).

Although no detectable amounts of HCN have been observed on Jupiter, the non-equilibrium conditions which prevail and the high CH_4 and NH_3 concentrations which exist in its upper atmosphere (Owen, 1975) would favor the gas-phase reaction

$$CH_4 + NH_3 \rightarrow HCN + 3H_2$$

It is likely, however, as Lewis (1969) has pointed out, that HCN cannot accumulate in the observable upper regions of the Jovian atmosphere due to the formation and further precipitation of NH_4CN, a process which yields a very low equilibrium pressure (less than 10^{-10} bars of HCN. Nevertheless, it should be added that HCN and CH_3CN play a prominent role in the synthesis of organic polymers in simulated Jovian atmospheres (Sagan and Miller, 1960; Ponnamperuma, 1976; Raulin *et al.*, 1979), thereby suggesting that hydrogen cyanide and its immediate derivatives may have been early constituents in the atmospheres of the outer planets and of some of their satellites.

From the standpoint of organic cosmochemistry, comets appear to be the least altered samples available of the primordial solar nebula, preserved in a more or less frozen state at the outskirts of the solar system. Cometary nuclei are small icy bodies of one to a few tens of kilometers radius, consisting of a mixture of ices of water and other compounds (CH_4, CO_2, NH_3), in addition to metals, silicates and other inorganic compounds. Table II presents more information on the chemical composition of comets, together with other cometary data. A more complete

Table II Chemical species detected in comets and other cometary data*

Organic	
	C, C_2, C_3, CH, CN, CO, CS, HCN, CH_3CN
Inorganic	
	H, NH, NH_2, O, OH, H_2O, S.
Metals	
	Na, Ca, Cr, Co, Mn, Fe, Ni, Cu, V, Si
Ions	
	C^+, CO^+, $CO_2{}^+$, CH^+, CN^+, $N_2{}^+$, OH^+, H_2O^+, Ca^+
Head and tail continuum including silicate particles (10 and 18 μm bands)	
Reported Negative Searches	
	H_2CO, CH_3OH, CH_3O-CH_3, CH_3-C≡CH, CH_4, HNC, HNCO, CH≡C-CN, CN-CH_2-CN, NH_3, SiO_2
Parameters of Cometary Nuclei	
Average Mass	$10^{18\pm3}$ grams (10^{18} gram minimum mass for Halley's comet)
Diameter	∿1 to a few tens of km.
Density	∿1 gm cm^{-3} to 1.5 gm cm^{-3}

*Adapted from Delsemme (1977) and Oró *et al.*, (1980).

treatment of the subject may be found in Delsemme (1977) and in Oró *et al.*, (1980).

As a comet approaches the Sun, bright emission lines of C_2, C_3, OH, CN and other simple chemical species appear in its spectrum, as a result of the dissociation and further excitation of the parent molecules present in the nucleus. In fact, the detection of the prominent cyanogen band in Halley's comet in 1910 led to public fear, and fortunes were made by selling "comet pills against the deadly cometary emanations". As quoted in a May, 1980, New York Times issue (Neugebauer *et al.*, 1979) "Chicago is terrified. Women are stopping up doors and windows to keep out cyanogen".

Recent radioastronomical observations of Comet Kohoutek have established the existence of HCN (Ulich and Conklin, 1974) and methyl cyanide (Heubner *et al.*, 1974), although cyanodiacetylene, which may be responsible for the observed cometary radical C_3, has not yet been detected.

Hydrogen cyanide is the most likely source of the cyanogen radical observed spectroscopically in comets. However, experiments in which frozen mixtures of CH_4, NH_3, and H_2O were irradiated with 5 Mev electrons (Oró, 1963b), and of HCHO, NH_3 and H_2O with high energy ^{14}C ions (Lemmon, pers.), yielded several non-volatile organic molecules, including amino acids, as well as hydrogen cyanide and cyanogen. This suggests that at least some of the cometary CN could be of secondary origin, being formed as the comet is intensely irradiated when it passes through its closest proximity to the Sun and further chemical reactions take place on its surface (Bar-Nun *et al.*, 1980).

The presence of HCN and other cyano derivatives in the material from which the parent bodies of the meteorites and the planets were formed is further indicated by the presence of amino acids (Miller *et al.*, 1976), adenine and guanine (Anders *et al.*, 1974), and urea, guanylurea, cyanuric acid and melamine (Hayatsu *et al.*, 1975), all of which are condensation and hydrolysis products of HCN and its immediate derivatives, like cyanamide (NH_2CN), in carbonaceous meteorites. Methyl cyanide has also been detected during the analysis of the Murchison (Holzer and Oró, 1977) and Allan Hills (Holzer and Oro, 1979) carbonaceous chondrites. Free HCN is not easy to detect in carbonaceous chondrites, as Chang (1979) has emphasized, a result which would be expected if liquid water were present in the parent bodies of the carbonaceous chondrites. Only minute traces of HCN resulting from the thermal decomposition of organic molecules have been detected during the 623 K volatilization by vacuum pyrolysis of a C2 type inclusion of the Jodzie meteorite (Bunch *et al.*, 1976), and similar results have been obtained with samples of the Murchison (Holzer and Oró, 1977) and Murray carbonaceous chondrites (Simoneit *et al.*, 1973; Wszolek *et al.*, 1973). Reviews on extraterrestrial organic analysis, carbonaceous chondrites and the formation of organic molecules in the solar system may be found in Oró (1972), Nagy (1975), Miller *et al.*, (1976) and Oró *et al.*, (1977).

IV. PREBIOTIC TERRESTRIAL ENVIRONMENT

The Earth does not contain large amounts of volatiles in proportion to refractory elements like Si, Na and Al (Rasool, 1972). This depletion, which probably occurred during the early accretionary phase of the planet as it was formed $\sim$4.5 x 10^9 years ago, does not imply however that the organogenic elements (H, C, N, S, O and P) were not available for primordial organic synthesis. In fact, the total amount of organic carbon in the sedimentary shell, 1.2×10^{22} grams (Schidlowski, 1978), is more than four orders of magnitude greater than the current estimates of $\sim 1 \times 10^{19}$ grams (Abelson, 1978) of living biomass present today on Earth.

It is likely that most of the organogenic elements were originally incorporated in the solid phase of the planet, from which they were liberated as relatively simple compounds (H_2, H_2O, CO_2, CO, N_2 and smaller amounts of CH_4 and NH_3) during an early degassing period (Walker, 1977, a,b) which led to the appearance of the secondary anoxic terrestrial atmosphere, the oceans and the volatile-rich sedimentary rocks. The amount of terrestrial surface volatiles, however, was significantly increased during the late accretion phase of the planet, when large amounts of chondritic (Owen and Anders, 1977) and cometary material (Oró *et al.*, 1978a, 1980; Chang, 1979) were captured by the Earth. The cometary matter thus captured was probably a significant prebiotic source of hydrogen cyanide and related chemical species directly incorporated into the primitive atmosphere. It is likely that some of the cometary carbon compounds were decomposed by the heat and shock waves of the cometary collision; however, such processes were probably an important source of highly reactive cyano derivatives, which upon quenching to low temperatures underwent further chemical reactions leading to the synthesis of a great variety of nitrogen containing products (Oró, 1961).

The trace amounts of HCN derived from carbonaceous meteorites (Bunch *et al.*, 1976) and its absence in contemporary volcanic eruptions (White and Waring, 1963) suggests that HCN was not a major volatile liberated during the early outgassing stage of atmosphere formation. However, several free-energy sources (Table III) in the prebiotic environment must have led to its synthesis from CH_4 and NH_3. As hydrogen was lost to space and less reduced gases dominated in the primordial atmosphere (Pollack and Yung, 1980), HCN was probably produced in relatively high yields from CO, H_2 and N_2 and other anoxic mixtures, as indicated by the experimental results of Abelson (1966).

The direct sources of energy available for prebiotic organic synthesis in the primitive Earth are listed in Table III. Although it should be emphasized that neither a single source of energy nor a single process can account for all the organic molecules in the primitive Earth (Oró *et al.*, 1977), the role and contribution of the different free-energy sources depended very strongly on their efficiency for producing HCN, a central intermediate in the prebiological formation of amino acids (Miller, 1957; Oró and Kamat, 1961), adenine and guanine (Oró, 1960; Oró and Kimball, 1962) and other compounds of prebiotic significance (Oró, 1976).

Table III Present sources of energy averaged over the Earth*

Source	Energy ($cal/cm^2/yr$)
Total radiation from sun	260,000
Ultraviolet light	
< 3000 Å	3,400
< 2500 Å	563
< 2000 Å	41
< 1500 Å	1.7
Electric discharges*	4
Cosmic rays	0.0015
Radioactivity (to 1.0 km depth)	0.8
Volcanoes	0.13
Shock waves*	1.1
Solar wind	0.2

From Miller *et al.*, 1976.

*Due to the collisional events occurring during the Earth's late accretion phase, the amounts of energy available as shock waves and electrical discharges were probably much higher than the values listed here.

The reader is referred to the review by Oró *et al.*, (1977) for a detailed discussion of the free-energy sources in the primitive Earth and the primordial solar nebula.

Although visible and ultraviolet light were probably the largest source of energy in the primitive Earth, they usually give poor yields of HCN. However electrical discharges and shock waves appear to be very efficient in synthesizing hydrogen cyanide from CH_4 and NH_3 or N_2, or less reduced mixtures (Miller and Orgel, 1974; Oró *et al.*, 1977). Another important product of electrical discharges is cyanoacetylene (H-C≡C-C≡N), which is an essential intermediate in the prebiotic synthesis of pyrimidines (Sanchez *et al.*, 1966). When a mixture of CH_4 and N_2 (but no NH_3) was subjected to the action of a spark by Sanchez *et al.*, (1966) HCN and cyanoacetylene were the first and second most abundant nitrogen containing products.

Electrical storms occur close to the surface of the Earth, so it is likely that the organic molecules and their intermediates could reach the oceans before being photodissociated (Miller and Orgel, 1974). Therefore, significant amounts of HCN must have existed in the anoxic atmosphere and in the primitive hydrosphere, although high concentrations of HCN and its immediate derivatives were probably attained in more localized environments, like rain drops, and in small ponds subject to low temperature during daily and seasonal climatic variations.

Regardless of the temperature at which the primitive Earth accreted, it is generally believed that the synthesis of most of the biochemical products took place under relatively moderate conditions (Oró, 1965, 1980) or otherwise the products formed would be destroyed. Such moderate conditions, which together with anoxic atmospheres and sources of free-energy are simulated in prebiotic organic synthesis experiments, include moderate temperatures, between 0°C and 100°C; aqueous environment; neutral or slightly basic pH (although in areas of volcanic emanations the pH could have been lower than 7 due to the presence of H_2S and SO_2), and appreciable concentration of organic compounds, the latter due to evaporation, absorption or phase separation processes (Oró, 1980).

V. ABIOTIC SYNTHESIS OF BIOCHEMICAL MONOMERS: AMINO ACIDS, PURINES AND PYRIMIDINES

The first successful synthesis of organic compounds under plausible prebiotic conditions was accomplished in the classical experiment of Stanley L. Miller (1953) by electric discharges. A gaseous mixture of CH_4, H_2, H_2O and NH_3 was subjected to an electric discharge for a week and then analyzed. Several amino acids, hydroxy acids and other molecules were formed. A more detailed study of the electrical discharge experiments (Ring *et al.*, 1972; Wolman *et al.*, 1972) demonstrated that all the protein and non-protein amino acids found in the Murchison meteorite were present among the products of the electric discharge. As shown in Table IV, perhaps one of the most remarkable results of this comparison is that the ratios of amino acids relative to glycine in the Murchison sample are quantitatively similar to those found in these experiments.

Laboratory simulations using CH_4, H_2O, NH_3 and less reduced mixtures, including CO, N_2, etc., with or without H_2 and different free-energy sources have also been successful in the abiotic production of amino acids and other compounds. A summary of the most important precursors for the synthesis of amino acids, purines, pyrimidines, sugars, and other molecules is given in Table I.

Miller (1957) has shown that the mechanism of synthesis of amino acids is the Strecker condensation, where the hydrogen cyanide and aldehydes formed by the electrical discharges condense with each other in the presence of ammonia, forming the amino nitriles which upon hydrolysis yield the amino acids,

Table IV Relative abundances of amino acids in the Murchison meteorite and in an electric discharge synthesis. Mol. ratio to glycine (= 100):0.05 - 0.5*); 0.5 - 5.**; 5 - 50***; > 50****

Amino Acid	Murchison Meteorite	Electric discharge
Glycine	****	****
Alanine	****	****
α-Amino-*n*-butyric acid	***	****
α-Aminosobutyric acid	****	**
Valine	***	**
Norvaline	***	***
Isovaline	**	**
Proline	***	*
Pipecolic acid	*	< *
Aspartic acid	***	***
Glutamic acid	***	**
β-Alanine	**	**
β-Amino-*n*-butyric acid	*	*
β-Aminoisobutyric acid	*	*
γ-Aminobutyric acid	*	**
Sarcosine	**	***
N-Ethyglycine	**	***
N-Methylalanine	**	**

From Miller *et al.* (1976).

$$R - CHO + HCN + NH_3 \rightleftarrows RCH(NH_2)CH + H_2O$$

$$RCH(HN_2)CN + 2H_2O \rightarrow RCH(NH_2)COOH + NH_3$$

while a similar mechanism can account for the synthesis of the reported hydroxy acids,

$$R - CHO + HCN \rightleftarrows RCH(OH)CN + H_2O$$

$$RCH(OH)CN + 2H_2O \rightarrow RCH(OH)COOH + NH_3$$

Although several other routes for the abiotic synthesis of amino acids in the primitive Earth have been suggested [see, for instance, Ponnamperuma and Woeller (1967) and Sanchez *et al.*, (1966)], a very important one appears to be the condensation of HCN from NH_4CN into polymers, which on hydrolysis, yield glycine, alanine and aspartic acid and several other amino acids (Oró and Kamat, 1961). The hydrolysis of the HCN tetramer, diaminomaleonitrile, yields glycine,

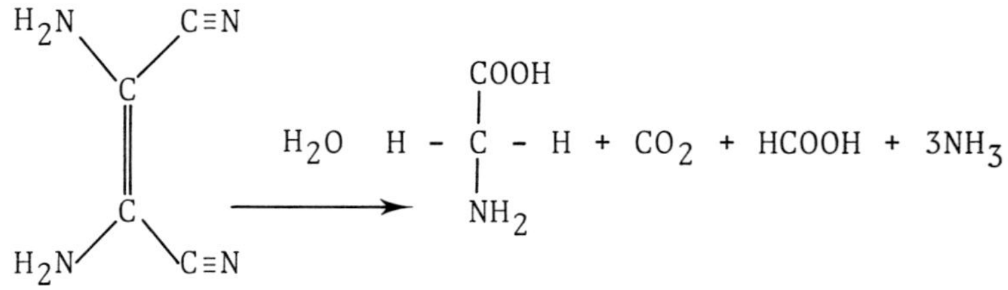

diaminomaleonitrile glycine

The base-catalysed condensation of HCN under the above conditions yields a very heterogeneous brown polymer. Hydrolysis of this polymer yields many of the α amino acids commonly found in proteins (Lowe *et al.*, 1963; Matthews and Moser, 1967; Moser and Matthews, 1968; Abelson, 1966; Labadie *et al.*, 1967, 1968; Harada, 1967; Friedmann and Miller, (1969)). Ferris *et al.*, (1978) have shown that at pH 9.2 dilute (0.1M) solutions of HCN condense into oligomers which on hydrolysis yield several protein and non-protein amino acids among other nitrogen bearing compounds. Moreover, Ivan and Zorica Draganic and their collaborators (Draganic *et al.*, 1978a,b; Draganic and Draganic, 1978) have extensively studied a long series of simple cyano compounds (HCN, NH_4CN, NaCN, KCN, CH_3CN, C_2H_5CN, NH_2CN, $NH_2C(=NH)NHCN$, $(CN)_2$ and $(CH_2CN)_2$) and have shown that the radiation-induced decomposition under primitive Earth conditions of some of these R-CN compounds forms oligomers exhibiting some peptide-like properties. These oligomers upon hydrolysis yield also several amino acids including glycine, alanine, glutamic acid, arginine, sarcosine and serine as well as non-protein amino acids.

Adenine, a purine which plays a central role in genetic processes and energy utilization, was first shown by Oró (1960) to form under primitive Earth conditions from HCN. When aqueous ammonia solutions containing large concentrations of hydrogen cyanide (1-10 M) are refluxed, adenine is formed as well as other purines and biochemical compounds, including amino acids and pteridines (Oró, 1960; Oró and Kimball, 1961, 1962). The synthesis of adenine is thought to take place by a series of condensation and cyclization reactions involving imidazole derivatives. A dimer of HCN is formed, and then another molecule of hydrogen cyanide added to it, forming a trimer (aminomalononitrile), followed by the condensation of this trimer with formamidine to 4-aminoimidazole-5-carbonitrile (AICN) or the corresponding amidine (AICAI). The cyclization into adenine is completed by condensation of either AICN or AICAI with formamidine. The net overall reaction can be represented simply as five molecules of HCN producing one molecule of adenine:

$$5\ HCN \rightarrow \text{Adenine}$$

There are other alternative pathways that have been suggested for the prebiotic synthesis of adenine. Namely, direct consecutive condensation of hydrogen cyanide (Oró and Kimball, 1962; Calvin, 19869), photochemical isomerization of the HCN-tetramer and condensation with formamidine (Sánchez *et al.*, 1966), as well as a more complex sequence of reactions in which no isomerization of the cis-diaminomaleonitrile is required to yield adenine (Voet and Schwartz, 1980). In fact, it is likely that more than one of these different pathways may have occurred under the presumably variable conditions of the primordial terrestrial environment.

Guanine and xanthine are formed by condensation of a 4-aminoimidazole-5-carboxamide with urea (Oró and Kimball, 1962). In fact, it should be noted that these imidazole derivatives can condense with monocarbon compounds to generate all biological purines (Oró, 1965). The prebiotic synthesis of adenine was confirmed by Lowe *et al.*, (1962), and indirectly by Ponnamperuma *et al.*, (1963), who found adenine after irradiating a CH_4, NH_3, H_2O and H_2 mixture with an electron beam at Berkeley. The kinetics and mechanisms of HCN oligomerization as well as the potential role of the HCN trimer and tetramer for purine synthesis have been extensively studied, particularly by Ferris and Orgel and their co-workers (1965) who have confirmed that the above sequence of reactions follows the same direction (first imidazole, then pyrimidine cyclization) as the biochemical synthesis of purines. It should be added that an industrial synthesis of adenine from anhydrous HCN and NH_3 has been reported (Wakamatsu *et al.*, 1966) and patented.

The pyrimidines can be synthesized under prebiotic conditions by condensation of cyanoacetylene with urea or cyanate (Sanchez *et al.*, 1966), a method which yields considerable amounts of cytosine. Cytosine is readily converted into uracil by deamination. Furthermore, Stephen-Sherwood *et al.*, (1971) have produced thymine in small yields from the reaction between uracil and formaldehyde in the presence of a reducing agent like hydrazine. More recently, Ferris *et al.*, (1978) have found that orotic acid, the common biochemical precursor of pyrimidine bases in living organisms, is released by the hydrolysis of HCN oligomers formed in dilute solutions.

VI. OLIGOMER SYNTHESIS

Several procedures have been studied for the polymerization of amino acids and nucleotides under prebiotic conditions. The simplest of all dehydrating mechanisms is the thermal condensation, which has been extensively studied for dry mixtures of amino acids by Fox and his co-workers (cf. Fox and Dose, 1977). However, these polypeptides have normal α-α bonds as well as abnormal α-β α-γ and other linkages not commonly found in proteins. The relatively large molecular weight and crosslinked nature of these polymers makes them quite inappropriate for biochemical information transfer processes between linear oligonucleotides and oligopeptides. Other approaches rely on the polymerization of activated monomers (such as aminoacyl adenylates and nucleoside 5'-triphosphates), the direct polymerization of certain precursors such as amino acid nitriles or amides, and polymerization using polyphosphate esters. The majority of these methods are applicable to the synthesis of both linear oligopeptides and oligonucleotides. One of the methods that has been more successful in recent years is the synthesis of oligomers under the abiotic conditions of an evaporating pond model using several prebiotic condensing agents. These include linear and cyclic polyphosphates and a number of reagents which contain a reactive CN bond or its tautomer. The prebiotic condensing molecules which have been studied more extensively are the following:

Cyanamide $N{\equiv}C-NH_2$

Carbodiimide $RN=C=NR$ (R is H or alkyl).

Dicyanamide 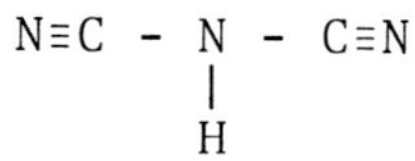

Dicyandiamide 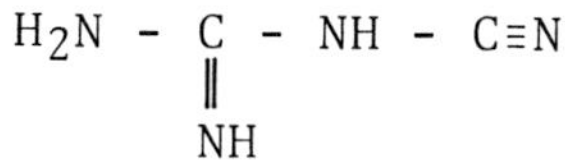

Cyanogen $N{\equiv}C-C{\equiv}N$

Cyanic Acid $HN=C=O$

Hydrogen Cyanide Tetramer 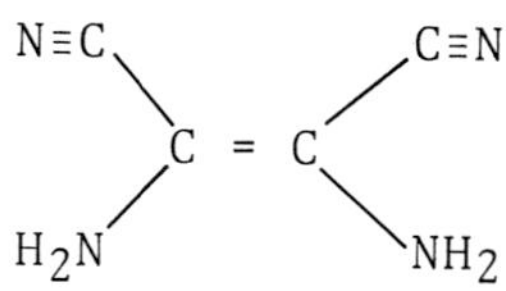

Reviews on these condensing agents and polymerization processes may be found elsewhere (Oró and Stephen-Sherwood, 1974, 1976; Hulshof and Ponnamperuma, 1976; Ponnamperuma, 1978).

Hydrogen cyanide, which has a large negative free-energy of hydrolysis, has not been used successfully as a condensing agent, whereas its tetramer, diaminomaleonitrile, is known to cause condensation of glycine into diglycine in solutions of neutral to basic pH solutions (Chang *et al.*, 1969). Of the several prebiotic condensing agents, cyanamide is the simplest and probably one of the most effective (Oró, 1963a). It has been found in interstellar space (Table I) and can be synthesized by ultraviolet irradiation of a HCN-containing solution (Schimpl *et al.*, 1965; Lohrmann, 1972). Under mild aqueous conditions, cyanamide (Ponnamperuma and Peterson, 1965), its dimer, dicyandiamide (Steinman *et al.*,1965a), and dicyanamide (Steinman *et al.*, 1965b), will cause condensation of amino acids to low molecular weight peptides. Recently Nooner *et al.* (1977) and Hawker and Oró (1980) have shown that when aqueous solutions of amino acids and cyanamide are evaporated and heated at 70°C for approximately one day, peptides of glycine, alanine, leucine, isoleucine, phenylalanine and other amino acids are readily obtained. The synthesized oligomers contain two to five amino acids, and are formed in relatively high yields.

Low yields of oligodeoxynucleotides have been reported when deoxythymine 5'-phosphate is heated in aqueous solutions with cyanamide (Ibanez *et al.*, 1971b,c). Imidazole also promotes the condensation of deoxythymidylic acid under aqueous conditions; oligomers of up to five units have been obtained containing mainly [3'→5']-phosphodiester bonds in yields of less than 1% (Ibanez *et al.*, 1971a). If the condensation of deoxythymidine-5'-triphosphate by means of cyanamide is carried out by evaporation and then heating at 70°C for one day, oligothymidylic acids containing two to eight monomers are obtained in reasonably good yields (Sherwood *et al.*, 1977). The enzymatic analysis of these oligonucleotides indicated that they contained primarily the biological [3'→5'] phosphodiester bonds, as in the case of DNA.

The yields of oligodeoxynucleotides can be further increased by the new addition of cyanamide and repetition of the evaporation and heating cycle (Odom and Oró, 1976). This and other experiments (Odom *et al.*, 1979) provide a simple and plausible prebiotic model for the repetitive synthesis of oligonucleotides in a primeval environment. It is conceivable that if similar reactions are carried out with mixtures of different deoxymononucleotides, for instance dAMP and dTMP, successive elongation and replication could be observed (Oró, 1976, 1980).

Recapitulating this section, we have seen that cyanamide and other HCN derivatives are efficient condensing agents for the formation of oligopeptides and oligonucleotides. We consider these results significant in the context of prebiological evolution, mainly because of the following factors. *Availability:* these condensing agents can be made readily from HCN and therefore they must have been synthesized continuously at a steady rate during the formation of the primitive atmosphere and hydrosphere. *Plausibility:* the evaporating pond model, involving the accumulation of water and organic compounds from the atmosphere followed by heating at moderate temperatures and evaporation is a realistic model for the primitive Earth. *Yields and nature of products:* the yields of linear oligomers obtained during only one cycle are substantial, ranging from a few percent to about 80% and they can be increased by repeating the cycle. The bonds synthesized are predominantly those present in biological molecules.

VII. SYNTHESIS OF NEUTRAL AND AMPHIPHILIC LIPIDS

Although the importance of lipids and membranes in the origin of life had been recognized previously by several workers in the field (Goldacre, 1958; Calvin, 1969; Shah, 1972) very little attention was paid until recently to the abiotic synthesis of complex neutral lipids, phospholipids and other amphiphilic molecules.

The positive results obtained in the prebiotic synthesis of oligopeptides and oligonucleotides by means of cyanamide, as shown in the previous section, prompted us to study the effect of cyanamide on the formation of complex lipids, including acylglycerols (neutral lipids), phospholipids (amphiphilic lipids) and related biochemical molecules which are involved in the formation of cellular membranes.

The precursors of complex lipids include normal fatty acids, glycerol and glycerol phosphate, and all have been synthesized under plausible prebiotic conditions (See Oró *et al.*, 1978b for a review). Normal fatty acids (C_6 to C_{18}) have been produced from CO and H_2 by Fischer-Tropsch-type reactions using meteoritic nickel-iron catalyst under conditions which may have occurred in the primordial solar nebula or during degassing of the primitive Earth (Nooner and Oró, 1979). It should be added, parenthetically, that fatty acids, hydrocarbons and other lipids are known to occur in carbonaceous chondrites (Oró, 1972; Nagy, 1975). Glycerol can also be produced by reduction of glyceraldehyde by any of these three compounds: hydrogen sulfide, hydrazine or formaldehyde (Epps *et al.*, 1979). Glyceraldehyde in turn is known to be formed from formaldehyde by base catalysts. The formation of glycerophosphates occurs when glycerol is heated with ammonium dihydrogen phosphate and either urea or cyanamide (Epps *et al.*, 1979).

Other work by Deamer coworkers (Hargreaves *et al.*, 1977; Hargreaves and Deamer, 1978) has shown that simple mixtures of fatty acid and glycerol give small yields of mono-, di- and triglycerides under mild conditions of dehydration (1 week at 60°C). Furthermore, if phosphate is present, together with fatty acid and a monoglyceride, three species of phospholipids can be found in the final reaction product. If these are isolated by acetone precipitation and mixed with aqueous solutions, they immediately produce highly stable membranous vesicles.

The relatively low yields obtained in the above studies in the absence of condensing agents can be significantly improved by means of cyanamide as shown in our laboratory. Thus, by reacting palmitic acid and glycerol, in the presence of cyanamide, under the moderate conditions described in the previous section, neutral lipids are formed in substantial amounts. The products include mono-, di- and tripalmitoyl derivatives of glycerol. They are obtained in total yields of up to 57% (Eichberg *et al.*, 1977). Phosphatidic acids, with one or two acyl groups, can be obtained by the condensation of glycerol-3-phosphate and palmitic acid by cyanamide (Epps *et al.*, 1978). The phosphatidic acids are obtained in yields of up to 45%. From recent work in our laboratory it appears that similar condensation reactions can produce most of the phospholipids of protoplasmic membranes as well.

On the basis of the above, it is reasonable to assume that in the primitive Earth atmosphere there was a steady synthesis of cyanamide (and other simple precursors) while complex lipids and biochemical oligomers were synthesized on the primitive Earth's surface by condensation processes. Under these conditions one can visualize the simultaneous synthesis of lipids, peptides and nucleotides, followed by the molecular association of amphiphilic lipid molecules into microvesicles, and the entrapment of hydrophilic peptides and nucleotides within the microvesicles.

VIII. PROTOBIOLOGICAL EVOLUTION

In the previous sections we have seen that with the exception of monosaccharides and other simple molecules, the prebiotic formation of most of the biochemical compounds (amino acids, purines, pyrimidines, oligopeptides, oligonucleotides, amphiphilic lipids, etc.) requires the direct or indirect participation of HCN or its derivatives. Thus from HCN and other simple molecules a complex system (primitive broth) was generated in which chemical and physical transformations led to the appearance of a heterogeneous mixture of monomeric and macromolecular organic compounds. However, the disordered nature of the changes which took place in it was essentially different from those occurring in living systems (Oparin, 1972). Indeed, the emergence of life must have involved the cooperative association of prebiologically synthesized oligomers within localized microenvironments. Although it is possible that rudimentary replication, transcriptional and translational processes involving oligonucleotides and oligopeptides evolved as a result of adsorption on clay surfaces, or from kinetic encounters in solution, the essential role of contemporary biomembranes and the recent synthesis of membranogenic amphyphilic molecules under plausible primitive Earth conditions suggests that the first living systems appeared as a result of the evolution of thermodynamically open, phase-separated multimolecular microsystems. This stage in the appearance of life, which provides a smooth transition between chemical and biological evolution is termed precellular or protobiological evolution (Oró, 1976, 1980).

The concept of protobiological evolution was first suggested by A. I. Oparin (1924 *et seq.*) in his pioneering work on the origin of life. He was able to show, using coacervate droplets as models of precellular structures, that macromolecular synthesis (polynucleotides, starch, etc.) and photoreduction processes mediated by activated chlorophyll, could occur inside the coacervate droplets at the expense of matter and energy from the external environment (Oparin, 1957, 1971, 1978).

Following this line several models of precellular structures have been proposed, including microspheres of thermal polypeptides (cf. Fox and Dose, 1977), Jeewanu (Bahadur, 1964), sulphobes and colpoids (Herrera, 1942) and organic microstructures (Folsome *et al.*, 1975). However, even though many of these models exhibit a superficial resemblance in shape and size to fossilized and living cells, many of them are typically gels or even solids, while others are made of macromolecular compounds of little or no prebiotic significance. Therefore as a result of the successful results on the prebiotic synthesis of amphiphilic lipids described in the previous section it would seem that these compounds would be more ideally suited to form the membranes of precellular structures (Deamer and Oró, 1980).

IX. MEMBRANES OF PRECELLULAR STRUCTURES

It is known that phospholipids and other amphiphilic lipids have the ability under appropriate conditions to become self-organized into liposomes. Liposomes are vesicular structures with bilayered or multilayered membranes. They are very stable and possess properties typical of the plasma cell membranes, such as semipermeability to certain ions and weak bases. They also have the ability to intercalate with hydrophobic peptides and to fuse with cell membranes and, in fact, they are used for the introduction of macromolecules into cells.

In the context of prebiotic evolution it is, therefore, conceivable that the simultaneous formation of lipids, peptides and nucleotides and their further accumulation in intertidal ponds and shallow lagoons in the primitive Earth led to the appearance of liposomes or microvesicles which could enclose biochemical monomers and oligomers (Deamer and Oró, 1980). This would have caused the entrapment of hydrophilic nucleotides and peptides (some with catalytic activity) in the inner vesicular cavity and the insertion of hydrophobic peptides within the hydrophobic region of the bilayered lipid membrane structure.

The major conclusion to be drawn from the work on the prebiotic formation of amphiphilic lipids and liposomes (Hargreaves *et al.*, 1977; Hargreaves and Deamer, 1978; Oró *et al.*, 1978b; Deamer and Oró, 1980) is that membrane structures resembling contemporary membranes are readily produced from lipid compounds likely to have been available on the prebiotic Earth. The presence of these prebiological membranes determined the preferential influx of weak bases, catalytic molecules, purines, pyrimidines and peptides and provided the high concentrations required for synthesis at higher rates. This in turn facilitated the cooperative interaction of biocatalytic peptides (protoenzymes), informational self-duplicating molecules (proto-DNA or proto-RNA), code translating molecules (proto-tRNA) and peptide synthesizing complexes (proto-ribosomes), within the internal microenvironment of the liposome (Oro, 1980).

The increasing complexity of such precellular systems, resulting from cooperative interaction and autocatalytic processes, eventually led to the duplication of these structures and the appearance of the first living cells. This precellular-cellular event is very little understood but certainly the most significant event in the evolutionary continuum since it marks the transition from chemical to biochemical evolution. In the words of J. B. S. Haldane "the critical event which may best be called the origin of life was the enclosure of several self-reproducing polymers within a semipermeable membrane". The degree of validity of Haldane's view will only be ascertained by future experiments following this line of inquiry. We feel that the prebiotic synthesis of amphiphilic lipids and of self-organizing liposomes, briefly described here, is a first step in this direction.

X. SUMMARY AND CONCLUSIONS

Aside from its interesting biological properties, HCN is a unique compound in the context of organic cosmochemistry, prebiotic evolution and the origin of life on Earth. Hydrogen cyanide is made of three of the most important elements to living systems (organogenic elements: H, C, N, O, S, P) which curiously enough are some of the most abundant elements in the Universe.

Thermonuclear reactions in the core of stars are responsible for the converstion of hydrogen into helium, helium into carbon and carbon into nitrogen. In the atmospheres of stars, carbon and nitrogen combine to form the CN radical which is one of the most thermally stable diatomic combinations known. Since there is a continuous transfer of stellar matter to interstellar space it is not surprising that cyanogen, hydrogen cyanide and its derivatives are widely distributed in the interstellar clouds of our Galaxy. Their presence in comets is a reflection of the composition of the solar nebula which gave rise to the formation of the solar system. Because of the collision of comets with the primitive Earth, HCN and its derivatives must have been present also in the primitive atmosphere and hydrosphere as primary or secondary products.

The reactivity of HCN and its ability to condense with itself and other compounds must have been responsible for the prebiotic formation of the majority of biochemical compounds necessary for life. Thus amino acids were probably formed by condensation of HCN with aldehydes; purines by the successive condensation of HCN oligome s and derivatives; pyrimidines by the condensation of cyanoacetylene with urea. Pteridines can also be formed from HCN. Amino acids can be condensed into oligopeptides by means of CN derivatives, especially cyanamide, and in a similar way mononucleotides can be converted into oligonucleotides. Neutral lipids and phospholipids can also be synthesized from their precursors by means of cyanamide. It is known that amphiphilic lipids have the ability of spontaneous self-organization into liposomes, or bilayered microvesicles, which show properties similar to those of cellular membranes. The inclusion of template-forming oligonucleotides and catalytic peptides within a liposome, could be a first step in the generation of a self-duplicating entity.

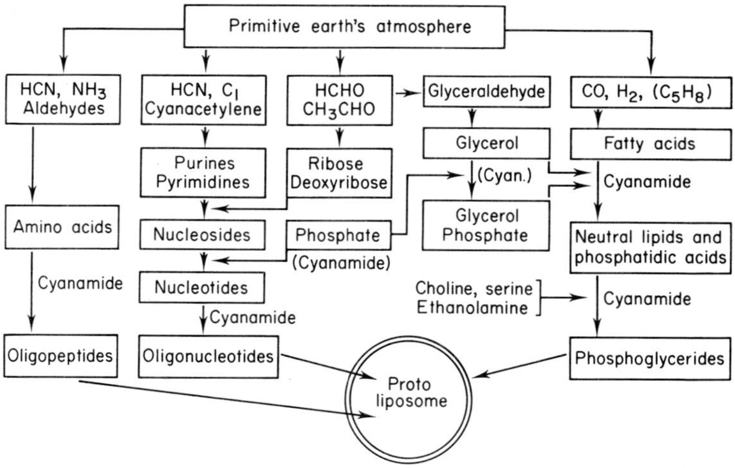

Fig. 1

Thus we can say that the origin of terrestrial life was very closely dependent on the synthetic capabilities of HCN and its derivatives, since it appears that all the above reactions and processes (summarized in Fig. 1) must have been very important for the emergence of the first living systems on Earth.

ACKNOWLEDGEMENTS

The experimental work summarized here has been supported in part by NASA Grant NGR 44-005-002. Support from CONACYT (Mexico) to one of us (ALA) is gratefully acknowledged.

REFERENCES

Abelson, P.H. (1966). *Proc. Nat. Acad. Sci. U.S.* 55, 1365-1372.

Abelson, P.H. (1978). *Ann. Rev. Earth Planet Sci.* 6, 325-351.

Adams, W.S. (1943). *Publ. Astron. Soc. Pacific*, 55, 217-225.

Anders, E., Hayatsu, R. and Studier, M.H. (1974). *In* "Cosmochemical Evolution and the Origins of Life" (J. Oró, S. L. Miller, C. Ponnamperuma and R. S. Young, eds), pp. 57-67, Reidel, Dordrecht.

Arrhenius, S. (1912). "Worlds in the Making", Harper and Bros., New York.

Awramik, S. (1977). *In* "Chemical Evolution of the Early Precambrian" (C. Ponnamperuma, ed.), pp. 111-131, Academic Press, New York.

Bahadur, K. (1964). *Zentrabl. Bakteriol.,Parasitenkd.* 118, 671-694.

Bar-Nun, A., Lazcano-Araujo, A., and Oró, J. (1981). *"Origins of Life"* (in press).

Beltran, E. (1978). *In* "El Origen de la Vida: Symp. en Homenaje a A. I. Oparin" (A. Lazcano-Araujo and A. Barrera, eds), pp.49-60 UNAM, Mexico.

Brown, R.D., Godfrey, P.S., Storey, J.W.W., Bassez, M.P., Robinson, B.J., Batchelor, R.A., McCulloch, M.G., Rydbeck, O.E.H. and Hjalmarson, A.G. (1979). *Monthly Not. Roy. Astr. Soc.* 186, 5P-8P.

Bunch, T.E., Chang, S., Neil, J.M. and Burlingame, A. (1976). *Meteoritics* 11, 260-261.

Calvin, M. (1969). "Chemical Evolution", Oxford Univ. Press, New York.

Cameron, A.G.W. (1959). *The Astrophys. J.* 129, 676-699.

Carracido, J.R. (1920). *Revue Scientifique* 11, 711.

Chang, S. (1979). *In* "Space Missions to Comets" (M. Neugebauer, D., K. Yeomans, J.C. Brandt and R.W. Hobbs, eds.), pp.59-111 NASA CP-2089, Washington, D.C.

Chang, S., Flores, J. and Ponnamperuma, C. (1969). *Proc. Nat. Acad. Sci. U.S.* 64, 1011-1015.

Deamer, D.W. and Oró, J., (1980). *BioSystems*, 784, 167-175.

Delsemme, A.H. (ed.) (1977). "Comets, Asteroids, Meteorites", The Univ. of Toledo Press, Toledo, Ohio.

Del Rio, C. (1978). *In* "El Origen de la Vida: Symp. en Homenaje a A. I. Oparin" (A. Lazcano-Araujo and A. Barrera, eds), pp.61-75 UNAM, Mexico.

Draganic, I.G. and Draganic, Z.D. (1979). *In* "Conferencias Plenarias del II Symp. Sobre Quimica Nuclear, Radioquimica y Quimica de Radiaciones" (C. Archundia, ed.), pp. 50-72, Publ. CEN-UNAM, Ser. Quim. 2-79, Mexico.

Draganic, I.G., Draganic, Z.D., Shimoyama, A. and C. Ponnamperuma. (1978a). *In* "Origin of Life" (H. Noda, ed.), pp.83-87, Japan Sci. Soc. Press, Tokyo.

Draganic, Z., Draganic I., Shimoyama, A. and Ponnamperuma, C. (1978b) *In* "Origin of Life" (H. Noda, ed.), pp. 129-133, Japan Sci. Soc. Press, Tokyo.

Eichberg, J., Sherwood, E., Epps, D.E. and Oró, J. (1977). *J. Mol. Evol.* 10, 221-230.

Epps, D.E., Sherwood, E., Eichberg, J. and Oró, J. (1978). *J. Mol. Evol.* 11, 279-292.

Epps, D.E., Nooner, D.W., Eichberg, J., Sherwood, E. and Oró, J. (1979). *J. Mol. Evol.* 14, 235-241.

Fernandez, O. (1964). *Rev. Real Acad. de Ciencias Exactas Fis. y. Mat. de Madrid,* LVIII, cuaderno 3°.

Ferris, J.P. and Orgel, L. (1965). *J. Am. Chem. Soc.* 87, 4976-4977.

Ferris, J.P., Joshi, P.C., Edelson, E.H. and Lawless, J.G. (1978). *J. Mol. Evol.* 11, 293-311.

Folsome, C.E., Allen, R.D. and Ichinose, R.K. (1975). *Precambrian Res.* 2, 263-275.

Fox, D.W. and Dose, K. (1977). "Molecular Evolution and the Origin of Life", Marcel Dekker, New York.

Friedmann, N. and Miller, S.L. (1969). *Nature* 221, 1152-1153.

Goldacre, R.J. (1958). *In* "Surface Phenomena in Chemistry and Biology" (J. P. Danelli, K. G. A. Pankhurst and A. C. Riddiford, eds.) pp. 278-298, Pergamon Press, New York.

Haldane, J.B.S. (1928). *Rationalist Ann.* 148, 3-10.

Harada, K. (1967). *Nature* 214, 479-480.

Hargreaves, W.R. and Deamer, D.W. (1978). *In* "Light Transducing Membranes" (D.W. Deamer, ed.) pp. 23-59, Academic Press, New York.

Hargreaves, W.R., Mulvihill, S.J. and Deamer, D.W. (1977). *Nature* 266, 78-80.

Hawker, J.R. and Oró, J. (1981). *In* "Origins of Life" (Y. Wolman, ed.) pp. 225-232, D. Reidel, Dordrecht.

Hayatsu, R., Studier, M.H., Moore, L.P. and Anders, E. (1977). *Nature* 266, 78-80.

Herrera, A. (1942). *Science* 96, 14.

Holzer, G. and Oró, J. (1977). *Organic Geochemistry* 1, 37-52.

Holzer, G. and Oró, J. (1979). *J. Mol. Evol.* 13, 265-270.

Huebner, W.F., Snyder, L.E. and Buhl, D. (1974). *Icarus* 22, 580-584.

Hulshof, J. and Ponnamperuma, C. (1976). *Origin of Life* 7, 197-224.

Ibanez, J.D., Kimball, A.P. and Oró, J. (1971a). *In* "Chemical Evolution and the Origin of Life" (R. Buvet and C. Ponnamperuma, eds.), pp.171-179, North-Holland Publ. Co., Amsterdam.

Ibanez, J.D., Kimball, A.P. and Oró, J. (1971b). *J. Mol. Evol.* 1, 112-114.

Ibanez, J.D., Kimball, A.P. and Oró, J. (1971c). *Science* 173, 444-446.

Ingmanson, D.E. and Dowler, M.J. (1981). *In* "Origins of Life" (Y. Wolman, ed.), pp. 129-134, D. Reidel, Dordrecht.

Labadie, M., Jensen, R. and Menzil, E. (1967). *Bull. Soc. Chem. Biol.* 49, 673-682.

Labadie, M., Jensen, R. and Menzil, E. (1968). *Biochim. Biophys. Acta,* 165, 525-533.

Lemmon, R.M. (1979), private comm.

Lewis, J.S. (1969). *Icarus* 10, 393-409.
Lohrmann, R.J. (1972). *J. Mol. Evol.* 1, 263-269.
Lowe, C.U., Rees, M.W. and Markham, R. (1963). *Nature* 199, 219-222.
Matthews, C.N. and Moser, R.E. (1967). *Nature* 215, 1230-1234.
Miller, S.L. (1953). *Science* 117, 529-529.
Miller, S.L. (1957). *Biochim. Biophys. Acta,* 23, 480-489.
Miller, S.L. and Orgel, L.E. (1974). "The Origins of Life on the Earth", Prentice-Hall, Englewood Cliffs.
Miller, S.L., Urey, H.C. and Oró, J. (1976). *J. Mol. Evol.* 9, 59-72.
Moser, R.E. and Matthews, C.N. (1968). *Experentia* 24, 658-662.
Nagy, B. (1975). "Carbonaceous Meteorites", Elsevier, Amsterdam.
Nooner, D.W. and Oró, J. (1979). *In* "Advances in Chemistry Series" No.178, (E. L. Kugler and F. W. Steffgen, eds.) pp. 159-166 Am. Chem. Soc., Washington, D.C.
Nooner, D.W., Sherwood, E., More, M.A. and Oró, J. (1977). *J. Mol. Evol.* 10, 211-220.
Odom, D.G. and Oró, J. (1976). *Fed. Proc.* 35, 661.
Odom, D.G., Lahav, N. and Chang, S. (1979). *J. Mol. Evol.* 12, 259-264.
Neugebauer, M., Yeomans, D.K., Brandt, J.C., Hobbs, R.W. (eds). (1977). "Space Missions to Comets", NASA Publication No. 2089.
Oparin, A.I. (1924). "Proiskhodenie Zhizni", Moscovksy Rabotchii, Moscow.
Oparin, A.I. (1957). "The Origin of Life on the Earth", Oliver and Boyd, Edinburgh.
Oparin, A.I. (1971). *In* "Prebiotic and Biochemical Evolution" (A.P. Kimball and J. Oró, eds.), pp. 1-7, North-Holland Publ. Co., Amsterdam.
Oparin, A.I. (1972). *In* "Exobiology" (C. Ponnamperuma, ed.), pp.1-15, North-Holland Publ. Co., Amsterdam.
Oparin, A.I. (1978). *In* "El Origen de la Vida: Symp. en Homenaje a A.I. Oparin" (A. Lazcano-Araujo and A. Barrera, eds.). pp. 137-144, UNAM, Mexico.
Oró, J. (1960). *Biochem. Biophys. Res. Comm.* 2, 407-412.
Oró, J. (1961). *Nature* 190, 389-390.
Oró, J. (1963a). *Ann. New York Acad. Sci.* 108, 464-481.
Oró, J. (1963b). *Nature* 197, 971-974.
Oró, J. (1965). *In* "The Origin of Prebiological Systems" (S. W. Fox, ed.), pp. 137-162, Academic Press, New York.
Oró, J. (1972). *Space Life Sci.* 3, 507-550.
Oró, J. (1976). *In* "Reflections on Biochemistry" (A. Kornberg, B. Horecker, L. Cornudella and J. Oró, eds.), pp. 423-443, Pergamon Press, Oxford).
Oró, J. (1980). *In* "The Origins of Life and Evolution" (H. O. Halvorson, Von Holde, K., eds.), pp. 47-63, Alan R. Liss, New York.
Oró, J. and Kamat, S.S. (1961). *Nature* 190, 422-423.
Oró, J. and Kimball, A.P. (1961). *Arch. Biochem. Biophys.* 94, 217-227.
Oró, J. and Kimball, A.P. (1962). *Arch. Biochem. Biophys.* 96, 292-313.
Oró, J. and Stephen-Sherwood, E. (1974). *In* "Cosmochemical Evolution and the Origin of Life" (J. Oró, S.L. Miller, C. Ponnamperuma and R.S. Young, eds.), pp. 159-172, Reidel, Dordrecht.

Oró, J. and Stephen-Sherwood, E. (1976). *Origin of Life* 7, 37-47.

Oró, J., Holzer, G. and Lazcano-Araujo, A. (1978a). *In* "Experimental Approaches to Comets" (J. Oró, Convenor), pp. 54-59.

Oró, J., Miller, S.L. and Urey, H.C. (1977). *In* "Living Systems as Energy Converters" (R. Buvet, M.J. Allen and J.P. Massue, eds.), pp. 7-19, North-Holland Publ. Co., Amsterdam.

Oró, J., Sherwood, E. Eichberg, J. and Epps, D. (1978b). *In* "Light Transducing Membranes" (D. W. Deamer, ed.), pp. 1-21, Academic Press, New York.

Owen, T. (1976). *In* "Chemical Evolution of the Giant Planets". (C. Ponnamperuma, ed.), pp. 49-58, Academic Press, New York.

Owen, T. and Anders, Ed. (1977). *Science* 198, 453-465.

Pflüger, E. (1875). *Arch. ges. Phisiol.* 10, 641-644.

Pollack, J.B. and Yung, Y.L. (1980). *Ann. Rev. Earth Planet. Sci.* (in press).

Ponnamperuma, C. (1976). *In* "Chemical Evolution of the Giant Planets" (C. Ponnamperuma, ed.), pp. 221-231, Academic Press, New York.

Ponnamperuma, C. (1978). *In* "Origin of Life" (H. Noda, ed.), pp. 67-81, Japan Sci. Soc. Press, Tokyo.

Ponnamperuma, C. and Peterson, E. (1965). *Science* 147, 1572-1574.

Ponnamperuma, C. and Woeller, F.H. (1967). *Currents in Mod. Biol.* 1, 156-158.

Ponnamperuma, C., Lemmon, R.M., Mariner, R. and Calvin, M. (1963). *Proc. Nat. Acad. Sci. U.S.* 49, 737-740.

Rasool, S.I. (1972). *In* "Exobiology" (C. Ponnamperuma, ed.), pp. 369-399, North-Holland Publ. Co., Amsterdam.

Raulin, F., Bossard, A., Toupance, G. and Ponnamperuma, C. (1979). *Icarus* 38, 358-366.

Ring, D., Wolman, Y., Friedmann, N. and Miller, S.L. (1972). *Proc. Nat. Acad. Sci. U.S.* 69, 765-768.

Sagan, C. and Miller, S.L. (1960). *Astron. Jour.* 65, 499.

Sanchez, R.A., Ferris, J. and Orgel, L.E. (1966). *Science* 154, 784-485.

Schidlowski, M. (1978). *In* "Origin of Life" (H. Noda, ed.), pp. 3-20, Japan Sci. Soc. Press, Tokyo.

Schimpl, A., Lemmon, R.M. and Calvin, M. (1965). *Science* 147, 149-150.

Shah, D.O. (1972). *In* "Exobiology" (C. Ponnamperuma, ed.), pp.235-265, North-Holland Publ. Co., Amsterdam.

Sherwood, E., Joshi, A. and Oró, J. (1977). *J. Mol. Evol.* 10, 193-209.

Simon, M.N. and Simon, M. (1973). *The Astrophys. Jour.* 184, 757-761.

Simoneit, B.R., Christiansen, J. and Burlingame, A.L. (1973). *Geochim. Cosmochim. Acta* 2, 1635-1650.

Snyder, L.E., Buhl, D., Zuckermann, B. and Palmer, P. (1969). *Phys. Rev. Lett.* 22, 679-681.

Steinman, G., Kenyon, D.H. and Calvin, M. (1965a). *Nature* 206, 707-708.

Steinman, G., Lemmon, R.M. and Calvin, M. (1965b). *Science* 147, 1574-1575.

Stephen-Sherwood, E., Oró, J. and Kimball, A.P. (1971). *Science* 173, 446-447.

Suess, H.E. and Urey, H.C. (1956). *Rev. Mod. Phys.* 28, 53-74.

Turner, B. (1980). *J. Mol. Evol.* 15, 79-101.
Ulich, B.L. and Conklin, B.K. (1974). *Nature* 248, 121-122.
Vennesland, B. and Pistorius, E.K. (this volume).
Von Helmholtz, H. (1871). *In* "Selected Writings of Hermann von Helmholtz", (R. Kahl, ed.), pp. 294, Weslayan Univ. Press, Middletown, Conn.
Wakanatsu, H., Yamada, Y., Saito, T., Kumashiro, I. and Takenishi, T. (1966). *J. Org. Chem.* 31, 2035-2038.
Walker, J.G.C. (1977a). *In* "Chemical Evolution of the Early Precambrian" (C. Ponnamperuma, ed.), pp. 1-11, Academic Press, New York.
Walker, J.G.C. (1977b). "Evolution of the Atmosphere", MacMillan, New York.
White, D.E. and Waring, G.A. (1963). "Volcanic Emanations", *U.S. Geological Survey Prof. Paper 440-K.*
Wolman, Y., Haverland, W.J. and Miller, S.L. (1972). *Proc. Nat. Acad. Sci. U.S.* 69, 809-811.
Wszolek, P.C., Simoneit, B.R. and Burlingame, A.L. (1973). *Geochim. Cosmochim. Acta,* 2, 1693-1706.

SUBJECT INDEX